AIRBORNE HAZARDS RELATED TO DEPLOYMENT

I can think of no higher responsibility than ensuring that the men and women who have served our nation in uniform are treated with the care and respect that they have earned.

Eric K. Shinseki
General (Retired), US Army
Secretary of Veterans Affairs

AIRBORNE HAZARDS RELATED TO DEPLOYMENT

Edited by

COLEEN P. BAIRD, MD, MPH
Program Manager
Environmental Medicine Program
US Army Public Health Command

and

DEANNA K. HARKINS, MD, MPH
Occupational Medicine Physician
Environmental Medicine Program
US Army Public Health Command

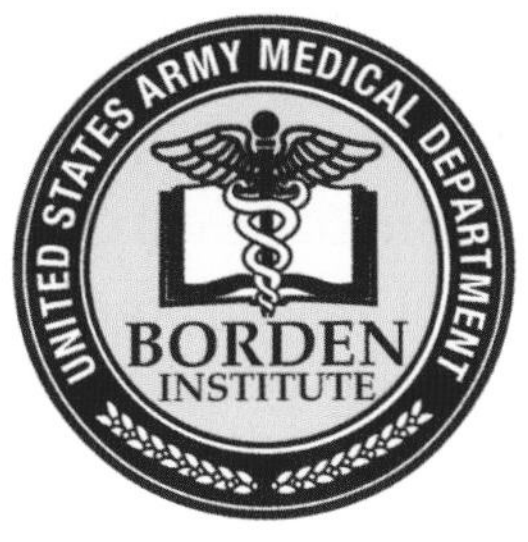

Borden Institute
US Army Medical Department Center and School
Fort Sam Houston, Texas

Office of The Surgeon General
United States Army
Falls Church, Virginia

2015

A Specialty Volume of the

TEXTBOOKS OF MILITARY MEDICINE

Published by the

Borden Institute

US Army Medical Department Center and School

Fort Sam Houston, Texas

Office of The Surgeon General

Department of the Army, United States of America

Editor in Chief

Daniel E. Banks, MD, MS, MACP

Lieutenant Colonel, Medical Corps, US Army

Director, Borden Institute

Timothy K. Jones, DDS

Colonel (Retired), Dental Corps, US Army

Assistant Director, Borden Institute

For sale by the Superintendent of Documents, U.S. Government Publishing Office
Internet: bookstore.gpo.gov Phone: toll free (866) 512-1800; DC area (202) 512-1800
Fax: (202) 512-2104 Mail: Stop IDCC, Washington, DC 20402-0001

ISBN 978-0-16-092762-1

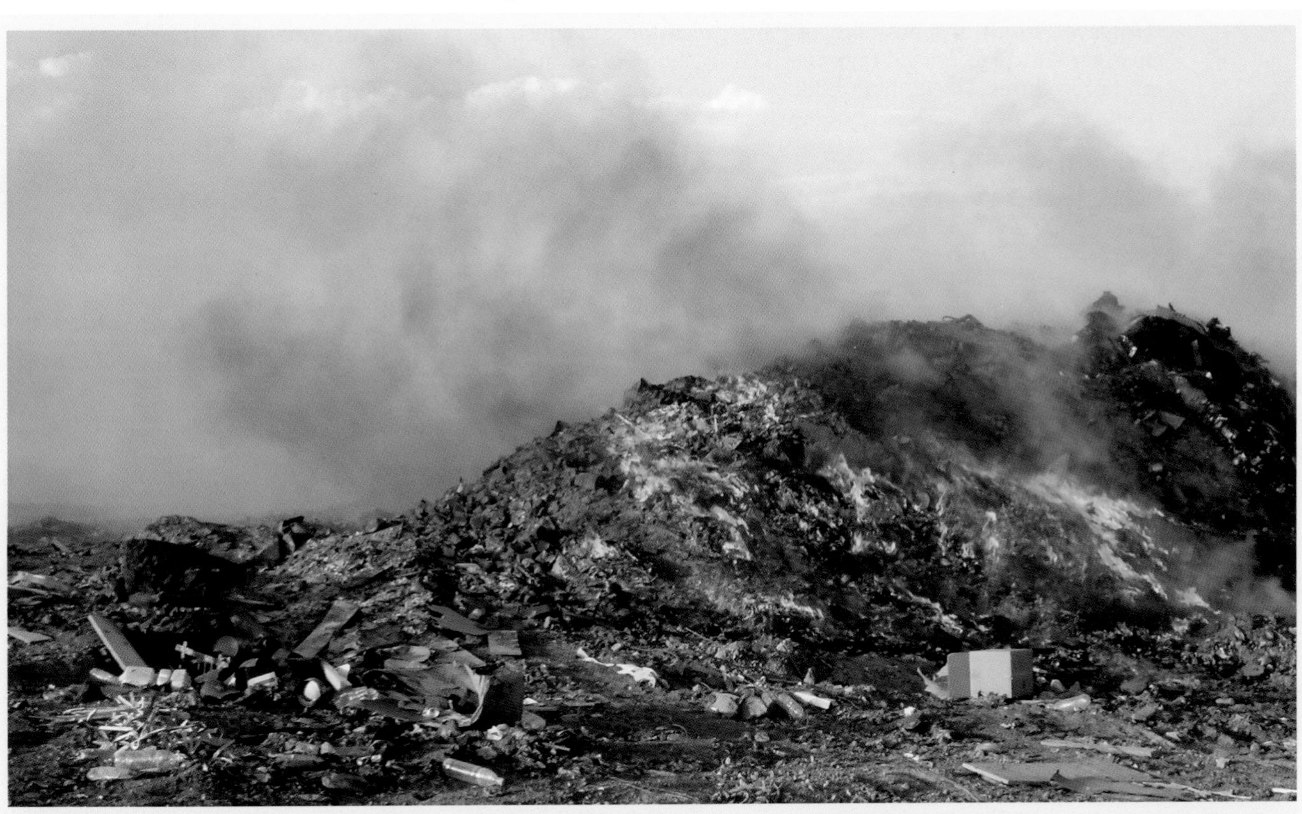

Burn pits have operated in the theater of war during Operation Enduring Freedom, Operation Iraqi Freedom, and Operation New Dawn.

Photograph: Courtesy of the US Army Public Health Command (Aberdeen Proving Ground, Maryland).

This volume was prepared for military medical educational use. The focus of the information is to foster discussion that may form the basis of doctrine and policy. The opinions or assertions contained herein are the private views of the authors and are not to be construed as official or as reflecting the views of the Department of the Army or the Department of Defense.

Dosage Selection:

The authors and publisher have made every effort to ensure the accuracy of dosages cited herein. However, it is the responsibility of every practitioner to consult appropriate information sources to ascertain correct dosages for each clinical situation, especially for new or unfamiliar drugs and procedures. The authors, editors, publisher, and the Department of Defense cannot be held responsible for any errors found in this book.

Use of Trade or Brand Names:

Use of trade or brand names in this publication is for illustrative purposes only and does not imply endorsement by the Department of Defense.

Neutral Language:

Unless this publication states otherwise, masculine nouns and pronouns do not refer exclusively to men.

Published by the Office of The Surgeon General
Borden Institute
Fort Sam Houston, TX 78234-6100

Library of Congress Cataloging-in-Publication Data

Airborne hazards related to deployment / edited by Coleen P. Baird and Deanna K. Harkins.
p. ; cm. -- (Textbooks of military medicine)
Includes bibliographical references and index.
I. Baird, Coleen P., editor. II. Harkins, Deanna K., editor. III. Borden Institute (U.S.), issuing body. IV. United States. Department of the Army. Office of the Surgeon General, issuing body. V. Series: Textbooks of military medicine.
[DNLM: 1. Air Pollutants, Occupational--adverse effects. 2. Lung Diseases. 3. Military Personnel. 4. Respiratory Function Tests. 5. Veterans. WA 450]
RC776.R38
616.2'4--dc23

2015009018

PRINTED IN THE UNITED STATES OF AMERICA

22, 21, 20, 19, 18, 17, 16, 15 5 4 3 2 1

Contents

Contributors

PAUL CIMINERA, MD, MPH
Co-Organizer, Joint DoD/VA Airborne Hazards Symposium
Director, Veterans Health Administration, Office of Public Health, Post-9/11 Era Environmental Health Program, US Department of Veterans Affairs, 810 Vermont Avenue, NW, Washington, DC 20420

WILLIAM ESCHENBACHER, MD
Co-Organizer, Joint DoD/VA Airborne Hazards Symposium
Pulmonologist, Veterans Health Administration, Pulmonary/Critical Care, Cincinnati VA Medical Center, 3200 Vine Street, Cincinnati, Ohio 45220; Professor of Medicine, Division of Pulmonary and Critical Care Medicine, Department of Internal Medicine, University of Cincinnati College of Medicine, 231 Albert Sabin Way, Cincinnati, Ohio 45229

JOSEPH H. ABRAHAM, SCD
Epidemiologist, Environmental Medicine Program, Occupational and Environmental Medicine Portfolio, Army Institute of Public Health, US Army Public Health Command, 5158 Blackhawk Road, Aberdeen Proving Ground, Maryland 21010-5403

COLEEN P. BAIRD, MD, MPH
Program Manager, Environmental Medicine Program, Occupational and Environmental Medicine Portfolio, Army Institute of Public Health, US Army Public Health Command, 5158 Blackhawk Road, Aberdeen Proving Ground, Maryland 21010-5403

DANIEL E. BANKS, MD
Lieutenant Colonel, Medical Corps, US Army; Professor, Department of Medicine, Uniformed Services University for the Health Sciences, 4301 Jones Bridge Road, Bethesda, Maryland 20814; Director and Editor in Chief, Borden Institute, 2478 Stanley Road, Fort Sam Houston, Texas 78234; Staff Physician, Department of Medicine, Brooke Army Medical Center, 3551 Roger Brooke Drive, Fort Sam Houston, Texas 78234

DAVID G. BELL, MD
Lieutenant Colonel, Medical Corps, US Army; Program Director, Pulmonary/Critical Care, San Antonio Military Medical Center, 3551 Roger Brooke Drive, Fort Sam Houston, Texas 78234

KELLEY ANN BRIX, MD, MPH
Deputy Director for the Defense Medical Research and Development Program, Office of the Assistant Secretary of Defense for Health Affairs, Force Health Protection and Readiness Defense Health Headquarters, 7700 Arlington Boulevard, Suite 5101, Falls Church, Virginia 22042-5101

PAUL CIMINERA, MD, MPH
Director, Veterans Health Administration, Office of Public Health, Post-9/11 Era Environmental Health Program, US Department of Veterans Affairs, 810 Vermont Avenue, NW, Washington, DC 20420

LESLIE L. CLARK, PhD
Senior Epidemiologist, General Dynamics Information Technology, Division of Epidemiology and Analysis, Armed Forces Health Surveillance Center, 11800 Tech Road, Suite 220, Silver Spring, Maryland 20904

NANCY F. CRUM-CIANFLONE, MD, MPH
Department Head, Deployment Health Research Department, Naval Health Research Center, 140 Sylvester Road, San Diego, California 92106-3521

BETHNEY A. DAVIDSON, BS
Health Risk Communication Specialist, Army Institute of Public Health, US Army Public Health Command, 5158 Blackhawk Road, Aberdeen Proving Ground, Maryland 21010-5403

WENDI J. DICK, MD, MSPH, MCRP
Senior Advisor to the Afghanistan Assistant Minister of Defense for Health Affairs, Office of the Command Surgeon, NATO Training Mission-Afghanistan, International Security Assistance Force, Kabul, Afghanistan; Former Director, Environmental Health Program, Pre-9/11 Era, Post-Deployment Health, Office of Public Health, Veterans Health Administration, US Department of Veterans Affairs, 810 Vermont Avenue, NW, Washington, DC 20420

DARREL W. DODSON, MD
Colonel, Medical Corps, US Army; Chief, Department of Medicine, Pulmonary / Critical Care Medicine, William Beaumont Army Medical Center, Fort Bliss, 5005 North Piedras Street, El Paso, Texas 79920

ANGELIA EICK-COST, PhD, SCM
Senior Epidemiologist, Henry M. Jackson Foundation for the Advancement of Military Medicine, Division of Epidemiology and Analysis, Armed Forces Health Surveillance Center, 11800 Tech Road, Suite 220, Silver Spring, Maryland 20904

WILLIAM ESCHENBACHER, MD
Pulmonologist, Veterans Health Administration, Pulmonary / Critical Care, Cincinnati VA Medical Center, 3200 Vine Street, Cincinnati, Ohio 45220; Professor of Medicine, Division of Pulmonary and Critical Care Medicine, Department of Internal Medicine, University of Cincinnati College of Medicine, 231 Albert Sabin Way, Cincinnati, Ohio 45229

MICHAEL J. FALVO, PhD
Research Physiologist, War Related Illness and Injury Study Center, Veterans Affairs New Jersey Health Care System, 385 Tremont Avenue, East Orange, New Jersey 07018; Assistant Professor, Rutgers University–New Jersey Medical School, 185 South Orange Avenue, Newark, New Jersey 07103

TERI J. FRANKS, MD
Senior Pulmonary and Mediastinal Pathologist, The Joint Pathology Center, Joint Task Force National Capital Region Medical, 606 Stephen Sitter Avenue, Silver Spring, Maryland 20910-1290

JOANNA M. GAITENS, PhD, MSN/MPH, RN
Research Nurse Associate, Baltimore Veterans Affairs Medical Center, 10 North Greene Street, Baltimore, Maryland 21201; Assistant Professor, Department of Medicine, Occupational Health Program, University of Maryland School of Medicine, 11 South Paca Street, Suite 200, Baltimore, Maryland 21201

JEFFREY R. GALVIN, MD
Professor, Departments of Diagnostic Radiology, Thoracic Imaging, and Internal Medicine, Pulmonary / Critical Care Medicine, University of Maryland School of Medicine, 685 West Baltimore Street, Baltimore, Maryland 21201

JOEL C. GAYDOS, MD, MPH
Colonel (Retired), Medical Corps, US Army; Science Advisor, Armed Forces Health Surveillance Center, 11800 Tech Road, Suite 220, Silver Spring, Maryland 20904

TEE L. GUIDOTTI, MD, MPH, DABT
Vice President for Health / Safety / Environment & Sustainability, Medical Advisory Services, PO Box 7479, Gaithersburg, Maryland 20898; Diplomate, American Board of Toxicology, PO Box 97786, Raleigh, North Carolina 27624

CARA HALLDIN, PhD
Epidemiologist, Division of Respiratory Disease Studies, National Institute for Occupational Safety and Health, Centers for Disease Control and Prevention, 1095 Willowdale Road, Morgantown, West Virginia 26505-2888

DEANNA K. HARKINS, MD, MPH
Occupational Medicine Physician, Environmental Medicine Program, US Army Public Health Command, 5158 Blackhawk Road, Aberdeen Proving Ground, Maryland 21010-5403

RUSSELL A. HARLEY, MD
Senior Pulmonary and Mediastinal Pathologist, The Joint Pathology Center, Joint Task Force National Capital Region Medical, 606 Stephen Sitter Avenue, Silver Spring, Maryland 20910-1290

VERONIQUE HAUSCHILD, MPH
Environmental Scientist, Injury Prevention Program, Epidemiology and Disease Surveillance Portfolio, Army Institute of Public Health, US Army Public Health Command, 5158 Blackhawk Road, Aberdeen Proving Ground, Maryland 21010-5403

ERIN N. HAYNES, DrPH, MS
Assistant Professor, Department of Environmental Health, Division of Epidemiology and Biostatistics, University of Cincinnati College of Medicine, 3223 Eden Avenue, Cincinnati, Ohio 45267-0056

DREW A. HELMER, MD, MS
Director, War Related Illness and Injury Study Center, Veterans Affairs New Jersey Health Care System, 385 Tremont Avenue, East Orange, New Jersey 07018; Associate Professor, Rutgers University–New Jersey Medical School, 185 South Orange Avenue, Newark, New Jersey 07103

STELLA E. HINES, MD, MSPH
Assistant Professor, University of Maryland School of Medicine, Department of Medicine Occupational Health Program and Division of Pulmonary & Critical Care Medicine, Baltimore Veterans Affairs Medical Center, 11 South Paca Street, Suite 200, Baltimore, Maryland 21201

EVA HNIZDO, PhD
Epidemiologist, Division of Respiratory Disease Studies, National Institute for Occupational Safety and Health, Centers for Disease Control and Prevention, 1095 Willowdale Road, Morgantown, West Virginia 26505-2888

ZHENG HU, MS
Biostatistician, Henry M. Jackson Foundation for the Advancement of Military Medicine, Division of Epidemiology and Analysis, Armed Forces Health Surveillance Center, 11800 Tech Road, Suite 220, Silver Spring, Maryland 20904

DAVID A. JACKSON, PhD
Director, Pulmonary Health Program, US Army Center for Environmental Health Research, 568 Doughten Drive, Fort Detrick, Maryland 21702-5010

MICHELLE KENNEDY PRISCO, MSN
Nurse Practitioner, Washington DC Veterans Administration Medical Center, US Department of Veterans Affairs, 810 Vermont Avenue, NW, Washington, DC 20420

LISA M. KIRK BROWN, DrPH
Adjunct Professor, Uniformed Services University of the Health Sciences, 4301 Jones Bridge Road, Bethesda, Maryland 20814

JEFFREY S. KIRKPATRICK, MS
Portfolio Director, Health Risk Management Portfolio, US Army Public Health Command, 5158 Blackhawk Road, Aberdeen Proving Ground, Maryland 21010-5403

KATHLEEN KREISS, MD
Field Studies Branch Chief, Division of Respiratory Disease Studies, National Institute for Occupational Safety and Health, Centers for Disease Control and Prevention, Mailstop H-2800, 1095 Willowdale Road, Morgantown, West Virginia 26505

MICHAEL R. LEWIN-SMITH, MB, BS
Senior Environmental Pathologist, The Joint Pathology Center, Joint Task Force National Capital Region Medical, 606 Stephen Sitter Avenue, Silver Spring, Maryland 20910-1290

JONATHAN LI, BS
Postbaccalaureate premedical student, Stony Brook University, 101 Nicolls Road, Stony Brook, New York 11794

SHARON LUDWIG, MD, MPH, MA
Captain, US Public Health Service/US Coast Guard; Director, Division of Epidemiology and Analysis, Armed Forces Health Surveillance Center, 11800 Tech Road, Suite 220, Silver Spring, Maryland 20904

CAMILLA A. MAUZY, PhD
Biomarker/Biomonitor Development Project Director, Aerospace Toxicology Program, Molecular Bioeffects Branch (RHDJ), 711th Human Performance Wing, Air Force Research Laboratory, Wright-Patterson Air Force Base, Ohio 45433

JENNIFER MBUTHIA, MD
Lieutenant Colonel, Medical Corps, US Army; Office of The Army Surgeon General, Defense Health Headquarters, 7700 Arlington Boulevard, Falls Church, Virginia 22042; Assistant Professor of Pediatrics, Uniformed Services University of the Health Sciences, 4301 Jones Bridge Road, Bethesda, Maryland 20814

CHARLES E. McCANNON, MD, MBA, MPH
Staff Physician, Environmental Medicine Program, Occupational and Environmental Medicine, US Army Public Health Command, 5158 Blackhawk Road, Aberdeen Proving Ground, Maryland 21010-5403

MELISSA A. McDIARMID, MD, MPH
Medical Director, Baltimore Veterans Affairs Medical Center, 10 North Greene Street, Baltimore, Maryland 21201; Professor of Medicine and Epidemiology & Public Health, and Director, Division of Occupational and Environmental Medicine, University of Maryland School of Medicine, 11 South Paca Street, Suite 200, Baltimore, Maryland 21201

RICHARD T. MEEHAN, MD
Captain (Retired), US Navy; Professor of Medicine, Department of Medicine and Rheumatology Division and Co-Director, National Jewish Health Deployment-Related Lung Disease Center, National Jewish Health, 1400 Jackson Street, Denver, Colorado 80206

ROBERT MILLER, MD
Associate Professor of Medicine, Vanderbilt University School of Medicine, Division of Allergy, Pulmonary, and Critical Care Medicine, 6134 Medical Center East, Nashville, Tennessee 37232-8288

YORK E. MILLER, MD
Thomas L. Petty Chair of Lung Research Professor, Department of Medicine, Division of Pulmonary Sciences and Critical Care Medicine, University of Colorado School of Medicine, Anschutz Medical Campus, 12700 East 19th Avenue, Aurora, Colorado 80045; Staff Physician and Chest Clinic Director, Denver Veterans Affairs Medical Center, Eastern Colorado Health Care System, 1055 Clermont Street, Denver, Colorado 80220

MICHAEL J. MORRIS, MD
Colonel (Retired), Medical Corps, US Army; Department of Defense Chair, Staff Physician, Pulmonary/Critical Care Medicine and Assistant Program Director, Internal Medicine Residency, San Antonio Military Medical Center, 3551 Roger Brooke Drive, Fort Sam Houston, Texas 78234

CORINA NEGRESCU, MD, MPH
Veterans Administration Chair and Medical Director, Veterans Benefits Administration, Contract Exams, US Department of Veterans Affairs, 810 Vermont Avenue, NW, Washington, DC 20420

MICHAEL R. PETERSON, DVM, MPH, DrPH
Chief Consultant, Post-Deployment Health, Office of Public Health, Veterans Health Administration, US Department of Veterans Affairs, 810 Vermont Avenue, NW, Washington, DC 20420

RONALD M. PRZYGODZKI, MD
Acting Director, Biomedical Laboratory Research & Development, Office of Research and Development, US Department of Veterans Affairs, 810 Vermont Avenue, NW, Washington, DC 20420

CONNIE RAAB, BA
Director, Public Health Communications, Office of Public Health, Veterans Health Administration, US Department of Veterans Affairs, 810 Vermont Avenue, NW, Washington, DC 20420

AARON I. SCHNEIDERMAN, PhD, MPH, RN
Deputy Director, Epidemiology Program, Post-Deployment Health Group (10P3A), Office of Public Health, Veterans Health Administration, US Department of Veterans Affairs, 810 Vermont Avenue, NW, Washington, DC 20420

JESSICA SHARKEY, MPH
Epidemiologist, Environmental Medicine Program, Occupational and Environmental Medicine Portfolio, Army Institute of Public Health, US Army Public Health Command, 5158 Blackhawk Road, Aberdeen Proving Ground, Maryland 21010-5403

ANTHONY M. SZEMA, MD
Assistant Professor of Medicine and Surgery, Stony Brook University School of Medicine, 101 Nicolls Road, Stony Brook, New York 11794; Chief, Allergy Section, Northport Veterans Affairs Medical Center, 79 Middleville Road, Northport, New York 11768

RONALD F. TEICHMAN, MD, MPH
Occupational and Environmental Medicine Specialist, War Related Illness and Injury Study Center, Veterans Affairs New Jersey Health Care System, 385 Tremont Avenue, East Orange, New Jersey 07018; Teichman Occupational Health Associates, 4 Forest Drive, West Orange, New Jersey 07052

CAROLE N. TINKLEPAUGH, MD, MBA
Occupational Medicine Physician, Environmental Medicine Program, US Army Public Health Command, 5158 Blackhawk Road, Aberdeen Proving Ground, Maryland 21010-5403

CAROLYN H. WELSH, MD
Professor, Department of Medicine, Division of Pulmonary Sciences and Critical Care Medicine, University of Colorado Denver School of Medicine, Anschutz Medical Campus, 12700 East 19th Avenue, Aurora, Colorado 80045; Staff Physician and Sleep Program Director, Denver Veterans Affairs Medical Center, Eastern Colorado Health Care System, 1055 Clermont Street, Denver, Colorado 80220

LISA L. ZACHER, MD
Colonel (Retired), Medical Corps, US Army; Chief, Department of Medicine, Orlando Veterans Administration Medical Center, 5201 Raymond Street, Orlando, Florida 32803

Additional Acknowledgments

COLONEL WILLIAM RICE
Director
Occupational and Environmental Medicine Portfolio
US Army Public Health Command

US ARMY PUBLIC HEALTH COMMAND PUBLICATIONS MANAGEMENT DIVISION
Val Buchanan
Jeannette England
John Eppinger
Audrey Gibson
Rachel Mitchell
Jessica Owens
Anne Quirin
Jody Rush
Joyce Woods

ADMINISTRATION

Patricia A. Gibbs
Tri-Service Vision Program Office Automation Technician
Occupational Medicine Program
US Army Public Health Command

Dinna J. Louissaint
Health Systems Specialist
Occupational and Environmental Medicine Portfolio
US Army Public Health Command

Foreword

I am pleased to present this volume, titled *Airborne Hazards Related to Deployment*, published by the Army Medical Department's Borden Institute. The Borden Institute, part of the Army Medical Department Center and School, is the primary outlet for scholarly and peer-reviewed publications describing observations made and science conducted by the healthcare providers who take care of our Nation's service members and veterans. The Borden Institute's publications do not necessarily represent Army doctrine or the opinion of the Department of Defense or the Army; nevertheless, they represent the best work of our providers as they seek to inform future policy and decision-making.

You are holding a unique book, one that demonstrates the commitment of the Army and the Nation to its soldiers. It was a decade in the making, following several special studies, the involvement of external subject matter experts, the development of strong interagency cooperation between the Department of Defense and the Department of Veterans Affairs, and the direct input of academic medical centers. Inside, the reader will find medical doctors and scientists reaching conclusions that are at odds with each other. This book puts these contradicting learned opinions under one cover, for it is important that readers absorb these writings and come to their own conclusions. Science itself exists on the border between what is known and what is not known, so we are constantly rewriting our medical library of knowledge, while recognizing there is no permanent certainty in science's conclusions. In spite of these difficulties, we are all seeking to understand and to intervene on the side of our soldier patients.

This book represents the state of the science in relation to postdeployment airborne hazards and illnesses. And what a Herculean effort! This work contains 33 chapters with 88 named authors. Although I thank the many authors for showcasing their work, the editors and editorial staff at the US Army Public Health Command—along with their counterparts at the Borden Institute—deserve special praise for their meticulous efforts to ensure the synchronization of many disparate parts into one harmonious whole. I am proud of the whole team!

Patricia D. Horoho
Lieutenant General, US Army
The Surgeon General and
Commanding General
US Army Medical Command

Washington, DC
October 2014

Preface

I join my US Department of Defense (DoD) colleague, Dr Karen Guice, in recognizing the pursuit of scientific truths as a fundamental obligation for US Veterans Affairs (VA) and military medical professionals. The substantial efforts of those who have contributed to this book are a clear signal of our combined commitment to this mission.

The VA asked the Institute of Medicine (IOM) to determine the health consequences of exposure to open burn pits in Iraq and Afghanistan. The IOM report[1] released in October 2011 was comprehensive and provided useful guidance for both the VA and DoD. The IOM endorsed our concern that open burn pits are just one source of potentially harmful exposures. The IOM report stated that, "the pollutants of greatest concern at Joint Base Balad (JBB) may be the mixture of chemicals from regional background and local sources—other than the burn pit—that contribute to high particulate matter . . . ."[1] These airborne exposures may lead to health consequences, especially in those with high exposures or special susceptibility. Particulate matter, which is ubiquitous in southwest Asia and Afghanistan, must be studied in the context of all potentially hazardous exposures.

The Airborne Hazards Symposium held in August 2012 provided an opportunity to discuss what *we know*, what *we need to know*, and what *can be done* to study and improve care for veterans and service members who might have suffered adverse health effects related to exposure to airborne hazards, including burn pit smoke and other pollutants.

We understand that service members and veterans are concerned about what may be causing their illnesses and that these illnesses may affect their future well-being. The VA and DoD are working to provide service members and veterans with the best possible care. For example:

- We are providing healthcare for deployment-related issues at no cost for at least 5 years after deployment. This allows the VA to provide care for veterans while we work to determine individual service connection for their health condition.
- We are providing consistent and seamless care between the DoD and VA by using the same screening and assessment guidelines associated with postdeployment respiratory disease.
- We are continuing to make use of existing studies, such as the 150,000-person Millennium Cohort Study led by the DoD and the 30,000-person National Health Study of a New Generation of US Veterans. These studies enable us to identify adverse health effects associated with deployment, including respiratory disease, and follow them over time.
- We are collaborating through our VA/DoD Deployment Health Working Group so that we can more easily share information, discuss the latest findings, and implement them quickly to serve our veterans.
- We are developing a proposal for a long-term prospective study. The VA's Office of Public Health, working with the VA's Office of Research and Development, is developing a proposal for long-term studies to examine the health effects of deployment to Iraq and Afghanistan and health outcomes among veterans of all eras.
- We developed an Airborne Hazards Joint Action Plan to respond to recommendations from the IOM and as directed by VA and DoD leadership. We are also implementing an Airborne Hazards and Open Burn Pit Registry as required by Public Law 112-260 enacted in January 2013.

The VA strives to care for veterans as a whole and is implementing Patient Aligned Care Teams (PACT) to maximize their total health. At the symposium, we brought together for the first time experts who could offer invaluable insight and expertise to address the environmental health concerns of veterans. Academicians, clinicians, and scientists from the civilian sector—along with representatives of veterans service organizations and veterans—shared their perspectives, experience, and expertise. This book captures those perspectives and scientific views and provides an unprecedented opportunity to make a difference in the lives of our veterans. This knowledge will be translated to better care for veterans through the VA's PACT and environmental health programs, thus ensuring that the combined commitment of the VA and DoD to scientifically understand the health effects of deployment translates to improved health for those who we serve—our service members and veterans.

Reference

1. Institute of Medicine of the National Academies. *Long-Term Health Consequences of Exposure to Burn Pits in Iraq and Afghanistan.* Washington, DC: National Academies Press; 2011: 1–9, 31–44, 117–129.

Madhulika Agarwal, MD, MPH
Deputy Under Secretary for Health for Policy and Services
Veterans Health Administration
US Department of Veterans Affairs

Washington, DC
June 2014

Prologue

The Sergeant Thomas Joseph Sullivan Center

The Sergeant Thomas Joseph Sullivan Center is named for a Marine Corps Sergeant who served in Iraq in 2004 and who suffered from severe postdeployment illnesses of the lung, heart, and musculoskeletal and gastrointestinal systems. Sergeant Sullivan's deployment health records indicate that he had been exposed to desert dust and smoke from burning refuse and chemical plants in theater. Sergeant Sullivan died in 2009 of complications related to postdeployment illness. His family founded The Sergeant Thomas Joseph Sullivan Center in his memory to improve postdeployment health outcomes through awareness, research, and connection, especially for those with complicated illness.

According to one analysis, 20% to 35% of military service members who served in our post-9/11 wars have been exposed to environmental hazards.[1] This potentially translates to as many as 800,000 personnel. The 2012 Joint Department of Defense/Department of Veterans Affairs Airborne Hazards Symposium, on which this book is based, highlighted that airborne hazards—especially dust and smoke (or particulate matter) inhalation—are deployment health risks with potentially serious long-term health consequences. It is important that available information about airborne hazards in the Middle East theater be conveyed to healthcare providers and patients (veterans and others) so that these risk factors may inform clinical practice and patient self-management while scientific research efforts proceed.

Ongoing research on the long-term health impacts of theater airborne hazards, especially dust and smoke inhalation, may yield explanations for respiratory, cardiovascular, immunological, neurological, and other mysterious illnesses that have plagued veterans since the 1991 Persian Gulf War. Research into the role that airborne exposures may play in causing such health problems is essential (as is rapid distribution of findings), even those that are as of yet inconclusive, to educate service members, veterans, and private and public sector healthcare providers.

Such research should be conducted in an open and transparent manner, with input sought from government and non-government centers of medical and scientific excellence and from veterans themselves. Information about ongoing research and lines of investigation, as well as data and findings, must be distributed to the broader medical and scientific communities through government-funded educational initiatives.

Beneath the data, theories, and findings are individuals and families searching for answers; and, in some cases, they are struggling for their lives. The Sergeant Thomas Joseph Sullivan Center stands firm in its support of robust research on the diagnosis, treatment, and prevention of postdeployment illness, including research on airborne hazards and other deployment exposures (environmental, metal, chemical, biological, etc) and the expeditious dissemination of theories and findings to those providing and receiving postdeployment healthcare. The guiding principle for this position is a belief that greater access to information about deployment health risks by providers and patients will improve the overall quality of care and facilitate better health outcomes for veterans and service members with complicated postdeployment illness.

Reference

1. Teichman R. Health hazards of exposures during deployment to war. *J Occup Environ Med.* 2012;54:655–658.

The Sergeant Thomas Joseph Sullivan Center
Washington, DC

Burnpits 360° Advocacy Group

After more than 20 years of military service, including deployment to southwest Asia, a US Army captain was medically retired earlier this year. His life had changed significantly following his redeployment to the United States. He experienced more than 100 medical visits, including encounters with various healthcare providers, numerous visits to emergency rooms, and multiple medical examinations. Also, he experienced first-hand the frustration felt by many who have found it necessary to explain their postdeployment health concerns repeatedly in an effort to obtain diagnosis and treatment. Additional challenges faced by these warfighters include the effects of time spent away from family members and time lost from civilian jobs and other pursuits. In the end, this soldier had to give up not one, but two careers that he loved.

This veteran's story is but one example. He speaks for many warfighters in expressing how extremely vital it is for the medical community of physicians and specialists to become aware of deployment-related health hazards, such as those examined in this book. **Medical education and research should be an uppermost priority for the Department of Defense and the Department of Veterans Affairs.** The medical community, governmental medical agencies, and others who care for warfighters need to work as a team. Cohesive action must be taken to establish protocols and clinics, and to continue to build and develop relevant websites and national registries to their maximum benefit. Veterans, active duty personnel, Department of the Army/Department of Defense civilians, and contractors should be made aware of potential postdeployment medical issues and should be kept up to date on the treatment options available.

We at Burnpits 360° ask that those who use this book join us in helping the community of warfighters achieve a better quality of life. May we work together to better understand and treat all who have been exposed to deployment-related airborne hazards.

Burnpits 360°
Robstown, Texas

Adrian Atizado/Disabled American Veterans

On behalf of Disabled American Veterans, we thank all of the book's contributors for the work that they have done and will continue to do to improve the health and well-being of veterans and service members. It is our hope that the information contained herein will be useful in improving the quality of life of the men and women who were exposed to hazards while serving in the military.

There is a well-documented history not only of toxic and hazardous exposures in the military, but also of the struggle to understand their effects on troops, and the battle to care for veterans, families, and dependents.

The association between deployment-related hazards and their specific resulting conditions often remains unresolved for both the veteran and the medical and research communities. Discussion about deployment-related hazards follows a well-worn path from World War II veterans concerned about ionizing radiation to today's generation of veterans concerned about exposures to airborne and other hazards.

One of the many lessons the Disabled American Veterans has learned from past experience with airborne hazard exposures is that **useful** information regarding their presence within military operating areas must be collected by the Department of Defense, transmitted, and acted on by the Department of Veterans Affairs as early as possible. For example, registries such as the Burn Pit Registry (described in this book), if designed and implemented effectively, can serve as tools for active outreach to concerned veterans and their families. Such registries offer a pathway into the Department of Veterans Affairs healthcare system—a system that is continually learning to provide better care for hazard-exposed veterans.

It is a privilege to be included in the prologue of this important and timely publication. We hope that the valuable information it provides will greatly assist the medical and research communities in their continuing efforts on behalf of our nation's veterans, service members, and their families.

Adrian Atizado
Assistant National Legislative Director
Disabled American Veterans
Cold Spring, Kentucky

Warren Goldstein/The American Legion

The American Legion has long been at the forefront of environmental exposures that have adversely affected our nation's service members and veterans during the Vietnam War, the Gulf War, Operation Iraqi Freedom, and Operation Enduring Freedom.

Agent Orange

After Vietnam, the American Legion announced its sponsorship of an independent study on the effects of exposure to Agent Orange on Vietnam War veterans. Congress received the results of the "American Legion–Columbia University Study of Vietnam-era Veterans" in 1989, which later led to the recognition of Agent Orange benefits. We applauded Secretary Shinseki's decision in 2010 to expand Agent Orange presumptives for veterans who served in Vietnam who currently have leukemia, Parkinson's disease, and hairy cell carcinoma.

Resolution Recommendations

- The American Legion continues to advocate for veterans currently afflicted by dioxins found in herbicides.
- The American Legion vigorously supports liberalization of the rules relating to the evaluation of studies involving exposure to dioxin, and we will continue to closely monitor the development of all ongoing research on the long-term effects of Agent Orange exposure.
- More recently, The American Legion has passed resolutions at national conventions relating to Agent Orange exposure sites within US Air Force C-123K Transport Aircraft and with Blue Water Navy Vietnam veterans.

Gulf War I and Gulf War II Illnesses

After the first Gulf War, The American Legion developed a Persian Gulf War Task Force and hired national staff to evaluate the undiagnosed environmental illnesses affecting these veterans. We have continued to work with the Department of Veterans Affairs through participation in advisory committees and development of several resolutions.

Resolution Recommendations

- It has been determined that thousands of Gulf War veterans will suffer from chronic, unexplained physical symptoms. Many service members who have served in the southwest Asia theater since the 1991 Gulf War, including those serving in Operation Iraqi Freedom, have also been exhibiting chronic, unexplained physical symptoms. The American Legion will present a resolution that extends the presumptive period for service connection for Gulf War veterans with undiagnosed illness.
- There has recently been some progress in research on the long-term health effects of many of the Gulf War veterans who were potentially exposed to environmental hazards during the war, but numerous health concerns experienced by these veterans are still not well understood. Additional research into the long-term health effects of exposures is needed.
- The American Legion recommends that the Department of Veterans Affairs not select a particular date for these undiagnosed symptoms to manifest. Currently, the date for presumptive conditions to manifest is December 3, 2016.

Although we still face ongoing challenges from environmental exposures today, The American Legion has also closely followed environmental exposures with the newest generations of veterans in Iraq and Afghanistan. Most of the focus has been on burn pits both abroad and stateside, but more environmental hazards exist—thus, The American Legion's passing of its resolution on environmental exposures.

The American Legion recommends that the Department of Defense provide a full listing of all environmental toxins. The American Legion believes in treating the veteran first, funding the necessary research, and ensuring that our nation's veterans are not subject to environmental exposures in the future. The American Legion will continue to publicly support and keep abreast of the ongoing Department of Defense and Department of Veterans Affairs research related to environmental hazards and exposures due to deployment. Examples of current research that is being closely monitored are from the War Related Illness and Injury Study Center, which is currently studying the effects of deployment as it relates to cardiopulmonary function and the medically unexplained autonomic functions of Gulf War veterans.

We applaud both the Department of Defense and the Department of Veterans Affairs's work with research and policy, and for supporting the environmental health needs of our nation's veterans. We look forward to sharing our resolutions and concerns with the proper offices and working together to improve health outcomes and treatment.

Warren Goldstein
Senior Field Service Representative
The American Legion
Indianapolis, Indiana

Introduction

One of our most fundamental obligations as military medical professionals is to follow the scientific facts, wherever they may lead, regarding the health status and health risks of the men and women who serve our country. This book honors that obligation. In the following chapters, we provide the scientific community and the public with the current state of our collective scientific knowledge about the long-term health consequences of exposure to airborne hazards in a deployed military environment. For several years, federal, academic, and private sector experts have explored one of the more complex scientific issues facing deployed service members: understanding the health risks from airborne particulates, including burn pit smoke in our deployments to Iraq and Afghanistan.

In October 2011, the Institute of Medicine (IOM), a prestigious and independent medical organization, released its report, *Long-Term Health Consequences of Exposure to Burn Pits in Iraq and Afghanistan*,[1] which examined the relationship of burn pit emissions and other possible airborne exposures to the health of the deployed force. Using measurements of airborne particulate matter, metals, volatile organic compounds, polycyclic aromatic hydrocarbons, dioxins, and furans, the IOM assessed possible exposures to burn pit emissions at Joint Base Balad, in Iraq, and possible health effects associated with those exposures.

Joint Base Balad had arguably the largest burn pit in the entire Iraq/Afghanistan theater. Still, most pollutants detected at Joint Base Balad were found at concentrations below those typical of urban areas outside of the United States and below US health-based reference values considered to be protective of the general population. Nonetheless, background levels of airborne particulate matter (PM) were measured well above US air pollution standards. The IOM noted increased respiratory and cardiovascular morbidity and mortality detected in many studies of other populations exposed to elevated PM levels. The IOM attributed the high PM levels at Joint Base Balad mostly to local and regional sources other than the burn pit emissions, and concluded that if any long-term health risks were associated with deployment to Iraq or Afghanistan, they most likely would be associated with high concentrations of airborne particulates rather than burn pit emissions. Information on health effects resulting from exposures to combinations of substances emitted from the burn pits was unavailable. In the end, the IOM's findings were inconclusive. More study is needed.

In response to the various challenges highlighted in the IOM report, the US Department of Defense (DoD) and the US Department of Veterans Affairs (VA) undertook a series of collaborative steps:

- We drafted an interagency Airborne Hazards Joint Action Plan to map out our objectives for the future. We will continue to address comprehensively the concerns about health effects of burn pit emissions and airborne particulates in theater, and enhance the follow-up medical care for all of our deployed populations at risk from possible airborne hazards.
- We asked the Defense Health Board, comprised of independent subject matter experts, to assess clinical protocols used in diagnosing symptomatic individuals who may have respiratory conditions related to deployment; determine how to establish clinical respiratory function baselines in future deployments; and recommend the types of registries we should consider establishing for tracking individuals with pulmonary symptoms or disease. We asked the Defense Health Board to help guide our research agenda by recommending future research for the DoD to address deployment-related pulmonary disease.

- We hosted the first-ever Joint DoD/VA Airborne Hazards Symposium in August 2012. It convened to help us better understand the possible health effects associated with a variety of inhalational exposures experienced by our military service members and veterans who deployed to Iraq and Afghanistan.

Airborne Hazards Related to Deployment captures the scientific information presented at that symposium. The chapters in this volume provide important background information, the past and present efforts in research and epidemiology, the clinical challenges, and the outreach and research initiatives for the future. I am confident that the scientific community will find them useful and informative.

The issues presented and discussed at this symposium are of great importance to many—our military community, veterans, deploying civilians, family members, contractors, the media, and our elected officials. All are interested in clarifying the long-term health consequences of military deployments, including the exposures to airborne substances in the current conflicts.

Over the last 10 years, the military public health community has overseen and achieved a remarkable outcome—the lowest disease and nonbattle injury rate ever recorded in warfare, despite our presence in some of the most inhospitable places on earth. Notwithstanding that success, our work is far from done. We will continue our efforts to reduce possible health effects of deployments that may not be detected until long after the deployment is over.

I thank everyone who took part in this symposium, whether as an invited speaker or as a participant in the discussions. We have a deep public, moral, and personal obligation to ensure that those who protect this nation are, in turn, protected. I am proud of the contributions of so many experts to advance the knowledge we have in support of these obligations and in support of the broader global health community.

Reference

1. Institute of Medicine of the National Academies. *Long-Term Health Consequences of Exposure to Burn Pits in Iraq and Afghanistan.* Washington, DC: National Academies Press; 2011: 1–9, 31–44, 117–129.

Karen S. Guice, MD, MPP
Principal Deputy
Office of the Assistant Secretary of Defense
Washington, DC

AIRBORNE HAZARDS RELATED TO DEPLOYMENT

Section I: Airborne Exposures and Characterization

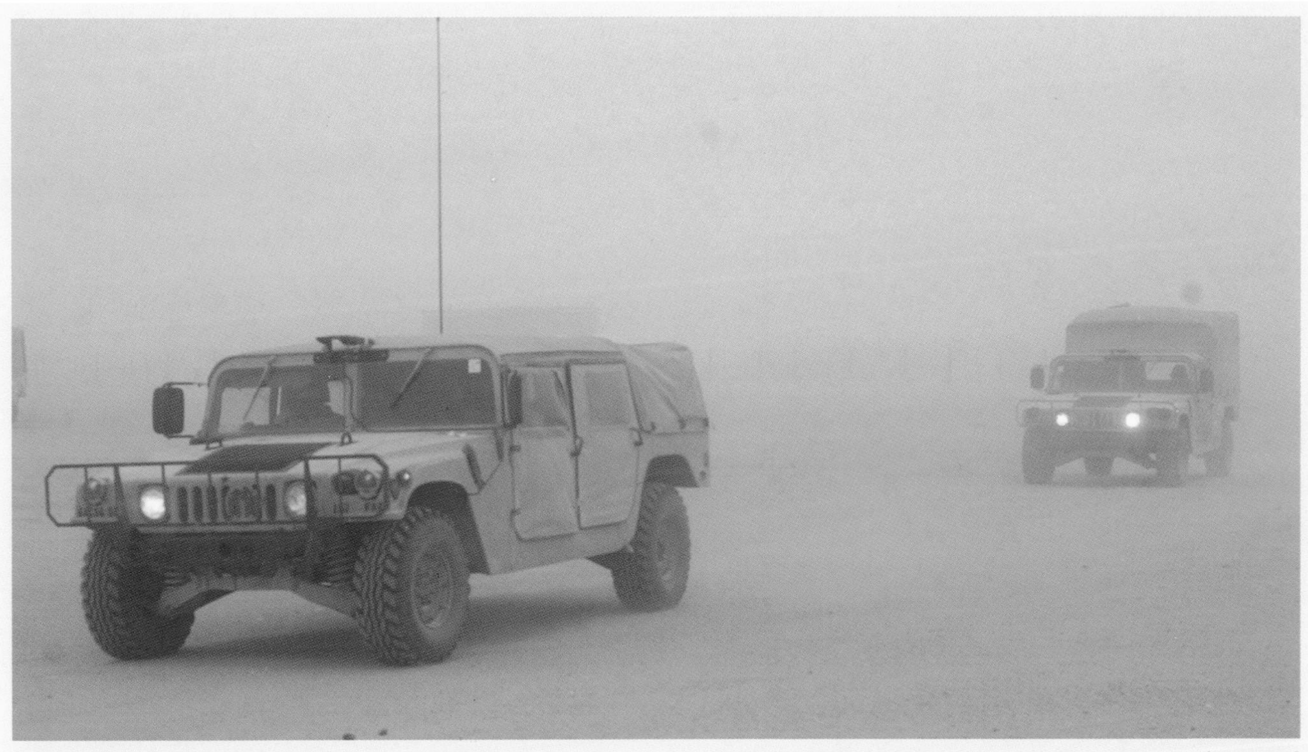

Humvees in the theater of war move cautiously during a dust storm with gusts of up to 29 knots, stirring up sand and cutting down visibility.

Photograph: Courtesy of the US Army Public Health Command (Aberdeen Proving Ground, Maryland). Photographer: Specialist Jacob Boyer.

Chapter 1

OVERVIEW OF AIRBORNE HAZARDS IN OPERATION ENDURING FREEDOM, OPERATION IRAQI FREEDOM, AND OPERATION NEW DAWN

PAUL CIMINERA, MD, MPH*; COLEEN P. BAIRD, MD, MPH†; WILLIAM ESCHENBACHER, MD‡; AND DEANNA K. HARKINS, MD, MPH§

*Director, Veterans Health Administration, Office of Public Health, Post-9/11 Era Environmental Health Program, US Department of Veterans Affairs, 810 Vermont Avenue, NW, Washington, DC 20420

†Program Manager, Environmental Medicine Program, Occupational and Environmental Medicine Portfolio, Army Institute of Public Health, US Army Public Health Command, 5158 Blackhawk Road, Aberdeen Proving Ground, Maryland 21010-5403

‡Pulmonologist, Veterans Health Administration, Pulmonary/Critical Care, Cincinnati VA Medical Center, 3200 Vine Street, Cincinnati, Ohio 45220; Professor of Medicine, Division of Pulmonary and Critical Care Medicine, Department of Internal Medicine, University of Cincinnati College of Medicine, 231 Albert Sabin Way, Cincinnati, Ohio 45229

§Occupational Medicine Physician, Environmental Medicine Program, US Army Public Health Command, 5158 Blackhawk Road, Aberdeen Proving Ground, Maryland 21010-5403

INTRODUCTION

The terrorist attacks of September 11, 2001 on the continental United States were quickly followed on October 7, 2001 by overseas military actions against Al-Qaeda and the supporting Taliban government in Afghanistan.[1] The initial deployment of US Special Forces was small compared with the peak number of service members who ultimately served in Iraq or Afghanistan. By late 2007, deployment of the US Army, the most represented service, peaked with a combined number of 150,000 personnel serving at the same time in Operation Enduring Freedom (OEF) and Operation Iraqi Freedom (OIF).[2] In total (as of June 2012), more than 2.4 million US service members were deployed to OEF, OIF, and Operation New Dawn (OND).[3] In addition to active duty service members, units of the National Guard and the US Army Reserve deployed frequently. The large number of personnel; the repeated individual deployments; the geographical span from southwest to south central Asia; and evolving missions, tactics, and equipment present a broad array of potential health risks. From occupational and environmental health perspectives, these items translate to an increased breadth of potential stressors and an increase in the potential for individuals with enhanced susceptibility to be present in the population at risk to those stressors.

In southwest and south central Asia, inhalational hazards (ie, airborne hazards that may enter the respiratory system) may be naturally occurring or manmade (anthropogenic). Naturally occurring dust from sandstorms caused by disruption of the crustal layer is ubiquitous. Manmade sources of inhalational hazards include local nation and military activities. Military activities and operations (eg, fuel combustion, propellant gases, and other activities) may generate additional inhalational hazards in locations with high levels of preexisting local and regional pollution. Military operations often place service members in locations with little foreign government oversight. These "failed states" lack the governmental services and infrastructure that are essential for the development and enforcement of environmental regulations, particularly regulations related to industrial and vehicle emissions. Military operations may also require emphasis on short-term mission requirements that must be balanced with public and occupational health priorities. The US Department of Veterans Affairs (VA) and the US Department of Defense (DoD) are addressing concerns raised by service members about the long-term health effects related to serving in Iraq and Afghanistan, most notably from exposure to emissions from open waste burning pits that are commonly used for trash disposal. Of note, airborne hazards were also a concern during Operation Desert Shield and Operation Desert Storm; veterans of the 1991 Gulf War expressed health concerns from exposure to smoke from oil well fires and burn pits.[4] These Gulf War concerns are among numerous environmental issues investigated in the context of Gulf War veterans' illnesses and were most recently evaluated in the National Academy of Sciences/Institute of Medicine's (IOM's) *Gulf War and Health*.[5] The two relevant summary findings from this report are (1) "insufficient/inadequate evidence to determine whether an association exists between deployment to the Gulf War and respiratory diseases," and (2) "limited/suggestive evidence of no association between deployment to the Gulf War and decreased lung function in the first 10 years after the war."[5(p149)]

POTENTIAL EXPOSURES OF CONCERN

High levels of ambient particulate matter (PM) were identified as a potential threat to respiratory health early in OIF.[6] Sampling conducted by preventive medicine personnel deployed to the US Central Command (USCENTCOM) area of operations typically demonstrated levels of PM (sometimes referred to as particle pollution in public communications) above those considered healthy by the US Environmental Protection Agency's (USEPA's) National Ambient Air Quality Standards (Exhibit 1-1).[7] In the United States, sources of coarse particles (2.5–10 μm in aerodynamic diameter) include resuspension of soil from roads and streets; disturbance of soil and dust by agricultural, mining, and construction operations; and ocean spray.[8] US sources of fine particles (<2.5 μm) include emissions generated by motor vehicles and coal-fired power plants. "In the Middle East, major sources of particles may differ from those in the United States and other industrialized regions where fossil fuel combustion and vehicle emissions are primary sources of PM."[8(p3)] Generally, the major contributor to PM in southwest Asia is resuspension of dust and soil from the desert floor. Open-air burn pits (hereinafter referred to as "burn pits") were alternate forms of waste disposal used by the US military to dispose of solid waste before incinerators became available during OEF and OIF (Exhibit 1-2). Burn pit emissions contributed to the total burden of pollutants, including gases and PM, to which deployed personnel were exposed. Emissions from open-air burn pits are likely to vary over time and between locations because

EXHIBIT 1-1

DEFINITION, SOURCES, AND GUIDELINES FOR PARTICULATE MATTER

Definition

Particulate matter (PM) pollutants are a complex mixture of extremely small solid particles and liquid droplets in the air. When breathed in, these particles can reach deep into the lungs and cause various health effects. There are generally two size ranges of particles in the air that pose a health concern: (1) particles with an aerodynamic diameter less than or equal to 10 μm (PM_{10}) and (2) even smaller particles, ie, those with a diameter of less than 2.5 μm ($PM_{2.5}$). The smaller particles ($PM_{2.5}$) have become an increasing concern, since medical research shows that they are most likely the particles responsible for the harmful health effects attributed to PM. Many variables influence the nature and probability of health outcomes. The key variables are the size fraction and chemical composition of the PM, the concentration levels, the duration of exposures, and various human factors (including age, health status, habits, genetics, and existing medical conditions). These variables, combined with scientific data gaps, limit the medical community's ability to estimate health impacts to relatively healthy troops, especially because most studies have been on older or less healthy groups.

Sources of Particulate Matter Air Pollution

PM emanates from both natural and manmade sources, including windblown dust, fires, construction activities, factories, power plants, incinerators, and automobiles. In the United States, the European Union, and certain other industrialized regions of the world, fossil fuel combustion and vehicle emissions are the primary sources of these pollutants. In some deployment regions, notably southwest Asia, the PM levels are higher and the sources of PM are different.

Exposure Guidelines

Most studies relate PM exposure data to respiratory and cardiopulmonary health effects in specific susceptible general population subgroups, including young children, the elderly, and especially those with existing asthma or cardiopulmonary disease. In addition, studies of PM-related health effects are primarily conducted in the United States and European urban settings where the PM particle size and composition tend to differ substantially from those of PM found in deployment settings in southwest Asia. As a result, direct use of the available data to estimate health effects on troops in southwest Asia has been problematic. In the interim, the US Army Public Health Command (USAPHC) recommends the use of Military Exposure Guidelines (MEGs) described in Appendix E to assess the severity of potential short-term (acute) and long-term (chronic) effects. These MEGs are based on criteria from the US Environmental Protection Agency (USEPA) National Ambient Air Quality Standards and the USEPA Air Quality Index reporting system (adjusted to reflect the generally healthy military population). The MEGs are based on professional judgment reflecting the current consensus opinion of USAPHC subject matter experts. Because of the substantial scientific uncertainty in estimating acute and especially chronic health outcomes among relatively healthy troops exposed to unique PM compositions, these MEGs are protective estimates about which there is relatively low confidence. They should be considered as such in any PM exposure health effects risk estimates.

of heterogeneity in fuel (trash), and may include PM, metals, volatile organic compounds, and polycyclic aromatic hydrocarbons.[9] Thus, individual exposure to burn pit emissions likely varies by personnel activity patterns and locations relative to the burn pit site, as well as meteorological conditions.

To identify the potential health risks associated with exposure to PM, the Assistant Secretary of Defense for Health Affairs chartered the Joint Particulate Matter Work Group (JPMWG) in 2005. The group included individuals from the three services and other governmental organizations. The JPMWG determined that health outcomes related to PM exposures were plausible, but also noted that there were limited data available to answer fundamental questions. One of the recommendations in the JPMWG report was to conduct enhanced PM surveillance and to conduct epidemiological studies of potential adverse health effects of exposures to PM in the southwest Asia area of operation. Although the risk of various adverse health outcomes, largely respiratory and cardiovascular, becomes greater with increased exposure to PM, the health effects of exposure to PM in the relatively healthy active military personnel deployed in the Middle East had not been well studied at the time of JPMWG analysis.[8]

EXHIBIT 1-2

DEFINITION OF AN OPEN-AIR BURN PIT

The Department of Defense defines an open-air burn pit as "an area, not containing a commercially manufactured incinerator or other equipment specifically designed and manufactured for burning of solid waste, designated for the purpose of disposing of solid waste by burning in the outdoor air at a location with more than 100 attached or assigned personnel and that is in place longer than 90 days."[1]

Data source: (1) US Department of Defense. *Use of Open-Air Burn Pits in Contingency Operations*. Washington, DC: DoD; February 15, 2011. DoD Instruction 4715.19.

ENHANCED PARTICULATE MATTER SAMPLING PROGRAM

Subsequent to the JPMWG recommendation, enhanced PM sampling (EPMS) was conducted every sixth day at 15 locations throughout Iraq and Afghanistan for 12 months (from 2006 to 2007). The final report of this effort is available online (http://phc.amedd.army.mil/PHC%20Resource%20Library/Final%20EPMSP%20Report%20without%20appx%20Feb08.pdf). Associating population health effects to these samples was difficult. In a retrospective manner, the EPMS data was compared with in-theater administrative health data to examine health outcomes for individuals who were at the sampling locations. The number of acute events (eg, asthma admissions or myocardial infarctions) was small, so the study had limited power to identify an association between any of the PM measurements (PM 10-µm or 2.5-µm concentrations) and health outcomes.[10] EPMS data were also used to examine the association between time-weighted average PM 2.5-µm and PM 10-µm samples, and postdeployment respiratory and cardiovascular health outcomes with increasing quartiles of exposure. After adjustment for a number of confounding factors, no statistically significant increases in diagnostic rates were noted, but data were limited by potential exposure misclassification and a relatively short follow-up period.

In 2009, the US Army asked the National Research Council (NRC) to review the EPMS report and its conclusions. Specifically, the NRC was asked to consider the potential acute and chronic health implications, as well as the epidemiological and health surveillance data collected in conjunction with the sampling, and to make recommendations for characterizing health risk. According to the 2010 NRC review, "Although interpretation of the epidemiological and health surveillance studies was encumbered by uncertainties regarding the actual exposures, the small number of study subjects, and the limited amount of exposure data, the EPMS results clearly document that military personnel deployed in the Middle East … are exposed to high concentrations of PM and that the particle composition varies considerably over time and space."[10(p6)] The committee concluded that, "it is indeed plausible that exposure to ambient pollution in the Middle East is associated with adverse health outcomes."[10] It also included a number of recommendations for improving the ability to discern an association between PM levels and health outcome, most specifically by means of more frequent (daily) sampling. Additionally, the committee recognized that the exposures were to a "complex mixture of pollutants."

POTENTIAL HEALTH EFFECTS IDENTIFIED IN EARLY POSTDEPLOYMENT STUDIES

A growing number of medical studies have investigated potential associations between deployment-related environmental exposures and postdeployment chronic respiratory conditions in service members and veterans. Considering the known exposures for deployed individuals, certain respiratory or pulmonary responses, primarily acute, are plausible-based. Specifically, for respirable PM and chemical pollutants, including airborne material from burn pits, previous research indicates that PM exposures can be an irritant and result in acute inflammatory changes in the airways of the lungs with acute decrements in lung function. This, in turn, can lead to development of certain airway diseases (eg, asthma) or worsening of those airway diseases if already present.

Thus far, studies of service members and veterans who have been deployed have shown a variety of clinical findings for specific respiratory conditions ranging from no significant association between PM and cardiorespiratory outcomes to increased respiratory symptoms and a possible increased number of individuals diagnosed with asthma.[11–13] One report suggests the finding of constrictive bronchiolitis (CB)—based on histology of lung tissue from open lung biopsy—in a high percentage of individuals who were evaluated for decreased exercise performance, but little evidence of other objective physiological or radiographic findings.[14] Reports of small numbers of individuals with severe respiratory symptoms, and some with CB, raise concerns regarding the completeness of case findings and appropriate diagnostic workups and resulting diagnoses. The lack of standard case definitions and medical codes may contribute to inconsistent research findings. Variability in the interpretation of radiological, pathological, and diagnostic testing results can also contribute to inconsistent findings of clinical conditions or disease.

To clarify this uncertainty, studies are either in progress or being planned to determine the prevalence of respiratory disease both after deployment and in comparison with nondeployed control groups. Routine clinical data are not sufficient to determine population levels of respiratory disease because neither the DoD nor the VA currently performs routine pulmonary medical monitoring, such as pulmonary function testing, on asymptomatic deployed service members. Chapter 8 (Pulmonary Function Testing—Spirometry Testing for Population Surveillance) and Chapter 9 (Discussion Summary: Recommendation for Surveillance Spirometry in Military Personnel) provide an in-depth discussion of the issues related to screening asymptomatic individuals. Researchers must contend with significant data gaps. It is difficult to evaluate the associations of exposures and health effects when an individual's exposures and potential confounding or contributing risks have not been characterized. Individual exposure data are limited in terms of type, frequency, and duration. Potential risk factors and risk modifiers (eg, smoking status and other personal behaviors, habits, activities, and unique susceptibilities) are not collected consistently, thus preventing the use of existing data to identify persons potentially at higher risk of adverse health outcomes.

HEALTH HAZARD EVALUATIONS OF OPEN-AIR BURN PITS

A notable burn pit existed at Joint Air Base Balad (JBB) in Iraq, the deployment location for many service members (more than 25,000 individuals during 2007 alone). The base generated large volumes of waste that was burned on site. Service members expressed concerns about the potential health risk associated with these operations. To assess exposures at JBB, DoD preventive medicine personnel conducted air sampling of emissions from the burn pit to measure PM, volatile organics, metals, polycyclic aromatic hydrocarbons, and polychlorodibenzodioxins/furans (dioxins and furans).[15] Sampling locations were selected to represent typical and maximum exposure levels for the general population. Samples were collected over multiple 24-hour periods to account for some of the operational and meteorological variabilities in exposure levels. One hundred sixty-three samples were collected, resulting in 4,811 individual analyte results. Data from the sampling effort were subsequently used in a quantitative screening human health risk assessment conducted by the Army and Air Force. Both noncancer and cancer risks were determined to be "acceptable" or "safe," utilizing the USEPA's methods and classification. A potential for short-term, reversible, noncancerous health effects and a "moderate" operational risk from PM were noted.[15(p13)]

The Defense Health Board (DHB), an independent committee comprised of experts from private industry and universities, reviewed the conclusions of the initial screening health risk assessment.[16] The DHB agreed with the conclusion that no long-term health effects should be expected as a result of exposure to dioxin or to the analytes measured and used in the risk assessment. However, that statement did not dismiss the potential for long-term health risk and did not specifically review PM. The DHB conclusions regarding long-term risk were limited by the short-term and intermittent nature of the sampling.

In 2009, to further address concerns that exposure to smoke produced by burn pit operations used to dispose of solid waste in the USCENTCOM contingency operations might be associated with acute and long-term health effects, the Assistant Secretary of Defense for Health Affairs tasked the Armed Forces Health Surveillance Center and the Naval Health Research Center to conduct expedient epidemiological studies using readily available data.[17] These studies were designed to assess whether a wide range of adverse health outcomes (respiratory and cardiovascular conditions, chronic multisystem illness, lupus erythematosus, rheumatoid arthritis, and birth outcomes for infants whose parents had been deployed) were potentially associated with deployment to a location where burn pit operations were known to have occurred. Based on those outcomes reviewed, it was determined that, "upon redeployment, service members from the USCENTCOM locations and the Korea cohort had either similar or significantly lower incidence rates of adverse health outcomes compared with the never-deployed continental US (CONUS)-based cohort, with the exception of 'signs, symptoms and ill-defined conditions' among the Arifjan cohort (a location with no burn pit)."[17(p3)] Comparisons of medical encounters between the USCENTCOM camps in theater did show a higher proportion of respiratory-related medical encounters at JBB (a location with a burn pit), compared with the other three camps, possibly indicating an association between acute respiratory effects and deployment to JBB. However, these effects did not persist upon redeployment. The authors concluded that, "the epidemiological approach used in these studies found no evidence that service members at burn pit locations are at an increased risk for most health outcomes examined."[17(p4)] However, the authors recognized the limitation posed by the lack of individual exposure data, unmeasured confounders, and the limited duration of surveillance. The Armed Forces Health Surveillance Center intends to periodically extend this analysis to longer durations.

In 2009, continued OIF service member and veteran concerns were reflected in letters to the VA from Senator Daniel Akaka (D-HI) and Congressman Tim Bishop (D-NY), along with six co-signers, asking the VA to describe its plans to track and evaluate possible long-term health problems among troops exposed to hazardous materials from open-waste burn pits.[18] Consequently, the Veterans Health Administration Office of Public Health (OPH) requested that an independent scientific body, the National Academy of Sciences/IOM, review the long-term health consequences of burn pit exposure in Iraq and Afghanistan. The IOM Committee report, *Long-Term Health Consequences of Exposure to Burn Pits in Iraq and Afghanistan*,[9] was a special report requested by the VA and was not required by law. This report was specifically requested to address both the veterans' concerns and the uncertainties in the exposure assessments taken from field monitoring data. The OPH presented its Charge to the IOM Committee during the latter's first public session (Exhibit 1-3). The IOM study began in November 2009 and was publicly released on October 31, 2011.

To accomplish its task, the IOM Committee used a wide range of data sources, including peer-reviewed literature, government reports, raw environmental monitoring data, public comment, and other government documents. The IOM Committee first assessed the "types and quantities of materials burned during the time of pit use."[18(p25)] Then, the IOM analyzed air monitoring data collected at JBB during 2007 and 2009. The Committee examined "anticipated health effects from exposure to air pollutants found at JABB"[18(p25)] (noted as JBB in this chapter) and studies of health effects in similar populations with similar exposures, thus grading the quality of those studies as key or supportive. After synthesizing information on potential long-term health effects in military personnel potentially exposed to burn pits, the Committee then developed the design elements and feasibility considerations for an epidemiological study.

The IOM Committee's synthesis on potential long-term health effects of burn pit exposure resulted in two conclusions:

1. limited/suggestive evidence of an association between exposure to combustion products and reduced pulmonary function in the populations studied; and
2. inadequate/insufficient evidence of an association between exposure to combustion products and cancer, respiratory diseases, circulatory diseases, neurological diseases, and adverse reproductive and developmental outcomes in the surrogate populations studied.

The IOM Committee also suggested six recommendations for further research:

1. "A pilot [feasibility] study should be conducted to ensure adequate statistical power, … to adjust for potential confounders, to identify data availability and limitations, and to develop testable research questions and specific objectives.
2. An independent oversight committee … should be established to provide guidance and to review specific objectives, study designs, protocols, and results from the burn pit emissions research programs. …
3. A cohort study of veterans and active duty military should be considered to assess potential long-term health effects related to burn pit emissions in the context of other ambient exposures at the JBB.
4. An exposure assessment for better source attribution and identification of chemicals associated with waste burning and other pollution sources at JBB should be conducted … to help the VA determine those health outcomes most likely to be associated with burn pit exposures.
5. Exposure assessment should include detailed deployment information, including distance and direction individuals lived and worked from the JBB burn pit, duration of deployment, and job duties.
6. Assessment of health outcomes is best done collaboratively using the clinical informatics systems of the DoD and VA."[18(p126)]

Reduced pulmonary function, even if found in returning service members or veterans, would not necessarily equate to the presence of disease, but it might

EXHIBIT 1-3

CHARGE TO THE INSTITUTE OF MEDICINE COMMITTEE[1]

As part of its formal contract with the Institute of Medicine, the Veterans Health Administration developed the following charge for the Committee on Long-term Health Consequences of Exposure to Burn Pits in Iraq and Afghanistan:

- Examine the potential exposures and long-term health risks arising from exposure to smoke created by open burning of solid waste and other materials in Iraq and Afghanistan.
- Use the Joint Air Base Balad (JBB) burn pit in Iraq as an example.
- Examine existing literature that has detailed the types of substances burned and their byproducts.
- Examine the feasibility and design issues for a possible epidemiological study of veterans exposed at the JBB (and other) burn pit(s).
- Explore the background and use of burn pits in the military. Areas of interest may include the following:
  - where burn pits are located,
  - the frequency of use of burn pits and average burn times, and
  - whether materials being burned at Balad are unique or similar to burn pits located elsewhere.
- Recognize if relevant evidence is available from other conflicts (most notably the 1991 Gulf War), the Committee can use that information.
- Note that for evaluation of long-term risks, review a wide range of sources, such as the following:
  - epidemiological studies conducted either by or under the auspices of Veterans Affairs or the Department of Defense;
  - other available epidemiological literature where it exists on
    - the exposed population in question and
    - the populations exposed to similar hazards;
  - environmental studies of relevant hazardous air quality events;
  - relevant toxicological studies;
  - clinical and pathological studies of veteran patients who may have been exposed to environmental hazards from burn pits regardless of conflict; and
  - effects related to short-term peak exposures, as well as chronic exposures (ie, measured as a time-weighted average).
- Recommend research initiatives for Veterans Affairs and the Department of Defense to further study potential long-term health effects.

Data source: (1) Veterans Health Administration. *Committee on Long-term Health Consequences of Exposure to Burn Pits in Iraq and Afghanistan*. Paper presented at: Institute of Medicine's Public Meeting 1; February 23, 2010.

indicate that health effects are occurring. However, as noted previously, the lack of routine pulmonary surveillance in asymptomatic service member and veteran populations limits the ability to detect accelerated pulmonary function decline.

It is important to note that the IOM Committee recognized that burn pits may not be the main cause of long-term health effects related to Iraq and Afghanistan deployment. The report states that, "service in Iraq or Afghanistan—that is, a broader consideration of air pollution than exposure only to burn pit emissions—might be associated with long-term health effects, particularly in susceptible (eg, those who have asthma) or highly exposed subpopulations (eg, those who worked at the burn pit). Such health effects would be caused mainly by high ambient concentrations of PM from both natural and anthropogenic sources, including military sources."[18(p114)] The IOM Committee's report also suggests the need for health outcome studies of those who deployed regardless of burn pit exposure, "preferably another deployed population unexposed to burn pits but exposed to PM and other chemicals identified at JBB from other sources."[18(p125)] This statement from the IOM, in conjunction with VA and DoD assessments that a multitude of inhalation hazards may require study, is best captured by the term *airborne hazards* to define the scope of potential exposures and stakeholders' concerns.

CLINICAL ASPECTS IN THE EVALUATION OF RETURNING SERVICE MEMBERS AND VETERANS

The IOM Committee's conclusion that there was inadequate/insufficient evidence of an association between exposure to combustion products and cancer, respiratory diseases, circulatory diseases, neurological diseases, and adverse reproductive and developmental outcomes is a population-level finding and may not adequately characterize an individual's risk for adverse health outcomes. Individuals may have experienced exposures or may have co-occurring conditions or predispositions that place them at additional risk. Population-level studies may not have sufficient power to recognize these variations. Veterans and service members are returning from deployment with symptoms they did not have during their predeployment screenings. Both the DoD and VA recognize the importance of proper clinical evaluation and risk communication for these symptomatic individuals. It is also important to inform those service members and veterans who are not currently symptomatic (a majority of the population) of evidence-based risk so that they can make informed health decisions with the available evidence, such as improving their overall health through smoking cessation and other prudent, healthy lifestyle modifications.

After appropriate clinical workups of the symptomatic populations within the Military Health System and the Veterans Health Administration, analysis of healthcare operations data revealed a spectrum of diagnoses (asthma, vocal cord dysfunction, obesity, hypersensitivity pneumonitis, and sarcoidosis), as well as individuals with dyspnea on exertion without a recognized cause. Unexplained dyspnea on exertion is not a condition unique to OEF/OIF/OND deployment. Previous studies have documented this finding in nondeployed, active duty populations.[19] As noted previously in this chapter, some service members were diagnosed with CB by means of open-lung biopsy. This finding in individuals with a positive biopsy who demonstrated little abnormality on radiological and physiological screening tests (eg, pulmonary function tests) is of concern. These cases were initially associated with proximity to the sulfur mine fire that burned in Iraq in 2003, but later cases had no such history and were attributed nonspecifically to deployment.[20] A review of the pathological samples from these and other cases is ongoing and expected to be available in late 2013.

A working group of VA and DoD clinicians is developing standardized recommendations for primary care health providers who encounter service members and veterans who have endorsed respiratory symptoms as a result of deployment. Criteria are being developed for the evaluation and referral of some of these patients to appropriate medical specialists for further evaluation. In addition, processes are being cultivated to help identify the number of cases of certain respiratory conditions that have developed during and after deployment, and have presented in patients being treated by DoD or VA medical specialists.

DISCUSSION OF RECOMMENDATIONS BY THE INSTITUTE OF MEDICINE FOR FUTURE EPIDEMIOLOGICAL RESEARCH

The VA-sponsored IOM report published in 2011 provided six recommendations (listed in the previous section on Health Hazard Evaluations of Open-Air Burn Pits) for future epidemiological research that have significant cross-cutting implications for both the VA and DoD. These recommendations are further discussed in Chapter 33 (Discussion Summary: Work Group E—Strategic Research Planning) with planned and potential VA and DoD responses. In light of exposure and long-term health outcome uncertainty, long-term prospective studies are needed to establish a scientific evidence base for further analysis. It is critical to perform these studies in the veteran and service member populations because the studies available to the IOM were surrogate populations whose exposures and risk factors may not represent actual deployed populations and deployment conditions. Respiratory and cardiovascular outcomes deserve the majority of research focus because the current body of evidence for health effects of PM points to these organ systems and to the field PM measurements that routinely exceeded the standards of both the USEPA and the military.

The VA and DoD are collaborating on existing studies (eg, the DoD's Millennium Cohort Study and the VA's National Health Study for a New Generation of US Veterans), and the VA has proposed additional long-term prospective epidemiological studies of potential long-term health effects that may be associated with military service to include deployments. History has shown that not all health effects can be predicted. Therefore, it is essential to develop studies that monitor the overall health status of the study populations rather than restricting the methods to a small list of postulated outcomes. The VA and DoD also recognize that there are concerns related to non-PM exposures (eg, gases containing carcinogens) and nonrespiratory outcomes (eg, cancers). Current exposure data suggest that gaseous exposure is not as ubiquitous as that of PM in OEF/OIF/OND and therefore requires different research methods. The VA and DoD continue to collaborate on current studies and the planning of additional studies to evaluate non-PM exposures and the health effects that may be associated with them.

DEPARTMENT OF DEFENSE AND DEPARTMENT OF VETERANS AFFAIRS ACTIONS

The VA and DoD have historically worked closely on environmental exposure-related health issues. Continuing this collaboration, the two departments developed an Airborne Hazards Joint Action Plan (included in this book as Appendix D) to improve the quality, efficiency, and effectiveness of postdeployment health services to veterans, service members, and military retirees with health concerns related to airborne hazards.[21] This plan was developed under the auspices of the Deployment Health Work Group, which is chartered under the joint Health Executive Council of the DoD and VA. The Airborne Hazards Joint Action Plan addresses not only the IOM Committee's conclusions and research recommendations on burn pits, but also the nonresearch operational matters necessary for the VA and the DoD to provide a comprehensive response. Focus areas in this plan include outreach, follow-up clinical care, population surveillance, and research aimed to improve the health of veterans and service members.

In November 2011, during the action plan's development phase, the VA OPH—with planning assistance from the US Army Public Health Command (Aberdeen Proving Ground, MD)—hosted a roundtable of invited subject matter experts from the VA, DoD, other federal agencies, and academia to collaboratively discuss the issue of airborne hazards and to explore possible "courses of action." Four subject areas were identified and discussed during the meeting: (1) trends in respiratory disease surveillance and their implications; (2) consideration of pulmonary function testing in service members; (3) case finding and workup of postdeployment respiratory disease; and (4) further research. Although the DoD and VA surveillance trends did not show high rates of respiratory disease in the postdeployment population, issues with surveillance using the *International Classification of Diseases, Ninth Revision, Clinical Modification*, codes were noted, and the potential merits of enhanced case findings were discussed.

As follow-up, the OPH and US Army Public Health Command held an Airborne Hazards Symposium in Washington, DC, on August 22, 2012. Through information sharing, this symposium advanced the issues identified during the previous roundtable. The symposium consisted of plenary sessions on relevant topics and working group discussions in seven specific areas:

1. diagnosis and workup of symptomatic individuals,
2. exposure characterization,
3. current epidemiology,
4. potential role of pulmonary function testing (spirometry) in surveillance,
5. strategic research planning,
6. clinical follow-up and registries, and
7. risk communication.

Of the many tangible outcomes from this conference, this book—developed from symposium presentations by a diverse group of scientific experts and with veteran perspectives—represents a compendium of what is currently known regarding the potential long-term health consequences of exposure to airborne hazards during OEF/OIF/OND deployments. This book presents a balanced, comprehensive approach to furthering the understanding of airborne hazards during deployments and other military operations, ultimately improving airborne hazard prevention, protection, and avoidance while improving healthcare and minimizing adverse health outcomes of our service members and veterans.

The DoD and VA are also coordinating closely to establish an Open Burn Pit Registry as required in Public Law 112-260 (Dignified Burial and Other Veterans' Benefits Improvement Act of 2012) that was enacted by President Obama on January 10, 2013. This law requires periodic outreach and requires the VA to work with an independent scientific organization to prepare a report on the activities of the secretaries. The VA will utilize the Open Burn Pit Registry to the maximum extent possible to improve understanding of the long-term health effects of deployment exposures, recognizing that the ability to determine robust scientific associations will be limited and given that participation in this voluntary health registry is self-selected. Unlike earlier environmental health registries that focused solely on in-person examinations, the planned Open Burn Pit Registry is a widely accessible self-assessment available through mobile Internet technologies. Optional in-person examinations will be available for symptomatic individuals and those who request an examination.

SUMMARY

Based on the available scientific and medical evidence presented in the IOM report—*Long-Term Health Consequences of Exposure to Burn Pits in Iraq and Afghanistan*—and other available scientific information, the Secretary of the VA made a determination (published in the *Federal Register* in February 2013) that the VA should further study the possible long-term adverse health effects of veterans of Iraq and Afghanistan who were potentially exposed to airborne hazards. This study was to include air pollution in general, as well as smoke from burn pits.[22] Specifically, the Secretary of the VA directed the Veterans Health Administration to conduct a longitudinal cohort study on all adverse effects related to military deployment to Iraq and Afghanistan (carefully considering the IOM's research recommendations). Realizing the importance of collaboration, the Secretary of the VA also sent a letter to the Secretary of Defense in late January 2013 describing the former's actions to date and highlighting the continued collaboration. The DoD and VA will continue their long-established clinical and research collaboration on this issue, specifically through the established joint work groups, to provide policy recommendations, clinical education, and outreach.

REFERENCES

1. Torreon BS. *U.S. Periods of War and Dates of Current Conflicts*. Washington, DC: Congressional Research Service; 2011. Report RS21405.

2. Bonds TM, Baiocchi D, McDonald LL. *Army Deployments to OIF and OEF*. Santa Monica, CA: Rand Corporation; 2010.

3. Epidemiology Program, Post Deployment Health Strategic Healthcare Group, Office of Public Health, Veterans Health Administration, Department of Veterans Affairs. *Analysis of VA Health Care Utilization Among Operation Enduring Freedom, Operation Iraqi Freedom, and Operation New Dawn Veterans, from 1st Qtr FY 2002 Through 1st Qtr FY 2012*. Washington, DC: Veterans Health Administration; 2012.

4. Institute of Medicine of the National Academies. *Gulf War and Health, Volume 1. Depleted Uranium, Sarin, Pyridostigmine Bromide, Vaccines*. Washington, DC: National Academies Press; 2000.

5. Institute of Medicine of the National Academies. *Gulf War and Health, Volume 8. Health Effects of Serving in the Gulf War*. Washington, DC: National Academies Press; 2010.

6. Desert Research Institute. *DoD Enhanced Particulate Matter Surveillance Program*. Reno, NV: DRI; 2008. Final Report.

7. US Environmental Protection Agency. *Integrated Science Assessment for Particulate Matter*. Washington, DC: USEPA; 2009. EPA/600/R-08/139F Final Report.

8. National Research Council. *Review of the Department of Defense Enhanced Particulate Matter Surveillance Program Report*. Washington, DC: National Academies Press; 2010: 10–11, 51–56.

9. Institute of Medicine of the National Academies. *Long-Term Health Consequences of Exposure to Burn Pits in Iraq and Afghanistan*. Washington, DC: National Academies Press; 2011: 1–9, 31–44, 117–129.

10. Teichman R, ed. Health effects of deployment to Afghanistan and Iraq. *J Occup Environ Med*. 2012;54;655–761.

11. Smith B, Wong CA, Smith TC, et al. Newly reported respiratory symptoms and conditions among military personnel deployed to Iraq and Afghanistan: a prospective population-based study. *Am J Epidemiol*. 2009;170:1433–1442.

12. Abraham JH, Baird CP. A case-crossover study of ambient particulate matter and cardiovascular and respiratory medical encounters among US military personnel deployed to southwest Asia. *J Occup Environ Med*. 2012;54:733–739.

13. Szema AM, Salihi W, Savary K, Chen JJ. Respiratory symptoms necessitating spirometry among soldiers with Iraq / Afghanistan war lung injury. *J Occup Environ Med.* 2011;53:961–965.

14. King M. Constrictive bronchiolitis in soldiers returning from Iraq and Afghanistan. *N Engl J Med.* 2011;365:222–230.

15. US Air Force Institute for Operational Health. *Screening Health Risk Assessment Burn Pit Exposures, Balad Air Base, Iraq and Addendum Report*. Brooks City-Base, TX: AFIOH; 2008. Report IOH-RS-BR-TR-2008-001.

16. Defense Health Board. *Defense Health Board Findings Pertaining to Health Risk Assessment, Burn Pit Exposures, Balad Air Base, Iraq.* Falls Church, VA: DHB; 2008. Memorandum.

17. Office of the Assistant Secretary of Defense for Health Affairs. *Evaluation of Potential Health Effects of Exposure to Smoke from Open Pit Burning During Deployment in the U.S. Central Command Area of Responsibility*. Washington, DC: OASDHA; 2009. Memorandum.

18. Shinseki EK. Burn pit toxic emissions. Letters from Veterans Affairs Secretary Eric K. Shinseki to Congressmen Bishop, Blumenauer, Delahunt, Ellison, Hinchey, Levin, and Schwartz. Washington, DC: Department of Veterans' Affairs; 2009.

19. Morris MJ, Grbach VX, Deal LE, et al. Evaluation of exertional dyspnea in the active duty patient: the diagnostic approach and the utility of clinical testing. *Mil Med*. 2002;167:281–288.

20. King MS, Miller R, Johnson J, et al. Bronchiolitis in soldiers with inhalational exposures in the Iraq War. Paper presented at: American Thoracic Society Conference; May 16–21, 2008; Toronto, Ontario, Canada.

21. Department of Defense / Department of Veterans' Affairs. *Draft VA/DoD Airborne Hazards Action Plan.* Washington, DC: DoD / VA; 2012.

22. Department of Veterans Affairs. Initial research on the long-term health consequences of exposure to burn pits in Iraq and Afghanistan. *Fed Regist*. 2013;78:7860–7861. Notice.

Chapter 2

BACKGROUND OF DEPLOYMENT-RELATED AIRBORNE EXPOSURES OF INTEREST AND USE OF EXPOSURE DATA IN ENVIRONMENTAL EPIDEMIOLOGY STUDIES

JEFFREY S. KIRKPATRICK, MS*; AND COLEEN P. BAIRD, MD, MPH†

**Portfolio Director, Health Risk Management Portfolio, US Army Public Health Command, 5158 Blackhawk Road, Aberdeen Proving Ground, Maryland 21010-5403*

†Program Manager, Environmental Medicine Program, Occupational and Environmental Medicine Portfolio, Army Institute of Public Health, US Army Public Health Command, 5158 Blackhawk Road, Aberdeen Proving Ground, Maryland 21010-5403

INTRODUCTION

Deployed US forces have faced several large- and small-scale airborne exposures from military operations since World War II. These forces have been deployed to worldwide locations that exhibit natural environmental conditions that create airborne exposures to particulate matter (PM) from sand and dust storms via the arid environment and active sand sheets. Examples of these locations include

- Northern Africa—World War II,
- Kuwait and Saudi Arabia—Operation Desert Storm,
- Afghanistan—Operation Enduring Freedom, and
- Iraq—Operation Iraqi Freedom and Operation New Dawn.

US forces have also been deployed to locations where operational aspects have inadvertently contributed to potential airborne exposures from chemical and combustion emissions. Examples of these include exposure to Agent Orange (Vietnam)[1]; low-level chemical agents (sarin/cyclosarin) in Khamisiyah, Iraq[2]; and airborne exposures to open-air burning and other local/regional pollution sources in Iraq and Afghanistan.[3]

The US Department of Defense (DoD) and the US Department of Veterans Affairs (DVA) remain diligent in protecting, maintaining, and improving the health of service members, veterans, and civilian employees. These departments strive to collaborate on understanding and sharing information and data on exposures that occur in deployed environments.

Over the past three decades, the DoD has worked to establish and focus proactive and retrospective efforts on deployment-related exposures. Past, current, and future populations of military personnel and veterans deserve the collaborative efforts of the DoD and DVA. Stakeholders need to understand and consider how airborne exposures can impact the health of these populations.

The DoD executed tactical-based operations in Vietnam, during which aerial spraying of tactical herbicide chemicals/Agent Orange—that contained 2,3,7,8-tetrachlorodibenzo-*p*-dioxin (TCDD)—defoliated jungle canopies to decrease the enemy's advantage of camouflage. Through the Vietnam conflict and postdeployment years, the military and veterans communities gained knowledge from toxicological and medical studies that exposure to chemicals comprising TCDD could have health implications.[1]

Over the past two decades, the DoD has deployed US forces to contingency locations exhibiting arid environments with predominant sand/dust surfaces. In addition, some of these environments contain natural resources (eg, crude oil) of strategic interest. Anthropogenic (combustion-related), naturally occurring (sand/dust storms), and mechanical/fugitive (tracked vehicles) sources contributed to an increase in the PM loading in the lower atmosphere. The DoD has extensively sampled, analyzed, characterized, and assessed the PM at forward and rear troop locations since 1991.[4] The Kuwait oil well fires in 1991, along with regional sand/dust storms and localized fugitive emissions, significantly contributed to increased ambient PM levels in Kuwait and Saudi Arabia.[5]

In southern Iraq, Kuwait, and Saudi Arabia, the period from February through October 1991 displayed measured PM levels with concentrations from tens to thousands of micrograms per cubic meter of air. Analysis of 1991 ambient PM samples showed that the particles were mostly sand-based materials that relate to the observed high levels of PM typically found in southwest Asia.[6] In addition, associated heavy metals analyses displayed vanadium (a component of Kuwaiti crude oil) and lead (from combustion of leaded gasoline) were not associated with any long-term health risks. Electron microscopy of the ambient particles revealed that sand-based particles accounted for the majority of the particle mass on the samples.

During Operation Desert Storm, chemical agent exposure from demolition activities in and around Khamisiyah, Iraq, posed a potential airborne hazard. In early March 1991, US forces used explosives to destroy captured munitions from the Khamisiyah Storage Depot (bunkers and open pit). In 1996, the DoD and US Central Intelligence Agency (CIA) determined that those demolition activities potentially released low levels of the sarin/cyclosarin chemical agent from destroyed 122-mm rockets. Extensive retrospective assessments culminated in July 1997 with the DoD's and the CIA's announcement that no US troops were in the area that was predicted to have association with noticeable health effects during the March 10, 1991 demolition event. However, the modeling results did indicate that troops in Iraq and Saudi Arabia were possibly exposed to low levels of nerve agent over a 4-day period from March 10 to 13, 1991. Using data on then-available unit locations, the DoD identified 98,910 soldiers within the potential hazard area predicted by the models. From late July through September 1997, the DoD sent written notices to two categories of veterans: (1) those who had served in the potential chemical agent hazard area; and (2) those who had received a letter and survey from the Deputy Secretary of Defense, but who had not served in the potential chemical agent hazard area. On September 4, 1997, the DoD/CIA team published the details of this modeling effort in the document *Modeling the Chemical Warfare Agent Release at the Khamisiyah Pit.*[2]

Concern regarding exposure to ambient PM for Operation Enduring Freedom and Operation Iraqi Freedom/Operation New Dawn continued in the mid-2000s. The DoD established a PM work group in 2005 to gather information and assess PM levels at 15 major base camps (troop locations) in the US Central Command area of responsibility.[7] Similar to those efforts conducted in 1991, extensive ambient air and surface soil sampling measures were completed. The samples characterized the mineralogy, particle size distribution, and geomorphological aspects of the ambient PM and surface soils at these locations. The primary conclusions from this study stated that,

> In general, we do not consider dust from the 2006–2007 studied areas in the Middle East to be out of the ordinary. Comparison of dust samples from the 15 Middle East sites to dust from the US, Sahara, and China shows similar chemical and mineralogical constituents in most cases. Mineralogical content, chemical composition, and to a lesser extent individual particle analysis of sieved and re-suspended dust as well as ambient samples from each site, bear the signature of that region's geology to some extent.[8(pii,7)]

Open-air burning of solid waste is a final example of an airborne hazard in a deployed environment. Open burning of solid waste materials and/or paper products has long been used by the DoD when other disposal options are not available.[3] During Operation Iraqi Freedom, open burning operations on various base camps increased in the mid-2000s because of the insurgency and the risks associated with offsite disposal. From 2007 to 2010, an ambient air sampling and surveillance effort was conducted at Joint Base Balad, Iraq, in response to concerns associated with solid waste burn pits. This proactive effort is an example of how sampling and information from occupational and environmental health site assessments were used to identify and assess inhalation hazards from a combination of the burn pits and other combustion sources, industrial activities, and natural PM. These air surveillance efforts provided enhanced data and information that helped to characterize the risk of possible acute and long-term health effects from degraded air quality and the effects of the measured pollutants.

In summary, the primary conclusions from these efforts showed that exposure levels of the receptors to carcinogenic chemicals of potential concern were within the exposure levels that the US Environmental Protection Agency (USEPA) generally considers acceptable excess lifetime cancer risk (1E-04 to 1E-06) and within which management of risk should be considered. The excess noncancer hazard indices exceed unity (ie, >1) primarily due to acrolein, indicating there may have been a concern for potential health effects. The associated health effects would primarily have been short-term, reversible, and possibly include irritation of the mucous membranes and dizziness or lightheadedness. Sensitive individuals, such as asthmatics, might have been more prone to develop worse, longer lasting symptoms (eg, wheezing and bronchitis), but these symptoms were expected to be reversible. Ambient particulate matter levels were typically elevated above respective military exposure guidelines. Because service members may be affected by longer term health effects—possibly from combined exposures (eg, sand, dust, industrial pollutants, tobacco, and other agents), as well as individual susceptibilities—studies continue.[4]

Since 1991, the DoD has extensively increased the amount of environmental sampling (ie, air, water, and soil) completed in deployed environments. It became apparent from evaluations of the Kuwait oil well fires and Operation Joint Endeavor (Bosnia) that the available environmental surveillance equipment for air, water, and soil sampling was complex, bulky, and expensive. In 1997, the US Army Center for Health Promotion and Preventive Medicine (now the US Army Public Health Command, Aberdeen Proving Ground, MD) initiated efforts to improve the environmental sampling equipment for military applications by obtaining available, commercial, and off-the-shelf sampling systems. Efforts were completed to make existing (garrison-based) equipment and sampling media lighter, smaller, simpler to operate, and more rugged. For ambient air sampling, efforts were completed to provide battery-operated, portable, commercial, off-the-shelf sampling equipment and media (along with needed training) to deploying and/or deployed personnel.[9]

The DoD has also enhanced exposure and health risk assessment processes so that predeployment or Phase I hazards assessment are completed for locations of interest.[4] This all-hazards analysis helps to identify the equipment, sampling media, and training required for "boots-on-the-ground" missions. When unique hazards or threats requiring special surveillance or sampling methods are identified, actions are taken to procure the special equipment and supplies needed by the deployed environmental health personnel to assess those hazards and threats. Sampling for dioxin levels near burn pit locations is an example. Risk is estimated using established health risk assessment methodologies from the USEPA and the DoD. The USEPA method summarizes exposure and toxicity data that are then integrated into expressions of risk. For potential noncarcinogenic effects, comparisons are made between projected intakes of substances and toxicity values. For potential carcinogenic effects, probabilities that an individual will develop cancer over a lifetime of exposure are estimated from projected intakes and chemical-specific, dose–response data. The DoD method uses health-based military exposure guidelines (ie, health-based chemical concentrations for various deployed military exposure scenarios representing levels at which no, some, or significant health effects could occur within the exposed, deployed population) for air, water, and soil to determine—via a military risk management framework—operational risk levels for deployed populations. In an iterative process, if results indicate that risk is high, the command is notified of mitigation options. Lower risks are prioritized and addressed with follow-on assessment and evaluation of mitigation methods. This ongoing effort has provided strong force health protection. This systematic and iterative assessment produces steady improvement in the understanding of risks.[4]

In addition, the DoD has developed and operates corporate databases that store field (administrative) data, analytical data, and health risk assessment reports. These corporate solutions for environmental health information and data are known as the Defense Occupational and Environmental Health Readiness System (DOEHRS) and the Military Exposure Surveillance Library (MESL). The DOEHRS maintains more than 24,500 samples collected worldwide since 1996, and the MESL maintains more than 30,000 environmental health/preventive medicine data, reports, and assessments.[4]

To advance health service support to future joint force commanders, the DoD is working strategic-level efforts through the Joint Capabilities Integration and Development System process that is used by the Joint Requirements Oversight Council to fulfill advisory responsibilities in identifying, assessing, validating, and prioritizing joint military capabilities documents.[10] Unique outputs of this process are used to facilitate doctrine, organization, training, materiel, leadership, education, personnel, facilities, and policy changes to the defense acquisition system to inform the planning, programming, budgeting, and execution process in the acquisition and budgeting systems. A recent accomplishment resulting from this process is the 2010 DoD *Joint Force Health Protection Initial Capabilities Document* that identified capability gaps and shortfalls, and recommended solution approaches for providing Joint Force Health Protection during the 2015–2025 timeframe.[11] In particular, the Joint Health Surveillance, Intelligence, and Preventive Medicine functional area outlines three capabilities:

1. providing comprehensive health surveillance,
2. enhancing medical intelligence preparation of the operational environment, and
3. providing full-spectrum preventive medicine support.

These capabilities feed the three lines of action that address the identified shortfalls and support the development of enterprise-wide solution sets for joint operational capabilities and improved support to the warfighter. A working example of the joint operational capability is the use of the DOEHRS to operate and maintain an environmental health surveillance registries website that contains the Operation Tomodachi Registry for the 2011 Japan radiation incident from the earthquake and tsunami.[12] The DoD is collaborating with the DVA to establish an individual longitudinal exposure record (ILER) that will be part of the integrated electronic health record (IEHR) rollout to improve the exchange of health data between the two departments. This effort is scheduled to "go live" in 2017, and the IEHR will be an integral component that identifies a single common health record for service members and veterans that can be accessed at any DoD or DVA medical facility.[13]

POTENTIAL USES OF ENVIRONMENTAL SAMPLING DATA

As previously described, efforts to characterize and address risk from environmental exposures have strengthened over the past two decades. The ultimate goal of environmental sampling is the protection of health or, barring that, the assessment of the health impact to those exposed either at the individual or population level.[14] Exposure assessment at the individual level may serve clinical needs, epidemiological research needs, or support policy considerations.[15] Characterization of individual exposure supports epidemiological studies, ideally with quantitative dose information useful for dose–response trend analysis. It may also address potentially confounding variables. Exposure information may assist in the determination of eligibility for registries, if criteria exist, and may enable physicians to establish service connection for medical compensation purposes.[16] Individual exposure characterizations are also used to support commanders' decisions related to risk prevention and mitigation—eg, removal of personnel from a site, work/rest cycles, or personal protective equipment use—to accomplish the mission as effectively as possible with the fewest casualties.

Uses of sampling data for epidemiological purposes can be problematic. Following the first Gulf War, the Institute of Medicine (IOM) noted that because very little personalized exposure information was available, defining relevant exposed and control groups was difficult. This lack of exposure data limited even the most expert and well-funded investigations to identify health outcomes linked to specific exposures or risk factors.[17] Similarly, the US Government Accountability Office noted that, "without accurate exposure information, the investment of millions of dollars in further epidemiological research on risk factors or potential causes for Veterans' illnesses may result in little return."[18] In the early 1990s, environmental sampling (apart from the testing of field drinking water) was not a traditional skill of environmental science officers. Appropriate equipment and methods included items that were not part of standard equipment sets, were complex to operate, had specific power requirements and were not field rugged, and often did not provide real-time results. In 2000, the IOM recommended a "systematic process to prospectively evaluate non-battle-related risks associated with the activities and settings of deployment."[19] Similarly, in an article addressing the IOM report, Lioy notes that, "a key to success … is the rapidity with which individuals, including exposure scientists and occupational hygienists, can identify the source(s) and agent(s) of concern, characterize exposure pathways, and implement controls. Thus, training in exposure science is a needed specialization within the Armed Forces."[20]

Although combatant commanders have recognized that a preventive medicine capability gap in the infectious disease realm can negatively impact current troop strength, most noninfectious environmental exposures pose a long-term risk of injury or illness, with the exception of acute, high-dose incidents (eg, chemical spills or releases). Despite the fact that DoD capabilities included environmental and occupational health specialists, many of these assets were not part of the typical deployment footprint, although this varies by service. Historically, forward-deployed preventive medicine assets focused on traditional public health activities, known as "field sanitation," which encompass food safety, vector control, water supply, and small scale waste management.[21] Traditional environmental exposure monitoring initiatives had been focused on chemical warfare agents, with a recent expansion into biological agent monitoring. This broadening followed key events, such as the anthrax exposures, as well as the increased availability of polymerase chain reaction technologies to identify agents. In light of the last decade's surge in global terrorist activities, commanders have expressed concern over the use of toxic industrial chemicals/toxic industrial materials (TICs/TIMs) as a cheap and effective way to induce casualties.[22]

Lioy[20] suggested that, for planning purposes, the military should consider the use of Acute Exposure Guideline Levels (AEGLs), established under the auspices of the USEPA, as short-term exposure guidelines when conducting health risk assessments in deployed settings. These AEGL values establish exposure levels for no-adverse effect, reversible effects, and as a lethal dose for specified time periods; this varies by chemical/material.[23] The military has used the AEGLs to serve as the starting point in the derivation of operationally specific Military Exposure Guidelines to address short-term exposures to highly toxic chemicals in deployed settings.[24] Long-term exposure levels have also been derived using other values, such as USEPA reference concentrations, as a starting point. Despite the available reference guidelines, there are technology gaps regarding the military's capability to monitor at those levels. The first AEGL chemical priority list included approximately 100 chemicals; the second list was several times as large. The development of field-rugged sensors for such an extensive list of hazards may be impractical. According to the National Research Council, improvements in military defense and preventive medicine material capabilities for chemical and biological exposures require a focused effort.[25] Although field gas chromatography/mass spectroscopy capability in deployed settings has become more widespread following post-9/11 concerns related to TIC/TIM releases, having the right equipment—at the right place and at the right time—remains a challenge.[14]

IMPLICATION OF DATA GAPS

Veterans who are injured as a result of their service, who become chronically ill while in service, or who (following their discharge) develop an illness whose origins are in their service have long been provided healthcare coverage and disability compensation. Any condition that develops while a service member is on military service is considered service-connected.[16] Whether his or her service caused or contributed to the condition or it occurred coincidentally while in service is not a factor if the service member did not have the condition upon entering the service, but does have it upon separation. The significance of the service connection is that it is necessary for awarding compensation to the service member. When a medical condition occurs after service, compensation may be provided if the condition is shown or "presumed" to be caused or aggravated by an exposure or event that occurred during military service. For example, asbestos-related disease in a service member with a known and documented past exposure to asbestos while in the military would be considered service-connected. Whereas it is recognized that service members may face a variety of exposures with the potential to affect their health, a presumption of service connection may be made when exposures are considered likely. Unfortunately, there is often limited documentation of exposure or uncertainty regarding who was exposed.[26] Presumption removes the need for the veteran to establish that the exposure occurred and that it contributed to a specific illness. The most well-known example of presumption addresses Agent Orange exposure during service in the Vietnam War.[16] Because of the uncertainty regarding the degree of exposure, the presumption is that all personnel with actual ground-based service in Vietnam were exposed.[27] Presumptions may result from limited records of the types and concentrations of environmental contaminants present in locations where service members served or difficulty in linking actual exposure data with individuals who spent time at those locations. However, potential exposure does not automatically equate to actual exposure or to a measurable risk of disease. During medieval times, physician and alchemist Paracelsus supposedly stated that, "Poison is in everything, and no thing is without poison. The dosage makes either a poison or a remedy."[28] This maxim recognizes that adverse health outcomes associated with exposure are dependent on the concentration (magnitude), frequency, and duration of exposure.

Using the specific diseases that are presumed to be related to Agent Orange exposure as an example, presumptions are based on the IOM's reviews of the scientific evidence and the DVA's assessment of those reviews. Since 1921, Congress and the Secretary of the DVA have made nearly 150 presumptions.[16] The DVA "now provides disability compensation to approximately 3,000,000 veterans and 342,000 beneficiaries (survivors of those who died as a result of their conditions), expending approximately $41 billion annually for this purpose."[16]

When an exposure is considered for presumption, the IOM conducts a systematic review of the available evidence regarding the exposure and assesses the weight of evidence and the strength of any associations. Under the Agent Orange model, four levels of evidence are identified:

1. Sufficient evidence of an association.
2. Limited/suggestive evidence of an association.
3. Inadequate/insufficient evidence to determine whether an association exists.
4. Limited/suggestive evidence of no association.

More recently, the IOM has added the category "sufficient evidence of a *causal* relationship."[3] Sufficient evidence of an association requires positive health outcomes in human studies in which bias and confounding have been ruled out with reasonable confidence. Sufficient evidence of *causality* requires the evidence to meet several of the Hill[29]criteria for causation:

- strength of an association,
- temporal association,
- dose–response relationship, and
- plausibility and specificity.

Following such a review, the DVA receives the report and determines whether particular health outcomes will be considered service-connected on a presumptive basis. Congress and the DVA generally "act to provide compensation so as to not exclude veterans deserving of compensation ('false negatives') while recognizing that some veterans with illnesses not caused by military service will be compensated as a result ('false positives')."[16] Therefore, evidence of a causal relationship is not necessary; indeed, consistent evidence of an association is not necessary because limited/suggestive evidence of an association has been found to be sufficient for presumption in some cases. This could be because of a statistically significant finding in one high-quality study. In the report on potential improvements to the presumptive disability decision-making process, the IOM recommended the preferred role of causation over association in evidence-based decisions.[16] It also recommended stakeholder input/nomination of illnesses and exposures for consideration (a transparent process), flexibility, and the consideration of the extent of a disease attributable to an exposure relative to other potential causes or contributors (eg, smoking).[26] The committee recognized that evidence might accumulate over time to alter the balance. To reduce uncertainty in assessing the relationship between health conditions and military service, the committee logically recommended better exposure information, but also recognized the complexity of exposures received during deployment and the complications from combat conditions. Exposures were broadly considered as complex physical, chemical, biological, and psychological stressors. It was recognized that feasibility and cost of data collection may be an issue, but these costs may be far less than those of presumptions made because of lack of data.

USE OF SAMPLING DATA FOR EPIDEMIOLOGY

Given the importance of human studies in the evidence base considered for presumptions, the use of available exposure information to conduct epidemiological studies is expected. Following the first Gulf War, modeled oil well fire smoke exposures were used to assess associations with hospitalizations, particularly for respiratory conditions.[30] The findings in these efforts were clouded by factors such as modeling based on limited sampling data points, limited access to unit location records, and the fact that hospitalization is an insensitive health outcome measure. In recent conflicts (Operation Enduring Freedom/Operation Iraqi Freedom/Operation New Dawn), likewise, available data have been leveraged in an attempt to assess exposure/outcome relationships. In the recent review of the long-term health consequences of exposure to burn pits, the IOM had five epidemiological studies of military personnel available for review.[3] These studies were conducted by the Armed Forces Health Surveillance Center, the Naval Health Research Center, and the US Army Public Health Command. All of them were contained in a report released by the Armed Forces Health Surveillance Center in 2010.[31] In these studies, exposure was defined as deployment to a site with an active burn pit because individual exposure data were not available. The report included one study of the respiratory health outcomes of individuals deployed to locations with and without burn pits, discussed elsewhere in this book. The four additional studies utilized a similar methodology and examined the rates of a variety of other outcomes. One study compared birth outcomes in infants of military personnel who were within certain distances from a burn pit or at a location without a burn pit before or during pregnancy. The other three studies utilized participants in the Millennium Cohort Study, comparing those who had deployed to locations with burn pits to those deployed to sites without burn pits. The outcomes examined included respiratory symptoms and conditions, birth outcomes, chronic multisystem illness, and physician-diagnosed lupus or rheumatoid arthritis. Although a discussion of the individual study findings and their strengths and limitations is beyond the scope of this chapter, taken as a whole, there were no consistent findings associated with past deployment to a site with an open burn pit. The IOM review noted that exposure misclassification was possible, and the IOM committee considered the studies important, but "supporting" versus "key" for the following reasons:

- because the follow-up period (36 months) was considered too short for some long-term outcomes to manifest, and
- because the studies lacked information on other hazardous environmental exposures common in the context of desert and war (eg, smoking, diesel exhaust, kerosene heaters, PM, and local and regional pollution).

The committee identified a variety of factors—such as job duties, specific locations, smoking status, activities, etc—that would enhance exposure characterization.[3] Acknowledging the limitations of the military studies, the IOM chose the approach of evaluating human health effects from exposure to combustion products.[3] These studies were evaluated for their quality and for their relevance to the situation and used in a weight-of-evidence approach. Studies on firefighters (those exposed to chemical and wildfires) and incinerator workers were most frequently relied upon, although studies of communities around incinerators were also reviewed. Outcomes in multiple organ systems, as well as cancer, were evaluated. On the basis of these reviews, the committee was "unable to say whether long-term health effects are likely to result from exposure to emissions." However, based on their review of the epidemiological literature, the committee concluded that there was limited/suggestive evidence of an association between exposure to combustion products and reduced pulmonary function in the populations studied. They also concluded that, "there is inadequate/insufficient evidence of an exposure to combustion products and cancer, respiratory disease, circulatory disease, neurologic disease, and adverse reproductive and developmental outcomes in the populations studied."

Regarding the military studies, while limitations due to length of follow-up are correctable as more time has elapsed, there is little accessible and available information to further evaluate other potential exposures. When base camp rosters are used to assess computerized coded health outcomes in large groups of interest and control groups, information on smoking status is not easily available, although it is certainly recorded somewhere within the actual medical record. Although the other hazards were known in some detail (PM levels and ranges at the base level), the magnitude of exposure to the other noted "hazards" would vary according to duties and location, and was not available for these cohorts.[8] Despite specific occupations, duties may change during deployments. For example, guard duty may be performed by a variety of individuals who have other typical duties, and these individuals likely had the highest exposure to burning trash. Information on local microclimates or specific areas on the camps is lacking.

It is interesting, however, to note that the committee stated that exposure misclassification was also a significant uncertainty/limitation in the key studies evaluated in addition to the military studies. "None of the studies ... have actual measures of inhalation to combustion products. Without measured individual exposure information, an individual might be assigned to the wrong level of exposure, thus masking the association between exposure and effect."[3] They also noted that most of these studies classified exposure qualitatively by employment status (yes/no), although a few attempted to quantify cumulative dose (duration of employment or number of fires fought) and distance from an incinerator for those studies of communities living around incinerators. In many of the epidemiological studies of respiratory effects potentially associated with deployment, exposure is defined as deployment, with nondeployed personnel serving as a comparison group.[32–37] Although some exposure data may be available, it is generally limited in scope, time, or space, and is rarely tied to an individual. It is difficult to assess dose–response trends without information on the frequency, magnitude, and duration of an exposure, ideally at the individual level. Data used comes from sampling that is conducted for hazard screening, not individual exposure assessment.

Despite these limitations, several additional attempts have been made to utilize the available data to perform epidemiological studies. Just as the committee relied on studies of populations exposed to combustion products lacking exposure measurements or data on other potential exposures, the study of deployment-related health conditions may never have the luxury of complete exposure information. Even so, if plausible health effects are demonstrated consistently in those deployed in excess of those who have not with no other explanation, this provides some evidence of association to airborne hazards, particularly for respiratory conditions. As the committee noted, these effects, if they occur, may be related to combustion products, PM exposure, air pollution, or other hazards alone or in combination. Conditions that occur more frequently in the broadly "exposed" that are plausibly associated with the potential exposures—after a time sufficient to cause disease, in the presence of clinical or laboratory findings compatible with that disease, and in the absence of other explanations for that disease—may be considered deployment-associated without complete information on exposure. Various studies have attempted to evaluate potential associations using available information, as discussed below.

Thus, in what ways are the IOM conclusions valid for a cause-and-effect relationship for burn pit exposure and lung disease? Consider, perhaps (among other notions), that the symptoms that developed in the exposed were the same. Then, those with greater exposures (nearer the burn pit or more time working at the burn pit) had more illnesses and recognition of the clearly toxic materials in the pits could explain the findings. We make this conclusion/diagnosis all the time—witness coal workers' pneumoconiosis and silicosis diagnoses. All that is made without personal sampling.

If we needed personal sampling to diagnose occupational/environmental illnesses, we would not diagnose many. To bring all this into the deployed environment is a grand expectation. Perhaps we should use a clinical definition for respiratory illness attributed to burn pit exposure to make the diagnosis (as we do for pneumoconiosis):

- exposure to the material in question for a time sufficient to cause disease;
- clinical features (including imaging if relevant) consistent with that disease; and
- the absence of other exposures that could be responsible for the illness.

AMBIENT PARTICULATE MATTER

During Operation Enduring Freedom/Operation Iraqi Freedom, ambient air sampling identified PM levels that were elevated, compared with US levels.[38] Data from epidemiological studies based in the United States had identified a number of acute and chronic health concerns, but these effects were identified in study populations to include children, adults over age 65, and those who had chronic conditions and, as such, were a somewhat different population than deployed forces.[39] Additionally, it was recognized that PM in southwest Asia was likely different in composition than the PM in the United States.[38] As a result, a more extensive, every-sixth-day sampling effort for PM was initiated and supported by forward-deployed preventive medicine assets. The samples were analyzed for PM concentration, as well as numerous other parameters (eg, heavy metals). Following this effort, two epidemiological studies were conducted to evaluate potential associations with measured PM levels and health outcomes.[40,41] One study attempted to correlate acute, in-theater health events with days during which PM levels were high. Individuals served as their own control by looking at acute visits for respiratory and cardiovascular events the day of and the day following high PM levels compared with other days. However, given the every-sixth-day sampling schedule, events that occurred on days when no samples were taken could not be evaluated. Because of this and the fact that the overall number of events was low, this effort suffered from low power to detect an association.[40] The other study identified populations at the base camp locations where sampling was conducted, and it compared postdeployment health outcomes by exposure levels. To do so, a variable associated with the PM exposure had to be created, and a decision was made to construct a time-weighted average based on the every-sixth-day sampling.[41] PM levels were divided into quartiles, and association between increasing quartiles of exposure and increased number of health events was assessed. Although this study also failed to identify a dose–response increase in health effects, it was noted that the every-sixth-day sampling may have been insufficient to characterize the exposure, and the constructed exposure variable may not have been sensitive for the outcome of interest. The PM sampling plan was primarily focused on characterization of the airborne PM because of concerns about its potential to cause a hazard; it had not been designed specifically to support epidemiological studies. However, when the studies attempted to utilize the data, it was recognized that there were data limitations. Health concerns in populations for which there is some exposure data often generate interest in utilizing the exposure data to assess health outcomes. Historically, in the field of occupational medicine, this approach was used to assess potential human health effects associated with occupational cohorts for whom limited sampling existed.[42] Then, as now, the generalizability of intermittent sampling—whether it represented peak or average exposures—remains an issue. Many of these occupational studies suffered from potential misclassification, were too small to have sufficient statistical power to detect elevated rates of significance, and lacked information on confounding variables (eg, smoking).[42] These limitations were evident in the studies utilizing deployment sampling data, as well. Regarding the use of the enhanced PM surveillance (EPMS) data for epidemiology, the Committee on Toxicology of the National Academy of Sciences reviewed the studies and noted that, "if the available exposure data are not sufficient to characterize adequately the likely exposures of people for whom health outcome data are collected, then an epidemiological study of associations between the exposure of interest and the outcome of interest will not provide valid results."[41] The committee concluded that the exposure data in the EPMS report, although informative, were insufficient to characterize the exposure of most deployed personnel during the period of monitoring for the purpose of linking exposure to health.

THE 2003 SULFUR MINE FIRE

Another effort to use limited environmental data for epidemiological purposes followed a 2003 sulfur mine fire. On June 24, 2003, US military field reports indicated a large fire had started at the state-run Al-Mishraq Sulfur Plant near Mosul, Iraq.[43] The fire burned continuously for almost a month—until approximately July 21, 2003—emitting dense clouds of sulfur dioxide (SO_2), a byproduct of the combustion of elemental sulfur piles.

The overall amount of SO_2 released into the atmosphere during the fire was later estimated at approximately 600 kilotons (Kt), with a daily average of approximately 21 Kt per day. In comparison with highly polluting plants in the United States that produce 20 Kt per year, the Mishraq sulfur fire was considered an exceptionally strong point source of SO_2.[44] At the time of the incident, thousands of US military personnel were deployed to the area in support of Operation Iraqi Freedom. Some of the troops in the area were called on to assist local Iraqis with fighting the sulfur fire. Others assisted with evacuating civilians from local towns nearby or continued various military missions and transport operations in the area. Military reports noted that odors characteristic of sulfur were reported at a base camp referred to as Q-West, which was 25 km southwest of Al-Mishraq, and also as far away as the Mosul International Airport area, approximately 50 km to the north. Medical personnel at Q-West reported that medical visits potentially associated with the fire, mostly associated with respiratory irritation, increased by approximately 20% during the period of the fire. Available direct-reading monitoring equipment was used to obtain a limited number of grab samples for SO_2 and hydrogen sulfide (H_2S); these samples demonstrated extremely variable concentrations over a broad area and time. Some of the grab sample concentrations were high enough to be consistent with significant acute effects, such as eye and respiratory tract irritation, and were compatible with some of the physical complaints reported by field personnel. Over long periods, these levels are potentially associated with chronic respiratory conditions. Because of the limited availability of equipment and personnel for this extensive area, these real-time samples were taken at only a few locations and only on a few days. Therefore, these sample results did not provide an adequate basis to characterize the exposure received by any particular person or group. Both SO_2 and H_2S can be acutely fatal at high levels of exposure, but no deaths were documented secondary to the fire.[43] High, but nonfatal, exposures can result in notable acute respiratory effects, as well as ocular and skin irritations. Neither SO_2 nor H_2S is a known carcinogen.[45–47]

A roster of individuals onsite to extinguish the fire was identified; a larger group was known to be within a 50-km radius of the site. These two groups were considered "exposed" and were followed to assess the impact of exposure to the smoke plume on the health of US Army personnel deployed to the area.[43] Self-reported, postdeployment health status and the occurrence of postdeployment medical encounters for respiratory health outcomes for these two groups were compared with corresponding data from two unexposed comparison groups. Postdeployment, self-reported health concerns were common in the population of interest, as were complaints of symptoms of difficulty breathing and shortness of breath. Medical encounter rates for chronic respiratory conditions increased not only in the two potentially exposed groups (firefighters, as well as personnel in the 50-km area), but also in both comparison groups when pre- to postdeployment time periods were compared.

The occurrence of postdeployment medical encounters for chronic respiratory conditions among the exposed group did not differ significantly from that expected, based on the unexposed comparison groups. In this study, postdeployment medical encounters for respiratory conditions were not associated with exposure to the sulfur fire. Troops deployed to the sulfur fire site well after the fire had been extinguished were more likely to have an initial, postdeployment respiratory disease medical encounter than did personnel exposed to the sulfur fire. All groups showed an increase in respiratory visits postdeployment compared with predeployment, although this increase was statistically significant in only one of the unexposed comparison groups. At least some of the increase in healthcare encounters after redeployment is expected because of referrals generated from self-reported symptoms and exposure concerns identified in the postdeployment health assessments. The limitations of this study were similar to those studies previously discussed, including a lack of individual exposure data and information on confounding variables. Unit location data might have placed some personnel at Q-West, for example, when they actually spent most of their time traveling the supply route to the north. Even when information regarding the base camp for a unit is available, the individual activity of the unit and its location patterns differ.

SUMMARY

Efforts to characterize the deployed environment have markedly increased in the last 15 years, and location data have improved as well. Although data identifying the exact location and activities of an individual are still lacking, the base camp locations of units are known. Much ambient sampling data are available; the lack of available individual data remains a concern. As previously described, the DoD has funded an electronic ILER for every service member to improve the availability of exposure information on individuals.[13] Conceptually, ILERs will be produced using a person-centric business intelligence strategy that connects person, time, place, event, and all available occupational and ambient environmental monitoring data with medical encounter information (diagnosis, treatment, and laboratory information, including biomonitoring where available). Information currently available to populate ILERs includes deployment dates and locations to the level of base camp, exposure concerns self-reported on the Post-Deployment Health Assessment, general location and time-specific ambient sampling data, and sampling information on specific exposure incidents that may have occurred (with rosters of those potentially exposed, where available). Utilizing individual identifiers, it is possible to tie base camp locations and sampling information to medical visit information codes (ICD [*International Classification of Diseases*] 9/10 revisions) either through direct connection of the systems or through data-use agreements between systems.[31] Because the current data are population-level data, all individuals at a location are considered equally exposed, which certainly has limitations. However, for PM at least, the exposure profiles, PM characteristics, and composition differ by base camp and might be used as a variable.

The ILER will facilitate the creation of exposure registries that can be assembled based on a multitude of parameters, including dates, locations, and types of exposure where such information exists. The Operation Tomodachi Registry, which includes more than 60,000 individuals who were in Japan at the time of the Fukushima nuclear reactor accident and their radiation doses, is such an example.[12] The value of the ILER will be enhanced with the fielding of technologies, including passive individual exposure dosimeters, occupational monitoring and the creation of similarly exposed groups in deployed settings, and validated biomarkers that may improve individual exposure assessment or serve as early indicators of effect. This knowledge can be used to enhance both the DoD's and DVA's medical care, medical surveillance, and disability evaluation and benefits determination processes. Characterizing deployed environments poses considerable challenges, but improvements in technological and information management systems will allow such characterizations to become more widely available. The challenge remains to improve them by means of selecting valid, reliable, and efficient exposure assessment tools for the most relevant exposures.

REFERENCES

1. Young AL, Cecil PF. Agent Orange exposure and attributed health effects in Vietnam veterans. *Mil Med*. 2011;176(suppl 7):29–34.

2. US Department of Defense. *Case Narrative: US Demolition Operations at the Khamisiyah Ammunition Storage Point, Final Report, April 16, 2002*. GulfLINK website. http://www.gulflink.osd.mil/khamisiyah_iii/. Accessed November 30, 2011.

3. Institute of Medicine of the National Academies. *Long-Term Health Consequences of Exposure to Burn Pits in Iraq and Afghanistan.* Washington, DC: The National Academies Press; 2011: 1–9, 31–44, 117–129.

4. Martin NJ, Richards EE, Kirkpatrick JS. Exposure science in U.S. military operations: a review. *Mil Med*. 2011;176(suppl 7):77–83.

5. US Department of the Army. *Final Report, Kuwait Oil Well Fires Health Risk Assessment No. 39-36-L192-91, 5 May–3 December 1991.* Washington, DC: US Army Environmental Hygiene Agency; 1994. Memorandum HSHB-ME-S(40).

6. Presidential Advisory Committee for Gulf War Veterans' Illnesses. *Presidential Advisory Committee for Gulf War Veterans' Illnesses: Final Report.* Washington, DC: US Government Printing Office; 1996.

7. US Department of Defense, Assistant Secretary of Defense for Health Affairs. *Joint Particulate Matter Work Group Charter; March 31, 2005.* Washington, DC: DoD.

8. Engelbrecht JP, McDonald EV, Gillies JA, Gertler AW. *Department of Defense Enhanced Particulate Matter Surveillance Program (EPMSP).* Reno, NV: Desert Research Institute; 2008. W9124R-05-C-0135/SUBCLIN 000101-ACRN-AB. Final Report.

9. Kirkpatrick JS. The impact of U.S. military operations in Kuwait, Bosnia, and Kosovo (1991–2000) on environmental health surveillance, *Mil Med*. 2011;176(suppl 7):41–45.

10. US Department of Defense. *Joint Capabilities Integration and Development System*. Washington, DC: Chairman of the Joint Chiefs of Staff (CJCS); 2012. CJCS Instruction (CJCSI) 3710.01H.

11. US Department of Defense. *Joint Force Health Protection Initial Capabilities Document.* Washington, DC: Joint Requirements Oversight Council (JROC); 2010. JROC Memorandum 113-10.

12. US Department of Defense. *Environmental Health Surveillance Registries.* Defense Health Services System website. https://registry.csd.disa.mil/registryWeb/DisplayHomePage.do. Accessed December 21, 2012.

13. US Department of Defense. *Electronic Health Record Milestone.* Washington, DC: Office of the Assistant Secretary of Defense (Public Affairs); May 2012. No. 408-12.

14. Baird C. The basis for and uses of environmental sampling to assess health risk in deployed settings. *Mil Med.* 2011;176(suppl 7):84–90.

15. Teichman R. Exposures of concern to veterans returning from Afghanistan and Iraq. *J Occup Environ Med.* 2012;54:677–681.

16. Samet JM, McMichael GH, Wilcox AJ. The use of epidemiological evidence in the compensation of veterans. *Ann Epidemiol.* 2010;20:421–427.

17. Institute of Medicine of the National Academies. *Consequences of Service During the Persian Gulf War: Recommendations for Research and Information Systems.* Washington, DC: The National Academies Press; 1996.

18. US Government Accountability Office. *Gulf War Illnesses: Improved Monitoring of Clinical Progress and Reexamination of Research Emphasis Are Needed.* Washington, DC: GAO; 1997. GAO/NSAID-97163.

19. Institute of Medicine of the National Academies. *Protecting Those That Service: Strategies to Protect the Health of Deployed US Forces.* Washington, DC: The National Academies Press; 2000.

20. Lioy PJ. Exposure science for terrorist attacks and theaters of military conflict: minimizing contact with toxicants. *Mil Med.* 2011;176(suppl 7):71–76.

21. US Department of the Army. *Field Hygiene and Sanitation.* Washington, DC: DA; 2000. Field Manual 21-10.

22. US Department of the Army. *Industrial Chemical Prioritization and Determination of Critical Hazards of Concern: Technical Annex and Supporting Documents for International Task Force (ITF)-40.* Aberdeen Proving Ground, MD: US Army Center for Health Promotion and Preventive Medicine; 2003. Report 47-EM-6154-0.

23. US Environmental Protection Agency. *Acute Emergency Guideline Levels Program (AEGLs).* EPA website. http://www.epa.gov/oppt/aegl/. Accessed December 21, 2012.

24. US Department of the Army. *Environmental Health Risk Assessment and Chemical Exposure Guidelines for Deployed Military Personnel.* Aberdeen Proving Ground, MD: US Army Public Health Command (Provisional); 2010. Technical Guide 230.

25. National Research Council. *Determining Core Capabilities in Chemical and Biological Defense Science and Technology (2012).* Washington, DC: The National Academies Press; 2012.

26. Institute of Medicine of the National Academies. *Improving the Presumptive Decision-making Process for Veterans.* Washington, DC: The National Academies Press; 2007.

27. Institute of Medicine of the National Academies. *Veterans and Agent Orange: Update 2010* (and prior reports). Washington, DC: The National Academies Press; 2010.

28. Paracelsus. About.com Medieval History website. http://www.egs.edu/library/paracelcus/biography. Accessed February 24, 2013.

29. Hill AB. The environment and disease: association or causation? *Proc Soc Med.* 1965;58:295–300.

30. Gray GC, Smith TC, Knoke JD, Heller JM. The postwar hospitalization experience of Gulf War veterans possibly exposed to chemical munitions destruction at Khamisiyah, Iraq. *Am J Epidemiol.* 1999;150:532–540.

31. US Armed Forces Health Surveillance Center, the Naval Health Research Center, and the US Army Public Health Command. *Epidemiological Studies of Health Outcomes Among Troops Deployed to Burn Pit Sites*. Silver Spring, MD: Defense Technical Information Center; 2010.

32. Sanders JW, Putnam SD, Frankart C, et al. Impact of illness and non-combat injury during Operations Iraqi Freedom and Enduring Freedom (Afghanistan). *Am J Trop Med Hyg*. 2005;73:713–719.

33. Smith B, Wong CA, Smith TC, et al. Newly reported respiratory symptoms and conditions among military personnel deployed to Iraq and Afghanistan: a prospective population-based study. *Am J Epidemiol*. 2009;170:1433–1442.

34. Smith TC, Leardman CA, Smith B, et al. Postdeployment hospitalizations among service members deployed in support of the operations in Iraq and Afghanistan. *Ann Epidemiol*. 2009;19:603–612.

35. Weese CB, Abraham JH. Potential health implications associated with particulate matter exposure in southwest Asia. *Inhal Toxicol*. 2009;21:291–296.

36. Roop SA, Niven AS, Calvin BE, et al. The prevalence and impact of respiratory symptoms in asthmatics and non-asthmatics during deployment. *Mil Med*. 2007;172:1264–1269.

37. Szema AM, Peters MC, Weissinger KM, et al. New-onset asthma among soldiers serving in Iraq and Afghanistan. *Allergy Asthma Proc*. 2010;31:67–71.

38. Engelbrecht JP, McDonald EV, Gillies JA, et al. Characterizing mineral dusts and other aerosols from the Middle East—Part 1: ambient sampling. *Inhal Toxicol*. 2009;21:297–326.

39. US Environmental Protection Agency. Part III: Environmental Protection Agency. Revisions to Ambient Air Monitoring Regulations. *Fed Regist*. October 17, 2006; 40 CFR §53 and §58. Final Rule, National Ambient Air Quality Standards.

40. Abraham JH, Baird CP. A case-crossover study of ambient particulate matter and cardiovascular and respiratory medical encounters among US military personnel deployed to southwest Asia. *J Occup Environ Med*. 2012;54:733–739.

41. Levy B, Wegman D, Baron SL, Sokas R. *Occupational and Environmental Health. Recognizing and Preventing Disease and Injury*. 6th ed. Oxford, England: Oxford University Press; 2010.

42. National Research Council. *Review of the Department of Defense Enhanced Particulate Matter Surveillance Program Report*. Washington, DC: The National Academies Press; 2010: 10–11, 51–56.

43. Baird CP, DeBakey S, Reid L, et al. Respiratory health status of US Army personnel potentially exposed to smoke from 2003 Al-Mishraq Sulfur Plant fire. *J Occup Environ Med*. 2012;54:717–723.

44. Carn SA, Krueger AJ, Krotkov NA, Gray MA. Fire at Iraqi sulfur plant emits SO_2 clouds detected by Earth Probe TOMS. *Geophys Res Lett*. 2004;31:1–4.

45. Agency for Toxic Substances and Disease Registry (ATSDR). *Toxicological Profile for Sulfur Dioxide*. Atlanta, GA: US Department of Health and Human Services, Public Health Service; 1998.

46. Agency for Toxic Substances and Disease Registry (ATSDR). *Toxicological Profile for Hydrogen Sulfide*. Atlanta, GA: US Department of Health and Human Services, Public Health Service; 2006.

47. National Research Council. *Acute Exposure Guideline Levels for Selected Airborne Chemicals: Volume 8*. Washington, DC: The National Academies Press; 2010.

Chapter 3

DEPLOYMENT TO AL ANBAR: A SEABEE BATTALION SURGEON'S PERSPECTIVE

RICHARD T. MEEHAN, MD*

Captain (Retired), US Navy; Professor of Medicine, Department of Medicine and Rheumatology Division and Co-Director, National Jewish Health Deployment-Related Lung Disease Center, National Jewish Health, 1400 Jackson Street, Denver, Colorado 80206

INTRODUCTION

The Naval Mobile Construction Battalion SEVENTEEN (NMCB-17) was mobilized in October 2007 to support Operation Iraqi Freedom. This reserve battalion underwent 4 months of rigorous military training at Port Hueneme Naval Base (Oxnard, CA) and at Fort Hunter Liggett (California) prior to deployment to southwest Asia (SWA). The vast majority of these deployed Seabees performed combat construction projects in Al Anbar Province, Iraq, from February to September 2008.

The medical department consisted of 3 Independent Duty Corpsmen, 14 Navy Corpsmen, and 1 Medical Officer (the author). The medical and command staffs were concerned about the potential negative impact of airborne hazards and dust exposure on the health and operations since measured particulate matter (PM) levels in Iraq frequently exceeded US Environmental Protection Agency standards.[1] There were also published cases of novel respiratory conditions, including eosinophilic pneumonia associated with military operations in this region.[2] Our Seabees might have been more susceptible to respiratory disorders because reservists tend to be older than their active duty counterparts, and military personnel also have higher smoking rates (32% vs 21%) than age-matched civilian controls.[3] Seabees might also have additional novel inhalation exposures unique to their construction duties, including welding, fueling, and vehicle equipment maintenance operations.

The NMCB-17 logged approximately 98,000 km of convoy operations to deliver Seabees and various construction materials to remote project sites. During combat outpost construction operations, Seabees engaged in diverse activities, including

- welding,
- building,
- plumbing,
- electrical work,
- vehicle and earth-moving equipment maintenance and operations,
- drilling,
- concrete work,
- bridge construction, and
- security.

The administration, planning, intelligence, communication, and supply personnel needed to support this high operational tempo of multiple simultaneous construction projects "outside the wire" were conducted by staff working in the Headquarters Company and Combat Operations Center at Al Asad Airbase, Iraq. The PM exposures varied greatly because some Seabees worked and slept exclusively in air-conditioned spaces while others manned gun turrets on convoys, often spending more than 60 hours a week exposed to very high levels of ambient and vehicle-generated dust. The extremely high temperatures, which often exceeded 120°F, made it very difficult to perform construction duties or convoy operations using any type of respirators or masks. As a result, most Seabees used issued cravats to cover their mouths and noses when working outside during dust storms, on high PM days, or in gun turrets.

PREDEPLOYMENT

All mobilized NMCB-17 personnel reported to the Navy Mobilization Processing Center at Port Hueneme Naval Base, and were screened by the author, who also monitored their health and performance during rigorous field exercises at Fort Hunter Liggett before allowing them to deploy to this combat zone. All Seabees were required to maintain Navy weight standards and pass the Physical Readiness Test, which included a timed 1.5-mile run. Only one member with a preexisting respiratory condition was permitted to deploy. This Seabee had recent-onset, well-controlled asthma with medication and was able to work exclusively in an air-conditioned space in Al Asad in close proximity to the Battalion Aid Station and the Combat Support Hospital.

RESPIRATORY CONDITIONS DURING DEPLOYMENT

More than 90% of NMCB-17 Seabees received their medical care at one of two Battalion Aid Stations by an Independent Duty Corpsman, the author, or a Navy Corpsman during convoy operations or at remote construction sites. During the first month of deployment, nonspecific respiratory complaints were frequently observed, including nonproductive cough and nasal congestion. During the first 1–2 months, these minor respiratory complaints were only exceeded by musculoskeletal injuries. However, those visits fell dramatically in subsequent months as these noninfectious maladies were not treated with medications. There were no medical evacuations, referrals to the Combat Support Hospital, confinement to quarters, or limited duty restrictions from respiratory conditions during this 7-month deployment to SWA. Only one Seabee developed new-onset asthma, which was documented using an EasyOne Spirometer (ndd Medizintechnik AG, Zurich Switzerland), and responded well to albuterol and glucocorticoid inhalers following a brief course of oral prednisone. However, the Seabee with preexisting, well-controlled asthma experienced no exacerbations in Iraq, during field exercises, or while at Port Hueneme. Following demobilization at Port Hueneme, no personnel were transferred to the Medical Hold Battalion in San Diego, California, because of any respiratory conditions.

AIR QUALITY STUDY

During this deployment, colleagues from the US Army Center for Health Promotion and Preventive Medicine (currently the US Army Public Health Command, Aberdeen Proving Ground, MD) supported NMCB-17 efforts to determine if air quality had any negative effect on operations. The PM_{10} levels (10 µm) were measured using a MiniVol Portable Air Sampler (Airmetrics, Eugene, OR; Figure 3-1) operating at 5 L/min for 24 hours at Al Asad Airbase. Samples were obtained and deposited onto quartz filter discs every 6 days from April through August 2008 on nine separate occasions when the author was not traveling outside the base and independent of weather conditions. Calibration of the MiniVol Portable Air Sampler and the collection techniques were identical to previously published methods and verified by Colonel Ron Ross, US Army Public Health Command scientist at Al Asad.[4] The author performed all of the sampling and shipped the filters in sealed plastic cassettes in two separate batches to the US Army's Aberdeen Proving Ground laboratories in Maryland. Metal analysis was performed by an acid extraction method of PM samples using inductively coupled plasma-mass spectrometry.[5,6]

RESULTS

The average and range of PM_{10} measurements from the separate samples were similar to results reported in other bases in Iraq previously by Englebrecht.[4] In addition to PM_{10} measurements, the following metals were also analyzed in the samples after acid digestion: antimony, arsenic, beryllium, cadmium, chromium, lead, manganese, vanadium, and zinc.

- PM (10 µm) concentrations averaged 190.92 µg/m^3 (range: 13.1–576.8 µg/m^3) ($n = 9$).
- Detection of the following metals from Al Asad Airbase Iraq was as follows:
  - ◦ <0.6980 µg/m^3 zinc;
  - ◦ <0.2792 µg/m^3 manganese and vanadium;
  - ◦ <0.1396 µg/m^3 antimony and lead; and
  - ◦ <0.0697 µg/m^3 arsenic, beryllium, cadmium, and chromium.

The "<" symbol indicates the lowest reliable level of detection for each group of metals. These low levels of metals measured in our PM_{10} samples were reassuring that inhalation exposure to these metals was unlikely to cause adverse health outcomes. The potential health hazards of these inhalation metal exposures is referenced in the Military Exposure Guidelines based on information also derived from US Environmental Protection Agency guidelines and workplace exposures.[7]

However, the National Research Council (Washington, DC) and the Institute of Medicine (Washington, DC) reviewed this method of measurement on PM_{10} samples that often exceed >150 µg/m^3 and raised concerns that these detection limits may have been set too high because most of the prior samples reported from southwest Asia (including Joint Base Balad) also had nondetectable levels of metals of interest.[8,9] The author also noted that, on days with poor visibility, after 24 hours the discs were overloaded with such a large volume of dust that the PM_{10} levels were likely be underestimated. In the future, replacing the discs every 6 hours on high dust days may yield more accurate PM_{10} results and metal measurement values.

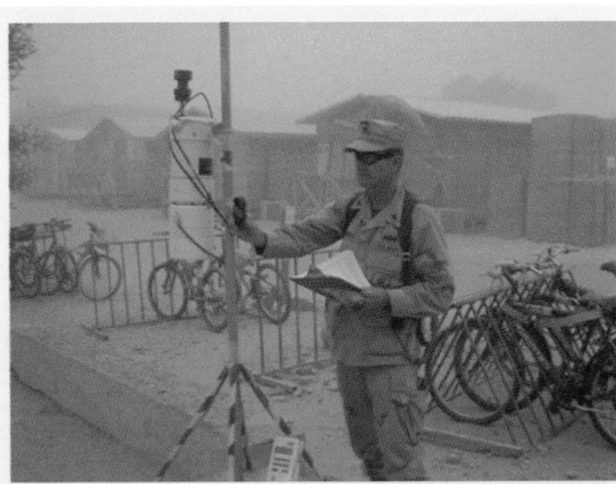

Figure 3-1. The author using the MiniVol Portable Air Sampler (Airmetrics, Eugene, OR) during a 2008 dust storm in Al Asad, Iraq.

SUMMARY

Despite high PM_{10} particulate exposures, which on average exceeded the 1990 Clean Air Act US Environmental Protection Agency guidelines of 150 μg/m^3 in 24 hours, no serious respiratory conditions were observed during this deployment that affected combat construction operations. The vast majority of construction workers in a Reserve Seabee unit may have also had prior industrial airborne toxicant exposures in their civilian construction or vehicle maintenance jobs, yet they still did quite well during this deployment.

The measured airborne metal exposures from Al Asad Airbase were negligible. However, these findings may differ from other bases within SWA because this sampling was from a single location. We planned on obtaining simultaneous PM samples from our other base in Camp Fallujah, but since the additional MiniVol air sampler could not be repaired, no samples from other regions in Iraq were obtained for analysis. We were also unable to obtain measurements from remote construction sites or during convoy operations that probably generated much higher PM levels than we measured from Al Asad Airbase. Furthermore, this air sampling was not performed in close proximity to factories or burn pits that could contribute to higher airborne contaminants.

This author's experience demonstrates that significant respiratory conditions during deployment were minimal among a well-screened, fit population exposed to these high dust levels. However, these findings may not be applicable to other populations (eg, civilian employees and contractors) or military units that allow members with undiagnosed or inadequately treated reactive airway disease to deploy.

Despite the lack of adverse health effects during this deployment from respiratory conditions, the long-term health effects of high $PM_{2.5}$ or PM_{10} exposures could prove more significant. Vanderbilt University Medical Center (Nashville, TN) investigators reported that 49 soldiers underwent video-assisted thoracoscopic lung biopsy that confirmed constrictive bronchiolitis in 38 soldiers who deployed to SWA. Ten of these cases were documented among soldiers who had no sulfur fire exposure.[10] Asthma rates have also been reported to be higher among deployed veterans (Operation Iraqi Freedom/Operation Enduring Freedom) versus nondeployed veterans from one Veterans Affairs medical center.[11] There is a long latency period from exposure to asbestos, beryllium, and the onset of respiratory symptoms among susceptible individuals. The $PM_{2.5}$-μm dust particles are small enough to penetrate the terminal airways and airspaces where they would require macrophage clearance by immune mechanisms.[12] Results from cohort-controlled epidemiology research studies, such as the Millennium Cohort Study, following deployers versus nondeployers should help identify the potential long-term respiratory health consequences of military deployment to SWA.

Acknowledgments

The author is indebted to the courageous Seabees of NMCB-17 with whom he had the privilege to serve, and the talented and dedicated Navy Corpsmen who provided outstanding care that allowed all Seabees to return home to their families. Deepest thanks to Naval Construction Force Surgeon, Captain Robert Alanso, MC, US Navy, for providing outstanding medical support and guidance throughout this deployment. This study would not have been possible without the generous support in time, resources, expertise, and guidance of US Army Public Health Command staff; Coleen Baird, MD, MPH; and Colonel Ron Ross, MD, PhD. Special thanks to Dr Cecile Rose, who is utilizing her expertise as a scientist and an Occupational Pulmonologist to improve the care of veterans afflicted with pulmonary disease by establishing a Center of Excellence on Deployment-Related Lung Disease at National Jewish Health.

REFERENCES

1. Weese CB, Abraham JH. Potential health implications associated with particulate matter exposure in southwest Asia. *Inhal Toxicol*. 2009;21:291–296.

2. Shorr AF, Scoville SL, Cersovsky SB, et al. Acute eosinophilic pneumonia among US military personnel deployed in or near Iraq. *JAMA*. 2004;292:2997–3005.

3. Research Triangle Institute. *2005 Department of Defense Survey of Health Related Behaviors Among Active Duty Personnel*. Research Triangle Park, NC: RTI; 2006. DTIC Accession Number ADA465678.

4. Engelbrecht JP. *Department of Defense Enhanced Particulate Matter Surveillance Program (EPMSP)*. Reno, NV: Desert Research Institute; 2008.

5. Office of Research and Development, US Environmental Protection Agency. *Determination of Trace Elements in Waters and Wastes by Inductively Coupled Plasma-Mass Spectrometry*. Cincinnati, OH: EPA; 1994. EPA Method 200.8 (Revision 5.4).

6. US Environmental Protection Agency. *40 CFR Appendix G to Part 50: Reference Method for the Determination of Lead in Suspended Particulate Matter Collected from Ambient Air*. Washington, DC: Government Printing Office; 2012.

7. US Army Public Health Command. *Environmental Health Risk Assessment and Chemical Exposure Guidelines for Deployed Military Personnel*. Aberdeen Proving Ground, MD: US Army Public Health Command; 2013. Technical Guide 230.

8. National Research Council. *Review of the Department of Defense Enhanced Particulate Matter Surveillance Program Report*. Washington, DC: The National Academies Press; 2010.

9. Institute of Medicine. *Long-term Health Consequences of Exposure to Burn Pits in Iraq and Afghanistan*. Washington, DC: The National Academies Press; 2011: 133–138.

10. King MS, Eisenberg R, Newman JH, et al. Constrictive bronchiolitis in soldiers returning from Iraq and Afghanistan. *N Engl J Med*. 2011;365:222–230.

11. Szema AM, Peters MC, Weissinger KM, et al. New-onset asthma among soldiers serving in Iraq and Afghanistan. *Allergy Asthma Proc*. 2010;31:67–71.

12. Provoost S, Maes T, Willart MA, et al. Diesel exhaust particles stimulate adaptive immunity by acting on pulmonary dentritic cells. *J Immunol*. 2010;184:426–432.

Chapter 4

PULMONARY RESPONSE TO AIRBORNE HAZARDS: INTERPRETING CASES OF SUSPECTED DEPLOYMENT-RELATED LUNG DISEASE

TEE L. GUIDOTTI, MD, MPH, DABT*

Vice President for Health/Safety/Environment & Sustainability, Medical Advisory Services, PO Box 7479, Gaithersburg, Maryland 20898; Diplomate, American Board of Toxicology, PO Box 97786, Raleigh, North Carolina 27624

INTRODUCTION

Respiratory complaints following deployment are common, and most are attributable to known risk factors. However, a small minority of cases in returning veterans of south Asia and the Middle East may suggest a novel or at least unexplained pathology. This chapter is directed largely at these cases and what they may tell us about the following:

- Exposures and pulmonary responses that we do not understand.
- Exposures of concern for future health that can be prevented during employment.
- Directions in which new technology or deployment management strategies may need to go.
- Sentinel cases, early clinical signs, biomarkers, and population-based indicators that can identify warriors and veterans who are at risk.
- Disease processes that might be addressed by appropriate and specific treatment rather than by general suppression of inflammation.
- Preventive measures (either primary, secondary, or tertiary) that reduce risk of disability among the deployed.

EXPOSURE CHARACTERISTICS

Some of these cases were associated with particular events that may have presented exposure to specific hazards, such as the Mishraq Sulfur Mine, in which sulfur dioxide would have been the relevant exposure. Others, however, were not. One universal in theater, however, was the presence of burn pits.[1] These are trenches in which combustible trash (undoubtedly with some noncombustible materials as well) is doused with diesel fuel and set on fire, producing emissions that consist of diesel fuel combustion products, products of combustion of the trash stream, and possibly entrained particles of dirt and other material of crustal origin.

Any consideration of the inhalation toxicology of combustion products begins with two phases: (1) particulate matter and (2) gases. However, particles should be understood not as a distinct and unrelated phase, but as a complex consisting of a particle core onto which is adsorbed other substances, including gases and volatile organic compounds. Emissions from burn pits are determined by several characteristics.

- Because burn pits are at or below ground level, their dispersion plumes are likely to spread laterally and to fumigate the area downwind, especially in the early morning, when an inversion would be expected.
- Burn temperatures are variable. Because of the use of accelerants (diesel fuel), they probably burn hotter than simple trash fires, but not as hot as diesel engines or furnaces.
- Efficiency of a burn pit is much less than that of an engineered incinerator, leading to production of carbon monoxide, more complex hydrocarbon species, and coarser particulate matter than might be expected from a more structured incineration process.
- In keeping with other combustion sources, toxic emissions are most likely to occur when the fire is beginning from a cold start and when it is cooling down, because this is when polycyclic aromatic hydrocarbons condense and are not consumed. Carbon monoxide is more likely to be formed from incomplete combustion, and thermal updrafts are less.
- Combustion of diesel fuel in the burn pit does not occur under pressure, as it would in a diesel engine. Thus, the emissions profile may be less rich in fine particulate matter compared with coarse particulate matter. Also, secondary fine particles from agglomerated sulfate are less likely to be an issue with emissions from burn pits compared with ambient air pollution derived from diesel engine exhaust.
- Content of the trash being burned—including plastic materials (such as vinyl chloride, which is a chlorine source for polychlorinated dioxins and furans), electronic components, human waste, and materials containing metals—may make the composition of emitted particulate matter variable in composition.

Toxic effects of particulate matter will be emphasized in this chapter because it is more complex, and toxicology is more consistent with longer term, subchronic health effects. Gaseous emissions from the burn pit are more likely to result in acute hazards and to be recognized at the time. Carbon monoxide, in particular, is a systemic poison rather than a pulmonary hazard. Therefore, it probably plays little if any role in open-air trash burning.

MODELS FOR UNDERSTANDING THE PULMONARY RESPONSE

There are several possible models for understanding the effects of particulate matter from burn pits on the lungs. They include learning from the following:

- occupational health experience of firefighters, including responders to the World Trade Center (WTC) tragedy;
- ambient air pollution;
- diesel engine exhaust studies;
- combustion of crude oil, as in oilfield fires; and
- cigarette smoking (this is both an important confounder for any study of combustion-related health effects and a model for effects of combustion products).

Table 4-1 describes the dominant chemical species for each of the two phases for each of these model pollution regimes.

These models overlap considerably and individually approximate exposures likely to occur from a burn pit. But none of them exactly replicates the exposure regime characteristic of a burn pit. Care should also be taken not to fall into the trap of *paradigm blindness*, wherein enthusiasm for an explanatory model that seems to fit the situation reduces awareness of differences and anomalies that may be significant in practice.

Firefighters Model

Firefighters represent an attractive model for healthy warriors because of their stringent selection for fitness. Obviously, the exposure profile of career firefighters is different from that of soldiers maintaining or downwind of burn pits, but the constituents of the smoke may not be much different. Firefighters are exposed to many inhalation hazards, most related to combustion products of fires, diesel exhaust, or airborne hazards from unusual fires (eg, pesticides) that occur on occasion throughout a firefighter's career, which of course is much longer than a tour of duty.[2,3]

It is well established that firefighters have an increased risk of myocardial infarction that persists about 24 hours or more after exposure to a fire.[4] It is not entirely clear, however, whether this is attributable to combustion products or to the stress response and catecholamine sensitization, because arrhythmias can be demonstrated from the stress of responding to the alarm alone. In terms of chronic disease, there appears to be an elevated risk of cancer for the kidney,

TABLE 4-1

CONSTITUENTS OF EMISSIONS FROM COMBUSTION IN FOUR MODEL EXPOSURE REGIMES AND CATEGORIES OF HEALTH EFFECTS

Phase	Firefighting	Ambient Air Pollution	Diesel Engine Exhaust	Cigarette Smoking
Particulate	Coarse and fine particulate matter with PAHs, chlorinated hydrocarbons	Coarse and fine particulate matter with PAHs, adsorbed metals	Coarse and fine particulate matter with PAHs	Coarse and fine particulate matter with PAHs, cadmium
Gas	Carbon monoxide, 1,3-butadiene, vinyl chloride	Carbon monoxide, oxidant gases* (air toxics)	(Carbon monoxide) Nitric oxide	Carbon monoxide, acrolein, numerous other gases
Health effects attributable to exposure	(Cardiovascular) Cancer	Cardiovascular respiratory cancer	(Acute lung inflammation) Cancer	Cardiovascular respiratory cancer

*Including oxidants that play no role in fresh diesel engine exhaust: ozone, peroxyacetyl nitrates, and aldehydes; nitrogen dioxide formed photochemically from nitric oxide.
PAHs: polycyclic aromatic hydrocarbons
Note: Parentheses indicate variability or uncertain associations.

bladder, and possibly the lung.[5] Lung disease, however, has proven elusive as an occupational association among firefighters, possibly reflecting a healthy worker effect of both selection and retention. Previous generations of firefighters tended to smoke less than the general population, and those in the current generation rarely smoke.

A population of particular concern has been surviving New York Fire Department members who responded to the WTC catastrophe. Their exposure profile was distinctly different from that of career firefighters and included heavy exposure to coarse particulate matter and heavier exposure to contaminants (eg, metals). Their exposure also most often occurred at the scene without personal protection.[6]

A disproportionately large number of these workers have experienced respiratory impairment in the years since, often diagnosed as asthma but reflecting a variety of conditions. At least some WTC responders, including firefighters who were athletic prior to exposure, subsequently developed serious, disabling disease as their underlying condition progressed. These have been attributed to asthma, but this explanation does not cover all cases.[6]

The known toxicology of the agents satisfactorily explains why WTC responders have experienced a high incidence of respiratory disease characterized by airways hyperreactivity. However, a progressive obstructive defect analogous to irritant asthma may not be the whole story. It does not explain why the frequency of symptoms appears to be getting worse in a subset of WTC responders or the anomalous findings that have emerged.

Many WTC responders are showing a decrease in forced vital capacity (FVC), which is usually indicative of restrictive disease, in the presence of a progressive decrease in forced expiratory volume in 1 second (FEV_1) that is more likely an indicator of air trapping in atypical obstructive airways disease.[6] The significance of the pattern and the importance of heterogeneity in the population as air trapping evolved may not have been appreciated at first because of the high level of statistical aggregation, wherein results were reported. Clinical deterioration has not been reported for the majority of surviving WTC responders, but a few have had unexplained disabling respiratory symptoms; the records of two responders came to the author's attention during preparation for litigation between the firefighters and the City of New York that ended with the settlement reached in 2010. Observations in these cases suggest findings at the bronchiolar (small airway) level that may or may not have their counterpart in cases of lung disease possibly arising from deployment and burn pit–associated exposures.

Constrictive bronchiolitis may be developing in at least some of the WTC cases, as suggested by findings consistent with air trapping at the bronchiolar level.[6] One case of bronchiolitis obliterans has already been reported among WTC responders, a possible sentinel event. The significance of these findings is that bronchiolar, or "small airway," disease may be more significant and more important as a response to toxic inhalation than previously appreciated, with implications for the deployed population in which constrictive bronchiolitis has already been reported.[7] Unfortunately, little is known of this condition in the context of toxic lung injury.

Constrictive bronchiolitis is characterized by a silent period, with latency depending on the underlying disease. It is possible that some WTC responders are in a silent period for the condition as the latency elapses. One reason for the silent period may be evolving inflammation, whereas cellular signals are released and stimulation of scar tissue is occurring. In this sense, latency would be similar to fibrogenic pneumoconioses (eg, asbestosis or silicosis), wherein proliferation of fibrosis takes at least 10 years until it can be seen on chest X-ray film. But a latency period can also be seen for toxic gases (eg, nitrogen dioxide) that result in interstitial fibrosis, thus presenting radiologically as *honeycombing*. Another reason for the silent period may be the time required for a sufficient number of functional units to be compromised enough to show a defect on testing. Functional reserve, in the form of numerous redundant units, preserves lung function until damage is advanced. Only when a sufficient and rather large number of bronchioles close down does an abnormality become apparent (eg, shortness of breath or pulmonary function testing). This logically would take longer for subjects whose bronchiolar walls are not weakened by smoking. Latency is not consistent with reactive airways dysfunction syndrome (RADS) or the onset of irritant asthma that provokes an airway response immediately after exposure that then persists. Firefighters other than WTC responders have not demonstrated apparent increased mortality from lung disease.[8]

Most of the functional disturbance that is a consequence of either conventional or WTC-related exposure of firefighters is likely to be reflected in changes in airways function, particularly airways' reactivity or inflammation, the major form of which is asthma. The cardinal symptoms of asthma are episodic: shortness of breath, wheezing, and coughing. The cardinal symptoms of bronchitis are cough and sputum production. However, these are not the only manifestations of hyperactive or inflamed airways. Other symptoms and signs may be present that interfere with daily life, especially fitness for duty as a firefighter or in another active job.

Monitoring pulmonary function is the most practical test to identify and track the evolution of this type of respiratory disease in this population. But care must be taken when interpreting the results. Firefighters, like healthy warriors, are a prescreened population, selected to be fit for duty in a strenuous occupation that favors strength and stamina. A firefighter who has supranormal pulmonary function (a vital capacity greater than the upper limit of that predicted in a big man) may have significant and progressive impairment that does not show up as abnormal on pulmonary function tests. A firefighter with a vital capacity of 120% predicted would have to lose 36% of lung function before reaching 80% of predicted, which is a conservative definition of abnormal, instead of 20% for a person who began at 100%. The individual trend may be more revealing than a comparison against population norms.

Urban Air Pollution Model

Urban air pollution has a number of similarities with burn pit emissions, specifically the health risk of particulate matter in ambient air pollution, especially derived from diesel emissions. Although the two situations share the characteristic that both have an admixture of pollutants from sources other than diesel, the sources of combustion products are not similar. The two differ in other important ways because exposure to burn pit emissions involves fresh emission of combustion products, and urban air pollution involves predominantly air pollutants that have "aged" in the atmosphere for a period, usually hours. The aging process in air pollution is important in the particulate phase for agglomeration of larger particles from fine particle nuclei and for increasing adsorption of volatile and aerosolized contaminants. The aging process is important in the gas phase for photochemical processes that lead to secondary pollutants (eg, ozone, nitrogen dioxide, and aldehydes). To the extent that these secondary processes modify the pathophysiological response, they render analogy to air pollution health effects less certain.

The epidemiological evidence for health effects is robust and provides clues to health outcomes of concern. However, the experimental evidence may be of greater value because of the acute high exposures that may be associated with burn pits.[1] Emissions from diesel engine exhaust are mixed with other air pollutants to produce a characteristic mix in urban air pollution. The composition of this mix is summarized in Table 4-1. It should be noted that, in addition to primary pollutants such as particulate matter, ambient air pollution contains many secondary pollutants that would not be expected to be present in emissions from burn pits. These include ozone, nitrogen dioxide, and other potent oxidizing photochemicals that are responsible for much of the effect of urban air pollution.

The particulate phase of urban air pollution is derived in part, and until recent changes in diesel technology, largely from diesel engine exhaust emissions. Fresh diesel engine exhaust produces coarse and fine particulate matter, nitric oxide (nitrogen dioxide is a secondary product not present in diesel exhaust), carbon dioxide, some carbon monoxide (much less than gasoline engines), and oxidized sulfur compounds (sulfur dioxide and sulfates), which vary depending on the sulfur content of fuels.

Ambient air pollution consists of particulate matter in three somewhat overlapping distributions characterized as cut points, but best understood as distinct particle populations: (1) coarse (£10 mm aerodynamic diameter, containing the bulk of the particulate mass); (2) fine (£2.5 mm); and (3) ultrafine (£0.1 mm, representing the largest number of individual particles). Each cut point represents a particular mode or population of particulate matter differentiated by composition and size. Particles in the coarse mode penetrate efficiently to the lower respiratory tract and are efficiently retained in the alveoli. However, they are also large enough to be deposited efficiently on the epithelial surface of bronchi and small airways, and are thus likely to have airways effects, alveolar effects (mediated in part by macrophage uptake), and systemic effects. Particles in the fine range penetrate to the alveoli efficiently, but are less likely to deposit in airways and more likely to migrate from the deep lung into the circulation and adjacent structures through intracellular junctions and cells.

Ultrafine particles behave more like gases than particles in their flow behavior and penetration to the deep lung. They migrate relatively freely, with the potential for systemic effects. However, evidence for significant health effects is weaker than for fine particulate matter.[9]

The smaller the particle size, the larger the surface area. Surface adsorption is critical to the biological effects of particulate matter because the surface of these particles has a high affinity for many biologically active chemicals. Fine and ultrafine particulate matter have many orders of magnitude greater capacity for binding volatile organic compounds in their surface and delivering them to deeper structures.

Coarse particulate matter predominantly consists of dust, particles of crustal origin (basically, very small dirt particles), bioaerosols, and, of interest in this context, carbonaceous particles formed by combustion on which are adsorbed a variety of volatile and organic materials. Ultrafine particles consist largely of aggregated or agglomerated structures of sulfate or nitrate, some with carbonaceous nuclei. These agglomerated particles tend to stick together when they touch, forming larger agglomerates over time. Fine particulate matter consists of both carbon-derived particles, on which are adsorbed volatile and organic materials, and agglomerated sulfate and nitrate ultrafine particles that build by accretion into the fine size range.

The adsorbed chemical species on both coarse and fine particles are biologically significant. The particle forms a carrier with a large surface area onto which are adsorbed many constituents, particularly

- volatile organic compounds,
- polycyclic aromatic hydrocarbons (PAHs) and nitroarenes,
- metals (particularly transitional metals and iron that may be proinflammatory),
- sulfate, and
- oxides of nitrogen.

Particulate matter in modern urban air pollution is closely associated on a population basis with mortality risk, the risk of cardiovascular and respiratory disease, pneumonia (indicating an effect on susceptibility), emergency department admissions for asthma, and lung cancer risk. On one hand, a few individual episodes of severe air pollution in the past (eg, the London fog [also known as the Great Smog of 1952] that occurred from December 4 to 9, 1952) have been so severe that mortality was obvious. On the other hand, the effect—although highly significant—is not readily apparent in short-term windows of observation, which resulted in it being overlooked for many years. To hear the signal against background noise, it is necessary to average out mortality and disease incidence data over long periods of time. It is convenient to report the data as attributable risk rather than relative risk because elevation is 5%. These effects, including and especially mortality, are linearly related to the concentration in air of fine particulate matter. (The relationship is not so clear for coarse or ultrafine particles.[9]) They are most apparent in the aged and chronically ill, but are also visible in healthy younger populations that have led to various theories of mechanism. One explanatory theory is that the timing of exposure is critical because people pass into and out of previously unrecognized stages of susceptibility for many factors, including and especially blood coagulability and thresholds for inflammation.[10] Figure 4-1, a schema for pathophysiology developed for the US Environmental Protection Agency (USEPA), integrates these factors into a model of how fine particulate air pollution may cause cardiovascular disease.

Based on the findings of the most recent studies, the USEPA recently dropped the air quality standard for fine particulate matter (level 2.5 or $PM_{2.5}$) from 15 to 12 mg/m^3, with an expected saving of thousands of lives, most of them from cardiovascular disease,[11] many of them from lung cancer,[12] and some from acute lung disease.

Diesel Engine Exhaust Model

Combustion of diesel fuel in a diesel engine takes place at high temperatures and under high pressure. Although probably different from the lower temperature, lower pressure combustion regime in a burn pit, the literature on toxic effects from diesel engine exhaust may suggest health outcomes and mechanisms of concern.

The International Agency for Research on Cancer (IARC) is a body of the World Health Organization that has as its primary purpose the evaluation of world knowledge to determine cancer risk from exposures to various agents. IARC is essentially universally considered authoritative in the field of cancer research, and its findings are accepted by agencies such as the USEPA. In June 2012, IARC reclassified diesel engine exhaust as a class 1 carcinogen, meaning that there is sufficient evidence to conclude that diesel exhaust causes cancer in humans, drawn from both epidemiology studying exposed populations and toxicology using animal studies. The evidence for concluding that diesel exhaust presents a human cancer risk will be summarized in the soon-to-be published IARC Monograph 105.

However, this finding was not a surprise. In 1988, IARC concluded that diesel exhaust was *probably* carcinogenic to human beings, but the evidence was not completely conclusive.[13] The case is made most strongly for lung cancer. Because of the putative exposure regime, the risk of other cancers is likely to be raised as well, specifically in the upper airway, kidney, and bladder that share many risk factors with the lungs.

It is well established that specific chemicals present in diesel exhaust cause cancer. In addition to many compounds already known to cause cancer, there are also PAHs and 1,3-butadiene. Evidence has accumulated that the class of compounds called nitroarenes are also present in diesel exhaust and are potently carcinogenic. Nitroarenes are nitrogenated versions of complex organic compounds called PAHs that are formed by combustion and comprise a mix of organic chemicals, several of them potently carcinogenic. It had long been known that diesel exhaust was rich in PAHs and their corresponding nitroarenes, several of which are potent carcinogens known to cause human cancers—such as lung, skin, and bladder cancer—and significantly for this case kidney and upper airway cancer (including nasopharyngeal cancer).

Several developments since 1988 persuaded IARC that the case for the carcinogenicity of diesel fuels had been fully made and was no longer speculative. The most important was the availability of studies that got around major methodological issues that limited earlier studies of occupations involving exposure to diesel engine exhaust. These earlier limitations had to do primarily with subtracting the obvious effect of cigarette smoking and determining an exposure–response

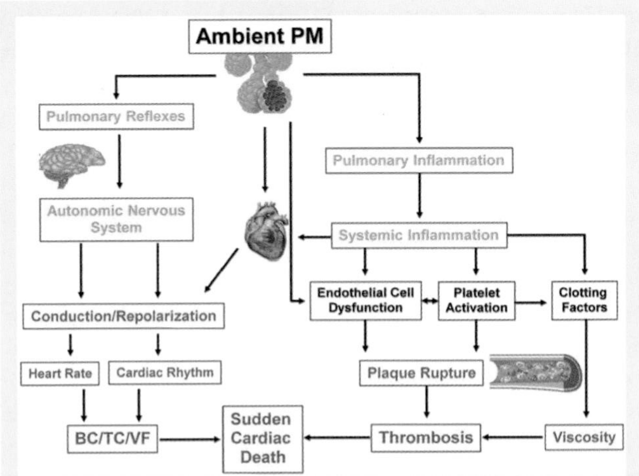

Figure 4-1. Plausible pathophysiological pathway.
BC: bradycardia (slow heart rhythm); PM: particulate matter; TC: tachycardia (fast heart rhythm); VF: ventricular fibrillation (chaotic rhythm)

relationship (basically asking the question: "Do more people get cancer the higher the exposure they experience?"). This gap was answered by a series of studies taking as their endpoint lung cancer, the cancer most likely to be caused by diesel engine exhaust. The populations studied were railroad workers, truckers, and underground miners who use diesel-powered equipment. Numerous studies were conducted, of which the most definitive version of the most important study for railroad workers[14] showed an excess risk of 1.40 (corresponding to a 40% elevation above expected). This level of risk was very similar to that found for the other two occupational groups in other studies. Thus, it is now firmly established that railroad workers have a 40% greater risk of developing lung cancer than they would otherwise, taking smoking into account. This number also means (mathematically) that approximately 29% of lung cancers in this population can be attributed to diesel exhaust, as opposed to tobacco or other causes.

Also, there has been resolution of a long-standing issue in inhalation toxicology over whether diesel exhaust itself was carcinogenic or whether diesel particles simply overloaded the protective cells of the lung and caused a sequence of events that induced cancer indirectly because these cells malfunctioned. It is now known that the particle overload problem is unique to mice and is not seen in human beings; thus, the findings of animal studies might not apply to human beings. The particle overload mechanism was therefore not so important in diesel exhaust toxicology and was not likely to be confusing to human studies. It is no longer questioned if the carcinogenic effect of diesel engine exhaust comes from chemicals in or on the surface of particles.

Stimulated by the attention to diesel brought by IARC's interest, the literature on diesel effects has grown for cancer risk, but not for acute and subchronic effects. Few studies are available for human beings on acute respiratory and cardiovascular responses to fresh diesel engine exhaust because this has not been seen as a pressing problem. However, it is clear that fresh diesel engine exhaust has potentially significant acute effects and small particles have effects distant from the lung and into kidney tissue.[14–18]

The gas phase of diesel exhaust may not contain secondary pollutants that are important in urban air pollution. However, depending on running conditions, they may be rich in formaldehyde (a potent respiratory and mucosal irritant and upper airway carcinogen) and acetaldehyde.[19]

The particle phase of diesel exhaust also has irritant potential and may induce inflammation. Recent subchronic and acute animal studies suggest that fresh (nonaged) diesel engine exhaust—administered in deployment-relevant time periods (1 month)—is associated with relatively mild, in context, proinflammatory and prothrombic effect. These effects overall were indicated by expired airway nitric oxide[20] and increased circulating cytokines that may paradoxically be attenuated by asthma-like airway reactivity. Of additional concern are findings that diesel engine exhaust may interfere with proliferation and remodeling of lung epithelial cells, thus setting the stage for subchronic and chronic health effects. Such studies require replication and integration into a hypothetical mechanism to be useful, but this is elusive in the absence of a specific respiratory outcome consistently observed with acute exposure.[10,21]

The conclusion from this still incomplete model is that inflammatory and thrombotic respiratory and cardiovascular effects are plausible with exposure to fresh diesel engine exhaust. This may be relevant to the effects of emissions from burning diesel fuel at open-fire temperatures and atmospheric pressure, but this has not been demonstrated. An experimental model using diesel fuel alone would not be complete, because the exposure was not confined to diesel fuel. The purpose of burn pits is to dispose of all types of trash, leading to diverse and variable composition in the emissions.

Oilfield Fires Model

The intentional oil fires set in Kuwait at the end of Operation Desert Storm have provided a conceptual model for exposure to burning oil products; but, because of the short duration of the problem, field conditions, and the difficulty in reproducing conditions, there is little empirical data available.[1] Elevations in circulating proinflammatory interleukin mediators (interleukin-8) have been reported and appear to be a good match to the linear response observed in particulate matter for healthy young people in exposure studies. Similarly, fine particulate matter from oil fires may reproduce the experimental effect in animal studies of fine particulate matter in urban air pollution with respect to accelerated atherosclerosis and induction of arrhythmias.

Oilfield flaring was a common practice and still exists as a safety measure in oil and gas installations. Emissions from flares have been extensively characterized and more than 200 organic chemicals are produced from gas flares, suggesting complicated combustion chemistry for the relatively simple input.[22] Extensive studies on the health effects of flaring emissions on human health are not available, but the literature on animals is now extensive as a result of two sets of studies conducted in western Canada.[23,24] Unfortunately, these studies may be of limited use because of species differences and difficulty characterizing burn pit exposures and isolating combustion products of interest.

PAHs remain the principal biologically active chemical class in oilfield exposures, especially in fires.[25]

Cigarette Smoking Model

The health effects of cigarette smoking are well characterized, and comparative pathology is readily available. However, the application of lessons from smoking to this problem is limited, in part because smoking is an important confounding exposure.

PATHOPHYSIOLOGY OF RESPONSE

Exhibit 4-1 summarizes the common lung responses to pulmonary injury after exposure to inhaled irritants. There are two components to such injury: (1) the toxic or irritant effect of the agent on tissue and (2) an injury that may result from the lung's response to the agent, which can be dysfunctional. For fibrogenic pneumoconioses, this is overexuberant fibrosis that—like the overexuberant response to tuberculosis—causes as much or more functional impairment as the agent itself. For airways disease, increased airways reactivity and structural remodeling of the airway wall may result in a greater and more chronic functional disturbance than that caused by the initial irritant exposure. Thus, consideration of the pulmonary outcomes of concern for the deployed population should include the possibility that clinically significant responses may not be a particular named disease or defined pathological condition, but the end result of host defense mechanisms that are stressed to the point of irreversible change.

Cases of respiratory illness in returning veterans include a subset with unexplained, but functionally disabling, symptoms and no obvious diagnosis. (These cases are summarized in other chapters in this book.) Most of these cases developed their illness over time after return, but a small number (two in the Vanderbilt series of cases) became symptomatic during deployment. There is a suggestion that those who developed their respiratory disorder early had a more rapid course of illness leading to impairment.

Cases were referred for dyspnea on exertion, wheezing, and productive coughing, with one case producing pigmented sputum. Physical examination was generally unremarkable. Imaging studies were not helpful except in one case where multiple nodules were apparent on the chest film and were found to represent small areas of consolidation (this case is also anomalous in other ways). Pulmonary function studies reported for the initial 38 soldiers seen at Vanderbilt University Medical Center (Nashville, TN) showed a strikingly preserved total lung capacity but reduced FVC, FEV_1 (in isolation and as the FEV_1/FVC ratio), and diffusing capacity. This pattern suggests air trapping and early airway closure. Exercise testing showed poor maximum ventilation. There was also anecdotal reference to desaturation in the case reports. Despite these findings, however, some of the soldiers responded at least partially to treatment for airways reactivity. Desaturation on polysomnography was reported, but this was a secondary phenomenon seen in many respiratory disorders. Although there was only one subject for which it was mentioned, methacholine challenge appeared to have been negative in that one relatively typical case.

In the four cases reported in detail by Welsh and Miller (Chapter 21, Denver Veterans Affairs Medical Center Experience With Postdeployment Dyspnea Case Report) and in the two cases each added by Miller (Chapter 14, Value of Lung Biopsy in Workup of Symptomatic Individuals) and Lewin-Smith et al (Chapter 19, Follow-up Medical Care of Service Members and Veterans: Case Reports—Usual and Unusual), the pathological findings are nonspecific and nondiagnostic, but clearly abnormal and in several cases permanently disabling. If a consistent picture of pathology emerges in the cases described in detail in this book, it is air trapping, chronic inflammation centered on bronchioles, and poorly formed granulomata, more reminiscent of hypersensitivity pneumonitis than sarcoidosis. (A subset of cases with eosinophilic granulomata is not included in this series.) Particle accumulation and subsequent inflammation centered on blood vessels and surrounding bronchioles are to be expected because of lymphatic drainage channels. Polarizable material, that would indicate silica exposure or be a marker for dust of crustal origin, is reported to be absent.

Thus, counting cases is difficult because the authors have not listed them uniquely, and references are often anecdotal. In addition to at least one of the cases reported in the more than 40 cases from Denver by Welsh and Miller (see Chapter 21, Denver Veterans Affairs Medical Center Experience With Postdeployment Dyspnea Case Reports), 52 of 65 cases seen at Vanderbilt University Medical Center between 2005 and 2012 are reported to show constrictive bronchiolitis, and four cases show respiratory bronchiolitis. Constrictive bronchiolitis is not reported consistently, but is reported to be present in at least one of the eight cases reviewed by a pathologist specializing in lung studies. One case showed clear intraluminal deposition of fibrin and hypertrophy of smooth muscle narrowing the caliber of an airway, but (to this author's eye) without bronchial gland hyperplasia that would be suggestive of bronchitis.

Exhibit 4-1 presents the common responses of the lung to an inhalation injury.[6,26] The lung, although a very complicated organ at the tissue or cellular level, has only a few stereotyped means of expressing injury. The expression of disease is restricted because the mechanical function of the lung is relatively simple compared with the function of some organs. Inhalation of irritant substances, either gases or particles, can produce effects on the upper airway (nose, pharynx, and throat), on the airways (trachea, bronchi, and small airways down to bronchioles), and on the tissue of the lung parenchyma, depending on the depth of penetration into the respiratory tract. Cough usually implies irritation of larger airways, although the symptom is entirely nonspecific. The role of smaller airways may be just as or more important in this population, however.[6,26]

For gases, the depth of penetration depends on the solubility of the gas in water because of clearance in the upper airway and the more proximal airways in the lower respiratory tract. The damage caused by toxic gases depends on

EXHIBIT 4-1

PULMONARY RESPONSE TO INJURY FOLLOWING AN INHALATION INJURY OR CHALLENGE

Functional airway abnormalities

- Upper airway
  - Reactive upper airways dysfunction syndrome
  - Voice problems (dysphonia)
  - Sleep apnea, obstructive
  - Aerodigestive disorders, such as gastroesophageal reflux (complex interactions with the epiglottis, esophagus, the lower esophageal sphincter, and reflux of stomach acid)
- Lower airway (airways hyperreactivity, acute and subacute inflammation)
  - Asthma-like wheezing (acute)
  - Asthma-like hyperreactivity to environmental irritants (eg, cigarette smoke, dust, smoke), cold, and exercise
    - Irritant-induced asthma
    - Reactive airways dysfunction syndrome
  - Bronchitis and sputum production
  - Fixed airways obstruction, including bronchiolitis
  - Bronchiectasis
  - Bronchiolitis
    - Constrictive bronchiolitis (progressive)
    - Bronchiolitis obliterans

Disorders of the tissue of the lung (parenchyma) other than airways

- Pulmonary edema (an extreme and lethal condition)
- Interstitial fibrosis (scarring of tissue in the parenchyma over time, with or without dust)
  - Nonpneumoconiotic (not associated with retained dust or reaction to its presence)
    - Granulomatous lung disease
    - Diffuse fibrotic lung disease ("honeycombing")
  - Pneumoconioses (specific disorders associated with dust retention and response)
- Disorders associated with particle overload in the lung
  - Impaired immune function
  - Oxidant stress injury

Migration of fine particles and secondary cardiovascular effects

Cancer

- Initiation of malignancy by a chemical carcinogen
- Promotion of a malignancy by a chemical promoter or co-carcinogen
- Facilitation or promotion of metastases

the irritation they produce on the way down (expressed as airways disease) and at the alveolar level (expressed as pulmonary edema and interstitial fibrosis), and the degree of toxicity to the body as a whole that occurs after they are absorbed. Highly toxic gases kill outright or cause acute illness. Gases that do not kill but instead primarily cause chronic lung problems—that may be permanently disabling—are usually not those that are most irritating or close to lethal concentrations, but are those that fall in the middle range of irritant potential.[26]

Medium-irritant gases may cause RADS, which is a form of irritant-induced asthma. Low-level irritant gases cause coughing and chronic lung irritation (eg, irritant-induced asthma or bronchitis) that may resolve. The usual variety of RADS (the term has been greatly overused), which follows an acute exposure to a gas or vapor, may take many years to resolve and may lead to sleep apnea, upper airway abnormalities, and other occlusive conditions.[26]

Size of the particle determines the location of maximal deposition, and particles in the predominant size range likely to be produced from burn pits would be expected to deposit more or less efficiently in the peripheral airways, where significant local effects may occur because of inflammation. Damage caused by irritant dusts depends on the degree of irritation they produce, their inherent toxicity (eg, asbestos), and the degree of toxicity to the body as a whole that occurs after they are absorbed (for particles that contain toxic materials such as fine particulate matter.) Irritating particles typically cause coughing and asthma-like symptoms appearing acutely at the time of the exposure.[26]

Air trapping is usually a consequence of advanced obstructive lung disease or acute asthma and as such occurs against a background of reduced airflow. However, air trapping may manifest itself mostly in a reduction in vital capacity, with relatively preserved ratios of airflow to vital capacity (FEV_1/FVC, %), which has been observed among WTC responders.[27] Air trapping has also been directly documented among WTC responders by imaging methods.[28] As discussed in the next section, this may be a sign of significant, progressive, and largely silent pathology at the level of bronchioles.

The time course of the cases presented in this chapter is puzzling because a few cases presented in theater, but most developed over some months or years after return. Irritant-induced asthma is sometimes acute, but often has a gradual onset resulting from subacute or repeated irritation; however, this must be sustained.[29] Interstitial disease primarily causes a restrictive defect that develops over time as a reduced vital capacity, but would be expected to result in a pure restrictive defect showing a reduced FVC, preserved flow rates, no air trapping, and a reduced residual volume. A nongranulomatous pneumoconiosis usually takes years to develop (acute silicosis being an exception). It generally requires either a dust load over a long period of exposure or an overwhelming acute exposure of a dust load with high fibrogenic potential (eg, silica) conditions unlikely to apply in the basic deployment situation, but more likely to apply in a construction or demolition scenario.

Role of Atopy and Airways Reactivity

Between 9% and 30% of the North American population has a hereditary predisposition to develop allergies, including asthma, as measured by atopic skin reactivity.[30,31] Asthma, skin rashes, allergies, and sinusitis or other manifestations are the common symptoms of atopy. When atopy preexists, there may be interactive effects with the irritant exposures leading to an exaggerated or worse condition than that expected from atopy alone. Aggravation of existing airways reactivity is a common and important mechanism for airways response following irritant exposure[26] and is now formally recognized as *work-exacerbated asthma*.[29] Lung injury that occurs in the presence of preexisting atopy is a work-related injury regardless of predisposing factors. When consequences are greater than that arising from the underlying condition alone, the additional injury would not have occurred *but for* the exposure at work.

These individuals almost universally have reactive airways and are prone to coughing, wheezing, choking, or symptoms of rhinitis (runny nose) when provoked by an irritant exposure. They are minor only in the sense that they are not part of the diagnosis and are usually not the endpoints for treatment. However, they are important in daily life and work, and should probably be called and thought of as *impairment factors* rather than minor symptoms. One important paper[32] on this topic makes the observation that, "It is widely acknowledged that the personal burden of illnesses, such as asthma, cannot be fully assessed by traditional clinical outcome variables, such as symptoms and lung function."

Constrictive Bronchiolitis and Bronchiolitis Obliterans

One pathological entity that has not been discussed much in the scientific literature on irritant exposure to combustion products is constrictive bronchiolitis. This condition is the result of inflammation at the level of small airways or bronchioles. It is very different from the more familiar small airways abnormality seen in cigarette smoking, which is what most physicians are used to when they look at an abnormal pulmonary function test. This pattern of pulmonary function is not consistent with most forms of asthma, where the airways reactivity affects somewhat larger airways.

Constrictive bronchiolitis is a less common form of intraluminal airway wall dysplastic repair. It shares with its more common form, *proliferative bronchiolitis* (perhaps more accurately called *intraluminal polypoid bronchiolitis*), a tendency to evolve into small airway effacement and destruction, leaving behind the familiar (and common) lesion of obliterative bronchiolitis. The terminology is confusing. Constrictive bronchiolitis and proliferative bronchiolitis are different processes that may follow their own pathways to arrive at similar end results, but do not necessarily progress to completion.[33–35]

Constrictive bronchiolitis is a form of bronchiolitis in which the clinical picture is dominated by inflammation in the bronchioles, abnormality of small airways function, and air trapping. Under a microscope, it looks like an inflammatory response of the smaller airways with the tissue around them relatively preserved (unlike the effect of cigarette smoking). In some of these bronchioles, the inflammation progresses to the point where the airway is completely obliterated by scar tissue and essentially disappears from where it ought to be under the microscope (its remnants can be found with special methods, specifically a stain for elastin), a condition known as bronchiolitis obliterans. Obliterative bronchiolitis is the end result of bronchiolar effacement, not a separate process.

Bronchiolitis has many causes and is often observed together with other pathology of the lung, such as asthma, cystic fibrosis, cigarette-induced emphysema, conventional pneumonia, or bronchiolitis obliterans organizing pneumonia (a distinct condition, unrelated to what is being discussed here). Bronchiolitis comes in many forms and is not at all the same as asthma, which is characterized by variable airflow reduction that may be associated with reversible inflammation and bronchoconstriction.[34] This is also RADS and affects larger airways.

Bronchiolitis is more familiar as a medical concept, common and noticeable in children because of the high frequency of respiratory syncytial virus in infancy, the increased risk of pertussis, and the dramatic functional effects on children's much smaller airways that disappear as they grow and their airways get bigger. There are many causes of acute bronchiolitis in adults, however, and the condition may accompany almost any lower respiratory tract infections. There are fewer causes of persistent (chronic) bronchiolitis and permanent alteration of the bronchiole structure in adults; but, in many adults, the causes are never identified and in such cases are called *cryptogenic* (Greek for "hidden cause"). The known causes unrelated to toxic exposure include

- adenovirus infection (specific strains of which are associated with persistent bronchiolitis),
- cancer (associated with a type called follicular bronchiolitis),
- mycoplasma infection,
- connective tissue disorders,
- eosinophilic lung diseases (there are several),
- inflammatory bowel disease,
- graft versus host reactions in lung transplantation, and
- several forms of autoimmune vascular disease.

There is also a form called diffuse panbronchiolitis, which is seen almost exclusively in Japanese men.[34]

The more familiar form of proliferative bronchiolitis is common and frequently associated with toxic inhalation exposures.[33] There has been almost no study of constrictive bronchiolitis as a pathological entity from toxic exposures. Most of the attention in the medical literature has been on nontoxic causes (eg, rheumatological disorders). Because of this, discussions on the functional implications of constrictive bronchiolitis are necessarily speculative. However, the relationship between proliferative bronchiolitis obliterans and irritant gases is well known, and there well may be overlap.

Bronchiolitis associated with toxic exposure includes most deeply penetrating irritant gases, but is characteristic of ozone and nitrogen dioxide, both highly oxidant gases that can progress to bronchiolitis obliterans.[26] Diacetyl provokes inflammation in the bronchioles that can result in a severe lung disorder trivialized by the name "popcorn lung" because it is a constituent of butter-tasting flavoring. It may be speculated that any irritant that can cause a bronchitis can probably cause a bronchiolitis if it penetrates to the bronchiolar level.

Invoking constrictive bronchiolitis as a process in some of these cases also explains another anomaly: latency period. It is striking that so few cases first became symptomatic during the period of deployment. An acute bronchiolitis is usually experienced by shortness of breath and coughing, followed by recovery. If they progress along the path to obliterative bronchiolitis, subjects experience the return of shortness of breath, in one form or another, and coughing months or years later. Some cases of toxic bronchiolitis (especially those associated with oxidant gases such as nitrogen dioxide and ozone) present minimal symptoms at the time of exposure, but may progress to classic hyperlucent lung over time. This time course would be inconsistent with RADS or irritant asthma, which provokes an airway response immediately after exposure. However, it would be consistent with advanced constrictive bronchiolitis.

Some of the apparently affected individuals show a pattern of pulmonary function that is consistent with air trapping. These are the firefighters who have a reduced FVC, but apparently well-preserved flow rates, of which the FEV_1 is the best understood. These cases present a puzzle because the net effect of the changes is to create a reduction in FVC that resembles a restrictive pattern, but that in reality is a form of obstruction. Air is trapped behind the obstruction, and the effect is as if the chest is filled with a tied-off balloon that is not emptying air.

Air trapping of this type occurs when pressure inside the chest (while breathing out) is greater than the air pressure within the airway, and it is pushed closed. In respiratory physiology, this effect is called a "Starling resistor," named after the physiologist who first described it. It shuts off the flow of air in the parts of the lung where it occurs. The bronchiolitis caused by cigarette smoking reduces the flow rate in small airways because tissue surrounding the airways disintegrates (from inflammation in the form of a focal alveolitis in tissue surrounding the small airway), and the airway loses the tethering effect that keeps it open. Thus, the airway collapses as soon as the air pressure around it in the lung exceeds the air pressure in the airway, which is the basis of emphysema. This occurs normally at the end of a breath; but where there is an abnormality of small airways, it occurs earlier before the breath out is finished and while there is still a relatively large amount of air in the lung.[36]

In a relatively isolated bronchiolitis, the structure of the airway is not weakened by inflammation around it with disintegration of supporting tissue; inflammation is confined to the airway itself. This means that, unlike in a heavy cigarette smoker, a person with constricted bronchioles close abruptly at a higher rate of flow, but not every small airway. This regularly occurs when a person is bearing down to blow hard, as in the FVC maneuver. Those small airways that remain open have normal flow rates and because resistance at that level is so low, there is no obvious sign of obstruction on most pulmonary function tests. This does not occur or occurs to a much lesser degree when a person breathes out more slowly, as in the *slow* vital capacity maneuver, because the pressure is not as great in the lung surrounding the airway.

The phenomenon is best explained by the idea of "communication," the term for whether an airway (in this case a bronchiole) is open and transferring air back and forth into the part of the lung where it leads. Bronchioles that shut down do not communicate and behave like the neck of a tied-off balloon, trapping air behind them. Normally, this trapping occurs at the end of a breath, when the remaining volume of air in the lung is low (called *closing volume*). When the bronchiole is abnormal, it may occur at higher lung volumes before it should. Those bronchioles that close at abnormally high closing volume (and so trap air behind them) shut off all flow abruptly and are therefore invisible in the flow rates of the pulmonary function study from that point on. Their net effect is to increase the residual volume that has the result of cutting flow out of the lung prematurely with an exhaled breath. Those bronchioles that allow flow permit it at a near-normal rate, so the flow in that part of the lung that *communicates* is not reduced. This is why flow rates could be preserved in the small airways as measured by midflows. (The correct test to show this is a seldom-used physiological test called the "closing volume" test, but it is not generally available and in this case would add nothing that is not already known.) In constrictive bronchiolitis, which has been much less studied, it would be expected that the small airway might remain patent for longer and that closing volumes might be heterogeneous. (No data on this are available.)

Anatomically, this early closure of small airways (<2 mm diameter) occurs mostly at the periphery of the lung, where resistance to flow is lower (beyond the first generation of bronchioles) and the pattern does not show up as obstruction. Instead, the air-trapping effect interferes with emptying of the lung and creates a pattern on pulmonary function testing resembling a restrictive defect, which is usually (but wrongly) thought to be the opposite of obstruction.

The underlying condition causing such abnormalities is inflammation of the smaller airways, occurring in a specific location in the respiratory tract where the airways are relatively small, but there are so many of them that resistance to flow is very low, especially compared with the larger airways where asthma exerts its effects. Because it is occurring in a part of the lung where resistance is very low, because it does not affect all parts of the lung, and because those parts of the lung that are affected are immediately sealed off when they close and no longer communicate air with the larger airways, the typical signs of airways obstruction (reduction in the FEV_1) are not visible in pulmonary function tests. Signs that this is happening, however, are that the FVC is much smaller than the *slow* vital capacity, which is obtained with less force and therefore results in a much lower closing volume and preserved airflow. Another sign is that there is little change with bronchodilators, which primarily act on the larger airways important in conventional asthma.

Whether constrictive bronchiolitis, or bronchiolitis in general, could play a role in cases of lung disease that may be associated with burn-pit exposures cannot be determined from the available evidence. Symptom monitoring[37] and systematic collection of pulmonary function data[37,38] would be required to sort out these issues, with close attention to whatever biopsy material becomes available on these subjects in the future. Unfortunately, the decentralized nature of healthcare for these subjects and, more fortunately, their relative youth and lack of other morbidity makes it unlikely that there will be a clear answer to this issue for some time to come.

SUMMARY

Deployment-related lung disease presents diagnostic and pathophysiological quandaries. It is not entirely clear whether these cases represent individual anomalies or a subset of postdeployed personnel who are demonstrating a disease syndrome. The potentially sentinel cases identified to date do show sufficient commonality of symptoms and a history suspecting a consistent pathological entity. This may or may not be a form of bronchiolitis and may or may not be an exaggeration of the normal host defense and physiological response to irritant exposure, including overexuberant airways repair.

There are several models that may inform analysis and interpretation going forward: firefighters, urban air pollution, diesel engine exhaust, and oilfield fires. None of them, however, exactly match the situation of exposure downwind from a burn pit, which is the most likely and consistent exposure scenario that may be associated with these cases.

Predeployment screening, postdeployment surveillance (targeted search for specific outcomes), and ongoing monitoring (broad observation to characterize the health experience of the population, such as the Millennium Study) will be required to determine what actually happens in warrior populations after deployment and to identify subsets that may have an anomalous experience. Specific, targeted investigation will be required to characterize these potentially sentinel cases. Protocols for clinical investigation and population monitoring are discussed elsewhere in this book. Research of a basic nature, focused on characterizing the exposures and toxicity under field conditions, may be necessary to answer the question of causation and therefore establish conditions for prevention.

REFERENCES

1. Institute of Medicine of the National Academies. *Long-Term Health Consequences of Exposure to Burn Pits in Iraq and Afghanistan.* Washington, DC: National Academies Press; 2011: 1–9, 31–44, 117–129.

2. Austin CC, Wang D, Ecobichon DJ, Dussault G. Characterization of volatile organic compounds in smoke at municipal structural fires. *J Toxicol Environ Health A.* 2001;63:437–458.

3. Guidotti TL, ed. Emergency services. In: Stellman JM, ed. *Encyclopaedia of Occupational Health and Safety.* 4th ed, vol 3. Geneva, Switzerland: International Labour Organization; 1996–1998:95.2–95.9.

4. Kales SN, Soteriades ES, Christophi CA, Christiani DC. Emergency duties and deaths from heart disease among firefighters in the United States. *N Engl J Med.* 2007;356:1207–1215.

5. Guidotti TL. Evaluating causality for occupational cancers: the example of firefighters. *Occup Med (Lond).* 2007;57:466–471.

6. Guidotti TL, Prezant D, de la Hoz RE, Miller A. The evolving spectrum of pulmonary disease in responders to the World Trade Center tragedy. *Am J Ind Med.* 2011;54:649–660.

7. King MS, Eisenberg R, Newman JH, et al. Constrictive bronchiolitis in soldiers returning from Iraq and Afghanistan. *N Engl J Med.* 2011;365:222–230.

8. Guidotti TL. Mortality of urban firefighters in Alberta, 1927–1987. *Am J Ind Med.* 1993;23:921–940.

9. HEI Review Panel on Ultrafine Particles. *Understanding the Health Effects of Ambient Ultrafine Particles: HEI Perspectives 3.* Boston, MA: Health Effects Institute; 2013.

10. Franchini M, Guida A, Tufano A, Coppola A. Air pollution, vascular disease and thrombosis; linking clinical data and pathogenic mechanisms. *J Thromb Haemost.* 2012;10:2438–2451.

11. Brook RD, Rajagopalan S, Pope CA 3rd, et al. Particulate matter air pollution and cardiovascular disease: an update to the scientific statement from the American Heart Association. *Circulation.* 2010;121:2331–2378.

12. Pope CA 3rd, Burnett RT, Turner MC, et al. Lung cancer and cardiovascular disease mortality associated with ambient air pollution and cigarette smoke: shape of the exposure-response relationships. *Environ Health Perspect.* 2011;119:1616–1621.

13. World Health Organization, International Agency for Research on Cancer (IARC). *Diesel and Gasoline Engine Exhausts and Some Nitroarenes.* Vol 46. IARC Monographs on the Evaluation of Carcinogenic Risks to Humans. Geneva, Switzerland: WHO/IARC; 1998.

14. Garshick E, Laden F, Hart JE, et al. Lung cancer in railroad workers exposed to diesel exhaust. *Environ Health Perspect.* 2004;112:1539–1543.

15. LaGier AJ, Manzo ND, Dye JA. Diesel exhaust particles induce aberrant alveolar epithelial directed cell movement by disruption of polarity mechanisms. *J Toxicol Environ Health A.* 2013;76:71–85.

16. Mcdonald JD, Doyle-Eisele M, Gigliotti A, et al. Part 1. Biologic responses in rats and mice to subchronic inhalation of diesel exhaust from U.S. 2007-compliant engines: report on 1-, 3-, and 12-month exposures in the ACES bioassay. *Res Rep Health Eff Inst.* 2012;166:9–120.

17. Nemmar A, Al-Salam S, Zia S, et al. Diesel exhaust particles in the lung aggravate experimental acute renal failure. *Toxicol Sci*. 2010;113:267–277.

18. Laks D, de Oliveira RC, de André PA, et al. Composition of diesel particles influences acute pulmonary toxicity: an experimental study in mice. *Inhal Toxicol*. 2008;20:1037–1042.

19. US Environmental Protection Agency. *Health Assessment Document for Diesel Engine Exhaust*. Washington, DC: USEPA; 2002. Report EPA/600/8-90/057F.

20. Hussain S, Laumbach R, Coleman J, et al. Controlled exposure to diesel exhaust causes increased nitrite in exhaled breath condensate among subjects with asthma. *J Occup Environ Med*. 2012;54:1186–1191.

21. Ghio AJ, Sobus JR, Pleil JD, Madden MC. Controlled human exposure to diesel exhaust. *Swiss Med Wkly*. 2012;142:w13597.

22. Strosher M. *Investigations of Flare Gas Emissions in Alberta*. Edmonton, Alberta, Canada: Alberta Research Council; 1996.

23. Scott HM, Soskolne CL, Martin SW, et al. Lack of associations between air emissions from sour-gas processing plants and beef cow-calf herd health and productivity in Alberta, Canada. *Prev Vet Med*. 2003;57:35–68.

24. Guidotti TL. The Western Canada study: overview and context. *Arch Environ Occup Health*. 2008;63:163–165.

25. Stellman SD, Guidotti TL. Polycyclic aromatic hydrocarbons and petroleum industry. In: Rom W, ed. *Environmental and Occupational Medicine*. 4th ed. Philadelphia, PA: Lippincott; 2006: 1240–1249.

26. Guidotti TL. Respiratory tract irritants. In: Rom W, ed. *Environmental and Occupational Medicine*. 4th ed. Philadelphia, PA: Lippincott; 2006: 543–555.

27. Weiden MD, Ferrier N, Nolan A, et al. Obstructive airways disease with air trapping among firefighters exposed to World Trade Center dust. *Chest*. 2010;137:566–574.

28. Mendelson DS, Roggeveen M, Levin SM, et al. Air trapping detected on end-expiratory high-resolution computed tomography in symptomatic World Trade Center rescue and recovery workers. *J Occup Environ Med*. 2007;49:840–845.

29. Henneberger PK, Redlich CA, Callahan DB, et al. An official American Thoracic Society statement: work-exacerbated asthma. *Am J Resp Crit Care Med*. 2011;184:368–378.

30. Rudikoff D, Lebwohl M. Atopic dermatitis. *Lancet*. 1998;351:1715–1721.

31. Larsen FS, Hanifin JM. Epidemiology of atopic dermatitis. *Immunol Allergy Clin North Am*. 2002;22:1–24.

32. Petersen KD, Kronborg C, Gyrd-Hansen D, et al. Quality of life in rhinoconjunctivitis assessed with generic and disease-specific questionnaires. *Allergy*. 2008;63:284–291.

33. Thurlbeck WM, Churg AM. *Pathology of the Lung*. 2nd ed. New York, NY: Thieme Medical Publishers; 1995.

34. Visscher DW, Myers JL. Bronchiolitis: the pathologist's perspective. *Proc Am Thorac Soc*. 2006;3:41–47.

35. Schlesinger C, Meyer CA, Veeraraghavan S, Koss MN. Constrictive (obliterative) bronchiolitis: diagnosis, etiology, and a critical review of the literature. *Ann Diagn Pathol*. 1998;2:321–334.

36. Howard P. The airway as a Starling resistor. *Bull Physiopathol Respir*. 1971;7:467–474.

37. Rose C, Abraham J, Harkins D, et al. Overview and recommendations for medical screening and diagnostic evaluation for postdeployment lung disease in returning US warfighters. *J Occup Environ Med*. 2012;54:746–751.

38. Szema AM, Salihi W, Savary K, Chen JJ. Respiratory symptoms necessitating spirometry among soldiers with Iraq/Afghanistan war lung injury. *J Occup Environ Med*. 2011;53:961–965.

Chapter 5

FUTURE IMPROVEMENTS TO INDIVIDUAL EXPOSURE CHARACTERIZATION FOR DEPLOYED MILITARY PERSONNEL

VERONIQUE HAUSCHILD, MPH*; AND JESSICA SHARKEY, MPH†

*Environmental Scientist, Injury Prevention Program, Epidemiology and Disease Surveillance Portfolio, Army Institute of Public Health, US Army Public Health Command, 5158 Blackhawk Road, Aberdeen Proving Ground, Maryland 21010-5403

†Epidemiologist, Environmental Medicine Program, Occupational and Environmental Medicine Portfolio, Army Institute of Public Health, US Army Public Health Command, 5158 Blackhawk Road, Aberdeen Proving Ground, Maryland 21010-5403

INTRODUCTION

Despite the substantial environmental exposure data collection described in Chapter 2, the evidence of a relationship between specific chronic respiratory conditions and environmental exposure(s) experienced by service members while deployed to southwest Asia is still inconclusive. Both the National Research Council (NRC) and the Institute of Medicine (IOM) acknowledge the plausibility of a relationship.[1,2] However, lack of granularity of the exposure data, especially the inability to synthesize large-scale ambient air sampling data into individual exposure profiles, is consistently identified as a limitation in epidemiological studies investigating the possible environmental exposure–respiratory disease relationship.[1–3] In addition to the substantial political, financial, and emotional implications that are not being adequately addressed, clinical and preventive measures are hindered by the lack of knowledge regarding specific hazards and dose-response characteristics. For example, whereas clinicians have criteria to assess, diagnose, and treat individuals' respiratory diseases, more definitive knowledge of disease relationships to deployment exposures could expedite diagnosis and even prevent cases of misdiagnosis (see Chapters 1, 4, 7, and 9; also see the chapters in Section III on Follow-up Medical Care of Service Members and Veterans). Although the military is reducing reliance on burn pits, this is primarily because of political pressures, as more specific source risk reduction practices cannot be directed without a clear link to specific exposures (Chapter 2, Background of Deployment-Related Airborne Exposures of Interest and Use of Exposure Data in Environmental Epidemiology Studies).

Despite inconclusive evidence, the Department of Defense (DoD) and the Department of Veterans Affairs (VA) have acknowledged that some previously deployed persons may experience persistent symptoms or develop chronic respiratory conditions because of their combined deployment exposures, unique experiences, and/or individual susceptibilities (eg, smoking, existing health conditions, or genetics).[2,3] However, it remains unclear who these persons are and what specific individual characteristics, activities, or exposure experiences might translate into a higher risk of chronic respiratory health outcomes. Unfortunately, at the present time, there is inadequate data to define the specific subgroups of personnel who may be or have been at greater risk. This includes those who may have experienced more significant exposures while deployed, as well as personnel who may have additional nondeployment exposures or susceptibilities that put them at greater risk.

As discussed in Chapter 2, air, soil, and water sample data have been routinely collected to support deployment base camp exposure and health risk characterizations (eg, Periodic Occupational and Environmental Monitoring Summaries).[4–6] Yet established base camps can be like small cities, where exposures to hazards in the air can depend on the time spent at specific locations and facilities in or around the camp, job tasks, and personal activities. Therefore, even if deployed to the same base camp, *individual* exposures can be quite different. As a result, these general population-level exposure summaries are of limited clinical use and have not been used in epidemiological studies to date.[3–8] Instead, epidemiological studies of the relationships between deployment exposures and adverse health outcomes have primarily used generic deployment status information (eg, number of deployments, timeframes, and occasionally base camp location) as a surrogate for actual exposure data. In fact, most published epidemiological studies use "deployment to southwest Asia" as a proxy for "exposure."[3] A few studies have compared the health outcomes of personnel from different locations for which exposure conditions are considered uniquely different; however, actual exposure data were not used in these studies.[2,9] One case-crossover study used particulate matter data from different locations, but data were limited temporally and spatially and did not address other types of airborne hazards present.[10] As a result, these studies do not adequately represent the unique exposures experienced by various persons deployed to Iraq and Afghanistan.

The impact of the potentially substantial variations in individual exposures, as well as personal confounding risk factors or inherent disease susceptibilities, has been acknowledged. The need to systematically collect individualized service member exposure assessment data has been repeatedly advocated for several years. Yet, this critical gap continues to plague military and VA deployment health research, surveillance, and clinical applications. This section summarizes identified benefits/applications and key disadvantages/limitations of specific approaches and tools as they relate to the characterization of individual military deployment exposures and associated risk factors.

HISTORY

The inability to capture information about individual military exposures has been repeatedly recognized in numerous past reviews. In 2000, nine years after the end of Operation Desert Shield and Operation Desert Storm (the Persian Gulf War), the IOM identified the need for individual-level exposure data in its recommendations titled *Protecting Those Who Serve: Strategies to Protect the Health of Deployed U.S. Forces*.[11] Although data obtained during the Persian Gulf War were of substantial limitations, their collection served as a basis for lessons to enhance exposure assessment in Operation Iraqi Freedom/Operation Enduring Freedom.[12] However, in 2010, the NRC concluded that, it "is plausible that exposure to ambient pollution in the Middle East theater is associated with adverse health outcomes."[1(p8)] However, the NRC noted that, "available data are not sufficient to characterize adequately the likely exposures of people for whom health outcome data are collected," and that "epidemiologic study of associations between exposures of interest and outcomes of interest will not produce valid results."[1(p52)] That same year, the DoD convened the symposium and workshop on "Assessing Potentially Hazardous Environmental Exposures Among Military Populations" to review the status of military and VA efforts to identify, assess, address, and communicate deployment exposure information gaps.[13] Participants agreed at the time that, "we must continue to improve our ability to link defined exposures to military members who may have been exposed."[14(p7)] It was acknowledged that, "sample data are not representative of individual exposures" and that "collecting area samples [ambient environmental data] would not define the exposures for individual service members [that] was needed to make informed judgments about risks to individuals."[15(p11)] Many of the other symposium articles and panel discussions repeated these concerns.[7,8,16–21] Finally, and most recently, the IOM[2] has recognized that burn pits may not be the main cause of long-term health effects related to Iraq and Afghanistan deployment. The IOM states that, "service in Iraq or Afghanistan—that is, a broader consideration of air pollution than exposure only to burn pit emissions—might be associated with long-term health effects, particularly in highly exposed populations (eg, those who worked at the burn pit) or susceptible populations (eg, those who have asthma), mainly because of the high ambient concentrations of PM [particulate matter] from both natural and anthropogenic, including military, sources."[2(p7)]

Susceptible subpopulations are known to exist in the deployed military population. Yet, little has been done to identify and describe these subpopulations. Several unique susceptibility or risk factors in the development of chronic respiratory conditions have been identified in scientific literature. For example, the scientific literature identifies or suggests that smokers,[22,23] males,[24] asthmatics,[23,25,26] and persons with various genetic differences[27] (eg, the α_1-antitrypsin deficiency that increases development of chronic obstructive pulmonary disease)[28] have higher risk for certain chronic respiratory conditions. Given repeated concerns regarding these unique subpopulations, identification of personnel who are "susceptible" (underlying disease or genetics) and/or who have "higher exposures" should be the focus of future enhancements to the military's exposure assessment process.

RETHINKING EXPOSURE ASSESSMENT

Exposure assessment has been defined as "the process of estimating or measuring the magnitude, frequency, and duration of exposure to an agent in a specific exposed population."[1(p51)] It is part of the risk assessment process that is used to characterize risks of disease to specific populations that may be associated with the exposure. The resulting information is used to direct policies to prevent and mitigate exposures, focus future research needs, and in some cases direct medical interventions or surveillance.[29] Even in controlled US occupational or civilian settings, the use of current technologies, tools, and scientific models to conduct exposure assessments is not without notable limitations and uncertainties. These problems tend to be amplified by the austere *work environment* during deployment and numerous variables that reflect the exposures of deployed military personnel.[8,12–17,20,21] However, "in addressing the relationship between exposures of military personnel deployed in the Middle East theater ... and the risk of adverse health effects, exposure assessment is a critical component."[1(p51)] For these reasons, the military has devoted substantial resources to the exposure assessment process over the past decade.[4,14–17,20,21]

The traditional exposure assessment process focuses on the exposure of a specific substance (eg, a chemical hazard) as experienced by an overall population. This construct ignores the numerous other external and internal factors that can impact the overall risk of a specific disease outcome that might be experienced by persons within a population (Figure 5-1). Current scientific models and data also do not tend to address the potential additive or synergistic impacts of these multiple hazards. Even when exposure assessment

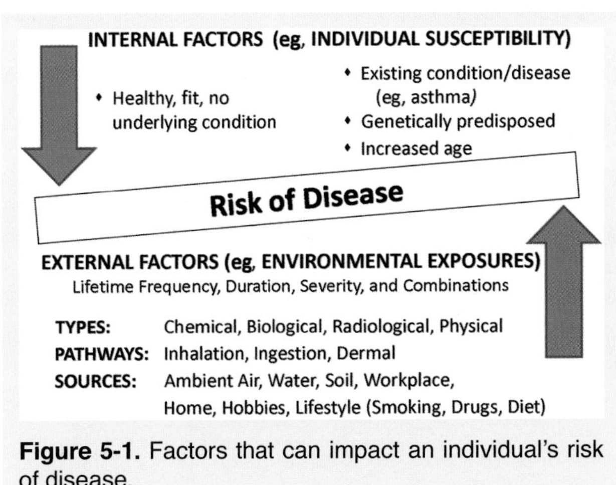

Figure 5-1. Factors that can impact an individual's risk of disease.

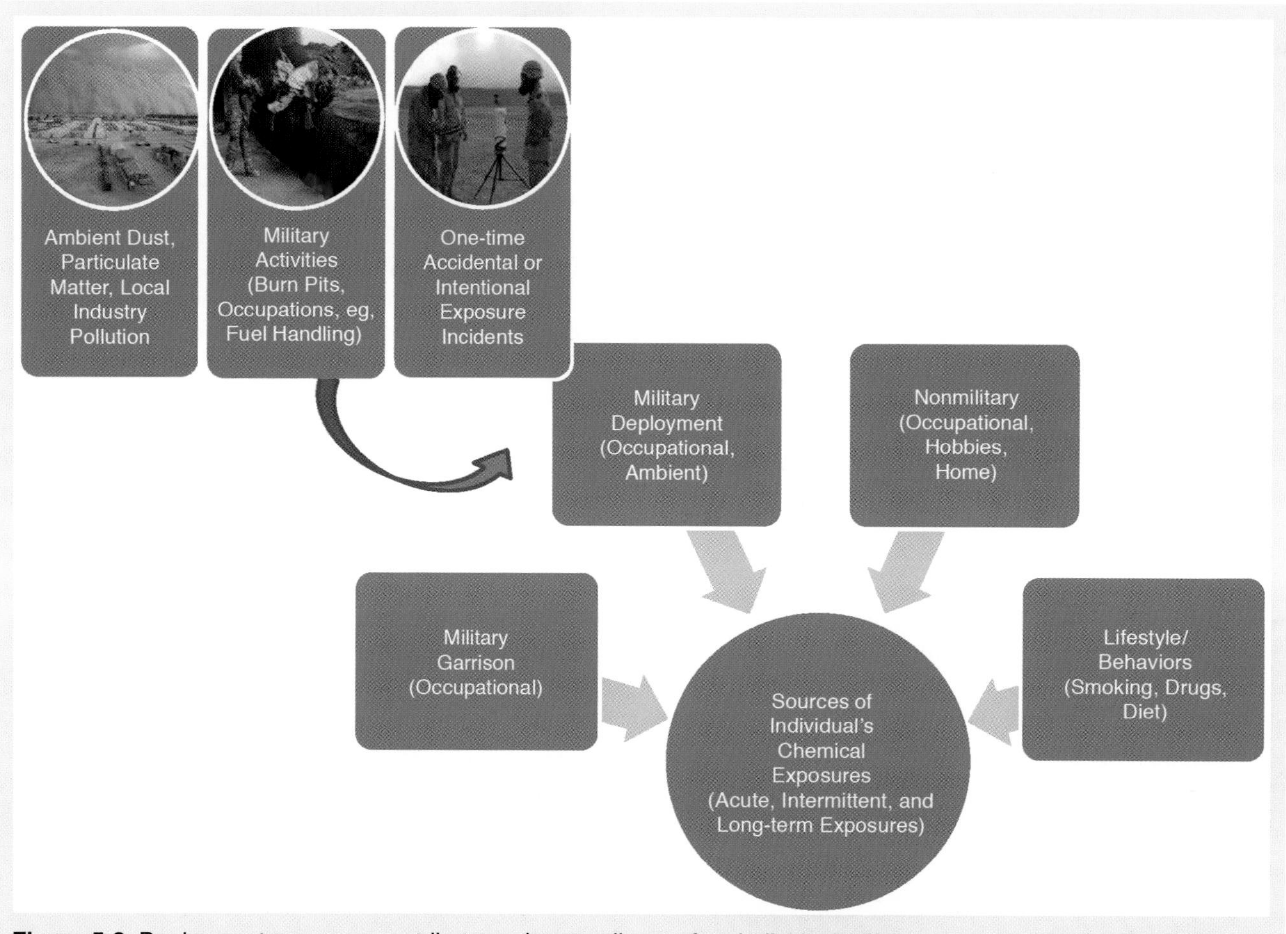

Figure 5-2. Deployment exposure contributes only a small part of an individual's lifelong chemical exposure profile.

attempts to address several hazards, there are numerous other types of prior, concurrent, and follow-on external stressors that may impact an individual's health condition. The environmental stressor may not reflect the combination of factors that results in an increased risk of disease. This need to consider tools that can provide information about the various contributing impacts to service members' health conditions has been previously identified[2,7,11,15,18] (Figure 5-2).

The traditional exposure assessment process itself cannot account for all factors that may influence individual health outcomes. However, the process should include identification of any subpopulations that are at higher risk of adverse health outcomes (eg, because of higher overall internal levels of the hazardous substance). Focus should shift from defining general population exposures to identifying the populations most likely to be at risk. This includes identifying and assessing the following subpopulations:

- Persons who experience hazardous exposures of greatest duration, frequency, and magnitude. Ideally, this would include consideration of key activities during *deployment* operations, as well as those experienced as part of military *garrison* occupational activities. These persons can be reflected by one or more similar exposure groups.
- Persons with lifestyle activities that may increase risk (eg, smoking history, physical fitness activities [such as poor aerobic conditioning, or alternately, frequent and high-intensity aerobic exercise that increases inhalation rate while deployed to areas with poor air quality], and/or exposures to chemicals from hobbies).
- Persons with unique susceptibilities to adverse health outcomes (eg, chronic pulmonary conditions).

The following section describes the benefits and disadvantages of different approaches for obtaining data to characterize individual exposures and relevant risk factors. Better individual data would help to identify subpopulations at greatest risk and possible prevention measures.

DATA COLLECTION APPROACHES AND TOOLS: BENEFITS AND DISADVANTAGES

Enhanced Environmental Monitoring

As described in Chapter 1, thousands of air, soil, and water samples have been collected during more than a decade of Operation Iraqi Freedom/Operation Enduring Freedom in southwest Asia. Data have been analyzed using peer-reviewed, state-of-the-art health risk assessment models[16,30,31] to provide summaries of typical ambient environmental exposures at deployment base camp locations.[5,6] Assessment of this environmental data has value as a screening tool to identify any substantial threats anticipated to have population-level impacts. The greatest limitation is that it cannot (or should not) be directly tied to individual service members.[1,2,4–6,14,15]Additionally, current military environmental data lack the scope and precision necessary to fully describe all the potential airborne chemical hazards and the associated temporal and spatial fluctuations. Because of the technology and resource limitations, environmental sampling also does not routinely include collection and analyses for volatile organic compounds or several irritating and acutely toxic industrial hazards, including those that represent primary US priority pollutants (eg, chlorine, ammonia, sulfur dioxide, and hydrogen sulfide). In addition, samples obtained from a larger area, such as a base camp, are generally limited in number and, therefore, cannot generally be used to describe temporal, spatial, geographic, or climate-related patterns.[2,5,14,15,20] Although improvements in this area could help to better identify major hazards or locations, these "area samples" will not provide information regarding individual exposure experiences. Furthermore, data associated with this approach would still be interpreted with a "single-hazard" assessment model.

Personal and Occupational Monitoring

Personal monitoring—including the use of passive chemical dosimeters, personal air sampling pumps, and portable real-time detection devices—has been repeatedly discussed as a means to obtain more specific exposure data from individuals and units during deployments.[1,2,8,15–17] However, limitations of current technologies, especially in the austere military operational environments, are a recognized problem with this approach.[2,8,16,17] Technologies today are only developed for a subset of the numerous hazards present in a military setting, have high detection level and/or low confidence in results, and have numerous logistical resource needs for accurate employment. Aside from limited use of chemical agent detectors,[32] portable field devices for chemical hazards have been extremely limited and the source of substantial evaluation over the years.[16,19,33]

For the last few years, however, the US Army has attempted to conduct occupational assessments of specific personnel in deployed settings and make use of available technologies. One example involved assessment of a security unit conducting missions near a brick factory.[34] Sampling was conducted by deployed military personnel who had received equipment and guidance from subject matter experts in the United States. Interpretations of results were hindered by problems with equipment and sample collection. A more recent, and still ongoing, industrial hygiene survey is assessing occupational exposures to members of a similar exposure group at Al Shuaiba Port of Debarkation/Embarkation, Kuwait. The initial survey was conducted by a specific team of experts with dedicated equipment from the US Army Public Health Command. According to one of the team's industrial hygienists (J. Cambre, oral communication, December 2012), personal air samples were collected using passive chemical dosimeters and a multigas analyzer to investigate chemicals that had been identified as potential exposure concerns during site industrial source assessments and prior environmental data collection. The chemicals included the following:

- ammonia,
- carbon monoxide,
- chlorine,
- hydrogen sulfide,
- nitrogen dioxide, and
- sulfur dioxide.

The potential exposure sources included the surrounding Kuwaiti industries and US Army vehicle and generator exhaust. The first phase is helping to highlight critical data gaps and equipment limitations, as well as to prioritize future efforts to enhance data confidence and detail through further sampling. Although efforts of this magnitude may not be feasible at other deployment locations, lessons learned may provide insights into activity-based exposures.

Finally, although not directly related to the feasibility of implementing field technologies to obtain individual-level, deployment-related exposure data, there is the question of how to factor in occupational exposures in garrison into the overall exposure assessment process. The long-term implications of daily occupational exposures experienced by Army personnel in nondeployed settings may be as important as those experienced during deployment. Military occupational tasks and associated exposures should be considered when identifying more highly exposed subpopulations. Occupational exposure data, such as that reported in the Defense Occupational and Environmental Health Readiness–Industrial Hygiene system, may be used to help identify priority hazards, personnel, and tasks/operations.

Biomonitoring

Biomarkers are broadly defined as measurements in biological systems or samples that are indicators of an event within the organism or compartment of the organism. There are three types of biomarkers: (1) exposure, (2) effect, and (3) susceptibility.[35] These are summarized in Table 5-1. Biomarkers are a tool to complement an overall exposure assessment process, especially where specific high-risk hazards, exposure sources, and populations have been identified. Whereas the Centers for Disease Control and Prevention reports results for more than 200 chemical biomarkers as part of its National Health and Nutrition Examination Survey, these data are for comparison reference purposes.[36] These data do not provide substantial information as to sources of exposure, the clinical significance of biomarker measurements, or actions to be taken. Because of these limitations, few public health and occupational applications require specific use of chemical biomarker data.

In military settings, biomonitoring procedures for certain exposures to lead and depleted uranium are required by policy.[37] In these cases, specific effects and medical actions are correlated to defined biomarker levels. Broader use of biomarkers by the military has been suggested.[5,14,38] The current DoD policy describes specific criteria to determine biomarkers that would be useful for military applications. Although no other biomarkers have met the criteria for assessment of deployment exposures, biomarkers that define deployment-related exposures have been attempted in several cases. Examples include the

- evaluation of Vietnam exposures to Agent Orange,[39,40]
- Gulf War assessment of depleted uranium and polycyclic aromatic hydrocarbon exposures,[16,41]
- Joint Base Balad dioxin assessment,[2,41] and
- medical assessment for chromium exposure during the Qarmat Ali chromium incident.[42]

In these cases, which all used biomarkers of exposure, the value of the results was questionable, especially given the many interpretive limitations[14,15,39,40,41] (see Table 5-1). Biomarkers of effect could facilitate medical intervention and/or provide a means for more concrete case definition. An example of a potential marker for disease that has been the subject of ongoing evaluation is the use of spirometry for lung function testing (Chapter 9, Discussion Summary: Recommendation for Surveillance Spirometry in Military Personnel). Of more recent scientific interest to the exposure science community has been the field of metabolomics and use of exposomic research to identify early indication of effect, disease, or susceptibility.[43,44]

The use of biomarkers of susceptibility has been a key area of pharmacological and medical research,[45–48] but has received lesser consideration by the military or VA.[15] Use of susceptibility biomarkers may have some relevance to better determine personnel at risk for chronic respiratory disease. Four broad types of susceptibility mechanisms particularly relevant to pulmonary health outcomes have been suggested:

1. toxicokinetic factors that affect the delivery and/or persistence of the chemical or particle in the lung,
2. regulation and resolution of inflammation and fibrogenesis,
3. immunological sensitization, and
4. biochemical (enzymatic and nonenzymatic) defense mechanisms to protect cells and tissues from oxidative stress.[27]

For example, the deficiency in the α_1-antitrypsin enzyme is a documented susceptibility factor in the development of chronic obstructive pulmonary disease in young adult nonsmokers.[28] Ideally, biomarkers of relevance to the military would be relatively low in cost, involve minimally complex procedures, be noninvasive, and ultimately provide discrete useable data that would support prevention and/or medical treatment and surveillance objectives.

Modeling

Modeling refers to computational air dispersion simulation tools that can be used to predictively or retrospectively estimate the direction and magnitude/extent of airborne hazards over time. Of critical importance, however, is that the air modeling tools can only be used to estimate specific substance(s) released from a known source. Current tools can incorporate satellite imagery, a variety of climate and geographic variables, and field sample results for validation or correction.[49] Tools can display results visually, for example, as plumes or wind rose plots. Air dispersion and/or plume estimation techniques and tools were used to estimate the 1991 Gulf War oil well fire plumes[16,17,50] and the 1991 Khamisayah exposures to agent sarin potentially released during munitions disposal operations.[16,51] The size of the plume exposure area investigated as part of the 2003 Al-Mishraq sulfur fire incident was determined by simplistic estimation drawn from satellite images of the smoke.[9] The use of wind rose plots to identify and prioritize sampling efforts of burn pit smoke at Joint Base Balad was evaluated by IOM.[2] The IOM discussed potential improvements to modeling of burn pits so that average concentrations could be estimated over time to describe possible exposure gradients. However, the quality of this information would depend on better knowledge of the types and quantities of materials burned, as well as more detailed individual activities and locations. Perhaps of greater consideration is that modeling of a burn pit would not address other possible sources of concurrent exposure. Furthermore, as concluded by the IOM, burn pits may not be the main cause of long-term health effects related to Iraq and

TABLE 5-1

SUMMARY OF BENEFITS AND ADVANTAGES

Approach/Tool	Applications/Possible Benefits to Improve Individual Assessments	Possible Disadvantages and/or Limitations
Environmental monitoring	Cost-effective approach to broadly assess population exposures to certain widespread hazards, such as particulate matter Use of continuous air monitoring systems at deployment locations has been employed at one location (SPOD/E, Kuwait)	Does not provide individual data Technology and resource limitations include gaps in hazards of concern (eg, VOCs, irritating and acutely toxic industrial hazards, priority pollutants [chlorine, ammonia, sulfur dioxide, and hydrogen sulfide]), and gaps in quantifying exposure variations (eg, temporal, spatial, geographic, or climate-related differences)
Occupational and personal monitoring	Can provide individual exposure data Recent/ongoing attempts pave the way for prioritizing follow-on assessment of personal occupational activities and/or hazards Helps focus priority needs for future military capabilities and technology improvements Garrison-based industrial hygiene surveys and exposure assessments may be used to help identify at-risk groups	Technology and resource limitations: • not available for many chemicals • detection levels not always quantifiable • low confidence in results (false-negatives and false-positives) • lack of criteria for interpretation of health impact • substantial cost and logistics to use in field
Biomarkers of exposure	Individual data (direct internal measurement of the chemical hazard or its metabolite[s], or indirect measurement of an interaction between the chemical and some target molecule[s] or cell[s]) Possibly could be used to identify subpopulations at higher risk for disease outcome and/or to categorize degree of exposure relative to US population norms or to other deployed personnel results Current military applications include lead and DU biomonitoring	Lack of inferable significance of measurement (generally cannot define exposure source OR indicate adverse effect or susceptibility) Measurements specific for a single chemical hazard Depending on the properties of the substance (eg, biological half-life) and environmental conditions, all or some of the substance and its metabolites may leave the body prior to sample collection Burden of a substance may be the result of exposures from more than one source External as well as internal (eg, essential mineral nutrients)

(**Table 5-1** *continues*)

Table 5-1 *continued*

Biomarkers of effect Measurements of biochemical, physiological, or other alteration within an organism that, depending on magnitude, can be recognized as an established or potential health impairment or disease	Individual data can possibly be used to identify subpopulations at higher risk for disease outcome Utility of lung function testing (spirometry) is an example being evaluated Can be used to support standard case definitions and diagnosis Can be used to identify effect that might be caused or influenced by multiple separate exposure types Would not need to be implemented in the field; greater time and logistics flexibility	Does not generally indicate specific exposures / not often substance-specific May not be directly adverse, but can indicate potential health impairment (eg, DNA adducts)
Biomarkers of susceptibility Indicators of an inherent or acquired limitation of an organism's ability to respond to the challenge of exposure to a specific substance	Individual data; can also be used to help identify subpopulations at higher risk for disease outcome Avoids need to infer impacts from single exposure pathway Would not need to be implemented in the field; greater time and logistical flexibility	Does not address specific exposures Knowledge of susceptibilities may be associated with legal or ethical concerns
Modeling	Can be used to estimate gradients of average levels resulting from a known source at various locations Can be enhanced by sample data	Not intended to define individual exposures, with the limited possible exception of case-specific use to rule out or verify the plausibility of substantial exposures to a specific source if adequate source and personal location data were available Hazard source-specific Requires accurate information regarding types and quantities of hazards (eg, materials in a burn pit) and release processes (eg, temperatures of fires) Many models exist and can produce different results
Self-reported data (questionnaires, surveys)	Mechanism design to capture individual data Can address many data gaps Flexibility for different applications Relatively inexpensive	Potential recall bias Data are subjective surrogate for objective measure of exposure Time and logistical constraints; ideally electronic system is needed Personal and privacy issues regarding collection, storage, and use of data

DNA: deoxyribonucleic acid; DU: depleted uranium; SPOD / E: Shuaiba Port of Debarkation / Embarkation; VOCs: volatile organic compounds

Afghanistan deployment, but the IOM states that, "service in Iraq or Afghanistan—that is, a broader consideration of air pollution than exposure only to burn pit emissions—might be associated with long-term health effects."[2(p7)]

Self-Reporting Tools

Self-reporting tools include questionnaires and surveys that are either provided to service members to complete or used by providers or researchers to ask patients/study participants about their past exposures. Benefits and key limitations, such as recall bias for use in military exposure assessments, have been assessed.[7,12] However, as described in Appendix A (A Self-Reporting Tool to Collect Individual Data for Respiratory Health Effects and Military Airborne Exposures) of this book, the use of self-reported exposure data in public health research and occupational applications has been long utilized by various national and international research and occupational entities. The military has also continuously relied on such tools; numerous questionnaires have been developed and used to collect exposure-related data with various cohorts of Gulf War veterans.[7,12,18,52–55] Current DoD policy requires use of Post-Deployment Health Assessment forms and Post-Deployment Health Reassessment forms that include questions about exposures experienced while deployed.[52] These forms, however, are for screening purposes and do not provide detailed information regarding magnitude, duration, and frequency of chemical exposures experienced or other relevant activities. Several studies of service members and veterans of the more recent and current operations have been conducted as part of the Millennium Cohort Study,[7] which utilizes self-reported occupational exposures as a source of *exposure assessment* information. Study investigators have noted the critical need for obtaining quantified measures of individual exposure and also that, "retrospective self-reported assessment of exposure is a viable option if designed in such a way that exposures and health outcomes are not collected simultaneously."[7(p60)] These Millennium Cohort Study investigators, as well as others,[2,56] have specifically recommended efforts to establish a standardized self-reported exposure assessment tool to be used across services and by the VA. Such a tool could improve case identification in clinical applications, as well as provide additional delineation of potentially higher risk factors and associated subgroup populations among deployed personnel. Appendix A provides a specific example of a library of questions that could be used to serve as a basis for future applications.

SUMMARY

The relationship between exposures experienced while deployed in southwest Asia and chronic respiratory effects is considered plausible, yet remains unproven. However, experts seem to agree that some persons may be at greater risk to develop these health outcomes because of their unique susceptibilities and exposures. Use of periodic, large-scale ambient environmental sampling will not help us identify these persons or their risk factors.

To better address the medical and deployment health issues faced by the DoD and the VA, the traditional concept of exposure assessment should be evaluated more broadly. Specifically, the collection of data that would help distinguish higher risk activities and/or susceptibilities to identified adverse health outcomes of interest should become a greater priority. No single approach or tool can address all the gaps in our understanding of an individual's unique exposure history. However, certain tools alone or in combination could be used to increase our understanding of individual military exposures, as well as key confounding factors and susceptibilities that may result in a higher risk of chronic respiratory conditions.

The approaches that would most effectively differentiate individual exposure variation and higher risk subpopulations should be priorities for future research, field work, and medical evaluation protocols. Areas of promise include the following:

- personal monitoring and occupational activity exposure assessment,
- biomarkers (especially of effect and susceptibility), and
- establishment and implementation of standardized self-reporting tools.

Ongoing field industrial hygiene efforts could be evaluated as a means to identify technological enhancements needed for personal monitoring and/or to help identify priority hazards or higher risk (exposure) military occupational activities. However, individual sample results for a single hazard from a single activity period will not adequately address the complex interaction of lifetime external stressors, and exposures and individual susceptibilities. Biomarker research has come a long way. Instead of biomarkers of exposure, research should perhaps focus more on applications and technologies for biomarkers of effect and susceptibility. Finally, use of a consistent set of standardized questions related to exposure and health history (such as those provided in Appendix E, Frequently Asked Questions About Military Exposure Guidelines) should be considered across services and agencies for future public health research, as well as clinical applications.

REFERENCES

1. National Research Council. *Review of the Department of Defense Enhanced Particulate Matter Surveillance Program Report.* Washington, DC: The National Academies Press; 2010.

2. Institute of Medicine. *Long-Term Health Consequences of Exposure to Burn Pits in Iraq and Afghanistan.* Washington, DC: The National Academies Press; 2011.

3. US Department of the Army. *Summary of Evidence Statement: Chronic Respiratory Conditions and Military Deployment.* Aberdeen Proving Ground, MD: US Army Public Health Command; 2011. Factsheet 64-018-1111.

4. Baird CP. The basis for and uses of environmental sampling to assess health risk in deployed settings. *Mil Med.* 2011;176(suppl 7):84–90.

5. US Department of the Army. *The Periodic Occupational and Environmental Monitoring Summary (POEMS)—History, Intent, and Relationship to Individual Exposures and Health Outcomes.* Aberdeen Proving Ground, MD: US Army Public Health Command; 2010. Technical Information Paper 64-002-1110.

6. US Department of the Army. *Documentation of Deployment Exposures and the Periodic Occupational Environmental Monitoring Summary (POEMS) Information for Preventive Medicine Personnel.* Aberdeen Proving Ground, MD: US Army Public Health Command (Provisional); 2010. Factsheet 64-010-0410.

7. Smith TC, Millennium Cohort Study Team. Linking exposures and health outcomes to a large population-based longitudinal study: the Millennium Cohort Study. *Mil Med.* 2011;176(suppl 7):56–63.

8. Riddle M, Lyles M. Panel 4: linking service members and exposure data to support determination of risk-proceedings of an educational symposium on assessing potentially hazardous environmental exposures among military populations. *Mil Med.* 2011;176(suppl 7):105–109.

9. Baird CP, DeBakey S, Reid L, et al. Respiratory health status of US Army personnel potentially exposed to smoke from 2003 Al-Mishraq Sulfur Plant fire. *J Occup Environ Med.* 2012;54:717–723.

10. Abraham JH, Debakey SF, Reid L, et al. Does deployment to Iraq or Afghanistan affect respiratory health of US military personnel? *J Occup Environ Med.* 2012;54:740–745.

11. Committee on Strategies to Protect the Health of Deployed U.S. Forces. *Protecting Those Who Serve: Strategies to Protect the Health of Deployed U.S. Forces.* Washington, DC: The National Academies Press; 2000.

12. Glass DC, Sim MR. The challenges of exposure assessment in health studies of Gulf War veterans. *Phil Trans R Soc Lond B Biol Sci.* 2006;361(1468):627–637.

13. US Department of Defense. Proceedings of the 2010 symposium "Assessing Potentially Hazardous Environmental Exposures Among Military Populations," May 19–21, 2010, Bethesda, Maryland. *Mil Med.* 2011;176(suppl 7):1–112.

14. Gaydos JC. Military occupational and environmental health: challenges for the 21st century. *Mil Med.* 2011;176(suppl 7):5–8.

15. Mallon TM. Progress in implementing recommendations in the National Academy of Sciences reports: "Protecting Those Who Serve: Strategies to Protect the Health of Deployed U.S. Forces." *Mil Med.* 2011;176(suppl 7):9–16.

16. Richards EE. Responses to occupational and environmental exposures in the U.S. military—World War II to the present. *Mil Med.* 2011;176(suppl 7):22–28.

17. DeFraites RF, Richards EE. Assessing potentially hazardous environmental exposures among military populations: 2010 symposium and workshop summary and conclusions. *Mil Med.* 2011;176(suppl 7):17–21.

18. Brix K, O'Donnell FL. Panel 1: medical surveillance prior to, during, and following potential environmental exposures. *Mil Med.* 2011;176(suppl 7):91–96.

19. Lioy PJ. Exposure science for terrorist attacks and theaters of military conflict: minimizing contact with toxicants. *Mil Med*. 2011;176(suppl 7):71–76.

20. Martin NJ, Richards EE, Kirkpatrick JS. Exposure science in U.S. military operations: a review. *Mil Med*. 2011;176(suppl 7):77–83.

21. Batts R, Parzik D. Panel 3: conducting environmental surveillance sampling to identify exposures. *Mil Med*. 2011;176(suppl 7):101–104.

22. Smith B, Ryan MA, Wingard DL, et al. Cigarette smoking and military deployment: a prospective evaluation. *Am J Prev Med*. 2008;35:539–546.

23. Global Initiative for Chronic Obstructive Lung Disease (GOLD). *Global Strategy for the Diagnosis, Management and Prevention of COPD.* Bethesda, MD: National Heart, Lung and Blood Institute; February 2013.

24. Yancey AL, Watson HL, Cartner SC, Simecka JW. Gender is a major factor in determining the severity of mycoplasma respiratory disease in mice. *Infect Immun*. 2001;69:2865–2871.

25. London SJ. Gene–air pollution interactions in asthma. *Proc Am Thorac Soc*. 2007;4:217–220.

26. Silva GE, Sherrill DL, Guerra S, Barbee RA. Asthma as a risk factor for COPD in a longitudinal study. *Chest*. 2004;126:59–65.

27. Nemery B, Bast A, Behr J, et al. Interstitial lung disease induced by exogenous agents: factors governing susceptibility. *Eur Respir J Suppl*. 2001;18:30s–42s.

28. Sandford AJ, Silverman EK. Chronic obstructive pulmonary disease. 1. Susceptibility factors for COPD the genotype–environment interaction. *Thorax*. 2002;57:736–741.

29. Abt E, Rodricks JV, Levy JI, et al. Science and decisions: advancing risk assessment. *Risk Anal*. 2010;30:1028–1036.

30. National Research Council. *Review of the Army's Technical Guides on Assessing and Managing Chemical Hazards to Deployed Personnel*. Washington, DC: National Academies Press; 2004.

31. US Department of the Army. *Environmental Health Risk Assessment and Chemical Exposure Guidelines for Deployed Military Personnel*. Aberdeen Proving Ground, MD: US Army Public Health Command (Provisional); 2010. Technical Guide 230.

32. Sferopoulos R. *A Review of Chemical Warfare Agent (CWA) Detector Technologies and Commercial-Off-The-Shelf Items*. Victoria, Australia: Human Protection and Performance Division, Defence Science and Technology Organisation; March 2009. Report DSTO-GD-0570.

33. US Department of the Army. *Health-Based Chemical Vapor Concentrations Levels for Future Systems Acquisition and Development*. Aberdeen Proving Ground, MD: US Army Center for Health Promotion and Preventive Medicine (now the US Army Public Health Command); February 2008. Technical Report 64-FF-07Z2-07.

34. US Department of the Army. *Medical Assessment of Air Quality at Narhwan Brick Factory and FOB Hammer in Iraq (2008-9)*. Aberdeen Proving Ground, MD: US Army Public Health Command; 2012. Factsheet 64-023-0412.

35. National Research Council. *Biological Markers in Pulmonary Toxicology*. Subcommittee on Reproductive and Neurodevelopmental Toxicology, Committee on Biologic Markers. Washington, DC: National Academies Press; 1989.

36. US Department of Health and Human Services. *Fourth National Report on Human Exposure to Environmental Chemicals, Updated Tables, March, 2013*. National Biomonitoring Program. Atlanta, GA: Centers for Disease Control and Prevention; 2013.

37. US Department of Defense. *Department of Defense Deployment Biomonitoring Policy and Approved Bioassays for Depleted Uranium and Lead*. Washington, DC: Under Secretary of Defense (Personnel and Readiness); February 2004. DOD Memorandum (HA Policy: 04-004).

38. May LM, Weese C, Ashley DL, et al. The recommended role of exposure biomarkers for the surveillance of environmental and occupational chemical exposures in military deployments: policy considerations. *Mil Med*. 2004;169:761–767.

39. Young AL, Cecil PF Sr. Agent Orange exposure and attributed health effects in Vietnam veterans. *Mil Med*. 2011;176(suppl 7):29–34.

40. Brown MA. Science versus policy in establishing equitable Agent Orange disability compensation policy. *Mil Med*. 2011;176(suppl 7):35–40.

41. Deeter DP. The Kuwait Oil Fire Risk Assessment Biological Surveillance Initiative. *Mil Med*. 2011;176(suppl 7):52–55.

42. US Department of the Army. *Health Assessment of 2003 Qarmat Ali Water Treatment Plant Sodium Dichromate Incident Status Update: May 2010*. Aberdeen Proving Ground, MD: US Army Public Health Command (Provisional); 2010. Factsheet 64-012-0510.

43. Rappaport SM. Implications of the exposome for exposure science. *J Expo Sci Environ Epidemiol*. 2011;21:5–9.

44. Lioy PJ, Rappaport SM. Exposure science and the exposome: an opportunity for coherence in the environmental health sciences. *Environ Health Perspect*. 2011;119:A466–A467.

45. Mayr M. Metabolomics: ready for the prime time? *Circ Cardiovasc Genet*. 2008;1:58–65.

46. Jian ZH, Rommereim DN, Minard KR, et al. Metabolomics in lung inflammation: a high-resolution ^{1}H NMR study of mice exposed to silica dust. *Toxicol Mech Methods*. 2008;18:385–398.

47. Aich P, Potter AA, Griebel PJ. Modern approaches to understanding stress and disease susceptibility: a review with special emphasis on respiratory disease. *Int J Gen Med*. 2009;2:19–32.

48. Lash LH, Hines RN, Gonzalez FJ, et al. Genetics and susceptibility to toxic chemicals: do you (or should you) know your genetic profile? *J Pharmacol Exp Ther*. 2003;305:403–409.

49. US Environmental Protection Agency. *Evaluation of Chemical Dispersion Models Using Atmospheric Plume Measurements from Field Experiments*. Research Triangle Park, NC: USEPA; September 2012. Final Report. EPA Contract EP-D-07-102.

50. Heller JM. Oil well fires of Operation Desert Storm—defining troop exposures and determining health risks. *Mil Med*. 2011;176(suppl 7):46–51.

51. US Department of Defense. *Case Narrative: US Demolition Operations at Khamisiyah*. Washington, DC: Assistant Secretary of Defense (Health Affairs) and Special Assistant to the Under Secretary of Defense (Personnel and Readiness) for Gulf War Illnesses, Medical Readiness, and Military Deployments; April 2002. Final Report.

52. US Department of Defense. *Post Deployment Health Assessment*. Washington, DC: Assistant Secretary for Defense (Health Affairs); March 2005. DOD Memorandum.

53. Helmer DA, Rossignol M, Blatt M, et al. Health and exposure concerns of veterans deployed to Iraq and Afghanistan. *J Occup Environ Med*. 2007;49:475–480.

54. Quigley KS, McAndrew LM, Almeida L, et al. Prevalence of environmental and other military exposure concerns in Operation Enduring Freedom and Operation Iraqi Freedom veterans. *J Occup Environ Med*. 2012;54:659–664.

55. Proctor SP. *Development of a Structured Neurotoxicant Assessment Checklist (SNAC) for Clinical Use in Veteran Populations*. Boston, MA: Department of Veterans Affairs, VA Boston Healthcare System; 2006.

56. Rose C, Abraham J, Harkins D, et al. Overview and recommendations for medical screening and diagnostic evaluation for postdeployment lung disease in returning US Warfighters. *J Occup Environ Med*. 2012;54:746–751.

AIRBORNE HAZARDS RELATED TO DEPLOYMENT

Section II: Population Surveillance

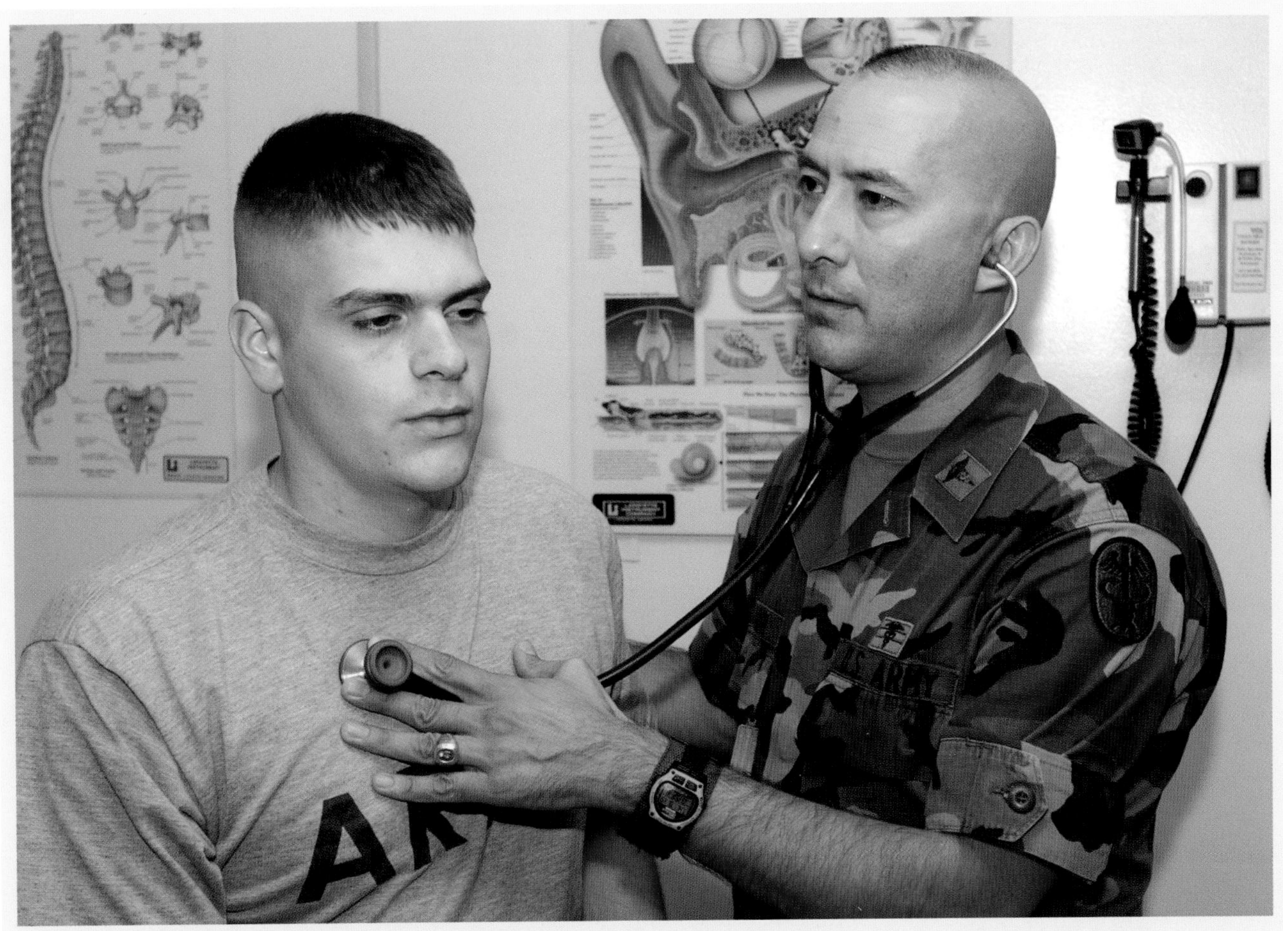

A service member receiving a medical evaluation at a military treatment facility.

Photograph: Courtesy of the US Army Public Health Command (Aberdeen Proving Ground, Maryland).

Chapter 6

EPIDEMIOLOGY OF AIRBORNE HAZARDS IN THE DEPLOYED ENVIRONMENT

JOSEPH H. ABRAHAM, SCD*; LESLIE L. CLARK, PHD†; AND AARON I. SCHNEIDERMAN, PHD‡

*Epidemiologist, Environmental Medicine Program, Occupational and Environmental Medicine Portfolio, Army Institute of Public Health, US Army Public Health Command, 5158 Blackhawk Road, Aberdeen Proving Ground, Maryland 21010-5403

†Senior Epidemiologist, General Dynamics Information Technology, Division of Epidemiology and Analysis, Armed Forces Health Surveillance Center, 11800 Tech Road, Suite 220, Silver Spring, Maryland 20904

‡Deputy Director, Epidemiology Program, Post-Deployment Health Group (10P3A), Office of Public Health, Veterans Health Administration, US Department of Veterans Affairs, 810 Vermont Avenue, NW, Washington, DC 20420

INTRODUCTION

Monitoring, maintaining, and promoting the health of current and former US military personnel is a priority of the US Department of Defense (DoD) and the US Department of Veterans Affairs (VA).[1,2] Deployed personnel are exposed to a vast array of airborne hazards, and it is plausible that these deployment-associated airborne hazards affect postdeployment respiratory health.[3] Some military personnel have returned from deployment to southwest Asia (SWA) with persistent respiratory symptoms, and a subset is being diagnosed with chronic respiratory illnesses.[4–6] Epidemiological evaluations of potential deployment-associated environmental health risks can detect trends in adverse respiratory health conditions, aid in quantifying the burden of postdeployment respiratory disease, and identify risk factors for respiratory diseases. The DoD and VA are conducting evaluations of the relationship between deployment and incidence of postdeployment respiratory symptoms and specific chronic lung conditions. In addition, the DoD and VA are evaluating investigations being conducted in the broader community.

Studies of veterans have assessed two different groups: (1) patients at VA facilities seeking care for conditions that may be related to their military service, and (2) veterans with no known specific service-related health concerns. In a VA-conducted study of exposure concerns among nontreatment-seeking US military personnel,[7] self-reporting of environmental concerns immediately after deployment in support of Operation Iraqi Freedom (OIF) and Operation Enduring Freedom (OEF) was low (less than 12% change relative to predeployment exposure), and chart reviews conducted in a separate analysis reported an average of less than three exposure concerns per veteran of OIF/OEF.[8] However, neither of these investigations surveyed exposure to air pollutants, perhaps because air pollutants are practically ubiquitous.[9,10] There is reason to be concerned about air pollution-related health effects,[11–13] but the risk in the deployed military population is not well characterized. The known potential health effects of chronic exposure to particulate matter (PM) include chronic obstructive pulmonary disease (COPD), increases in lower respiratory symptoms, reduction in lung function, and reduction in life expectancy, primarily from cardiorespiratory-specific mortality. The effects of air pollution are population-specific, with most effects observed among the very young, the elderly, and those with underlying conditions that increase susceptibility to air pollution health effects.[12]

At the outset of both OIF and OEF, the DoD began conducting environmental sampling in the Central Command Area of Operations to characterize the deployment environment.[14] The most widespread air pollutant documented by ambient air sampling was PM.[10] Particulate levels varied by location, although average levels were uniformly high across SWA relative to levels typically encountered in the United States. The sources of PM air pollution in SWA are many, including blowing sand and dust, combustion of fossil fuels from vehicles and industry, and fires. Although levels of PM on average are higher in SWA, compared with the US, the composition of PM in samples from US military bases in SWA is generally similar in terms of chemical and mineralogical constituents to samples from the US, the Sahara, and China.[10,15] PM samples typically contain mixtures of silicate minerals, carbonates, oxides, sulfates, and salts in various proportions. Differences lie in the relative proportions of these minerals and chemical components in different soils. In comparison with the Sahara, China, and the US, the SWA samples had lower proportions of silicon dioxide and higher proportions of calcium oxide and magnesium oxide.[10,15] Extremely high PM levels in the region have been attributed to short-term dust events exacerbated by dirt roads, agricultural activities, and disturbance of the desert surface by motorized vehicles.

Exposure to smoke from burning waste has been of particular concern to OIF- and OEF-deployed military personnel.[3,16,17] Disposing of solid waste in large, open "burn pit" operations has been common practice at US camps in Iraq and Afghanistan. A burn pit is defined as an area, not containing a commercially manufactured incinerator or other equipment specifically designed and manufactured for burning of solid waste, designated for the purpose of disposing of solid waste by burning in the outdoor air at a location with more than 100 attached or assigned personnel and that is in place longer than 90 days.[18]

Burn pit emissions likely vary because of heterogeneity in the trash stream and combustion characteristics. Individuals' activity patterns and meteorological conditions additionally influence exposures to burn pit emissions.

Several studies either describing deployment-related environmental conditions or seeking to establish an association of exposure to this environment and the subsequent health outcomes among troops have been completed or are under way.

The purpose of this chapter is to summarize the epidemiological evaluations being conducted by the US Army Public Health Command (USAPHC), the Armed Forces Health Surveillance Center (AFHSC), the Department of VA Post-Deployment Health Epidemiology Program, as well as by other US government and nongovernment research centers. Trends in select health conditions—primarily chronic respiratory diseases—and their relationship to deployment experiences are presented, followed by a discussion of the issues and implications of the findings of these studies, particularly in the context of a recent Institute of Medicine report on the long-term health consequences of exposure to burn pits in Iraq and Afghanistan.[3]

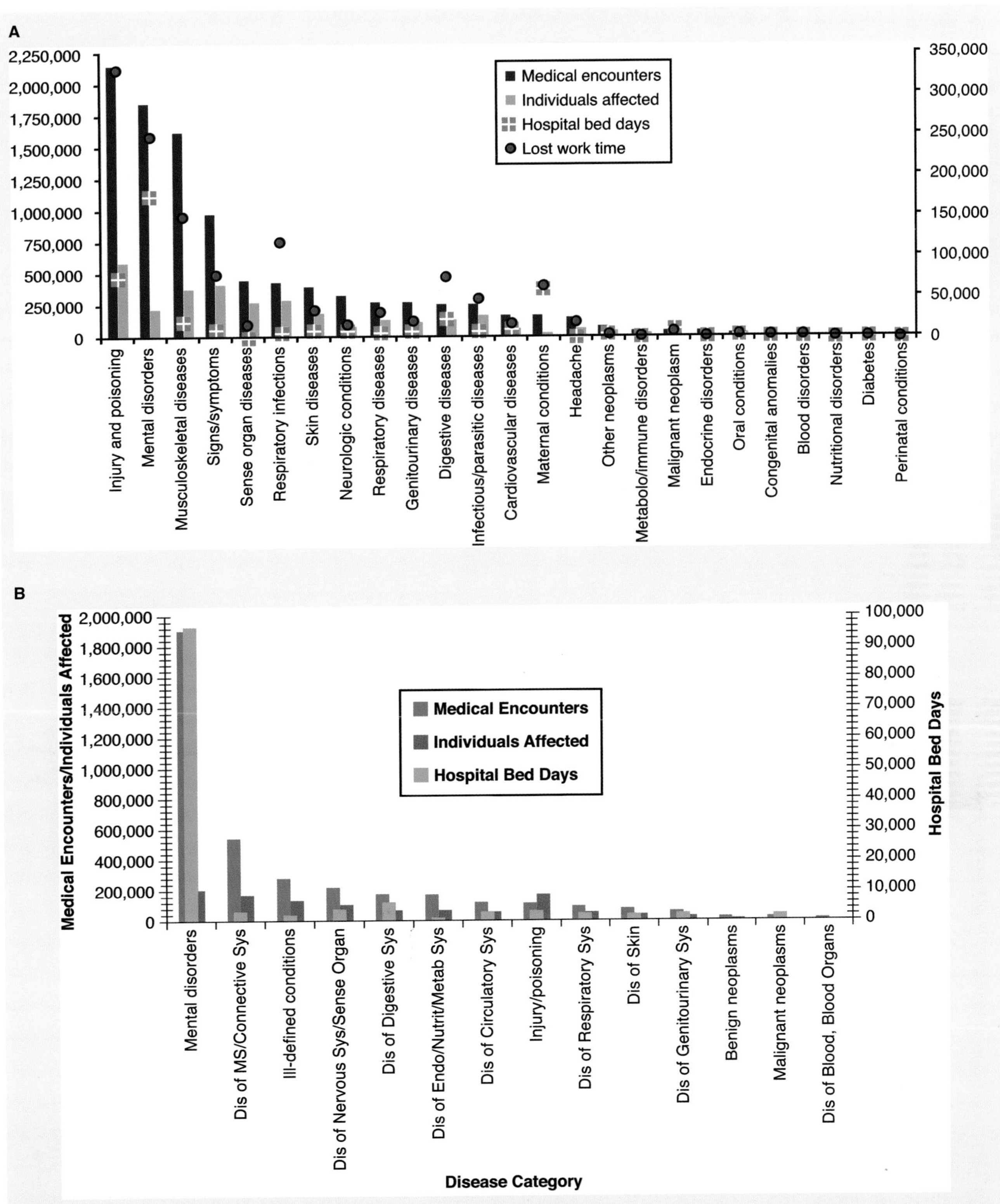

Figure 6-1. (**A**) Department of Defense Burden of Disease Data, 2011. (**B**) Veterans Affairs Burden of Disease Data, 2011. Dis: disease; Endo: endocrine; Metab: metabolism; MS: musculoskeletal; Nutrit: nutrition; Sys: system

BURDEN OF DISEASE AND SURVEILLANCE TRENDS

Figure 6-1 presents the 2011 burden of disease data for the DoD and VA, respectively. Respiratory disease ranks far below the major drivers of healthcare utilization; for example, in the DoD, the number of medical encounters for respiratory diseases (250,000) was seven times less than medical encounters for injuries (more than 2 million). Among VA beneficiaries, the roughly 100,000 medical encounters for diseases of the respiratory system are dwarfed by almost 1.9 million medical encounters for mental disorders. However, respiratory diseases account for a substantial portion of medical encounters, ranking ninth in terms of healthcare utilization among both the DoD and VA populations.

In 2012, the AFHSC conducted a comparison of ambulatory medical encounters and hospitalizations among active duty US military personnel during prewar (January 1998–August 2001) and wartime periods (October 2001–June 2012).[19] The rate of medical encounters for respiratory diseases increased from 149.7 encounters per 1,000 person-years prewar to 173.2 encounters per 1,000 person-years during the war period (incidence rate ratio = 1.16; 95% CI [confidence interval]: 1.08–1.24). However, hospitalizations for respiratory diseases decreased from 1.4 hospitalizations per 1,000 person-years to one hospitalization per 1,000 person-years (incidence rate ratio = 0.71; 95% CI: 0.28–1.73) over the same period.

Between 2000 and 2011, rates of medical encounters for asthma (ICD [International Classification of Diseases]-9 diagnosis code 493) and COPD (ICD-9 diagnosis code 491 and ICD-9 diagnosis code 492) decreased in all branches of the military (Figure 6-2). However, medical encounter rates for respiratory symptoms (ICD-9 diagnosis code 786) and bronchitis not specified as acute or chronic (ICD-9 diagnosis code 490) have increased (see Figure 6-2). Medical encounter rates for respiratory symptoms,

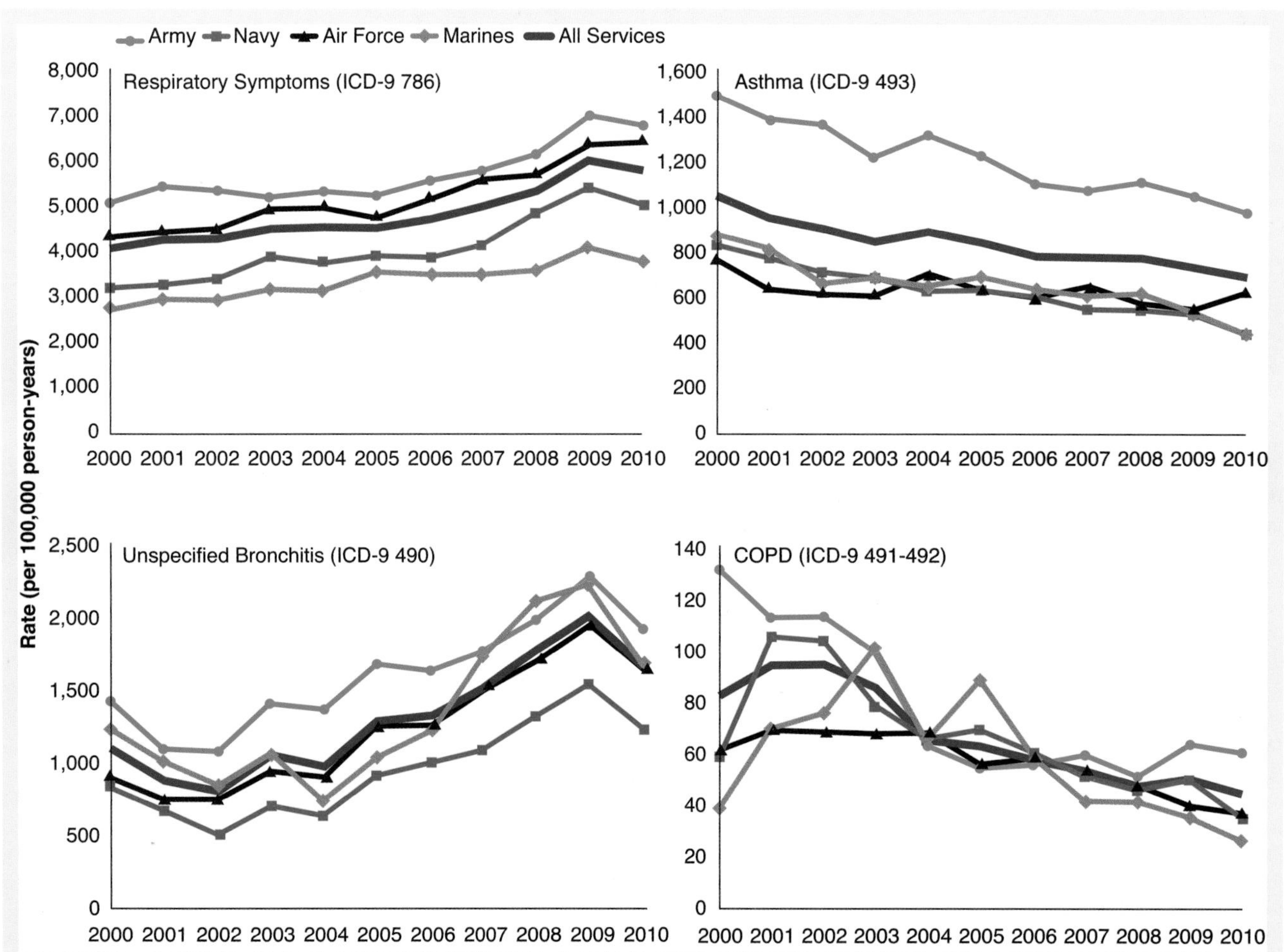

Figure 6-2. Rates of respiratory symptoms and diseases among the services, 2000–2010.
COPD: chronic obstructive pulmonary disease; ICD: *International Classification of Diseases*

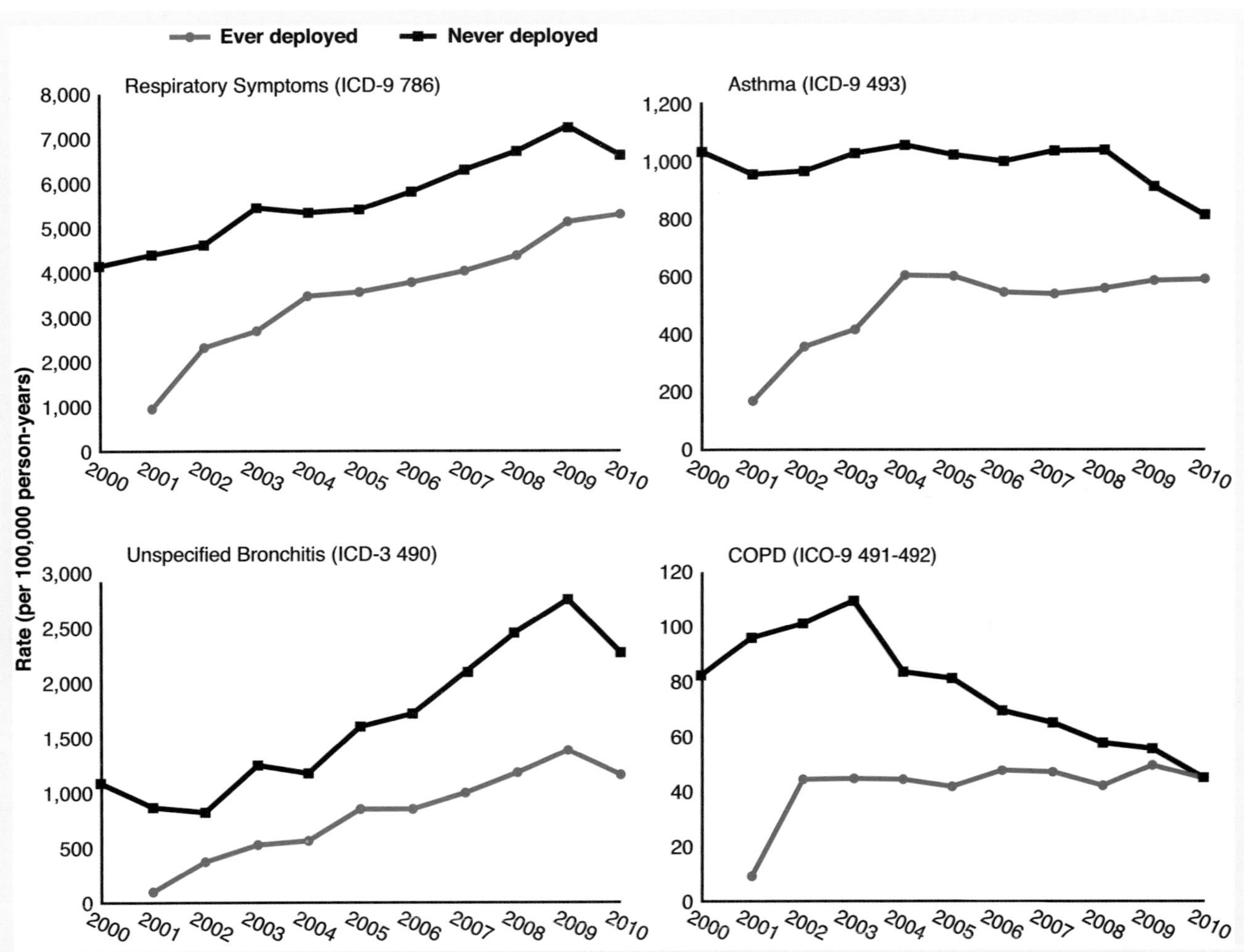

Figure 6-3. Rates of respiratory symptoms and diseases among ever-deployed and never-deployed service members, 2000–2010.
COPD: chronic obstructive pulmonary disease; ICD: *International Classification of Diseases*

asthma, and bronchitis not specified as acute or chronic were uniformly lower among personnel who had deployed at least once (*ever-deployers*), compared with personnel who had no history of deployment (*never-deployers*), although annual incidence trends generally followed the same pattern among ever-deployers as never-deployers (Figure 6-3). These data provide evidence that nondeployed (ie, "unexposed") personnel may not be exchangeable[20] with deployed (ie, "exposed") personnel with respect to baseline health status. Therefore, caution is urged regarding the use of nondeployed personnel as a comparison group for estimating relative and absolute risks in epidemiological studies. Medical encounter rates for chronic bronchitis and emphysema are a possible exception; rates for these conditions appear to be decreasing after 2003, whereas they are stable or slightly increasing among ever-deployed personnel. In 2010, the most recent year for which data were analyzed, COPD medical encounter rates among never- and ever-deployers were approximately the same. Among the VA beneficiary population, rates of asthma, bronchitis, COPD, and chronic bronchitis have been relatively stable over a similar time period (Figure 6-4).

SUMMARY OF EPIDEMIOLOGICAL STUDIES

A summary of the investigations summarized below can be found in Table 6-1. In 2004, Sanders et al[21] initiated a Naval Medical Research Center survey designed to assess the impact of illness and injury during OIF and OEF deployments. The investigators administered a questionnaire to consenting military personnel leaving Iraq or Afghanistan at the end of their deployments. Among 15,459 respondents, 69% self-reported having a respiratory illness during their

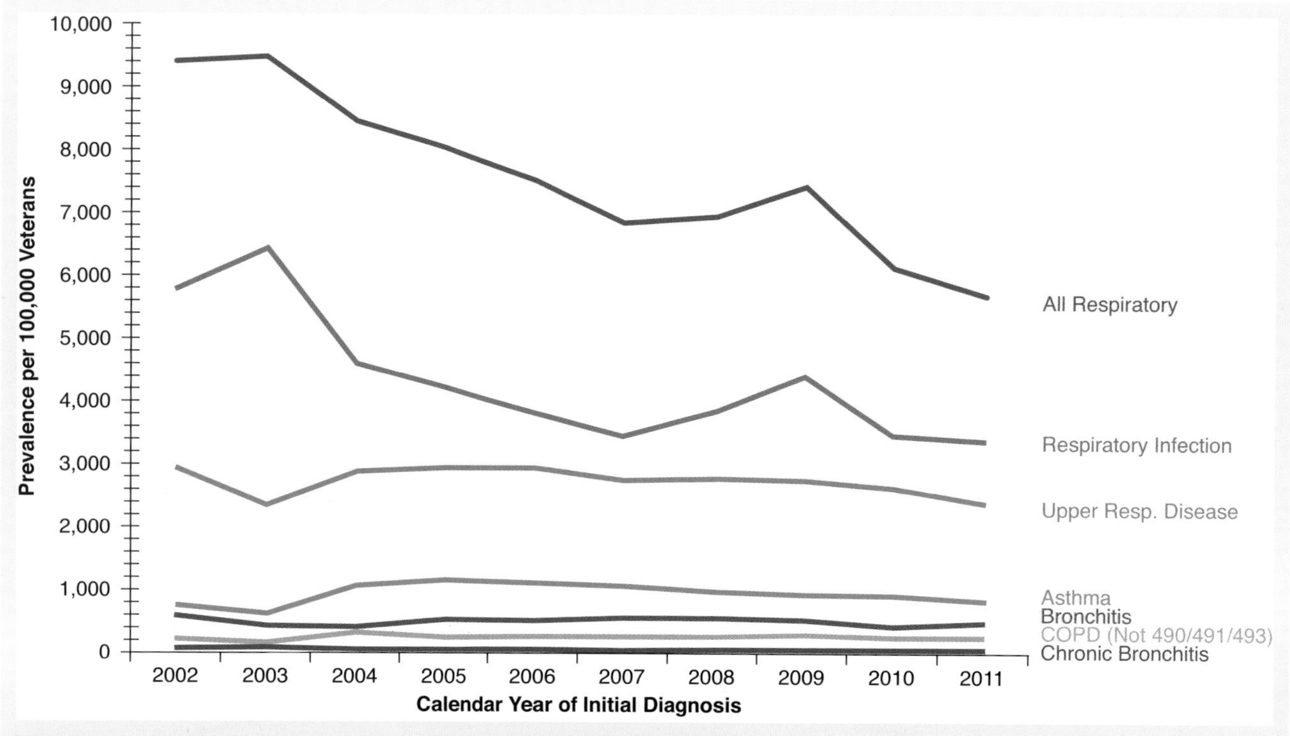

Figure 6-4. Rates of respiratory diseases among the Veterans Affairs beneficiary population, 2002–2011. COPD: chronic obstructive pulmonary disease; Resp: respiratory

deployment. Twenty-two percent of those surveyed reported having an allergy attack, and almost 4% reported having an asthma attack. Greater than one-third (39%) of all respondents reported smoking at least one-half pack of cigarettes per day. Among the self-identifying smokers, 48% either began smoking or restarted smoking during their deployment. The cross-sectional design of the study captured prevalent rather than incident disease, and the survey design was dependent on accurate and reliable self-reporting of conditions. Those who agreed to participate in the study may not have been representative of the larger pool of redeploying military personnel, which would serve to limit generalizability of the prevalence figures.

In 2007, Roop et al[22] reported on a survey designed to assess the prevalence and severity of respiratory symptoms among asthmatics and nonasthmatic active duty Army personnel and DoD contractors returning from OIF and OEF deployments.[22] The prevalence of respiratory symptoms (wheezing, cough, sputum production, and chest pain/tightness) and allergy symptoms following deployment were statistically significantly increased relative to predeployment. Thirty-one percent of the survey respondents were former or current smokers.

In 2009, investigators at the Naval Health Research Center (NHRC) conducted a prospective study designed to assess the relationship between deployment to Iraq and Afghanistan and newly reported respiratory symptoms and respiratory conditions. This study by Smith et al[4] found no difference in the rate of chronic bronchitis, emphysema, or asthma when comparing deployers to nondeployers. However, they observed statistically significant increases in the odds of newly reported respiratory symptoms among formerly deployed Army and Marine Corps personnel compared with nondeployers. Strengths of the study include its prospective design, measurement and adjustment for demographic characteristics and behaviors (including smoking status), and inclusion of personnel from all branches and components of the military in the cohort. The study utilized data garnered from self-administered questionnaire surveys; it lacked the precise information necessary to evaluate associations between specific exposures and pathologies. Its follow-up period was relatively short (2.7 years on average), which precluded elucidation of associations between deployment and diseases characterized by long latency periods.

In 2010, a collaboration of researchers at AFHSC, NHRC, and USAPHC produced a report (*Epidemiological Studies of Health Outcomes Among Troops Deployed to Burn Pit Sites*) in response to a tasking from the Office of the Assistant Secretary of Defense for Health Affairs to conduct expedient evaluations of health effects potentially related to exposures to burn pits at deployment locations.[23] The AFHSC conducted a retrospective evaluation of postdeployment

TABLE 6-1

SUMMARY OF EPIDEMIOLOGICAL REPORTS OF DEPLOYMENT-ASSOCIATED RESPIRATORY HEALTH OF US MILITARY PERSONNEL AND VETERANS

Reference	Study Design	Summary of Findings
Abraham and Baird *J Occup Environ Med* 2012;54:733–739	Case crossover	No evidence of an association between in-theater PM2.5 and acute cardiorespiratory medical encounters
Abraham et al *J Occup Environ Med* 2012;54:740–745	Retrospective cohort	Increase in postdeployment respiratory symptoms and medical encounters for obstructive pulmonary diseases, relative to predeployment rates, in the absence of an association with cumulative deployment duration or total number of deployments
Szema et al *J Occup Environ Med* 2011;53:961–965	Retrospective cohort	Rates of respiratory symptoms leading to a diagnosis requiring spirometry are high among veterans formerly deployed to SWA
Szema et al *Allergy Asthma Proc* 2010;31:67–71	Retrospective cohort	Deployment to Iraq was associated with a higher prevalence of asthma compared with nondeployed soldiers (6.6% vs 4.3%)
AFHSC DoD report, 2010	Retrospective cohort	Deployment to bases in SWA is associated with signs, symptoms, and ill-defined conditions, but is not associated with encounters for respiratory diseases, respiratory infections, circulatory system diseases, and respiratory symptoms; findings are not specific to burn pit locations
NHRC DoD report, 2010	Prospective cohort	Deployment to a base camp with a burn pit was not associated with increased risk of respiratory outcomes, chronic multisymptom illness, lupus, rheumatoid arthritis, birth defects, or preterm birth
Smith et al *Am J Epidemiol* 2009;170:1433–1442	Prospective cohort	Deployment was associated with respiratory symptoms in the Army and Marine Corps, but not associated with respiratory disease diagnoses
Smith et al *Am J Epidemiol* 2009;170:1433–1442	Cross-sectional survey	Prevalence of respiratory symptoms increased during deployment, compared with predeployment for both asthmatics and nonasthmatics
Sanders et al *Am J Trop Med Hyg* 2005;73:713–719	Cross-sectional survey	Prevalence of respiratory illness among deployed personnel is high (69%); prevalence of respiratory infections doubled from precombat to combat phases

AFHSC: Armed Forces Health Surveillance Center; DoD: US Department of Defense; NHRC: Naval Health Research Center; PM: particulate matter; SWA: southwest Asia

respiratory diseases, circulatory diseases, cardiovascular diseases, and sleep apnea in response to the tasking. The AFHSC found no increase in the rates of medical encounters for these conditions among active duty US Army and Air Force personnel formerly deployed to US military bases with burn pit operations in Iraq, compared with personnel stationed in the continental US without a history of OIF/OEF deployment (see Chapter 30, Review of Epidemiological Analyses of Respiratory Health Outcomes After Military Deployment to Burn Pit Locations With Respect to Feasibility and Design Issues Highlighted by the Institute of Medicine). Similar or significantly lower incidence rates were also observed among personnel deployed to locations in Kuwait that operated without burn pits relative to the nondeployed reference group. The AFHSC used deployment to a base camp as a proxy for ambient environmental exposures, including burn pit emissions. The design did not include each deployed individual's actual environmental exposures. This approach allows the potential for errors in the assigning of exposure among the deployed study subjects (ie, differential exposure misclassification). It also precluded the ability to determine study-specific associations between many deployment-related exposures (environmental and otherwise) and postdeployment health status. In addition, the study lacked data on potential confounders and effect modifiers, the most important of which is smoking. Although these analyses did control statistically for age and other demographic characteristics of the population, the negative findings may also have been because of the use of a never-deployed reference group that differed systematically from the exposed groups with respect to baseline health status. The health outcomes defined in the study were based on ICD-9–coded inpatient and outpatient medical encounters pulled from military medical records. It is possible that such medical encounters are imperfect proxies for incident disease, instead, for example, representing preexisting disease. It is also possible that individuals with incident disease either do not present, or have not yet presented, for medical care related to their condition, and therefore are not represented in the medical record. The study focused on health conditions among personnel presenting with respiratory complaints shortly after deployment; as a consequence of the limited follow-up time (a maximum of 3 years postdeployment), the study has almost no power to assess associations between military deployment and diseases of longer latency (eg, emphysema, chronic bronchitis, and lung cancer). Finally, the generalizability of the AFHSC results may also be limited, because they included only active duty components of the Army and Air Force.

In the same 2010 report, the NHRC assessed adverse birth outcomes, respiratory illnesses, chronic multisymptom illness, lupus, and rheumatoid arthritis in relationship to the deployment histories of participants in the Millennium Cohort Study (MCS). The NHRC studies included active duty, Reserve, and National Guard personnel of all services.[23] Overall, deployment to a base camp with a burn pit was not associated with increased risk of respiratory outcomes, chronic multisymptom illness, lupus, or rheumatoid arthritis. However, odds of newly reported lupus were elevated among cohort participants with a history of deployment to one of the locations with a burn pit (Joint Base Balad in Iraq). In the primary analysis, the potential burn pit emissions exposure was not associated with an increase in birth defects or preterm birth. However, the NHRC investigators did observe an increase in the odds of birth defects among a subset of infants whose fathers were exposed more than 280 days prior to the estimated date of conception. In contrast to the AFHSC evaluation, the NHRC study collected information on, and adjusted for, smoking status and physical activity among other demographic, behavioral, and military characteristics of the MCS participants. However, similar to the AFHSC study, the NHRC study used deployment to a military base camp location as a proxy for environmental exposures and is, therefore, similarly susceptible to bias caused by differential exposure misclassification and limited in its ability to resolve specific deployment-associated exposure effects. The NHRC analyses are also susceptible to confounding by unmeasured occupational and behavioral factors that are determinants of postdeployment health status. The health outcomes in the NHRC study are self-reported by MCS participants and may be subject to differential errors in reporting (ie, differential health outcome misclassification), although the NHRC researchers reported that previously conducted investigations of such bias indicate that the MCS participants provide reliable data with responses unaffected by their health status prior to enrollment.[24,25]

Two retrospective studies by a research group at the Veterans Administration Medical Center (VAMC) in Northport, New York, have investigated the relationship between deployment and respiratory health among veterans receiving care at the VAMC's OIF and OEF clinics, comparing them with veterans receiving care at the same medical center but who were not deployed in support of OIF or OEF. In the first study, Szema et al[26] found that 6.6% of veterans deployed to Iraq or Afghanistan had received an asthma diagnosis compared with 4.3% of veterans who were stationed in the United States. The study also reported a statistically significant age- and gender-adjusted estimated increase in the odds of asthma (88%), comparing OIF/OEF deployed veterans to their nondeployed counterparts. In the second study, Szema et al[27] conducted a medical record review of former active duty military personnel registered at the Northport VAMC to assess the relative frequency of respiratory symptoms indicating follow-up spirometric assessment among veterans formerly deployed in support of OIF or OEF compared with veterans who did not deploy to SWA. More than 14% of veterans with a history of OIF/OEF deployment were found to have respiratory symptoms and a follow-up spirometric evaluation compared with fewer than 2% among personnel without a history of OIF/OEF deployment. The inference from this finding is limited by the potential confounding bias; the prevalence of smoking was higher among the formerly deployed group of veterans (16.1%) compared with the nondeployed veterans (3.3%). Despite this observed difference, investigators did not adjust their findings for confounding by smoking status. The authors did not observe differences in clinical disease between veterans with and without a history of deployment, spirometric results were very similar between the two groups, and lung function following either bronchoprovocation or bronchodilation was not assessed. It is not clear from the published reports of either of these studies if attempts were made to exclude prevalent cases of respiratory disease. Neither of the studies evaluates specific environmental or other exposures, relying instead on history of OIF/OEF deployment as a nonspecific proxy for environmental and other exposures that may affect risk of respiratory conditions, similar to the AFHSC and NHRC studies discussed previously. Finally, the representativeness of the Northport VAMC patients with respect to the larger veteran population is not evaluated in these studies. Although the authors draw general conclusions from the results of these studies, their generalizability may be limited to veterans who have a baseline risk of respiratory disease similar to those veterans seen at the Northport VAMC.

In 2012, USAPHC investigators reported on a case-crossover study of ambient PM levels and cardiorespiratory conditions among US active duty military personnel deployed to 15 locations in SWA.[28] The study found no statistically significant associations between daily PM levels and daily rates of in-theater cardiovascular and respiratory-related medical encounters. Strengths of the study included restriction of confounding by design with respect to factors that do not exhibit day-to-day variability (eg, smoking) and the use of measured exposure levels. However, the assessment evaluated every-sixth-day ambient PM levels rather than personal exposures, allowing for the possibility of nondifferential exposure measurement error. The study was also limited in statistical power by its relatively small sample size (2,838 cases) and short duration (1 year). Finally, the study design limited the outcome assessment to potential acute effects of PM.

This same USAPHC group conducted a retrospective assessment examining the relationship between deployment history and postdeployment respiratory health among a random sample of active duty US military personnel formerly deployed in support of OIF or OEF.[5] They observed no statistically significant elevation in the frequency of medical encounters for obstructive pulmonary diseases (asthma, COPD, and allied conditions) among personnel with a history of multiple deployments relative to those with a single deployment. Cumulative duration of deployment was also not significantly associated with medical encounters for obstructive pulmonary diseases. However, they did observe an increase in the rate of medical encounters for respiratory symptoms and encounters for obstructive pulmonary diseases (predominantly asthma and bronchitis) in the postdeployment period relative to a 6-month period prior to deployment. The study shares many of the same limitations as the NHRC and AFHSC studies discussed previously; the authors did not assess specific exposures. The short follow-up period prevents the assessment of associations between deployment and diseases with longer latency. The investigators did collect and adjust for relevant demographic characteristics, but they did not adjust for smoking behaviors. The health outcomes were defined using ICD-9 medical encounter data and are imperfect proxies for incidence of disease. The authors did not assess the Reserve and Guard components of the military, which may limit the generalizability of the findings.

DISCUSSION

The epidemiological evidence to date is inconclusive regarding any definitive associations, or lack thereof, between deployment in support of US contingency operations in SWA (OIF, OEF, and Operation New Dawn) and respiratory health among deployed and formerly deployed military personnel. Findings from different scientific studies include the following:

- no evidence of an association between deployment and respiratory conditions;
- an association between specific lung disease and deployment;
- an association between deployment and increased respiratory symptoms, but not of specific, physician-diagnosed disease; and
- increased frequency of asthma in the VA healthcare system, which is a driver of overall healthcare utilization.

As discussed elsewhere in this chapter, case series have also described particular conditions generating hypotheses regarding a link between environmental exposures encountered while deployed and postdeployment respiratory health[1] (see Chapter 14, Value of Lung Biopsy in Workup of Symptomatic Individuals). All of these studies have methodological limitations that constrain the strength of the drawn conclusions, including limitations in the study methods and regarding exposure, health outcome, and confounder assessment.

No single study can provide or present a definitive answer. The significance of a study's contribution to the overall body of evidence should be based on a consideration of both its strengths and limitations. Findings should be balanced against limitations regarding study design, including

- adequacy of comparison groups,
- exposure assumptions,
- how outcomes are assessed,
- latency periods,
- confounding and other epidemiological biases, and
- low statistical power.

Arriving at an evidence-based conclusion regarding associations between deployment-associated environmental exposures and long-term respiratory health of military personnel is challenging for several reasons. This is a relatively new area of scientific investigation. As discussed, a small but growing number of assessments evaluating associations between military deployment to SWA and subsequent health status of military personnel and veterans have been published in the peer-reviewed scientific literature. The current body of evidence includes multiple studies putatively assessing the same relationship, but with inconsistent findings. Multiple, well-conducted studies with consistent results are typically needed to support a strong conclusion regarding an exposure–disease relationship. Current work is ongoing to fulfill this need.

The epidemiological studies assessing health effects of inhalational hazards in deployed environments are susceptible to the sources of bias common to all epidemiological studies, including selection bias, wherein the baseline health status of comparison groups is not necessarily comparable. Information bias is from errors in the assignment of exposure and health outcome status, and confounding.

Bias from confounding by factors that are both predictive of deployment exposures and determinants of respiratory health is a particular weakness of the investigations reviewed previously. Most notably, smoking behaviors, which increase with deployment[21] and are among the strongest known behavioral determinants of respiratory health, are often not known to researchers. Even when smoking data were available, they were not consistently used to adjust for confounding. In addition, changes in smoking behaviors that occur during deployment (eg, initiation of smoking and increasing frequency among current smokers) may be intermediate determinants of postdeployment health conditions.

Errors in the characterization of exposures present a substantial limitation of the current literature. Although conceptually one may be interested in exposure to specific pollutants and their sources, most of the studies reviewed herein use OIF/OEF deployment or deployment to a specific location as a proxy for environmental exposures. Thus, operationally, the indicators or surrogates of the exposures of interest are assessed. The primary impact of this limitation is twofold. These methods almost certainly misclassify the inhalational exposures whose impact is the aim of the assessment. Such measurement error can result in biased associations and corresponding estimates of uncertainty. In general, these biases attenuate the estimates of associations. In addition, it is plausible that changes in behaviors, occupational exposures, or other nonenvironmental exposures coincide with deployment. In addition to smoking, other potential determinants of observed respiratory disease risk include massing of personnel in confined spaces, changes in chronic stress levels, combat-related exposures, and bias from changes in medical attention-seeking behaviors that are both associated with deployment and predictive of subsequent frequency of respiratory and other medical encounters and conditions. With the exception of the case-crossover study by Abraham and Baird,[28] that was limited to assessments of acute associations, none of the studies reviewed previously can discriminate between the impacts of myriad environmental exposures or between the effects of environmental exposures and the impacts of coincidental, nonenvironmental exposures. For those studies that identify an association between deployment and subsequent health conditions, one can only speculate as to the underlying exposure or exposures that are responsible for the observation. As a result of this limitation, there has been no epidemiological evidence to date that specifically implicates any specific exposure (eg, burn pit emissions) as a necessary or sufficient cause of postdeployment chronic respiratory symptoms or disease incidence.

Health outcomes assessed in these studies are also likely to be measured with error. Again, the potential consequence of such errors is an attenuation of observed associations if the errors are not related to exposure status.

A further practical limitation of many of these studies is heterogeneity in the definition of the outcomes. For example, case definitions of COPD or asthma have not been consistently applied from study to study. Although there are, at times, legitimate reasons for such heterogeneity, researchers should endeavor to decrease these differences across various research groups to the extent possible.

The relatively short length of follow-up common to the cohort studies reviewed precludes statistically powerful assessments of associations between deployment-associated exposures and diseases of long latency, such as emphysema, chronic bronchitis, and many cancers. Because military personnel commonly separate from the service within a few years of deployment, assessments that leverage DoD medical data will remain limited in this respect. The VA, in contrast, is in a unique position to establish long-term follow-up of former service members. The representativeness of the VA beneficiary population with respect to the larger population of formerly OIF-/OEF-/Operation New Dawn-deployed US military personnel is imperfect, however, which may impact the generalizability of future assessments set in this population.

Reports of individual cases may be newsworthy, but can also easily distort or distract from the interpretation of available scientific evidence. Such cases are often compelling and deserving of the public's attention and may serve as clues to the scientific community for their hypothesis-generating potential. However, individual case reports alone do not provide strong scientific evidence of an association between deployment-related exposures and the condition. Further studies are needed to explore any potential relationships.

Findings from the Institute of Medicine report *Long-Term Health Consequences of Exposure to Burn Pits in Iraq and Afghanistan*[3] indicate that service in Iraq or Afghanistan—ie, a broader consideration of air pollution than exposure only to burn pit emissions—might be associated with long-term health effects, particularly in highly exposed or susceptible populations that are mainly from the high ambient concentrations of PM from both natural and anthropogenic (including military) sources. Indeed, the epidemiological evidence has not identified specific risk factors for postdeployment chronic respiratory health conditions. In the few studies that have examined specific exposures, no associations were observed. More often, epidemiological studies have used nonspecific indicators of exposure. Such studies, by design, cannot inform questions about specific exposures. The DoD and VA are working to expand the evidence base using more refined methods.

SUMMARY

The epidemiological evidence to date does not support definitive conclusions regarding associations, or an absence thereof, between deployment-associated environmental exposures and chronic respiratory conditions among service members and veterans. Epidemiological methods are being implemented to improve understanding of the potential impacts of deployment on the health of those who have been deployed. It should be noted that no matter how refined the methodology, no epidemiological study can prove that a causal association does not or cannot exist. Rather, an epidemiological study merely provides one data point: that an association of a given magnitude was or was not observed. This piece of evidence must then be taken together with evidence from all other sources, put in the context of mission requirements, and used to inform military policy and public health practice. Completely avoiding exposure to airborne hazards in the deployed environment is not feasible. However, steps can be taken to maximize postdeployment respiratory health. As suggested by the National Research Council Committee that reviewed the DoD's report titled *Enhanced Particulate Matter Surveillance Program*,[15,29] exposures should be minimized if and when possible; emissions sources (eg, burn pits and generator banks) can be located downwind from areas of personnel locations, and burning of waste, if necessary, should be conducted when meteorological conditions support dispersion of emissions. Perhaps, most importantly, antismoking and smoking cessation programs should focus on deploying and deployed personnel. Finally, the health and research community serving military personnel and veterans would be well served to extend its research focus beyond burn pits when evaluating sources, exposures, and health effects. Both the DoD and VA will no doubt continue to prioritize the identification and care of current and former military personnel who fall ill. Future research and public health efforts should focus on minimizing the known behavioral determinants of respiratory health conditions (eg, smoking among deployed personnel), mitigate exposures to environmental hazards and their sources, and identify individual-level determinants of warfighter and veteran susceptibility to, and resiliency against, austere and inhospitable environmental conditions.

REFERENCES

1. Morris MJ, Zacher LL, Jackson DA. Investigating the respiratory health of deployed military personnel. *Mil Med.* 2011;176:1157–1161.

2. Baird C. The basis for and uses of environmental sampling to assess health risk in deployed settings. *Mil Med.* 2011;176(suppl 7):84–90.

3. Institute of Medicine of the National Academies. *Long-Term Health Consequences of Exposure to Burn Pits in Iraq and Afghanistan.* Washington, DC: The National Academies Press; 2011:1–9, 31–44, 117–129.

4. Smith B, Wong CA, Smith TC, et al. Newly reported respiratory symptoms and conditions among military personnel deployed to Iraq and Afghanistan: a prospective population-based study. *Am J Epidemiol.* 2009;170:1433–1442.

5. Abraham JH, DeBakey SF, Reid L, et al. Does deployment to Iraq and Afghanistan affect respiratory health of US military personnel? *J Occup Environ Med.* 2012;54:740–745.

6. Rose C, Abraham J, Harkins D, et al. Overview and recommendations for medical screening and diagnostic evaluation for postdeployment lung disease in returning US warfighters. *J Occup Environ Med.* 2012;54:746–751.

7. Quigley KS, McAndrew LM, Almeida L, et al. Prevalence of environmental and other military exposure concerns in Operation Enduring Freedom and Operation Iraqi Freedom veterans. *J Occup Environ Med.* 2012;54:659–664.

8. Helmer DA, Rossignol M, Blatt M, et al. Health and exposure concerns of veterans deployed to Iraq and Afghanistan. *J Occup Environ Med.* 2007;49:475–480.

9. Brown KW, Bouhamra W, Lamoureux DP, et al. Characterization of particulate matter for three sites in Kuwait. *J Air Waste Manag Assoc.* 2008;58:994–1003.

10. Engelbrecht JP, McDonald EV, Gillies JA, et al. Characterizing mineral dusts and other aerosols from the Middle East—part 1: ambient sampling. *Inhal Toxicol.* 2009;21:297–326.

11. Davidson CI, Phalen RF, Solomon PA. Airborne particulate matter and human health: a review. *Aerosol Sci Technol.* 2005;39:737–749.

12. Pope CA 3rd. Epidemiology of fine particulate air pollution and human health: biologic mechanisms and who's at risk? *Environ Health Perspect.* 2000;108(suppl 4):713–723.

13. Pope CA 3rd, Dockery DW. Health effects of fine particulate air pollution: lines that connect. *J Air Waste Manag Assoc.* 2006;56:709–742.

14. Weese CB, Abraham JH. Potential health implications associated with particulate matter exposure in southwest Asia. *Inhal Toxicol.* 2009;21:291–296.

15. Engelbrecht JP, McDonald EV, Gillies JA, Gertler AW. Final report. *Department of Defense Enhanced Particulate Matter Surveillance Program (EPMSP).* Reno, NV: Desert Research Institute; 2008. Contract W9124R-05-C-0135/SUBCLIN 000101-ACRN-AB.

16. Smith B, Wong CA, Boyko EJ, et al. The effects of exposure to documented open-air burn pits on respiratory health among deployers of the Millennium Cohort Study. *J Occup Environ Med.* 2012;54:708–716.

17. Taylor G, Rush V, Deck A, Vietas JA. *Screening Health Risk Assessment: Burn Pit Exposures Balad Air Base, Iraq and Addendum Report.* Aberdeen Proving Ground, MD: Army Center for Health Promotion and Preventive Medicine; 2008. Technical Report 47-MA-08PV-08.

18. US Department of Defense. *Use of Open-Air Burn Pits in Contingency Operations.* Washington, DC: DoD; 2011. DoD Instruction 4715.19.

19. Armed Forces Health Surveillance Center. Costs of war: excess health care burdens during the wars in Afghanistan and Iraq (relative to the health care experience pre-war). *MSMR.* 2012;19:2–10.

20. Greenland S, Robins JM. Identifiability, exchangeability, and epidemiological confounding. *Int J Epidemiol.* 1986;15:413–419.

21. Sanders JW, Putnam SD, Frankart C, et al. Impact of illness and non-combat injury during Operations Iraqi Freedom and Enduring Freedom (Afghanistan). *Am J Trop Med Hyg.* 2005;73:713–719.

22. Roop SA, Niven AS, Calvin BE, et al. The prevalence and impact of respiratory symptoms in asthmatics and non-asthmatics during deployment. *Mil Med.* 2007;172:1264–1269.

23. Armed Forces Health Surveillance Center. *Epidemiological Studies of Health Outcomes Among Troops Deployed to Burn Pit Sites.* Silver Spring, MD: Naval Health Research Center/The U.S. Army Public Health Command (Provisional); 2010.

24. Leardman CA, Smith B, Smith TC, et al. Smallpox vaccination: comparison of self-reported and electronic vaccine records in the Millennium Cohort Study. *Hum Vaccin.* 2007;3:245–251.

25. Smith B, Chu LK, Smith TC, et al. Challenges of self-reported medical conditions and electronic medical records among members of a large military cohort. *BMC Med Res Methodol.* 2008;8:37.

26. Szema AM, Peters MC, Weissinger KM, Gagliano CA, Chen JJ. New-onset asthma among soldiers serving in Iraq and Afghanistan. *Allergy Asthma Proc.* 2010;31:67–71.

27. Szema AM, Salihi W, Savary K, Chen JJ. Respiratory symptoms necessitating spirometry among soldiers with Iraq/Afghanistan war lung injury. *J Occup Environ Med.* 2011;53:961–965.

28. Abraham JH, Baird CP. A case-crossover study of ambient particulate matter and cardiovascular and respiratory medical encounters among US military personnel deployed to southwest Asia. *J Occup Environ Med.* 2012;54:733–739.

29. National Research Council. *Review of the Department of Defense Enhanced Particulate Matter Surveillance Program Report.* Washington, DC: The National Academies Press; 2010:10–11, 51.

Chapter 7

DISCUSSION SUMMARY: DEFINING HEALTH OUTCOMES IN EPIDEMIOLOGICAL INVESTIGATIONS OF POPULATIONS DEPLOYED IN SUPPORT OF OPERATION IRAQI FREEDOM AND OPERATION ENDURING FREEDOM

JOSEPH H. ABRAHAM, SCD*

Epidemiologist, Environmental Medicine Program, Occupational and Environmental Medicine Portfolio, Army Institute of Public Health, US Army Public Health Command, 5158 Blackhawk Road, Aberdeen Proving Ground, Maryland 21010-5403

INTRODUCTION

Identifying potential health implications associated with environmental conditions experienced during military deployment in support of Operation Enduring Freedom, Operation Iraqi Freedom, and Operation New Dawn is an ongoing effort of the US Department of Defense (DoD) and the US Department of Veterans Affairs (VA) researchers. Epidemiology is a primary tool used in this endeavor.[1] Epidemiology is "the study of the distribution and determinants of health-related states or events in specified populations, and the application of this study to control health problems."[2] Epidemiological research often involves assessing the relationship between an event or trait (an exposure) and another event or trait (an outcome). Defining and ascertaining information on an outcome are primary tasks in the design and conduct of epidemiological studies. The outcome of an epidemiological study is a broad term representing a defined disease, state of health, or health-related event. Measurement and classification of health outcomes in epidemiological studies are an exercise in balance: minimizing errors and maximizing efficiency. Evaluating outcomes used in epidemiological assessments of airborne hazards was the primary focus of a work group at the VA/DoD Airborne Hazards Symposium held in August 2012. The work group identified limitations in current data systems (Exhibit 7-1), then focused on the question of whether the DoD and VA could, and should, standardize outcome definitions.

This chapter expands on the workshop discussion by reviewing concepts and consequences of outcome definitions used in epidemiological investigations of the health effects of airborne hazards among deployed and formerly deployed military personnel and veterans. The first section introduces concepts that could be helpful in formulating outcome definitions for use in epidemiological studies, as well as in evaluating a study's quality vis-à-vis outcome assessment. Consequences of operational outcome definitions on both individual study results and on inferences to be drawn from the body of epidemiological evidence regarding airborne hazards health effects are also discussed. The second section reviews outcome definitions used in selected published research studies relevant to the epidemiology of health effects potentially associated with airborne hazards in the deployment environment. Improving the state of science with respect to outcome definitions, including a discussion of the pros and cons of standardizing outcome definitions across studies being conducted by VA and DoD researchers, is the topic of the third section.

EXHIBIT 7-1

LIMITATIONS IN CURRENT DATA COLLECTION SYSTEMS IDENTIFIED DURING THE WORKSHOP

- Lack of integration between medical record systems (eg, AHLTA,* JMeWs†) and administrative medical encounter databases (eg, DMSS‡)
- Misclassification of health conditions and missing data
- Inaccuracy of health outcome data
- Subjective nature of health outcome assignment
- Imperfect or incomplete models of disease etiology
- Lack of clinical corroboration of symptom outcomes

*The Armed Forces Health Longitudinal Technology Application (AHLTA) is the electronic medical record system used by US Department of Defense medical providers.
†The Joint Medical Workstation (JMeWS) is the theater medical surveillance system that integrates medical information from separate health data collection systems for the US Army, Navy, Air Force, and Marine Corps.
‡The Defense Medical Surveillance System (DMSS) is the central repository of medical surveillance data for the US Armed Forces.

CONCEPTS OF HEALTH OUTCOME DEFINITION FOR EPIDEMIOLOGICAL STUDIES

Epidemiological study outcomes must be defined in advance of the conduct of the study, and they should be clear, specific, and measurable. These outcomes are often based on a combination of signs and symptoms, physical examinations, pathology, and diagnostic test results. Typically, outcome data consist of physical measurements, laboratory results, responses to self-administered questionnaires or interview questions, information garnered from medical record reviews, or diagnostic codes abstracted from administrative databases.

In the textbook *Essentials of Epidemiology in Public Health* by Aschengrau and Seage,[3] they suggest that "it is best to use all available evidence to define with as much accuracy as possible the true cases of disease." An accurate measurement is one that is close to the true value. From a theoretical viewpoint, maximizing the accuracy of an outcome definition should be a primary objective because inaccurate outcome assessment can induce bias in both estimates of measures of association (eg, relative risks) and estimates of the precision of those measures (eg, confidence intervals). Practically speaking, however, the salient part of Aschengrau and Seage's phrase *with as much accuracy as possible* is *as possible*. Conducting gold standard tests in epidemiological studies, if such tests exist, may not be feasible based on logistical, technical, and ethical reasons.

For practical purposes, a number of elements (Exhibit 7-2) must be *jointly* considered in defining a health outcome for an epidemiological study. The researcher and those wishing to evaluate an epidemiological study must consider what is required of the measurement in judging its appropriateness. True health outcome status is often ambiguously defined and poorly measured in the context of an epidemiological study.

EXHIBIT 7-2

FEATURES TO CONSIDER IN DEFINING A HEALTH OUTCOME FOR USE IN AN EPIDEMIOLOGICAL STUDY

- Study hypothesis
- Objectives of the study
- Conceptually relevant health condition given a mechanistic, biological, or social model
- Accuracy of the outcome measurement:
  - Probability and magnitude of misclassification or measurement error
  - Consequences of misclassification or measurement error on estimated measures of association
  - Previous validation of the measurement
- Feasibility:
  - Logistical constraints
  - Available resources
  - Ethical considerations
  - Time constraints
- Magnitude of the hypothesized association
- Incidence versus prevalence as the appropriate metric of outcome frequency

Validity

Like all epidemiological investigations, epidemiological assessments of deployed and formerly deployed military personnel are susceptible to bias. In epidemiology, bias is defined as the difference between an expected estimate (eg, the average value of association estimates over many hypothetical study repetitions) and the true value, or the processes leading to such deviation.[4] Bias arises from systematic errors in the selection of study participants, confounding of exposure–outcome relationships, and errors in the ascertainment (measurement) of exposures and outcomes. Both measures of association and measures of variability can be biased. In the absence of bias, an epidemiological study is valid. On average, valid studies will produce an estimate of the true underlying association being assessed.

Sensitivity, Specificity, and Misclassification

In epidemiology, outcomes are often classified dichotomously (ie, individuals either have the outcome or they do not have the outcome). Such binary outcome measures are susceptible to two types of systematic error: (1) outcome-free individuals incorrectly classified as having the outcome (false positives); and (2) individuals having the outcome, but incorrectly classified as being free of it (false negatives). Two statistical measures of a binary classification function—sensitivity and specificity—correspond to these two types of errors in assessments of an outcome in epidemiological studies.[5] For example, consider a health condition of interest (D), for which individuals can have a disease (D+) or not (D–). Consider an epidemiological classification function of the disease status (O) that divides individuals into two groups: (1) positive for the outcome (O+) or (2) negative for the outcome (O–). Consider a study assessing the risk of developing asthma (D) and defined as self-report of a physician's diagnosis of asthma (O).

Sensitivity refers to the proportion of individuals with the disease (D+) who are correctly identified as having the outcome (O+); it is the probability of individuals being classified as having the outcome among those who truly have it (Sensitivity = Prob[O+|D+]). An outcome metric with high sensitivity has minimal false negatives. In the asthma example, it is the percentage of individuals with asthma who are correctly identified as having asthma and are considered as having asthma for the purpose of the study. Sensitivity less than 100% implies that a proportion of individuals with asthma (1 – Sensitivity) will be incorrectly classified as not having asthma in the study (false-negative proportion).

Specificity refers to the proportion of those who are truly free of the disease (D–) and are correctly identified as negative for the outcome (O–). It is the probability of individuals being classified as not having the outcome among those who truly do not have it (Specificity = Prob[O–|D–]). An outcome metric with high specificity has minimal false positives. In the asthma example, it is the percentage of individuals who do not have asthma who are correctly identified as nonasthmatic. Specificity less than 100% implies that a proportion of individuals who are free of asthma (1 – Specificity) will be incorrectly classified as having asthma in the study (false-positive proportion).

For any given classification function of disease status, there is usually a trade-off between sensitivity and specificity. For example, increasing the proportion of asthmatic individuals correctly classified as asthmatic results in a decrease in the proportion of nonasthmatic individuals correctly classified as nonasthmatic.

Error in disease classification of a study outcome is referred to as *outcome misclassification*. The consequences of outcome misclassification on study results are two-fold: (1) bias in the observed measures of association and (2) bias in the estimates of the variance of the observed measures of association (eg, confidence intervals). The magnitude of bias from outcome misclassification depends on the sensitivity, specificity, outcome prevalence, and the magnitude of the true association. Some epidemiologists[6,7] have argued that specificity is more important in evaluating bias in relative risks resulting from misclassified health outcome data. However, sensitivity is also important, and bias in relative risk is actually dependent on a third property of a classification function of disease status: the positive predictive value (or PPV). The PPV = Prob[D+|O+], which, in contrast to sensitivity and specificity, is dependent on the prevalence of the disease in the population being assessed.[8]

Note that estimating sensitivity, specificity, and the PPV all require knowledge of true disease status (although for the latter, true disease status must be known only among the subgroup of participants who are deemed positive by the classification function O+). Although it is preferable, in many cases it is not possible to obtain estimates of sensitivity, specificity, and PPV in a population of interest, primarily because information on true outcome status is unobtainable. Thus, critical readers of epidemiological studies are most often not privy to this validation data. Nonetheless, one can use the concepts of sensitivity, specificity, and PPV as heuristics to better understand the potential strengths and weaknesses of an outcome metric with respect to validity in the context of a given epidemiological study.

If the probability of misclassifying a study subject's outcome is independent of exposure status, the classification error is referred to as *nondifferential* or *random* outcome misclassification. In contrast, differential (nonrandom) outcome misclassification occurs when the probability of incorrectly assigning outcome status is *not* independent of exposure status. A paradigmatic example of differential misclassification occurs in case-control and retrospective studies when there is a greater level of accuracy in reporting outcome status among exposed study participants relative to unexposed subjects. A recall bias may occur because individuals who have the health condition under study may have more thoroughly considered their exposure history in an attempt to answer the question, "Why me?" The bias of observed estimates of association from differential misclassification can generate either overestimates or underestimates of the true association. The direction of bias of observed estimates of association from nondifferential misclassification is discussed herein. As a general rule, outcome assessment should be conducted in such a manner that is comparable with all exposure levels (ie, independent of exposure). Often, this maxim is implemented by "blinding" those who are responsible for outcome assignment to the exposure status of the study participants, especially when the outcome measure is subjective in nature.

Under certain circumstances, the bias from outcome misclassification is theoretically predictable.[9,10] If the misclassification of a dichotomous outcome is exactly nondifferential, and, additionally

- the misclassification error is independent of errors in other variables in the analysis,
- there is no interaction between the misclassification and other sources of bias (eg, selection bias, confounding), and
- there is no random sampling variability,

then nondifferential outcome misclassification will result in a bias of measures of association toward the null value for the association (eg, toward 1 for the relative risk). Technically, the direction of the bias from nondifferential misclassification refers to the average error across hypothetical study repetitions, (ie, ignoring random variability in the misclassification). Because these conditions are rarely met in practice, nondifferential outcome misclassification does not always lead to an underestimation of measures of association. In practice, an observed measure of association estimated in the presence of nondifferential misclassification is a joint function of the misclassification error, the true association, other sources of bias, and random sampling variability.

Bias in estimated measures of association from outcome misclassification is arguably less of an issue in assessing the strong effects of environmental exposures. However, as epidemiologists attempt to evaluate associations of increasingly small magnitude, the importance of preventing or decreasing classification errors increases.[11]

Repeatability

Repeatability is important in the assessments of outcomes that are not expected to change over time (eg, outcomes for chronic diseases). Assessing repeatability may be useful in characterizing an outcome metric in the absence of a gold standard (diagnostic) test wherein one can compare an epidemiological outcome indicator. Therefore, an outcome that is repeatable is not necessarily valid. The repeatability of an outcome assessment, also known as test-retest reliability or stability, is a joint function of intrasubject variability, interobserver variability, and intraobserver variability. An outcome measure with no variability arising from these sources is repeatable. If, however, an outcome measure is random in nature (ie, independent of exposure status), its departure from perfect repeatability will result in an attenuation of relative measures of association.

Incidence, Prevalence, and Mortality

In planning a study, epidemiologists are often faced with a choice regarding whether to assess incidence or prevalence of the outcome, and, at times, they additionally consider whether or not to assess mortality as the outcome of interest. Generally speaking, incidence measures of outcome are more useful in investigating outcome etiology, as both prevalence and mortality can be influenced by determinants of outcome duration and survival in addition to causes of the outcome.[12] This limitation must be considered against the logistical efficiency gained by assessing prevalence or mortality as outcomes and the fact that—depending on the circumstance—prevalence and mortality may be able to be measured with less error, relative to the corresponding measure of incidence.

Objective Versus Subjective Outcome Measurements

In evaluating outcome assessment in epidemiological studies, epidemiologists often distinguish between assessments that are objective in nature and those that are subjective in nature. Objective assessments are often preferred for the following reasons, both of which are plausible, but neither of which is necessarily true: (1) objective measures are less susceptible to misclassification; and (2) misclassification of objective measures, compared with that of subjective measures, is less likely to be influenced by the exposure status of the study subjects. For example, survey respondents may self-report their health differently, depending on their understanding of the survey question, other questions asked in the survey, their health-related aspirations and expectations, their access to and use of health care, as well as their social and socioeconomic context. All of these may be associated with the exposure under study. In addition, respondents' answers may be directly influenced by their exposure status.

In many instances, however, subjective outcome assessment measures are preferred, often for their logistical efficiency. In many contexts, subjective measures have been validated to be strong predictors of logistically more complex objective outcome measures. Moreover, it is often *perceived* health that drives the use of healthcare resources. Finally, it is worth reiterating that objective assessments are not immune to measurement error, both differential and nondifferential.

Balancing Advantages With Costs

As alluded to earlier, it is often not feasible to implement an ideal outcome assessment (eg, a diagnostic evaluation with perfect sensitivity, specificity, and reliability) in the context of a large-scale epidemiological study. A more practical strategy to outcome assessment may include the use of gold standard outcome assessments in a subset of the larger study population. This strategy has the dual advantages of providing evidence of the degree to which the less resource-intensive outcome assessment methodology misclassifies true outcome status and providing information to facilitate analytic techniques to correct for the bias induced by the misclassification. Another strategy for balancing advantages with costs is to use a combination of outcome indicators (eg, signs and symptoms), examination results, medication use, and test results to increase the accuracy of outcome measurement.[3]

Evaluating Health Outcome Measurement

Consider the following three questions when critiquing a study's outcome assessment:

1. What is the conceptual outcome (ie, the outcome of true interest to the researchers)?
2. What is the operational outcome definition (ie, how the researchers define and ascertain information on the outcome)?
3. What impact does any discrepancy between the conceptual outcome and the operational outcome definition have on the estimates of association and the inference that can be drawn from the study?

The first question relates to the conceptually relevant outcome. The second question relates to the operational definition of the outcome as it is implemented in the study. The third question invites the individual evaluating the study to consider the impact of the outcome definition on internal validity (from bias) and external validity (limitations regarding generalizability).

Consider the following research question: Does exposure to particulate matter (PM) air pollution increase the risk of asthma (outcome) among deployed military personnel? The outcome (asthma) is readily understood by the reader. Asthma is a chronic inflammatory disorder of

EXHIBIT 7-3

EXAMPLES OF ASTHMA* DEFINITIONS USED IN EPIDEMIOLOGICAL STUDIES

- A postbronchodilator response of 12% improvement in either FEV_1 or FVC relative to baseline spirometry
- Appearance of ICD-9 diagnosis code 493 in a medical record
- Reported presence of persistent respiratory symptoms (cough, wheezing)
- Spirometric evidence of airway obstruction
- A positive answer to the question, "Do you have asthma?"
- A positive answer to the question, "Has a doctor ever told you that you have asthma?"
- Self-report of the presence of asthma symptoms (eg, recurrent cough and wheeze, apart from upper respiratory illness)
- Identified use of asthma-control medications
- Reported improvement of asthma symptoms with use of asthma-control medications
- Combinations of the above definitions

*According to the National Heart, Lung, and Blood Institute and the National Asthma Education and Prevention Program, asthma is defined as a chronic inflammatory disorder of the airways with generally reversible airflow obstruction and airway hyperresponsiveness causing episodic respiratory symptoms.
FEV_1: forced expiratory volume in 1 second; FVC: forced vital capacity; ICD-9: *International Classification of Diseases*, Ninth Revision
Data source: National Asthma Education and Prevention Program, NHLBI, National Institutes of Health. *Asthma Expert Panel Report 3. Guidelines for the Diagnosis and Management of Asthma.* Bethesda, MD: National Institutes of Health; 2007. NIH Publication 08-5846.

the airways with generally reversible airflow obstruction and airway hyperresponsiveness causing episodic respiratory symptoms.[13] However, asthma is variously defined for use in epidemiological studies. Although partially a reflection of the fact that asthma is a heterogeneous outcome, the number of definitions is also an indication of the trade-offs inherent in using different approaches to identify asthma as a health outcome (Exhibit 7-3).[14] A Danish study comparing three of these operational definitions (participant report of doctor diagnoses of asthma, hospitalization diagnosis codes for asthma, and use of antiasthmatic medication) observed kappa statistics in the range of 0.21–0.38, indicating only fair agreement.[15,16] One can think of these, and other, operational definitions as outcome metrics. They are *indicators* of true, underlying asthma. There is no one correct outcome metric, because each has its advantages and disadvantages in the setting of a given epidemiological study. Some may be more accurate than others, some more specific, some more sensitive, and some more efficient to implement.

HEALTH OUTCOMES USED IN DEPLOYMENT EPIDEMIOLOGY

This section provides a summary and discussion of the health outcomes used in a select group of six recently published articles on the topic of epidemiological assessments of health effects of airborne hazards in the deployment environment. The appropriateness of each study's health outcome was evaluated by considering the following:

- the conceptually relevant health condition;
- logistical constraints;
- previous validation of the measurement;
- probability and magnitude of misclassification;
- consequences of misclassification on estimated measures of association; and
- scientific context of the study, including standardization with outcome definitions and methods used in previous work.

Selected Studies

This section reviews the health outcomes of the six major studies.

Study 1

Smith B, Wong CA, Smith TC, et al. Newly reported respiratory symptoms and conditions among military personnel deployed to Iraq and Afghanistan: a prospective population-based study. Am J Epidemiol. *2009;170:1433–1442.*

The Millennium Cohort Study (MCS), the largest DoD prospective cohort study ever conducted, has enrolled more than 150,000 military personnel.[17] Launched in 2001, prior to the September 11 terrorist attacks, the MCS was designed to investigate the effects of military service, specifically deployment-related exposures, on long-term health.[18] The study relies on mailed and web-based questionnaires to ascertain self-reported medical conditions.

In 2009, Smith et al published an assessment of respiratory symptoms and conditions among MCS participants who deployed to Iraq and Afghanistan.[19] The objective of the study was to assess whether respiratory symptoms and conditions were associated with deployment among MCS participants. The conceptually relevant health conditions were incident respiratory symptoms, incident asthma, and incident chronic bronchitis or emphysema (ie, chronic obstructive pulmonary disease or COPD). To ascertain disease status at baseline, participants were asked, "Has your doctor or other health professional ever told you that you have any of the following conditions?" Asthma, chronic bronchitis, and emphysema were listed as possible responses, and the question was repeated on annual follow-up assessments. To identify respiratory symptoms at baseline, participants were asked, "During the last 12 months, have you had persistent or recurring problems with any of the following?" Cough and shortness of breath were offered as possible responses. On follow-up assessments, participants were asked the same questions, but with the timeframe extended from "during the last 12 months" to "in the last 3 years." The study outcomes were defined as a positive endorsement regarding the corresponding symptom or condition on a follow-up assessment without such indication on the baseline questionnaire.[19]

As with many survey-based research initiatives, this study relies heavily on participants' ability to correctly recall their medical history. In this study, it is possible that respondents' errors in recall of their health conditions are likely, but independent of their deployment status (ie, nondifferential misclassification). If, however, previously deployed MCS participants more accurately recall incidence of respiratory symptoms relative to their nondeployed peers, the resulting differential misclassification would result in an upward bias of the association between deployment and respiratory symptoms.

In 2008, MCS researchers published an article identifying some of the challenges of using self-reported medical conditions in the conduct of epidemiological studies.[20] After considering using the kappa statistic and measurements of sensitivity and specificity to evaluate agreement between self-reported and diagnostic codes in the medical record, the authors decided to use measures of positive and negative agreement.[21] In comparisons of self-report of medical conditions to electronic medical record data, they observed "near-perfect negative agreement and moderate positive agreement" for 38 diagnoses of "less-prevalent conditions."[20,21] Positive agreement (percentage) among self-reported diagnoses for asthma, emphysema, and chronic bronchitis was 42.0%, 2.7%, and 12.9%, respectively; negative agreement among self-reported diagnoses for asthma, emphysema, and chronic bronchitis was 97.1%, 99.6%, and 96.7%, respectively. The high negative agreement percentages indicate that self-report of health conditions may be an effective means of ruling out a history of a particular condition—a finding similar to a classification scheme with high specificity and low false-positive proportion. However, the low positive-agreement percentages suggest that the self-reporting had low sensitivity and a high proportion of false negatives. In their discussion, the authors conclude that their results speak to the importance of using multiple data sources, when possible, to assess health outcomes.

Study 2

Szema AM, Peters MC, Weissinger KM, et al. New-onset asthma among soldiers serving in Iraq and Afghanistan. Allergy Asthma Proc. *2010;31:67–71.*

In 2010, researchers at the Northport Veterans Affairs Medical Center (VAMC) in Long Island, New York, published a study using medical record data.[22] The objective of the study was to assess whether former US military personnel with a history of deployment to Iraq or Afghanistan have higher risk of asthma compared with veterans who did not deploy to these regions. The conceptually relevant health condition was incidence of asthma among US military veterans. This contrasts with the outcome metric used to evaluate the hypothesis: the appearance of an *International Classification of Diseases*, Ninth Revision (ICD-9), diagnostic code for asthma (ICD-9 code 493) in a veteran's VAMC medical record. The authors enumerated the three clinical guidelines used by the VAMC clinic to diagnose asthma: (1) evidence of recurrent episodes of respiratory symptoms (cough, wheezing, dyspnea, and exercise-induced shortness of breath), (2) spirometric evidence of airway obstruction, and (3) improvement of symptoms after administration of a bronchodilator. These guidelines differ from those of the National Institutes of Health and the National Heart, Lung, and Blood Institute (NHLBI), which recommend that an asthma diagnosis be based on a combination of clinical symptoms consistent with airway obstruction, spirometric evidence of reversible airway obstruction (rather than control of symptoms), and exclusion of alternative diagnoses.[23] Consistent with the NHLBI criteria for diagnosis of asthma, the authors presented spirometric results, including data on reversibility of airway obstruction (and not improvement of symptoms) after bronchodilator administration.

The authors identified 290 veterans with asthma for inclusion in the study. Although the VAMC clinic guidelines for asthma diagnosis include spirometry, lung function data were presented for only 45 patients (approximately 16% of the veterans identified as having asthma based on the presence of an asthma diagnosis code in their medical record). The authors did not explain why lung function data were only available for such a small subset of subjects in the study, nor did they deliberate on the representativeness of the spirometry results they did obtain. They did note that spirometric measurements were obtained while patients were taking medication to control their asthma.

In the discussion, the authors identify reliance on ICD-9 diagnosis codes as a limitation of the study, although they do not discuss the potential impact of the use of ICD-9 codes on the study results. They do suggest that more sensitive outcome measures—including methacholine challenge, cardiopulmonary exercise testing, impulse oscillometry, exhaled breath condensate nitric oxide levels, and skin prick testing for aeroallergens—may be helpful, but did not elaborate on the point. These outcomes may have better sensitivity in identification of pulmonary (and other) impairments, relative to outcomes defined on the presence of ICD-9 diagnostic codes in medical records.

The authors identify a lack of baseline (predeployment) spirometry measurements as a limitation of the study. The utility of longitudinal assessments of lung function among military personnel is currently a matter of debate,[24] and studies of longitudinal changes may inform this discussion. Longitudinal changes in lung function parameters that incorporate predeployment assessments may serve as potentially sensitive markers of exposure to deployment-associated airborne hazards. No longitudinal assessments of lung function that incorporate baseline testing among military personnel who deploy to southwest Asia have been published. Without baseline spirometry, evaluations of lung function often rely on comparisons of lung function among those with a history of deployment to a nondeployed reference population that may not be comparable with the exposed population. As performed in this study, such comparisons often use general population average lung function values. Similarly, lung function parameters can be expressed as a percentage of gender-, age-, and race-specific predicted values[25] and then used in conjunction with a cut-point (eg, 80% of predicted values) to indicate impaired lung function. The sensitivity and specificity of these methods depend on the definition of the cut-point. They are generally less sensitive, relative to measures of longitudinal change in pulmonary function.

The ICD-9 code-based outcome assessed in the study is subject to several sources of misclassification. Misdiagnosis of asthma because of reliance on evidence of symptom control after bronchodilator use as specified by the diagnostic criteria used by the VAMC clinic—rather than spirometric evidence of reversibility of airway obstruction—is possible (although likely not substantial), especially considering the authors reported evidence of reversibility (not control of symptoms) in their results. The discrepancy between the number of asthma outcomes identified and the number of patients with lung function data are potential evidence of a larger problem: the asthma diagnoses, as evidenced by the appearance of asthma ICD-9 codes in the medical records, may not have been based on functional parameters (ie, indicators of airway obstruction) assessed by spirometry, despite the diagnosis guidelines used by Northport VAMC.

The probability of outcome misclassification may not be independent of exposure if deployment itself was an indication for referral in the mind of the diagnosing physician. This differential misclassification would result in an upward bias of estimated odds ratios.

Study 3

Szema AM, Salihi W, Savary K, Chen JJ. Respiratory symptoms necessitating spirometry among soldiers with Iraq/Afghanistan war lung injury. J Occup Environ Med. *2011;53:961–965.*

The same researchers at the Northport VAMC conducted a follow-on study to evaluate the hypothesis that US military veterans with a history of deployment to Iraq and Afghanistan have higher rates of respiratory symptoms compared with veterans who had not deployed to those regions.[26] The conceptually relevant health condition is the incidence of persistent respiratory symptoms that indicate possible lung injury or pulmonary disease. To operationalize the conceptual outcome, the authors reviewed the Northport VAMC patient records to identify individuals referred for spirometric evaluation. The authors also presented lung function parameters assessed by spirometry, although these later data were not used to classify study subjects with respect to health outcome.

The authors focused on asthma as a condition potentially underlying respiratory symptoms. In this study, the indication for referral for spirometry was the presence of clinical symptoms consistent with a diagnosis of asthma. The set of qualifying symptoms was not specified.

In their discussion, the authors conflate evidence of clinical symptoms indicating referral for spirometry with the presence of pulmonary disease or injury; this is an unsupported inference rather than an actual outcome misclassification. However, if the conceptual outcome of interest was lung injury or disease, rather than respiratory symptoms, the outcome misclassification error is greatly exacerbated, primarily from false positives. Ambiguity in the relevant conceptual outcome definition may be fostered by the following three factors:

1. The VAMC physicians referring patients for spirometry must *specify the relevant symptoms* prior to the pulmonary function testing.
2. The VAMC physicians referring patients for spirometry must *specify a diagnosis* prior to the pulmonary function testing.
3. The clinical guidelines used by VAMC clinicians to diagnose asthma rely on clinical symptoms, rather than functional (lung function) parameters, to assess reversibility of airway obstruction.

Although they discuss the clinical guidelines for a diagnosis of asthma, the authors do not elucidate the set of diagnoses given to patients by the referring physician, nor do they provide the reader with an analysis of the diagnoses made following the spirometric assessments.

The study presents an interesting opportunity to contrast the findings of analyses drawn on medical records data with the assessments of functional parameters. The conclusions of the study, based on a higher proportion of previously deployed veterans presenting with respiratory symptoms and being referred for spirometric evaluations relative to veterans without a history of deployment, contrasts with the spirometric findings presented. The average forced expiratory volume in 1 second and the forced vital capacity parameters were higher among veterans with a history of deployment relative to veterans who had not deployed to Iraq or Afghanistan. The mean forced expiratory volume in 1 second and the forced vital capacity ratios between the two groups were not statistically different.

The authors did not report any validation of the diagnostic code-based outcome, either by evaluating faithfulness to the clinics' diagnostic guidelines or other guidelines that combine clinical assessment of symptoms with measurements of lung function and exclusion of other diagnoses.

Findings of the study are likely biased because the outcome classification (referral for spirometry) was not independent of the exposure of interest (deployment to Iraq or Afghanistan). Veterans with a history of deployment were sourced from VA clinics catering specifically to veterans of Operation Iraqi Freedom and Operation Enduring Freedom, and the referring physicians were (appropriately, from a clinical standpoint) aware of the exposure status of their patients. The authors' coining of the term "Iraq/Afghanistan War Lung Injury" to refer to the pulmonary complaints evaluated in the study may be an inadvertent allusion to this source of bias; the exposure is implicit in the definition of the outcome. The authors did not report their having evaluated the degree to which the history of deployment was an indication for referral for lung function testing, nor did they discuss the impact of this potential source of bias.

The outcome for the study was defined using an easily accessible, preexisting database. Correspondingly, the primary advantage of the outcome metric is logistical efficiency. Additional strengths include the fact that the administrative diagnostic codes culled from the patient record database correspond to both prespecified diagnostic criteria and clinically assessed functional parameters (ie, lung function); however, these strengths are more theoretical in nature than realized.

In 2012, researchers at the US Army Public Health Command (including the author) published three original research papers in the *Journal of Occupational and Environmental Medicine.*[27–29] All three evaluations leveraged diagnostic code data obtained from military medical records systems.

Study 4

Abraham JH, Baird CP. A case-crossover study of ambient particulate matter and cardiovascular and respiratory medical encounters among US military personnel deployed to southwest Asia. J Occup Environ Med. *2012;54:733–739.*

The aim of this study[27] was to evaluate the hypothesis that acute PM exposure precipitates the incidence of acute cardiovascular or respiratory events such as myocardial infarctions or severe asthma attacks. Both the occurrence and timing of the health event with respect to exposure were of interest in evaluating the hypothesis. The conceptually relevant health condition is the incidence of a serious cardiovascular or respiratory health event. This contrasts with the outcome metric used: the appearance of any one of a set of ICD-9 diagnostic codes in either of two medical record databases (the Joint Medical Workstation, and the Transportation Command Regulating and Command & Control Evacuation System). Case status was defined as having any one of the qualifying cardiovascular (ICD-9 diagnosis codes 390–459, Diseases of the Circulatory System) or respiratory (ICD-9 diagnosis codes 460–519, Diseases of the Respiratory System) outcomes. The date of the medical encounter was defined as the incidence of the health event. The case definition was not validated as part of this study, nor has it been validated in other studies of military personnel.

The outcome assessed in this study is subject to several sources of misclassification. Health events that otherwise may have qualified for inclusion in the study may not have appeared in the medical records obtained, either because personnel did not seek medical attention or because medical encounters were not entered into the electronic medical record. These situations result in false negatives. Case status was defined to *cast a wide net* to increase case ascertainment (ie, to increase sensitivity and decrease the number of false negatives). However, some of the diagnostic codes may indicate encounters for conditions that are not biologically relevant; any cases with these codes could be considered false positives. Misclassification of the health event's *timing* is also likely, because the date of the medical encounter may not have been the date of incidence of the conceptually relevant health condition.

The probability of outcome misclassification resulting from both design choices and imperfect capture of otherwise qualifying medical events was likely independent of exposure. If an association between acute PM exposure and acute cardiovascular events truly exists, bias from this nondifferential outcome misclassification would have attenuated odds ratios in the direction of no association.[6,30] This study was unable to reject the null hypothesis of no association between ambient PM levels and cardiorespiratory medical encounters. Nondifferential outcome misclassification in this study is thus a potential noncausal explanation for the null findings.

Study 5

Abraham JH, DeBakey SF, Reid L, et al. Does deployment to Iraq and Afghanistan affect respiratory health of US military personnel? J Occup Environ Med. *2012;54:740–745.*

Another article published in the same issue of the *Journal of Occupational and Environmental Medicine* presented the results of a study that assessed the impact of deployment on the respiratory health of US military personnel.[28] The researchers' aim was to evaluate the association between postdeployment respiratory conditions and deployment to Iraq or Afghanistan. The conceptually relevant outcomes include the incidence of respiratory symptoms (eg, cough, wheezing, and shortness of breath) and a set of respiratory health conditions (eg, asthma, chronic bronchitis, and emphysema) after deployment. These outcome contrast with the outcome metrics assessed in the study: the appearance (postdeployment) of any one of a set of ICD-9 diagnostic codes in the hospitalization and outpatient medical encounter records of TRICARE beneficiaries. Specifically, the respiratory symptom outcome was defined as a single instance of "symptoms involving respiratory system and other chest symptoms" (ICD-9-CM [Clinical Modification] diagnosis code 786) in the medical record. Respiratory outcomes were similarly defined as a single instance of any diagnosis code in the broad category of "diseases of the respiratory system" (ICD-9-CM diagnosis codes 460–519). They were further categorized into six narrower ranges of diagnostic codes corresponding to healthcare encounters for

1. acute respiratory infections: ICD-9-CM diagnosis codes 460–466,
2. other diseases of the upper respiratory tract: ICD-9-CM diagnosis codes 470–478,
3. pneumonia and influenza: ICD-9-CM diagnosis codes 480–487,
4. COPD and allied conditions: ICD-9-CM diagnosis codes 490–496,
5. pneumoconiosis and other lung diseases due to external agents: ICD-9-CM diagnosis codes 500–508, and
6. other diseases of the respiratory system: ICD-9-CM diagnosis codes 510–519.

Sources of outcome misclassification are similar to those discussed for the in-theater assessment of cardiorespiratory encounters discussed previously, with some notable differences. The existence of false negatives is plausible because of, for example,

- individuals not seeking medical care,
- errors in the medical record,
- failure of medical providers to record health care encounters, and
- medical care received and paid for outside the TRICARE system.

The recording of medical conditions occurring in garrison is regarded as having much higher fidelity, relative to the systems used to record healthcare encounters during deployment. Miscoding of diagnoses and failure to record encounters likely occurred at lower frequencies in the medical systems that provided the outcome data in this study.

Usual patterns of healthcare utilization are disrupted during military deployment. Following troops' redeployment to garrison, it is likely that healthcare utilization, in general, spikes for a period of time. This is because personnel seek healthcare for conditions not addressed during their deployment (before returning to its normal level), except for the potential increase in healthcare required as a consequence of deployment experiences. This study did not discriminate between healthcare encounters that could be considered as part of the redeployment spike and those that are indicative of persistent increases in the respiratory health conditions of interest.

Regarding misdiagnoses and potential false-positive case assignment, this study found that 50% of diagnoses within the "COPD and allied conditions" category fall into the diagnostic code category of "bronchitis, not specified as acute or chronic" (ICD-9-CM diagnosis code 490). For reasons that can only be speculated on, military healthcare providers are frequently making use of this relatively uninformative, nonspecific diagnostic category. Furthermore, as discussed in Chapter 6 (Epidemiology of Airborne Hazards in the Deployed Environment) of this volume, the rate of medical encounters coded as "unspecified bronchitis" has increased in the military population (among both deployed and nondeployed personnel) from 2000 to 2011. It is as yet unclear whether personnel with encounters for unspecified bronchitis have true COPD conditions, such as asthma or chronic bronchitis.

Study 6

Baird CP, DeBakey S, Reid L, et al. Respiratory health status of US Army personnel potentially exposed to smoke from 2003 Al-Mishraq Sulfur Plant fire. J Occup Environ Med. *2012;54:717–723.*

Researchers in Study 3 assessed the postdeployment respiratory health of US Army personnel potentially exposed to smoke from a large sulfur fire in Iraq.[29] Again, outcomes were defined based on ICD-9 diagnosis codes abstracted from military medical records databases. Outcomes consisted of the following large diagnostic code categories:

- diseases of the circulatory system: ICD-9 diagnosis codes 390–459;
- diseases of the respiratory system: ICD-9 diagnosis codes 460–519; and
- symptoms, signs, and ill-defined conditions: ICD-9 diagnosis codes 780–799.

The authors also focused on the following smaller categories of respiratory disease diagnostic codes:

- COPD and allied conditions: ICD-9-CM diagnosis codes 490–496,
- asthma: ICD-9 diagnosis code 493,
- other chronic bronchitis: ICD-9 diagnosis code 491.8,
- pneumoconiosis and other lung disease from external agents: ICD-9 diagnosis codes 500–508,
- ischemic heart disease: ICD-9 diagnosis codes 410–414,
- other forms of heart disease: ICD-9 diagnosis codes 420–429,
- cerebrovascular disease: ICD-9 diagnosis codes 430–438,
- symptoms involving the cardiovascular system: ICD-9 diagnosis code 785, and
- symptoms involving the respiratory system: ICD-9 diagnosis code 786.

These outcome definitions are subject to the same errors (primarily nondifferential misclassification) as those discussed for Studies 4 and 5. However, outcome misclassification in this study may have been differential with respect to exposure if healthcare utilization among personnel exposed to the fire increased as a result of exposure concerns.

In addition to the case definitions based on diagnostic codes, the study also leveraged characterizations of health status as self-reported on DoD-mandated postdeployment health assessments (PDHAs). Errors in recalling health conditions on PDHAs likely occurred because of lapses in memory and complex determinants of respondents' motivation to report health concerns accurately. It has thus been wisely suggested that PDHA results be interpreted with caution.[31] Because differential misclassification bias would be induced if the quality (accuracy and completeness) of postdeployment survey data was not independent of exposure to the sulfur fire in this population. In light of evidence that rates of survey completion differed between exposure groups, the authors of this study chose not to compare the PDHA results between exposed and unexposed groups.

The length of the follow-up period in this study (and others) is limited. The historical proximity of the deployments of interest to the time when the study was conducted places an obvious limit on the amount of postdeployment person-time that can be accrued by formerly deployed military personnel. However, there are other limitations that are surmountable. In this study, subjects' postdeployment person-time accrued only while they remained in military service and did not again deploy; follow-up was discontinued when subjects separated from military service or had a subsequent deployment. These study design decisions were implemented because a subject, once redeployed, is not served by TRICARE. Therefore, the administrative database used to identify medical encounters does not collect medical encounter data in such instances. Linking with other medical record databases (eg, in-theater medical encounter databases, VA databases, and databases of large private insurance/healthcare providers) can facilitate the extension of follow-up for health outcome incidence beyond the service connection. This improvement in outcome capture is particularly important in evaluations of the relationship between deployment-associated hazards and diseases of long latency (eg, many types of cancers).

IMPROVING THE STATE OF SCIENCE BY IMPROVING OUTCOME ASSESSMENT

Measurement and classification of health outcomes in epidemiological studies are exercises in balance: minimizing errors and maximizing efficiency. Although challenges will persist, epidemiologists assessing potential health effects of deployment-associated airborne hazards can better align their operational outcome definitions with conceptually relevant outcomes. Doing so requires not only adherence to epidemiological principles, but also ingenuity, cleverness, and hard work on the part of the investigators, in addition to their having adequate resources to conduct high-quality studies.

Exhibit 7-4 summarizes identified weaknesses in epidemiological studies of deployment-associated airborne hazards' health effects with respect to the health outcome assessment. There will always be health outcome measurement and classification errors in epidemiological studies, just as there will remain technical, logistical, ethical, and financial barriers to implementing better outcome assessment methods. For any given assessment instrument, a trade-off between sensitivity and specificity in defining outcomes will be present. Despite these realities, steps can be taken in the design of a study, the analysis of study data, and the discussion of study results that can either reduce bias because of outcome misclassification or at least diminish the impact of imperfect outcome classification on the inferences drawn from a study (Exhibit 7-5).

The best way to overcome bias in epidemiological measures of association and estimates of precision from errors in

EXHIBIT 7-4

SUMMARY OF IDENTIFIED WEAKNESSES IN EPIDEMIOLOGICAL STUDIES OF DEPLOYMENT-ASSOCIATED AIRBORNE HAZARDS' HEALTH EFFECTS WITH RESPECT TO THE HEALTH OUTCOME ASSESSMENT

Assessment Methods

- Failure to ascertain and compare multiple sources of health outcome information
- Absence of efforts to validate outcome classification within the context of a given study
- No efforts to correct for bias in measures of association from outcome misclassification
- Inadequate use of sensitivity analyses to evaluate impact of misclassification on inference
- Inadequate discussion of the sources of outcome misclassification in published papers
- Insufficient discussion of prior validation of outcome assessment instrument(s)
- Insufficient discussion of the impacts of outcome misclassification on estimated measures of association and associated measures of precision
- Overreliance on administrative sources of outcome data

outcome classification is to avoid the errors in the design of the study. This can be achieved by using the most valid and reliable outcome assessment methods available. In designing a study, researchers should ask themselves the following questions:

- Is the measured outcome to be used in the study a valid and reliable indicator of the conceptually relevant health outcome?
- What are the potential sources of error in outcome classification?
- Are the sources of error in outcome classification independent of subjects' exposure status?
- Can outcome be assessed in different ways, potentially using a gold standard assessment method to classify outcomes in at least a subset of the study population?

Health outcome metrics should be empirically tested for validity and reliability, ideally in the setting of a pilot study conducted in advance of a large-scale investigation. As discussed, avoiding errors entirely is rarely possible. In designing a study, investigators should take steps to prevent, in particular, outcome classification errors that are not independent of subjects' exposure status. In defining outcomes, investigators should further acknowledge the trade-off between sensitivity and specificity, and weigh the advantages and disadvantages of false-positive and false-negative outcome assignments.

Statistical methods have been developed to correct for bias of measures of association from outcome misclassification, in conjunction with validation parameters. If appropriate steps are taken to parameterize outcome misclassification in the study design, analytic techniques can be used to reduce bias of measures of association and correct spurious estimates of precision from misclassification.[32–35] These methods rely on validation data and/or a set of assumptions that may or may not apply in a given study setting. In the absence of formal correction for bias from outcome misclassification, sensitivity analyses should be performed to assess the impact of outcome misclassification errors on the estimated measures of association.[36,37]

EXHIBIT 7-5

RECOMMENDATIONS FOR IMPROVEMENT OF USE OF ADMINISTRATIVE DATABASES

- Reduce outcome misclassification and measurement error in the study design phase
- Conduct validation of outcome measures
- Correct for outcome misclassification
- Coordinate health outcome definitions across research groups
- Acknowledge and evaluate outcome misclassification and measurement error and resulting bias in estimated measures of association
- Increase funding for research efforts and technologies development for outcome assessment

Finally, the discussions of study limitations published in the literature do not sufficiently enumerate the potential sources of errors in health outcome assessment and the impact of these errors on the validity of study results. Robust discussion of the limitations and impacts of imperfect outcome assessment should be included in the reports of epidemiological investigations. Such disclosure facilitates the reader's task of drawing an appropriate inference from the study.

The epidemiological studies of deployment-associated airborne hazards' health effects published to date rely disproportionately on administrative health record databases as the sole source of outcome classification data. Although the advantages are clear in terms of costs and logistical efficiency, such reliance is not without consequences. The result of this overreliance is persistence of sources (and impact on inference) of outcome misclassification across the literature. Inference would be strengthened if different research groups arrived at consistent results after having assessed the same hypothesis using different methods of outcome ascertainment.

To the extent that different research groups rely on the same sources of outcome data, the strategies they use to define outcomes (using medical record data, for example) could be better coordinated within or between research groups. The symposium work group identified a need to establish a follow-on working group to develop outcome definition criteria. At the very least, the use of standard outcome definitions facilitates comparability across research efforts conducted at different institutions. At best, such standardization can ensure that outcomes are appropriately defined for a given research goal. As a starting point, the Armed Forces Health Surveillance Center (AFHSC) has developed a set of outcome definitions for medical surveillance to "facilitate comparisons of case counts performed in different populations by different public health agencies" and to "harmonize health surveillance and epidemiologic analyses throughout the Department of Defense."[38] These outcome definitions are being adopted by researchers at the AFHSC and the US Army Public Health Command. Several research groups have begun to incorporate evidence of persistence of chronic disease into case definitions, and this practice should be adopted by other groups if appropriate to their investigations. Requiring evidence of persistence, such as requiring two or more diagnostic codes for a related condition observed in a prespecified time period for a given individual, will increase the specificity of the case assignment scheme and correspondingly decrease the proportion of false positives. Note, however, that this comes at a cost, namely a decreased sensitivity of the outcome classification scheme and a relatively greater proportion of false negatives.

Although resource-dependent, researchers need to advocate for initiatives to develop and validate novel indicators of outcomes and adopt the use of such indicators as they can. Adopting more refined outcome assessment technologies and strategies can reduce outcome measurement errors and the associated bias of measures of association.

SUMMARY

It is incumbent upon researchers conducting epidemiological studies to minimize sources and impacts of bias, where feasible, and to be aware of and disclose factors that impact the validity of their work. Sources of bias can be, at times, obvious and at other times obscure; engaging with an epidemiologist to evaluate the health outcome in the design phase may be a cost-efficient step in improving the quality of a study. Making inference using epidemiological study results requires an evaluation of the impacts of these errors. Prudent use of epidemiological study results then proceeds by contextualizing the results within the larger set of evidence, epidemiological and otherwise. As often as possible, the goal should be to measure what matters and measure it well.

REFERENCES

1. Weese CB, Abraham JH. Potential health implications associated with particulate matter exposure in deployed settings in southwest Asia. *Inhal Toxicol.* 2009;21:291–296.

2. Last JM, Spasoff RA, Harris, SS, eds. *A Dictionary of Epidemiology.* 4th ed. New York, NY: Oxford University Press; 1998.

3. Aschengrau A, Seage G, III. *Essentials of Epidemiology in Public Health.* Sudbury, MA: Jones & Bartlett Publishers; 2003.

4. Rothman KJ, Greenland S, Lash T. *Modern Epidemiology.* 3rd ed. Philadelphia, PA: Lippincott Williams & Wilkins; 2008.

5. Altman DG, Bland JM. Diagnostic tests. 1: Sensitivity and specificity. *BMJ.* 1994;308(6943):1552.

6. Copeland KT, Checkoway H, McMichael AJ, Holbrook RH. Bias due to misclassification in the estimation of relative risk. *Am J Epidemiol.* 1977;105:488–495.

7. White E. The effect of misclassification of disease status in follow-up studies: implications for selecting disease classification criteria. *Am J Epidemiol.* 1986;124:816–825.

8. Brenner H, Gefeller O. Use of the positive predictive value to correct for disease misclassification in epidemiologic studies. *Am J Epidemiol.* 1993;138:1007–1015.

9. Jurek AM, Greenland S, Maldonado G, Church TR. Proper interpretation of non-differential misclassification effects: expectations vs observations. *Int J Epidemiol.* 2005;34:680–687.

10. Wacholder S, Hartge P, Lubin JH, Dosemeci M. Non-differential misclassification and bias towards the null: a clarification. *Occup Environ Med.* 1995;52:557–558.

11. Rothman KJ, Poole C. A strengthening programme for weak associations. *Int J Epidemiol.* 1988;17:955–959.

12. Hatch M, Thomas D. Measurement issues in environmental epidemiology. *Environ Health Perspect.* 1993;101(suppl 4):49–57.

13. Expert Panel Report 3 (EPR-3). Guidelines for the Diagnosis and Management of Asthma—Summary Report 2007. *J Allergy Clin Immunol.* 2007;120(suppl 5):S94–S138.

14. Pekkanen J, Pearce N. Defining asthma in epidemiological studies. *Eur Respir J.* 1999;14:951–957.

15. Hansen S, Strøm M, Maslova E, et al. A comparison of three methods to measure asthma in epidemiologic studies: results from the Danish National Birth Cohort. *PLOS ONE.* 2012;7:e36328.

16. Altman DG. *Practical Statistics for Medical Research.* London, England: Chapman and Hall; 1991.

17. Gray GC, Chesbrough KB, Ryan MAK, et al. The Millennium Cohort Study: a 21-year prospective cohort study of 140,000 military personnel. *Mil Med.* 2002;167:483–488.

18. Smith TC, Jacobson IG, Hooper TI, et al. Health impact of US military service in a large population-based military cohort: findings of the Millennium Cohort Study, 2001–2008. *BMC Public Health.* 2011;11:69.

19. Smith B, Wong CA, Smith TC, et al. Newly reported respiratory symptoms and conditions among military personnel deployed to Iraq and Afghanistan: a prospective population-based study. *Am J Epidemiol.* 2009;170:1433–1442.

20. Smith B, Chu LK, Smith TC, et al. Challenges of self-reported medical conditions and electronic medical records among members of a large military cohort. *BMC Med Res Methodol.* 2008;8:37.

21. Cicchetti DV, Feinstein AR. High agreement but low kappa: II. Resolving the paradoxes. *J Clin Epidemiol.* 1990;43:551–558.

22. Szema AM, Peters MC, Weissinger KM, et al. New-onset asthma among soldiers serving in Iraq and Afghanistan. *Allergy Asthma Proc.* 2010;31:67–71.

23. National Asthma Education and Prevention Program, NHLBI, National Institutes of Health. *Asthma Expert Panel Report 3. Guidelines for the Diagnosis and Management of Asthma.* Bethesda, MD: National Institutes of Health; 2007. NIH Publication 08-5846.

24. Rose C, Abraham J, Harkins D, et al. Overview and recommendations for medical screening and diagnostic evaluation for postdeployment lung disease in returning US warfighters. *J Occup Environ Med.* 2012;54:746–751.

25. Hankinson JL, Odencrantz JR, Fedan KB. Spirometric reference values from a sample of the general U.S. population. *Am J Respir Crit Care Med.* 1999;159:179–187.

26. Szema AM, Salihi W, Savary K, Chen JJ. Respiratory symptoms necessitating spirometry among soldiers with Iraq/Afghanistan war lung injury. *J Occup Environ Med.* 2011;53:961–965.

27. Abraham JH, Baird CP. A case-crossover study of ambient particulate matter and cardiovascular and respiratory medical encounters among US military personnel deployed to southwest Asia. *J Occup Environ Med.* 2012;54:733–739.

28. Abraham JH, DeBakey SF, Reid L, et al. Does deployment to Iraq and Afghanistan affect respiratory health of US military personnel? *J Occup Environ Med.* 2012;54:740–745.

29. Baird CP, DeBakey S, Reid L, et al. Respiratory health status of US Army personnel potentially exposed to smoke from 2003 Al-Mishraq Sulfur Plant fire. *J Occup Environ Med.* 2012;54:717–723.

30. Greenland S. The effect of misclassification in the presence of covariates. *Am J Epidemiol.* 1980;112:564–569.

31. Mancuso JD, Ostafin M, Lovell M. Postdeployment evaluation of health risk communication after exposure to a toxic industrial chemical. *Mil Med.* 2008;173:369–374.

32. Duffy SW, Warwick J, Williams AR, et al. A simple model for potential use with a misclassified binary outcome in epidemiology. *J Epidemiol Community Health.* 2004;58:712–717.

33. Lyles RH, Tang L, Superak HM, et al. Validation data-based adjustments for outcome misclassification in logistic regression: an illustration. *Epidemiology.* 2011;22:589–597.

34. Magder LS, Hughes JP. Logistic regression when the outcome is measured with uncertainty. *Am J Epidemiol.* 1997;146:195–203.

35. Luo S, Chan W, Detry MA, Massman PJ, Doody RS. Binomial regression with a misclassified covariate and outcome. *Stat Methods Med Res.* 2012;March 15 [e-pub ahead of print].

36. Greenland S. Basic methods for sensitivity analysis of biases. *Int J Epidemiol.* 1996;25:1107–1116.

37. Lash TL, Fink AK. Semi-automated sensitivity analysis to assess systematic errors in observational data. *Epidemiology.* 2003;14:451–458.

38. Armed Forces Health Surveillance Center. *AFHSC Surveillance Case Definitions.* Silver Spring, MD: AFHSC; 2013. http://www.afhsc.mil/caseSurveillanceDefs. Accessed August 22, 2013.

Chapter 8

PULMONARY FUNCTION TESTING—SPIROMETRY TESTING FOR POPULATION SURVEILLANCE

WILLIAM ESCHENBACHER, MD*

**Pulmonologist, Veterans Health Administration, Pulmonary/Critical Care, Cincinnati VA Medical Center, 3200 Vine Street, Cincinnati, Ohio 45220; Professor of Medicine, Division of Pulmonary and Critical Care Medicine, Department of Internal Medicine, University of Cincinnati College of Medicine, 231 Albert Sabin Way, Cincinnati, Ohio 45229*

INTRODUCTION

Spirometry is a test of respiratory function that measures the volume of air that an individual can inhale and exhale, usually in a forceful manner. After the individual fills his or her lungs to maximal capacity, he or she is asked to exhale forcefully while the exhaled volume is measured over time until the expiration is complete. This volume–time relationship as graphed is known as a *spirogram*. The device used for the measurement is referred to as a spirometer. The important parameters determined by this test include the following:

- the total volume that is exhaled forcefully;
- the forced vital capacity (FVC);
- the volume of air that is exhaled in the first second of time;
- the forced expiratory volume in 1 second (FEV_1); and
- the ratio between these two values: FEV_1/FVC.

Spirometry is considered a screening test that is useful in the evaluation of a patient who presents with respiratory symptoms (eg, dyspnea, cough, sputum production, chest tightness, and wheezing). Thus, the results of spirometry can be interpreted according to specific patterns of normality or abnormality, including airflow obstruction, possible lung restriction, or a mixed pattern of obstruction and possible restriction. If the spirometry test results are interpreted as abnormal, the individual may then be referred for more complete testing and other evaluation.

TECHNICAL ASPECTS OF SPIROMETRY

The spirometers used for testing can either directly measure the volume of air exhaled (volume spirometers) or indirectly measure volume by integrating expiratory flows over time (flow spirometers). When volume spirometers are computerized, the change in volume can be quantified over time to determine the instantaneous rates of air exhaled. For flow spirometers, the flow rates of air are integrated over time to obtain measures of the expiratory volume of air. All spirometers used in clinical and research settings must have passed standards for accuracy, precision, and graphical display size as established by the American Thoracic Society (ATS).[1] In addition, because the test depends on the maximal effort of each individual being tested, the technician

- must be appropriately trained to explain the test to the subject,
- should coach the subject to help produce his/her maximal efforts, and
- be able to review each maneuver to determine if the effort was maximal and acceptable.

Each technician must have completed training provided by courses such as those approved by the National Institute for Occupational Safety and Health,[2] and demonstrate continued good testing technique when reviewed for technical quality by pulmonary specialists with feedback for the technician. Figure 8-1 shows an individual performing spiromety while being coached by an experienced technician.

Each spirometry maneuver must meet specific criteria established by ATS-recommended guidelines for acceptability. For a valid spirometry test session, there should be three acceptable maneuvers, with consistent (repeatable) results recorded for both the maximal FVC and the maximal FEV_1.[1] Trained technicians can identify maneuvers that meet acceptability and repeatability criteria.

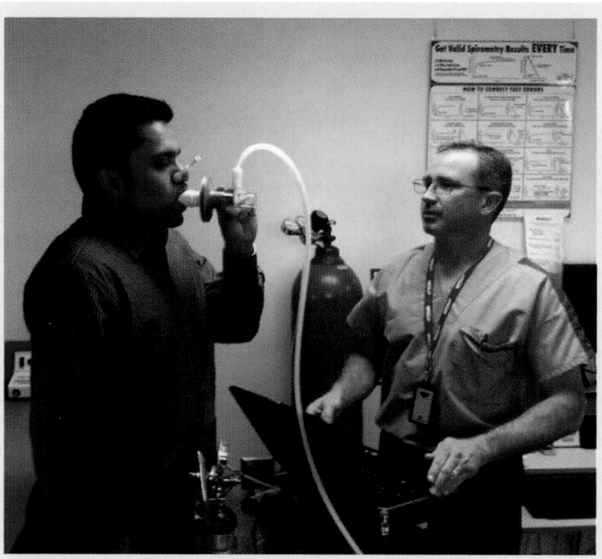

Figure 8-1. Individual performing spirometry.

PROBLEMS WITH POOR QUALITY TESTING

If the spirometry testing maneuvers are not performed with adequate quality (meeting acceptability and repeatability criteria), then it is possible that false-positive or false-negative results may be reported. If so, unnecessary additional testing may be performed or necessary medical follow-up may not be conducted. Both of these errors can eventually add to the expense of a spirometry surveillance program.

INTERPRETATION OF RESULTS AND USE OF REFERENCE EQUATIONS

To permit confident interpretation of spirometry results, valid tests should be conducted whenever possible, meeting acceptability and repeatability criteria. Measured results are compared with reference equations to determine if the measured results are normal or abnormal. Abnormality is present if the values fall below the 5th percentile lower limit of normal[3] (LLN) based on the reference equations chosen. Reference values most often recommended for comparison were derived from spirometry testing performed as part of the Third National Health and Nutrition Examination Survey (NHANES III).[4,5] These reference values—derived from high-quality spirometry test results from healthy, randomly selected nonsmokers aged 17 and older from across the United States—would be the most appropriate reference values for use with service members and veterans.

SPIROMETRY IMPAIRMENT PATTERNS

Spirometry testing results can be interpreted as normal, showing airflow obstruction, possible restriction, or indicating a mixed impairment (both airflow obstruction and possible restriction). If an acceptable and repeatable testing session reveals an abnormal pattern (obstruction, possible restriction, or a mixed impairment pattern), then additional tests may be indicated to further evaluate the presence of a possible respiratory condition.

Airflow obstruction is based on the finding that the FEV_1/FVC ratio is below the LLN for that ratio. Airflow obstruction can be seen in pulmonary conditions, such as asthma, chronic obstructive pulmonary disease, bronchiolitis obliterans, and constrictive bronchiolitis.

Possible restrictive lung defect is suggested by spirometry testing when the FVC is below the LLN for that parameter. Restrictive patterns can be seen in any condition that limits the ability of the lungs and/or chest wall to expand: obesity, chest wall abnormalities (as might occur after trauma), pleural disease, or pulmonary interstitial/parenchymal disease. Spirometry can only indicate possible restrictive lung defect. To confirm the presence of restriction, additional testing—including measurement of lung volumes—is usually indicated.

SURVEILLANCE SPIROMETRY: WHO SHOULD BE TESTED?

Surveillance programs for respiratory disease must first determine which individuals should have spirometry testing. Because the development of a respiratory disease may be identified by the presence of respiratory symptoms and the finding of abnormal spirometry results, then individuals who present with persistent symptoms of dyspnea, cough, sputum production, chest tightness, and/or wheezing should have spirometry testing performed. It is also possible that the individuals without overt symptoms may have decrements in lung function from exposures that could eventually be diagnosed as a respiratory disease. To adequately measure significant decrements or declines in lung function as a result of environmental or occupational exposures, it would be necessary to have baseline lung function testing prior to exposures. For those in military service, this would mean testing all individuals who enter the service because it may not be known at that time if the individual would subsequently be exposed to adverse environmental/airborne toxic agents.

The cost of performing spirometry testing for every service member upon entering into service would be considerable. Estimated costs for testing all 2,255,100 service members upon entry are shown in Table 8-1.

DISADVANTAGES AND CONCERNS FOR PERFORMING BASELINE SCREENING SPIROMETRY FOR EVERY SERVICE MEMBER

In addition to the significant cost for performing baseline screening spirometry for every service member, there are also other considerations. One important issue is that the normal range of pulmonary function values is designed to exclude one in twenty normal healthy individuals since the LLN is set at the 5th percentile for all examined spirometry measurements, as discussed previously. Therefore, when large numbers of healthy service members are tested, a significant number of false positives should be expected. Because spirometry is an effort-driven test, false-positive results may also be seen in individuals with less than maximal efforts if not identified by the technician as unacceptable. All false-positive test results may lead to further evaluation with associated additional costs.

Identification of abnormal test results for an individual who may have no symptoms may limit that individual's ability for future employment or career choice. For those individuals who may have a previous diagnosis of a pulmonary impairment, identification of the severity of impairment may limit their ability for some assignments, including deployment.

There are also concerns for establishing a department-wide testing program:

- Who would assume leadership for this program?
- Where logistically would the testing be done?
- At what point in the early career of the service member would he or she be tested?
- Who would be assigned the task of reviewing, interpreting, and reporting all the results? Where would the data be stored?

Other concerns would be the effort and cost for other proposed surveillance procedures, including symptom questionnaires and other routine medical diagnostic testing results.

TABLE 8-1

ESTIMATED COST FOR TESTING ALL SERVICE MEMBERS UPON ENTRY INTO SERVICE*

Item	Cost
1,000 spirometry technicians, salaries	$50,637,000
Training for technicians	$2,000,000
Spirometers (one per technician)	$5,000,000
Cost of server and databases	$200,000
Cost to review and interpret tests	$27,061,000
Cost for follow-up of abnormal results	$169,132,500
Administration of program	$200,000
Supplies	$11,275,500
Total cost of program	$265,506,000

*Total number of service members: 2,255,100. One technician can test 2,200–2,400 service members / year (need 1,000 technicians). Salary for one technician: GS-06, Step 5, $39,560 + 28% benefits ($11,077) = $50,637. Spirometry training, including travel: $2,000 / technician. Cost to review and interpret each spirometry test: $12 / test. Percentage of abnormal tests (true- and false-positive test results): 15%. Cost for follow-up of each abnormal test (further testing and medical evaluation): $500.

COMPARISON OF BASELINE SPIROMETRY WITH POSTDEPLOYMENT SPIROMETRY TESTING

As described previously, identification of a deployment-related respiratory condition would include evaluation of an individual who presented with respiratory symptoms and was then found through additional testing to have either abnormal lung function test results or significant decrements in lung function when compared with baseline test results. Less consensus exists about the criterion for a significant decrement in spirometry test results than has occurred for the cross-sectional interpretation of pulmonary function results relative to the normal range. Since 1991, the ATS has stated that a 15% decline in FEV_1 would be considered to be a significant change, even if that postvalue by itself was found to be in the normal range based on a reference equation.[3] Thus, the individual's test results may have been above average (ie, high in the normal range) to begin with. More recent reports using regression analysis would suggest that, depending on the technical quality of the test and the resulting precision of the data being examined, smaller decrements in lung function might be considered to be significant.[6]

Another option would be to test service members pre- or postdeployment who present with respiratory symptoms.

SUMMARY

Surveillance spirometry performed on every individual who enters military service has the advantage that, if deployment-related respiratory illnesses did occur, having accurate baseline values would allow comparison to test results obtained after deployment. The logistics and costs for performing such baseline testing are considerable, as described previously, which may make such testing prohibitive. In addition, there are other concerns for such testing, including limiting the career choices for asymptomatic individuals who were found to have abnormal results from this baseline testing. The advantages and disadvantages of such baseline testing, including the expected false positives associated with using the 5th percentile LLN, would have to be examined closely before deciding on implementation.

REFERENCES

1. Miller MR, Hankinson J, Brusasco V, et al. Standardisation of spirometry. *Eur Respir J.* 2005;26:319–338.

2. Centers for Disease Control and Prevention, National Institute for Occupational Safety and Health. Spirometry Training Program. http://www.cdc.gov/niosh/topics/spirometry/training.html. Accessed August 28, 2013.

3. Pelligrino R, Viegi G, Brusasco V, et al. Interpretative strategies for lung function tests. *Eur Respir J.* 2005;26:948–968.

4. Hankinson JL, Odencrantz JR, Fedan KB. Spirometric reference values from a sample of the general U.S. population. *Am J Respir Crit Care Med.* 1999;159:179–187.

5. Townsend MC. Spirometry in the occupational health setting—2011 update. *J Occup Environ Med.* 2011;53:569–584.

6. Hnizdo E, Sircar K, Glindmeyer H, Petsonk E. Longitudinal limits of normal decline in lung function in an individual. *J Occup Environ Med.* 2006;48:625–634.

Chapter 9

DISCUSSION SUMMARY: RECOMMENDATION FOR SURVEILLANCE SPIROMETRY IN MILITARY PERSONNEL

MICHAEL J. MORRIS, MD*; WILLIAM ESCHENBACHER, MD†; AND CHARLES E. MCCANNON, MD, MBA, MPH‡

*Colonel (Retired), Medical Corps, US Army; Department of Defense Chair, Staff Physician, Pulmonary/Critical Care Medicine and Assistant Program Director, Internal Medicine Residency, San Antonio Military Medical Center, 3551 Roger Brooke Drive, Fort Sam Houston, Texas 78234

†Pulmonologist, Veterans Health Administration, Pulmonary/Critical Care, Cincinnati VA Medical Center, 3200 Vine Street, Cincinnati, Ohio 45220; Professor of Medicine, Division of Pulmonary and Critical Care Medicine, Department of Internal Medicine, University of Cincinnati College of Medicine, 231 Albert Sabin Way, Cincinnati, Ohio 45229

‡Staff Physician, Environmental Medicine Program, Occupational and Environmental Medicine, US Army Public Health Command, 5158 Blackhawk Road, Aberdeen Proving Ground, Maryland 21010-5403

INTRODUCTION

In the March 2012 issue of the *Journal of Occupational and Environmental Medicine* an article was published titled "Overview and Recommendations for Medical Screening and Diagnostic Evaluation for Post-Deployment Lung Disease in Returning US Warfighters."[1] This paper contained the proceedings of a one-day meeting held at National Jewish Health (Denver, CO) in February 2010 by a group of Department of Defense (DoD), Department of Veterans Administration (VA), and civilian physicians and environmental scientists.[1] At issue was the question of whether US military personnel deployed to Iraq and Afghanistan were at risk for respiratory symptoms and chronic lung disease resulting from exposure to airborne contaminants from open-air burn pits, geological dusts, industrial fires and emissions, and vehicular exhaust. The discussion at the meeting was based on environmental studies conducted in the theaters of operation and limited clinical data on lung disease compiled by civilian researchers. One general recommendation listed in the *Journal of Occupational and Environmental Medicine* article pertained to the role of pre- and postdeployment medical surveillance. According to Table 9-1 in that paper, the recommendation includes the following:

- a standardized questionnaire eliciting smoking history, pertinent medical history, and respiratory symptoms;
- spirometry (pre- and postbronchodilator); and
- an exercise-capacity evaluation (Physical Readiness Test), including 1- or 2-mile run times.

A work group at the National Jewish Health meeting addressed the need for medical surveillance using spirometry as part of a deployment evaluation and for the military population as a whole.

INDICATIONS FOR MEDICAL SURVEILLANCE FOR OCCUPATIONAL LUNG DISEASE

According to an American College of Occupational and Environmental Medicine position statement published in 2000, there are three main indications for the use of spirometry in the workplace.[2] The *first indication* is the primary prevention of respiratory disease in preemployment or fitness-for-duty examinations. Included are those individuals with a demanding physical job, such as firefighters, who require a high level of cardiopulmonary fitness and have a potential occupational respiratory exposure. An additional role of primary prevention is population screening for the potential effects of occupational respiratory exposures. In both these situations, identification of an abnormal spirometry may indicate the need to obviate their potential exposure or change occupations as a secondary prevention.

The *second indication* is that repeated spirometry is used in medical surveillance programs when workers are at risk of developing occupation-related respiratory disorders. Surveillance spirometry can detect the slowly developing or delayed losses of function that are characteristic of work-related respiratory disorders. Many healthy individuals may be tested to detect early excessive declines in the pulmonary function of a subgroup of sensitive workers, even though the spirometry test results of these workers may still remain in the normal range. Current regulations from the Occupational Safety and Health Administration recommend periodic spirometry for the following exposures:

- asbestos,
- cadmium,
- coke oven emissions,
- cotton dust,
- benzene,
- formaldehyde, and
- silica.[3]

An additional 25 respiratory exposures are recommended for screening spirometry by the National Institute for Occupational Safety and Health.[4] Screening needs to be done on a longitudinal basis to identify a 15% decline in forced expiratory volume at 1 second (FEV_1) based on initial recommendations by the American Thoracic Society and the American College of Occupational and Environmental Medicine.[5] A limit of approximately 10% decline in FEV_1 appears appropriate for quality workplace monitoring programs, whereas a limit of about 15% appears appropriate for clinical evaluation of individuals with an obstructive airway disease.[6]

The *third indication* is that spirometry is used in the clinical evaluation of symptomatic individuals because many pulmonary diseases manifest themselves as restrictive, obstructive, or combined ventilatory defects. Spirometry allows some quantification of the severity of lung function loss and is one of the pulmonary function tests used in assessing respiratory impairment to determine disability. This is the most common use of spirometry in physician clinics as part of an overall symptomatic evaluation.

SURVEILLANCE SPIROMETRY IN THE GENERAL POPULATION

The two most common chronic respiratory diseases in the United States are (1) asthma and (2) chronic obstructive pulmonary disease (COPD). Asthma is reported to affect as much as 10% of the population, whereas COPD has been diagnosed in approximately 12 million persons and is currently the fourth leading cause of death. These two affected populations with asthma and COPD are substantially much larger than the population with occupation-related exposures. Occupation-related asthma accounts for 10% to 15% of all asthma cases and overall may affect only 1% to 2% of the general population.[7] Contrasted with many other diseases where there is recommended surveillance, such as

- cancer (breast, colon, prostate, and cervical),
- diabetes mellitus,
- hypertension,
- hyperlipidemia,
- aortic aneurysms, and
- osteoporosis,

no current recommendations exist for routine screening of asymptomatic populations for either COPD or asthma. Two major scientific organizations do not recommend using routine screening for COPD in smokers: the American College of Physicians and the US Preventive Services Task Force. The American College of Physicians recommended in 2007 that "spirometry should not be used to screen for airflow obstruction in asymptomatic individuals," including those with known COPD risk factors.[8] The US Preventive Services Task Force also recommended against routine screening for COPD in smokers in the absence of clinical symptoms.[9]

The burden to the healthcare system of overdiagnosis in older patients, the accuracy of spirometry, and the lack of clinical benefit from earlier diagnosis were cited as reasons. Because spirometry is used as a confirmatory test, as well as a screening test for COPD, no gold standard exists for comparing precise estimates of sensitivity and specificity. Two cross-sectional studies that performed spirometry tests in adults with no history of tobacco use or respiratory disease suggest that spirometry yields some false-positive results and that the number of false-positive results increases in patients older than 70 years of age.[10,11] Further studies on asthma screening in children also found it to be not cost-effective compared with use of a questionnaire.[12]

INCIDENCE OF DEPLOYMENT-RELATED LUNG DISEASE

An excellent example of the use of surveillance spirometry is the World Trade Center (WTC) Worker and Volunteer Medical Screening Program. Of approximately 40,000 rescue and recovery workers exposed to the ambient particulate matter from the site, nearly 10,000 responders participated in the program. Notably, 59% of the workers in this cohort reported persistent respiratory symptoms. Evaluations using spirometry found a decrease in forced vital capacity in 21% of the workers and evidence of obstruction in 5% of the workers compared with preexposure values.[13] Among nonsmokers, 27% in the WTC population had abnormal spirometry compared with the reported 13% in the general US population (data taken from the Third National Health and Nutrition Examination Survey [NHANES III] data).[14] Additionally, the prevalence of low forced vital capacity among nonsmokers was five-fold greater than in the US population (20% vs 4%). Respiratory symptoms and spirometry abnormalities were significantly associated with early arrival at the site. A variety of reports identified pulmonary diseases as

- increased bronchial hyperreactivity,
- asthma,
- reactive airway dysfunction syndrome,
- chronic sinusitis,
- vocal cord dysfunction,
- eosinophilic pneumonia,
- granulomatous pneumonia, and
- bronchiolitis obliterans.[13]

A separate study involved 12,781 workers with the Fire Department, City of New York, who participated in a longitudinal study of spirometric measurements over 7 years. The average decline in FEV_1 was 439 mL during the first year with persistent declines and no recovery in the 6-year follow-up.[15]

How does exposure in the WTC workers, some with acute inhalational exposures and others with chronic exposure, relate to the issue at hand involving deployed military personnel? There is limited exposure data available in the military setting, but the symptomatic population is relatively small in comparison with the WTC cohort. In general, there are reported increases in respiratory symptoms, such as cough and dyspnea, during deployment. Reporting on the health effects of the Kuwaiti oil fires of 1991 among US troops, survey research by Army investigators found an increase in reported symptoms of upper respiratory tract irritation, shortness of breath, and cough associated with proximity to the Kuwaiti oil fires. The effects, however, were generally short-lived and resolved after leaving Kuwait.[16]

Researchers from the Naval Medical Research Center (Silver Spring, MD) conducted a one-time survey of 15,000 redeploying military personnel from Iraq and Afghanistan, and estimated that 69.1% reported experiencing acute respiratory illnesses, of which 17% required medical care.[17] Long-term postdeployment survey data on respiratory symptoms from the Millennium Cohort Study conducted by the Naval Health Research Center (San Diego, CA) found that deployed personnel had a higher rate of newly reported respiratory symptoms than nondeployed personnel (14% vs 10%), with similar rates of chronic bronchitis/emphysema (1% vs 1%) and asthma (1% vs 1%) observed. The authors suggested that specific, but unidentified, exposures rather than deployment may be a determinant of postdeployment respiratory illness.[18]

In terms of common respiratory diseases, such as COPD and asthma, these rates also tend to be lower than the general population. Roop et al[19] surveyed deploying Army personnel and found that 5% of troops deployed to southwest Asia reported a previous diagnosis of asthma. In this study, there were no differences between asthmatics and nonasthmatics because both groups reported significantly increased respiratory symptoms during deployment compared with symptoms preceding deployment. A retrospective chart review of more than 6,000 VA medical records (based solely on the *International Classification of Diseases*, Ninth Revision [ICD-9] diagnostic codes) found higher rates of new-onset asthma in deployed US military personnel between 2004 and 2007 compared with nondeployed military personnel stationed in the US (6.6% vs 4.3%).[20] The lack of predeployment data and spirometry values in this cohort makes the determination of new-onset asthma suspect. Recent studies conducted at Brooke Army Medical Center (Fort Sam Houston, TX) evaluated the medical records of military personnel with diagnosed asthma undergoing a medical evaluation board, diagnosis of COPD or emphysema, and new-onset asthma. In each group, approximately 70% of the cohort had no history of deployment, and nearly 20% had an inadequate evaluation without documented spirometry to confirm evidence of obstructive airway disease.[21,22]

WORK GROUP DISCUSSION ON SURVEILLANCE SPIROMETRY

Numerous questions were presented to the work group to discuss general recommendations on the use of spirometry for military personnel. The following issues were discussed throughout the course of the workshop:

- Should surveillance spirometry be initiated in the DoD?
- Should a screening questionnaire be administered first?
- Would all military personnel or only specific individuals be tested?
- Should individuals be tested (at what point in a military career)?
- Should testing be completed once or repeated periodically?
- What are implementation issues across the DoD?
- What are the cost/benefit considerations?
- How will the evaluation of abnormal studies be handled?
- What information technology is required to store and retrieve results?
- What impact could an abnormal spirometry have on a military career?

CURRENT LIMITATIONS FOR IMPLEMENTATION

One major factor for consideration is the cost related to performance of surveillance spirometry across the DoD. The US Army Public Health Command provided an in-depth analysis for consideration of a single spirometry examination. Making an assumption that the cost of a single examination would be $15 per service member (if done in military facilities) and there are currently 2.2 million service members within the DoD, the start-up costs alone would be nearly $35 million. Additional costs would be incurred for repeat testing, further evaluation of abnormal testing, and other issues related to the conduct of quality spirometry. Given that the DoD system would not be able to undertake this added testing, costs would also increase if spirometry examinations were performed in the civilian healthcare system.

The primary issues in periodic spirometry evaluation are to establish good baseline measurement, maintain spirometry quality and low within-person variability, and identify individuals with excessive decline in lung function.[23] Longitudinal evaluation of spirometry data can be best tracked through the analysis software that can interpret periodic spirometry data, screen for individuals with abnormal spirometry results, and maintain spirometry precision and quality. An example of software that can be used is the Spirometry Longitudinal Data Analysis (SPIROLA) software that is freely available on the Internet. An essential component for obtaining spirometry in a large group, such as a military population, would be a central database to collect, store, and track information aside from the current electronic medical record. Although many tracking systems exist for other military health issues, it would be burdensome to establish such a system for spirometry. Current electronic medical records in both DoD and VA do not allow the direct uploading of spirometry or other pulmonary test results into a predesignated section. Results are generally scanned in with PDF (Portable Document Format) files and located in different places in the medical record, severely limiting searching for results.

Because the main concern for respiratory disease is linked to deployment, should surveillance be limited to pre- and postdeployment spirometry? Additionally, there may be added value in use of a screening questionnaire for respiratory symptoms or preexisting respiratory disease (asthma,

EXHIBIT 9-1

SURVEILLANCE SPIROMETRY ALGORITHM

Indications for Testing Military Personnel

- Postdeployment (in the presence of respiratory symptoms only)
- Physical fitness test run failure (screening for subclinical lung disease)
- History of childhood asthma (rule out asthma recurrence)
- Military specialties with increased occupational exposures (annual testing)
- Evaluation of persistent respiratory symptoms as part of clinical evaluation

Requirements for Testing

- Trained technician—NIOSH spirometry course or higher
- Certified spirometer—meets American Thoracic Society standards
- Use of nose clips and patient in seated position
- Three reproducible efforts within 5% based on expiratory effort
- Minimum expiratory time of 6 seconds
- Reference values—NHANES III

Testing Documentation

- Demographics; age, gender, ethnicity, measured height, weight
- Smoking history
- Pulmonary history
- Active seasonal allergic rhinitis within 4 weeks
- Active upper respiratory infection within 4 weeks
- Current allergy and pulmonary medications (should perform spirometry off medications for 1 week if feasible)

Testing Outcomes

- Normal—no further evaluation
- Restrictive indices
  - Repeat study in 2–4 weeks
  - If study unchanged and FVC <70%, refer for full pulmonary function testing
  - Obtain chest radiograph to evaluate for interstitial lung disease
  - Refer for evaluation if full pulmonary function testing confirms restrictive defect (TLC <70%) or chest radiograph is abnormal
- Obstructive indices
  - Repeat study in 2–4 weeks
  - If study unchanged and FEV_1 <70%, refer for spirometry with postbronchodilator testing
  - If FEV_1 postbronchodilator response >8%, refer for further evaluation
- Abnormal flow volume loop
  - Interpretation of the FVL is required for an adequate spirometry
  - Truncation or flattening of the inspiratory flow volume curve (below the 0 axis) should prompt referral for formal spirometry
  - Repeatability of two-thirds abnormal FVLs confirms possible upper airway obstruction
- Technically inadequate study—repeat study in 2–4 weeks

FEV_1: forced expiratory volume in 1 second; FVC: forced vital capacity; FVL: flow volume loop; NIOSH: National Institute for Occupational Safety and Health; NHANES III: Third National Health and Nutrition Examination Survey; TLC: total lung capacity

COPD) prior to deployment. Those with a positive response to exposure questions could then have baseline spirometry testing prior to deployment and repeat testing upon return. Although this approach may better identify those patients with demonstrable reduction in pulmonary function post-deployment due to underlying lung disease, many deployed personnel may not complete the questions honestly because of the perception that it may prevent deployment or compensation for deployment-related lung disease. Even pre- and postdeployment spirometry would have significant logistic implications given the numbers (>2.5 million) deployed and the numerous locations to which personnel are deployed.

Another significant question raised was the true incidence of new pulmonary disease in deployed or nondeployed service members. If the percentage is small, as currently suggested by epidemiological data, will there be any advantage in having baseline measurements for the vast majority of military personnel who will not develop symptoms or disease? Should we continue to evaluate current available data to better estimate more precise incidence of deployment pulmonary disease development? There are problems with analyzing current data, including use of ICD-9 codes to establish a true incidence of new and existing pulmonary disease.

SUMMARY

Is there a role for surveillance spirometry in the military population? Current evidence suggests that the military population reflects the general population as a whole, with respect to rates of pulmonary disease. Potentially, there is increased workplace exposure for certain military occupational specialties, and current deployment locations have documented increases in environmental ambient particulate matter from sand/dust, as well as burn pit smoke. However, no evidence suggests any significant increase in respiratory disease over the general population. The following recommendations are outlined in Exhibit 9-1:

- DoD policy at present should not require routine surveillance spirometry in all military personnel. The burden of evaluating asymptomatic personnel with pulmonary function testing abnormalities would outweigh any benefit from early disease detection. No such recommendations exist for asthma and COPD screening for the general population, and the incidence of other chronic lung diseases is extremely small.[24]
- Predeployment surveillance (baseline) spirometry should be evaluated in a feasibility pilot study. A research study is currently being conducted at Fort Hood, Texas, to obtain pre- and postdeployment spirometry (with chest radiographs) in deploying military personnel to Afghanistan. It is anticipated that the change in postdeployment spirometry will likely be minimal (<5% of FEV_1) and more prominent in smokers. Additionally, a feasibility study is being conducted in new soldiers at Fort Sam Houston to evaluate the number of abnormal baseline studies in an asymptomatic population.
- The use of bronchodilators (short-acting beta-agonists, such as albuterol or levalbuterol) is not warranted as part of routine surveillance spirometry. The use of bronchodilators outside of a clinical setting logistically complicates and prolongs the conduct of a spirometry examination. Information from recording postbronchodilator values is minimal unless the screening examination is strictly for asthma symptoms or detecting occupational asthma.
- Surveillance spirometry should be considered in those military occupational specialties with the potential for increased exposure to respiratory hazards, such as firefighters.[25] Additionally, some consideration should be given to spirometry for those persons who fail the aerobic event of a physical fitness test to rule out subclinical lung disease as part of an overall evaluation. However, use of physical fitness testing as the sole criterion fails to understand the complexities of dyspnea and cardiovascular fitness.

REFERENCES

1. Rose C, Abraham J, Harkins D, et al. Overview and recommendations for medical screening and diagnostic evaluation for post-deployment lung disease in returning US warfighters. *J Occup Environ Med*. 2012;54:746–751.

2. Townsend MC, Lockey JE, Velez H, et al. ACOEM position statement. Spirometry in the occupational setting. American College of Occupational and Environmental Medicine. *J Occup Environ Med*. 2000;42:228–245.

3. US Department of Labor. Medical Screening and Surveillance. Occupational Safety and Health Administration, 2011. http://www.osha.gov/SLTC/medicalsurveillance/index.html. Accessed October 16, 2012.

4. National Institute for Occupational Safety and Health. *Proposed National Strategy for the Prevention of Occupational Lung Diseases*. Atlanta, GA: NIOSH; 1986. DHHS (NIOSH) Publication 89-128.

5. Hankinson JL, Wagner GR. Medical screening using periodic spirometry for detection of chronic lung disease. *Occup Med*. 1993;8:353–361.

6. Hnizdo E, Sircar K, Yan T, et al. Limits of longitudinal decline for the interpretation of annual changes in FEV_1 in individuals. *Occup Environ Med*. 2007;64:701–707.

7. Balmes J, Becklake M, Blanc P, et al. American Thoracic Society Statement: occupational contribution to the burden of airway disease. *Am J Respir Crit Care Med*. 2003;167:787–797.

8. Qaseem A, Snow V, Shekelle P, et al. Clinical Efficacy Assessment Subcommittee of the American College of Physicians. Diagnosis and management of stable chronic obstructive pulmonary disease: a clinical practice guideline from the American College of Physicians. *Ann Intern Med*. 2007;147:633–638.

9. U.S. Preventive Services Task Force. Screening for chronic obstructive pulmonary disease using spirometry: U.S. Preventive Services Task Force Recommendation Statement. *Ann Intern Med*. 2008;148:529–534.

10. Hardie JA, Buist AS, Vollmer WM, et al. Risk of over-diagnosis of COPD in asymptomatic elderly never-smokers. *Eur Respir J*. 2002;20:1117–1122.

11. Vedal S, Crapo RO. False positive rates of multiple pulmonary function tests in healthy subjects. *Bull Eur Physiopathol Respir*. 1983;19:263–266.

12. Abramson JM, Wollan P, Kurland M, Yawn BP. Feasibility of school-based spirometry screening for asthma. *J Sch Health*. 2003;73:150–153.

13. Herbert R, Moline J, Skloot G, et al. The World Trade Center disaster and the health of workers: five-year assessment of a unique medical screening program. *Environ Health Perspect*. 2006;114:1853–1858.

14. Mannino DM, Ford ES, Redd SC. Obstructive and restrictive lung disease and functional limitation: data from the Third National Health and Nutrition Examination. *J Intern Med*. 2003;254:540–547.

15. Aldrich TK, Gustave J, Hall CB, et al. Lung function in rescue workers at the World Trade Center after 7 years. *N Engl J Med*. 2010;362:1263–1272.

16. Sanders JW, Putnam SD, Frankart C, et al. Impact of illness and non-combat injury during Operations Iraqi Freedom and Enduring Freedom (Afghanistan). *Am J Trop Med Hyg*. 2005;73:713–719.

17. Smith B, Wong CA, Smith TC, et al. Newly reported respiratory symptoms and conditions among military personnel deployed to Iraq and Afghanistan: a prospective population-based study. *Am J Epidemiol*. 2009;70:1433–1442.

18. Petruccelli BP, Goldenbaum M, Scott B, et al. Health effects of the 1991 Kuwait oil fires: a survey of US army troops. *J Occup Environ Med*. 1999;41:433–439.

19. Roop SA, Niven AS, Calvin BE, et al. The prevalence and impact of respiratory symptoms in asthmatics and non-asthmatics during deployment. *Mil Med*. 2007;172:1264–1269.

20. Szema AM, Peters MC, Weissinger KM, et al. New-onset asthma among soldiers serving in Iraq and Afghanistan. *Allergy Asthma Proc*. 2010;31:67–71.

21. Delvecchio S, Zacher L, Morris M. Correlation of asthma with deployment in active duty military personnel [abstract]. *Chest*. 2010;138:145A.

22. Matthews T, Morris M. The effect of deployment on COPD in active duty military [abstract]. *Chest*. 2011;140:581A.

23. Townsend MC, the Occupational and Environmental Lung Disorders Committee. Spirometry in the occupational health setting—2011 update. *J Occup Environ Med.* 2011;53:569–584.

24. Zacher LL, Browning R, Bisnett T, et al. Clarifications from representatives of the Department of Defense regarding the article "Recommendations for medical screening and diagnostic evaluation for postdeployment lung disease in returning US warfighters." *J Occup Environ Med.* 2012;54:760–761.

25. US Department of Defense. *Occupational Medical Examinations and Surveillance Manual.* Washington, DC: DoD; 2007. DoD Manual 6055.05-M.

Chapter 10

SPIROMETRY MONITORING AND PREVENTION USING SPIROLA SOFTWARE

EVA HNIZDO, PhD*; AND CARA HALLDIN, PhD†

*Epidemiologist, Division of Respiratory Disease Studies, National Institute for Occupational Safety and Health, Centers for Disease Control and Prevention, 1095 Willowdale Road, Morgantown, West Virginia 26505-2888

†Epidemiologist, Division of Respiratory Disease Studies, National Institute for Occupational Safety and Health, Centers for Disease Control and Prevention, 1095 Willowdale Road, Morgantown, West Virginia 26505-2888

INTRODUCTION

Several medical and case studies indicate a potential association between military deployment-related environmental exposures and postdeployment chronic respiratory conditions among US Army service members. Pulmonary conditions and diseases of concern include obstructive airways disease, symptom of breathlessness, asthma, bronchiolitis, and interstitial pulmonary disease.[1,2] Suspected attributable exposures include high concentrations of particulate matter generated by various sources, including smoke from oil well fires,[3] sand exposure from sandstorms,[4,5] smoke from burn pits, and smoking.[6,7] Data from the Millennium Cohort Study suggest a >25% increase in chest symptoms among US Army service members after deployment compared with predeployment.[8] Nevertheless, there is still lack of conclusive epidemiological evidence on an association between adverse respiratory health effects and deployment airborne exposure and on the severity of the associated respiratory outcomes, especially their longer term effect on pulmonary function and general fitness. The lack of conclusive evidence is at least in part from lack of systematic data on baseline (predeployment) and postdeployment respiratory health status in individuals and on respiratory exposure to particulate matter during deployment.

Prevention of environmental and lifestyle exposures that may lead to chronic airway diseases, such as chronic obstructive pulmonary disease (COPD) and asthma, are important because these diseases often profoundly diminish the affected individual's quality of life and are associated with premature functional impairment and disability, early retirement from work, and increased future morbidity and mortality.[9–13] Fortunately, most respiratory diseases can be prevented through early recognition of the risk and effective interventions directed at controlling known risk factors, including environmental, occupational, and lifestyle exposures.[14–18]

In general, the respiratory health status of a population at risk can be established using respiratory questionnaires and spirometric measurements of pulmonary function. Although baseline and periodic spirometry for the whole deployed military population may be logistically challenging, periodic evaluation by spirometry and questionnaire could be done for groups or individuals a priori known to be likely at risk of exposure to harmful respiratory agents. This would help to identify hazardous exposures, establish their effect on the prevalence and severity of respiratory conditions, and provide information for prevention. Also, to ensure that there are no longer term consequences of the observed adverse respiratory health effects, the exposed or affected individuals, or smaller representative groups, may be included in a postdeployment periodic spirometry monitoring for at least 5 years to investigate the longer term consequences of the various exposures or deployment-related respiratory conditions.

Computerized spirometry data and appropriate software can be used to assist healthcare providers manage and interpret periodic spirometry data and thus help in achieving the full potential of spirometry monitoring in disease prevention and management. In this chapter, an easy-to-use visual and analytical tool known as SPIROLA (Spirometry Longitudinal Data Analysis) software (Morgantown, WV)[19]—designed for use by healthcare providers as an aid in spirometry monitoring—is described. The SPIROLA methodology and functions are outlined, and results from its application in ongoing monitoring programs are presented. Software and instructions for use can be downloaded free of charge from the Internet.[19]

RESPIRATORY HEALTH EVALUATION AND SPIROMETRY MONITORING

Monitoring of spirometric measurements in occupational settings is widely accepted as a key step in recognizing the early (preclinical) obstructive and restrictive lung diseases and in maintaining respiratory and general fitness to wear respiratory protection.[20,21] Spirometric measurements of forced expiratory volume in 1 second (FEV_1) and forced vital capacity (FVC), as well as the ratio of FEV_1:FVC are most commonly used for establishing and monitoring respiratory health in at-risk populations (eg, firefighters, cotton dust-exposed workers, miners, construction workers exposed to silica dust, and diacetyl-exposed workers[22]). Professional recommendations emphasize several key steps in achieving the full potential of spirometry monitoring in disease prevention and management. These recommendations include

- maintaining acceptable spirometry quality and accuracy through adherence to American Thoracic Society (ATS) and European Respiratory Society (ERS) standards;[23]
- maintaining acceptable longitudinal data precision (ie, low variability of lung function measurements over time in individuals);[24–26]
- applying interpretative strategies that have good sensitivity, yet sufficient specificity, to identify individuals at risk of experiencing excessive loss of lung function and developing functional impairment;[25] and
- using health monitoring results (including symptoms) to target and monitor intervention, including medical treatment.[20,21,27]

METHODS OF LONGITUDINAL SPIROMETRY DATA EVALUATION

Generally, the main objective of spirometry monitoring is to identify individuals at risk of developing lung function impairment (ie, those with abnormally low lung function or those with excessive decline in lung function). Identification of individuals with low lung function has been described elsewhere in detail[23] and will not be covered here. In healthy working populations, including the military, most individuals are likely to have normal lung function, but may develop—in response to hazardous exposures—adverse changes in the lungs that may lead to excessive decline in lung function and long-term consequences. Thus, one of the objectives in workplace spirometry monitoring is to characterize the time-related pattern of lung function decline to identify individuals whose lung function decline is excessive and may be at risk of developing lung function impairment. This section briefly describes methods recommended to identify individuals whose decline in lung function is greater than expected and the method for monitoring longitudinal spirometry data precision and quality.

The most suitable of the spirometry measures for evaluation of lung function changes over time is FEV_1 because it is least prone to measurement error and is decreased in both obstructive and restrictive impairment. In healthy adults who never smoked and have normal body weight, FEV_1 declines at about 27 mL/yr (starting at around 27 years of age), and the decline appears to be linear over the working lifetime.[28]

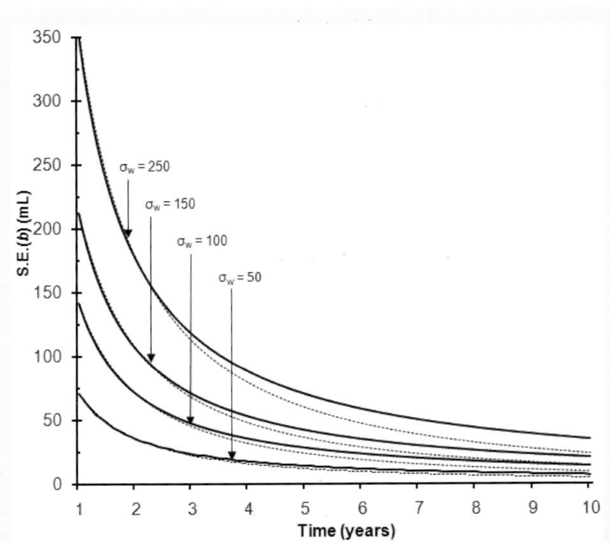

Figure 10-1. Decline in SE(b) in relation to follow-up time and varying within-person variation s_w. *Solid line* is based on two measurements (ie, baseline and a measurement at a specific year). *Dotted line* is based on all annual measurements.
SE: standard error

However, because of inherent within-person variability in the spirometry measurements, it generally takes 5 or more years to establish the rate of lung function decline in individuals reliably.[25,26,29]

It can be shown with simple linear regression model statistics why at least 5 years of follow-up are needed, and how the longitudinal data variability affects the duration of follow-up needed to estimate the rate of decline with sufficient precision. The rate of decline in FEV_1 with age can be estimated using a simple linear regression model:

$$(1) \quad FEV_1 = a + b \times \text{age},$$

where slope b represents the rate of FEV_1 change (eg, mL/yr).[28,29] In addition, the variability of longitudinal FEV_1 measurements around the predicted line, as measured by its standard error, SE(b), then determines the precision of the estimated rate of decline (b). Figure 10-1 shows how the estimated SE(b), shown for four individuals with varying inherent within-person variation (from a low of 50 mL to a high of 250 mL), decreases with increasing years of follow-up. The solid line is based on two measurements (ie, baseline and a test taken at a specific year), and the dotted line is based on annual measurements. The one-sided 95% upper confidence limit (95% UCL) for the person's rate of decline measured by slope b is then calculated as

$$(2) \quad 95\% \text{ UCL} = b + 1.645 \text{ SE}(b).$$

Given that the rate of decline usually ranges from about 20 to 90 mL/yr, it takes approximately 5 to 8 years to estimate an individual's rate of decline with sufficient precision, depending on the magnitude of the individual's within-person variation.

Figure 10-1 demonstrates two important aspects in longitudinal spirometry data evaluation. First, it is important to maintain good quality of the spirometry tests to keep the longitudinal data variability as low as possible so that the signal from the effect of environmental exposure or disease process can be detected. Second, in prospectively collected spirometry data where testing is done on an annual or less frequent basis, the slopes provided by the linear regression model during the first 5 years are generally imprecise and may not provide a reliable estimate of the "true" rate of decline which, on average, ranges around 30 mL/yr in healthy people who never smoked.[25,29–32] Nevertheless, during the early period of spirometry monitoring from 0 to 5 years, there is a need to determine whether a person's observed decline in lung function exceeds what would be predicted based on an expected rate of decline and expected FEV_1 data variability.[30,31,33] The ATS recommends a limit of annual

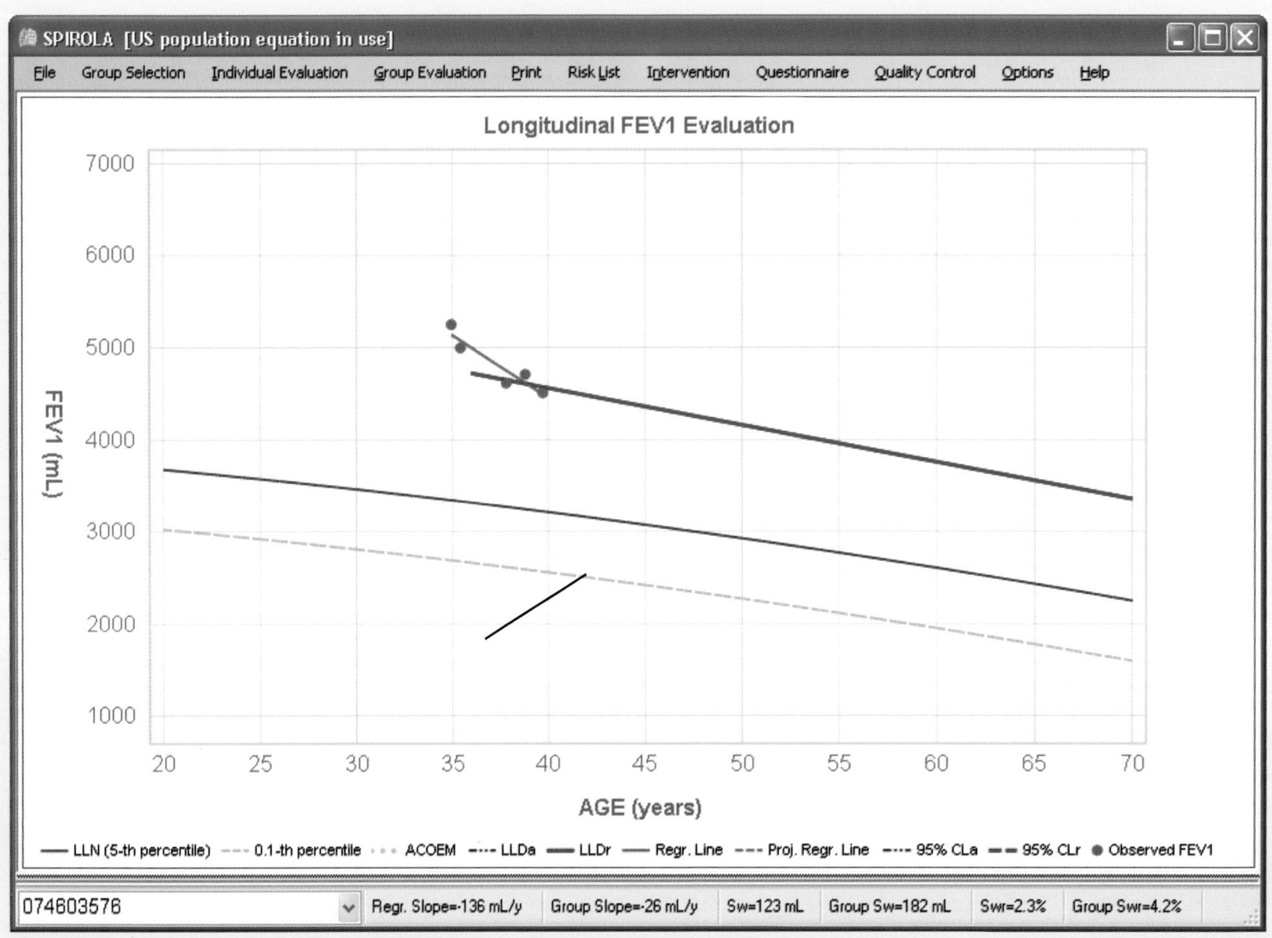

Figure 10-2. Screen capture of a SPIROLA chart that shows longitudinal FEV_1 data for an individual plotted against age, in relation to cross-sectional lower limit of normal (LLN; *purple line*), the limit of longitudinal decline (LLD; *blue line*), and the lower 0.1th percentile (approximately comparable to 60% predicted; *yellow line*).
ACOEM: American College of Occupational and Environmental Medicine; CLa: absolute confidence limit; CLr: relative confidence limit; FEV1: forced expiratory volume in 1 sec; LLDa: absolute limit of longitudinal decline; LLDr: relative limit of longitudinal decline; Proj.: projected; Regr.: regression; Sw: within-person variation; Swr: relative within-person variation; y: year

decline for FEV_1 of 15% as a clinically significant decline.[33] The American College of Occupational and Environmental Medicine (ACOEM) has proposed a longitudinal reference limit based on a 15% annual FEV_1 decline for working populations.[21] However, the fixed limit of 15% may be too wide for maintaining acceptable data precision in a relatively healthy workforce, and has low sensitivity to detect acute adverse effects in some workplace situations where excessive decline over a short period of time has been observed (eg, diacetyl-exposed workers).[34,35]

Computer software, such as SPIROLA, helps to maintain acceptable longitudinal data precision through monitoring of longitudinal data variability. Knowing the variability of the existing data also allows the user to tailor the limit of longitudinal decline (LLD) so that it reflects existing data precision. With increasing data precision, the longitudinal limit can be made more sensitive than the ACOEM recommended 15%. If an individual's FEV_1 decline exceeds LLD, a first step in the evaluation should include an increase in precision of the longitudinal measurements by review of data quality or retesting in the near future, before further steps are taken. Generally, after 5 to 8 years of follow-up, the individual's own regression slope reaches sufficient precision and can be used for decision-making.[25,29,34] Figure 10-2 shows a screen capture from SPIROLA with an example of longitudinal spirometry data for an individual with 5 years of follow-up data, plotted in relation to the estimated lower 5th percentile (lower limit of normal or LLN) for a person of the same age, height, gender, and race, and in relation to the LLD. Although the observed FEV_1 values are within the "normal" range (ie, they are above the LLN), the decline in FEV_1 is excessive when evaluated in relation to LLD.

SPIROLA SOFTWARE FUNCTIONS AND METHODS OF EVALUATION

SPIROLA provides functions for group and individual data evaluation. Group data evaluation is designed to help maintain good spirometry data quality, low within-person variation for the longitudinal FEV_1 and FVC data, and stable mean lung function values for the group over time. Individual data evaluation helps to identify individuals with low lung function values or those with excessive lung function decline or variability.

The following sections demonstrate each function and usefulness of SPIROLA to healthcare providers and provide examples of the application of SPIROLA to data from several ongoing monitoring programs.

Functions for Evaluation of Data at a Group Level

Monitoring Longitudinal Data Precision

Monitoring the program's within-person variation, overall and by individual technicians or centers, helps to maintain longitudinal data precision at an acceptable level and allows prompt investigation into the source of increased variation (eg, instrument malfunction, procedural errors, effects of exposure on lung function, and technician-related errors).[36,37] The program's data variation can be monitored on an annual basis using the absolute or relative pair-wise, within-person variation statistics.[34]

Example Data. Application of SPIROLA in 2005 for the evaluation of data precision in a monitoring program conducted on about 2,500 firefighters prompted concerns about spirometry quality. Figure 10-3 shows that the annual values of absolute (left axis) and relative (right axis) pair-wise, within-person variation for FEV_1 had declined gradually from the program's inception in 1988 until 1999—indicating improving data quality and precision—but then the statistics indicated a marked increase in data variability from 2000. At that time, a volumetric spirometer, used since 1988, had been replaced by a new flow-based spirometer. Usage of the new spirometer resulted in a marked increase in spirometry data variability after 2000. Application of SPIROLA in 2005 led to recognition of the problem and prompted intervention to improve spirometry quality and involved the following measures:

- replacing a flow-based spirometer with a volumetric spirometer in December 2005;
- using a computerized central-quality control by a senior technician from September 2006; and
- monitoring of SPIROLA's indicators of spirometry quality and data variability from January 2008.

Taken together, the interventions resulted in a substantial decrease in the relative within-person variation from 2006 to 4%. The relative within-person variation of about 4% from 2006 to 2011 (Figure 10-3, red line and right axis) signifies acceptable data precision and corresponds to an annual LLD value of $\approx$10%.[19]

Monitoring Spirometry Quality Control

Monitoring test quality grades assigned by a spirometer at a testing session indicates what percentage of tests adheres to the ATS/ERS recommendations. To help optimize the spirometry quality control for the monitoring program and individual technicians, SPIROLA analyzes the quality grades assigned by a spirometer at a testing session[19,38,39] and monitors on a quarterly basis the percentage of tests that meets the ATS/ERS criteria for acceptability and repeatability, and the percentage of tests that meets repeatability criteria only (ie, $\leq$150 mL between the two best FEV_1 and FVC measurements).[19]

Example Data. Figure 10-4 shows a SPIROLA chart generated from the analysis of the firefighters' data: quality indices as assigned by a spirometer; within-test repeatability; and relative pair-wise, within-person variation. The figure shows the percentage of tests of acceptable quality (ie, grades A, B, and C); the unacceptable quality includes grades D and F. In this example, data are summarized across all technicians by quartiles. The charts of individual technicians can also be shown. From the onset, a large percentage of FVC tests did not meet the ATS/ERS criteria of quality. Additional training in 2008 helped to improve acceptability of FVC measurements by 2010; most of the unacceptable tests failed to fulfill the end-of-test criteria. Reviewing the charts of individual technicians prompted technician-specific tailored guidance toward improvements.[36]

Monitoring the Group Mean Forced Expiratory Volume in One Second and Forced Vital Capacity Values

Time trends in mean FEV_1 and FVC are displayed to help identify effects taking place at a group level (eg, because of an occupational hazard or a smoking cessation program). To adjust for time-related changes in a group's demographics, SPIROLA also monitors the mean-predicted values estimated from standard or user-supplied reference equations and the z-score. The z-score reflects the mean difference between the observed and predicted values in standard deviation units.

Example Data. Improved spirometry quality and longitudinal data precision resulted in more accurate and precise

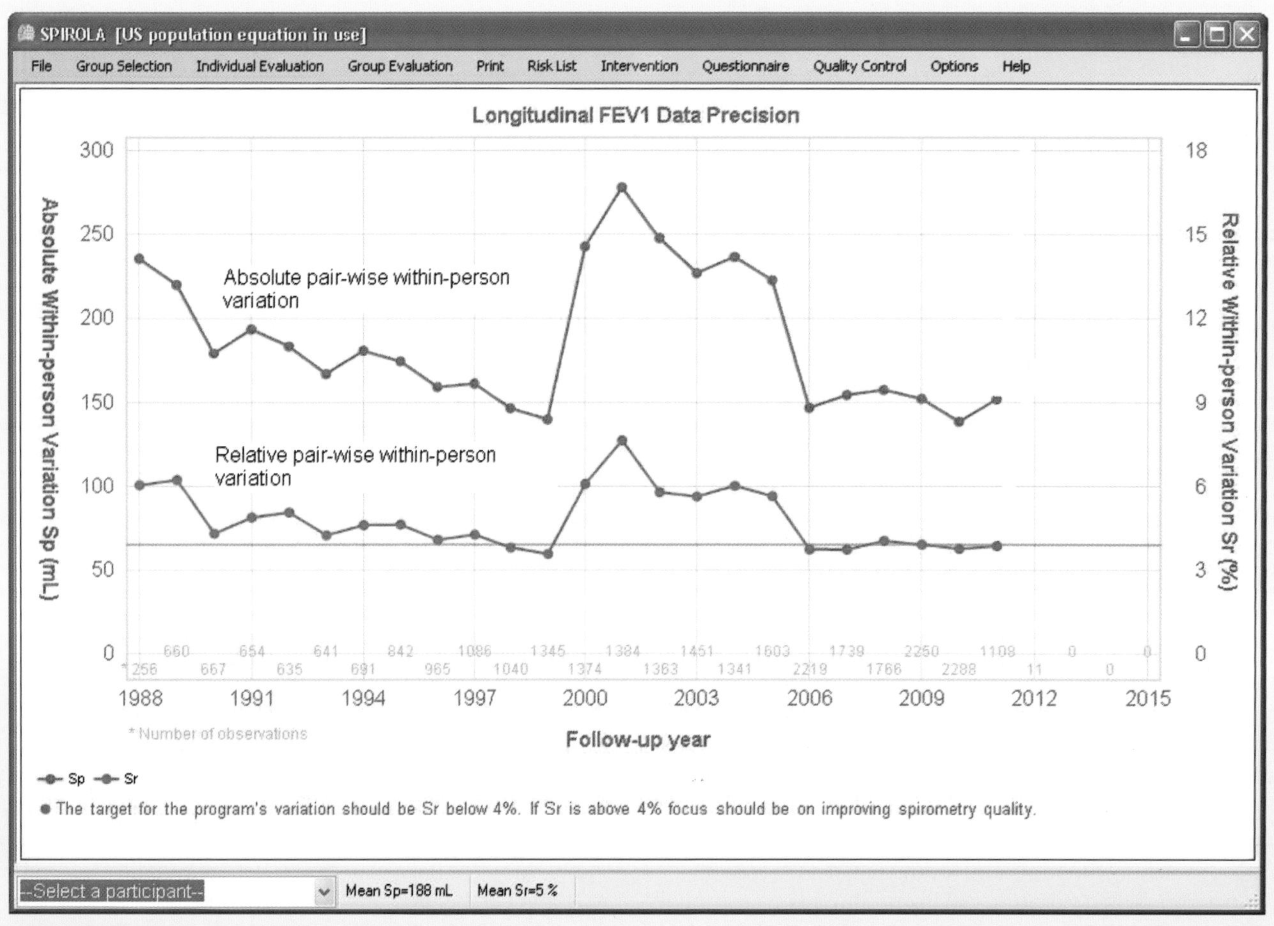

Figure 10-3. Screen capture of a SPIROLA chart for evaluation of longitudinal FEV_1 data precision measured by pair-wise, within-person variation (absolute in mL, *green line*; relative in %, *red line*). Within-person variation of 4% is the desirable level of precision.
FEV1: forced expiratory volume in 1 sec; Sp: absolute within-person variation; Sr: relative within-person variation

lung function values. Figure 10-5 shows the observed mean FVC values plotted against time (green line) in relation to the mean predicted values (yellow line) and the z-score (red line). Because there were no changes in the employment or hiring pattern since the intervention onset in 2005, the increase in the observed means in relation to the predicted means and the increase in the z-scores (red line) was mainly from the improvement in spirometry quality.

Screening for Individuals With Abnormal Results

The individuals identified to have abnormal lung function results appear in the Risk List function, which provides summary statistics on the number screened and found with a specific type of abnormal results. The summary results from one of the monitoring programs (Figure 10-6) show that there were 5,632 workers who had at least one spirometry test during the screening period. The Risk List then shows the number of workers identified with a potential abnormality in lung function: the last observation below LLN, and excessive decline or variation in FEV_1 or FVC. The healthcare provider can then choose participants with a selected condition and click on the "Evaluate" button to assess data for the chosen individuals.

Functions for Evaluation of Data at an Individual Level

Evaluating the Most Recent Spirometry Test Results

As recommended by the ATS, ERS, and ACOEM, the most recent best FEV_1, FVC, and FEV_1/FVC values are compared with US population-based reference values (default)[21,23,40] or with user-defined reference values. Individuals whose values are below the LLN (ie, values that have a 5% probability of being normal in a healthy nonsmoker population) are identified for further evaluation and recorded in the Risk List.

Evaluating Longitudinal Changes in Forced Expiratory Volume in One Second and Forced Vital Capacity

Time trends for FEV_1, FVC, and their percentage of predicted values and the FEV_1/FVC ratio are displayed graphically. During the first 7 years of follow-up, SPIROLA applies the LLD criterion to identify FEV_1 and FVC measurements that decline excessively from the baseline measurement(s). The LLD can be specified in absolute values or in relative values as percentage, or as the ACOEM limit based on the annual limit of 15%.[20,21] Beginning with 4 years of follow-up, changes in the rate of FEV_1 decline from each longitudinal data point are monitored graphically. The latter function is useful in monitoring the effect of intervention or identification of events leading to deterioration in the rate of decline. Beginning with 8 years of follow-up, SPIROLA evaluates whether an individual is at risk of developing FEV_1 values that have a low probability of being normal (ie, <0.1 percentile, which is comparable with 60% predicted, as defined by ATS as moderate impairment), based on the level of FEV_1 and the rate of FEV_1 decline.

Evaluating Longitudinal Forced Expiratory Volume in One Second and Force Vital Capacity Data Variability

Within-person variation in FEV_1 and FVC is calculated when there are three or more longitudinal measurements and evaluated for the probability of being normal.

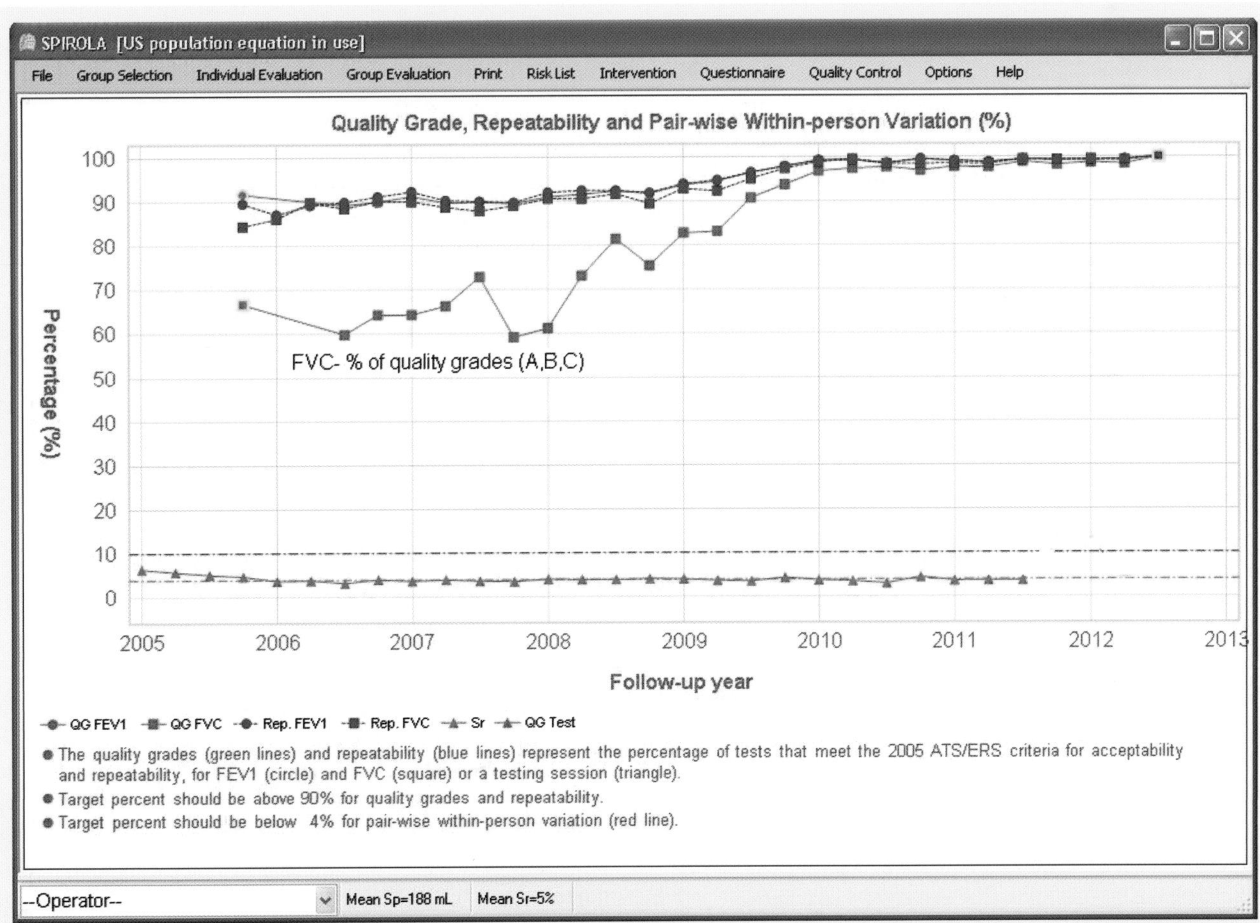

Figure 10-4. Screen capture of a SPIROLA chart that shows the percentage of tests that meet the ATS/ERS criteria for acceptability and repeatability for FVC (*green squares*) and FEV_1 (*green circles*); repeatability (respective *blue lines*); and relative pair-wise, within-person variation (*red line*). This is also a summary chart by all technicians and quartiles. ATS: American Thoracic Society; ERS: European Thoracic Society; FEV1: forced expiratory volume in 1 sec; FVC: forced vital capacity; QG: quality grade; Rep: repeatability; Sp: absolute within-person variation; Sr: relative within-person variation

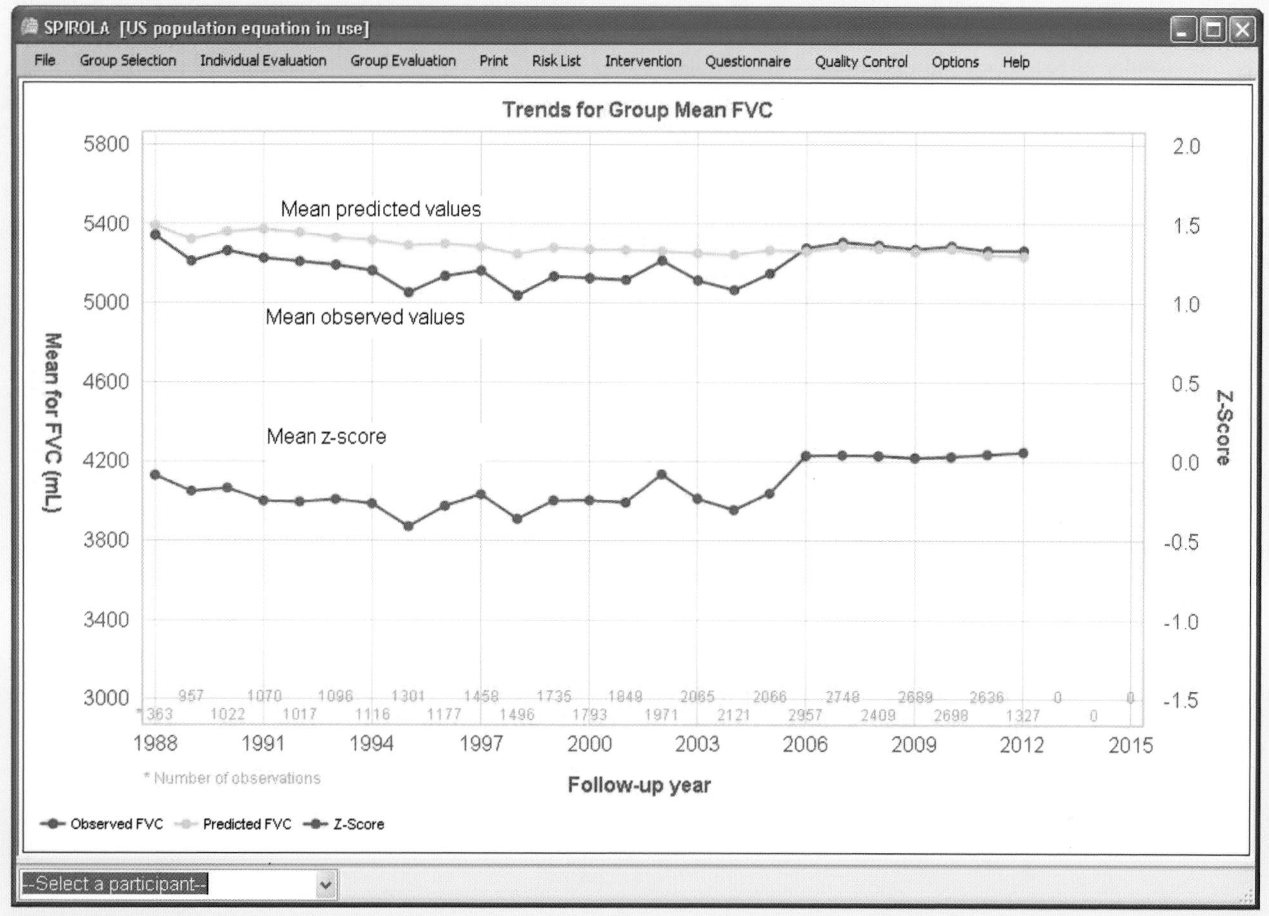

Figure 10-5. Screen capture of a SPIROLA chart that shows group means for observed FVC data (*green line*) and the predicted (*yellow line*) and z-scores (*red line*), by year.
FVC: forced vital capacity

Reporting an Individual's Results

An individual's reports display results of data analyses together with demographic data. If there are abnormal findings, the individual report suggests steps to be considered in further evaluation. These steps include the following:

- assessment of the individual's longitudinal data—obvious outliers can be excluded temporarily from the analysis;
- review of the baseline and most recent spirometry tracings and test quality;
- retesting in the near future to confirm the results; and
- recommendation of further steps, such as medical evaluation and intervention on potential risk factors, but only if abnormal test results are confirmed.

Tagging Individuals for Further Evaluation

The SPIROLA software enables the user to create a list of individuals for quality control or retesting and intervention.

Examples of an Individual's Data Evaluation

The first step in the evaluation of an individual's data is to view the longitudinal trends. Figure 10-7 shows SPIROLA's multiple charts of longitudinal data for FEV_1, FVC, and the FEV_1/FVC ratio for an individual with less than 8 years of follow-up. Although the most recent lung function values were above the LLN (ie, the lung function levels are within normal limits), the FEV_1 and FVC are below LLD for the last two measurements, indicating excessive decline for both FEV and FVC.

Figure 10-8 shows longitudinal data for an individual with

8 or more years of follow-up. The individual was identified as having an excessive decline based on the regression slope and an increased risk of developing moderate impairment (ie, FEV_1 value that has <0.1% probability of being normal when compared with the US population of healthy nonsmokers). The 0.1% corresponds to 60% predicted (ie, moderate impairment).

The first step in the evaluation is to confirm the results by reviewing the longitudinal data, the quality of the baseline and last tests, and retesting, if needed, to increase longitudinal data precision. If an obvious outlier is observed, a data point can be temporarily deleted from the analysis. If the abnormal findings are confirmed, the individual should be referred for further medical evaluation to investigate whether there is respiratory abnormality because of a specific condition or disease and, if needed, intervention on potential risk factors should be initiated. Results should be discussed with an individual to motivate participation in interventions directed at controlling occupational and nonoccupational risk factors. Because of confidentiality issues, an individual's results should not be made available to the employer; only group summary findings should be provided to the healthcare provider to motivate preventive measures in the workplace.

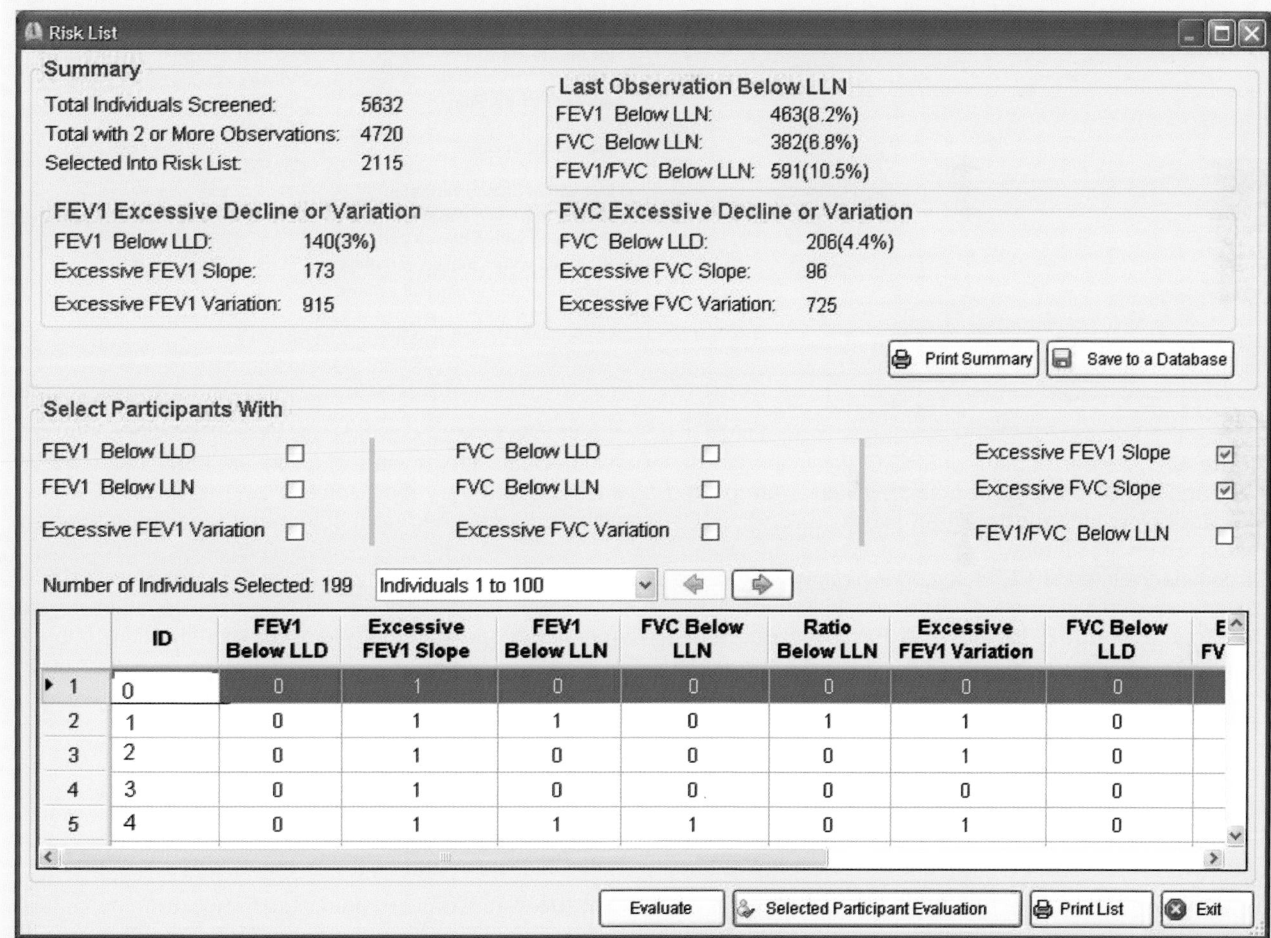

Figure 10-6. Screen capture of the SPIROLA Risk List function. Summary results from automatic screening for individuals at risk for having abnormal lung function or excessive decline in lung function. De-identified data obtained from spirometry monitoring program conducted on firefighters.

FEV1: forced expiratory volume in 1 sec; FVC: forced vital capacity; ID: identification; LLD: limit of longitudinal decline; LLN: lower limit of normal

Data source: Hnizdo E, Hakobyan A, Fleming J, Beeckman-Wagner L. Periodic spirometry in occupational setting: improving quality, accuracy, and precision. *J Occup Environ Med.* 2011;53:1205–1209.

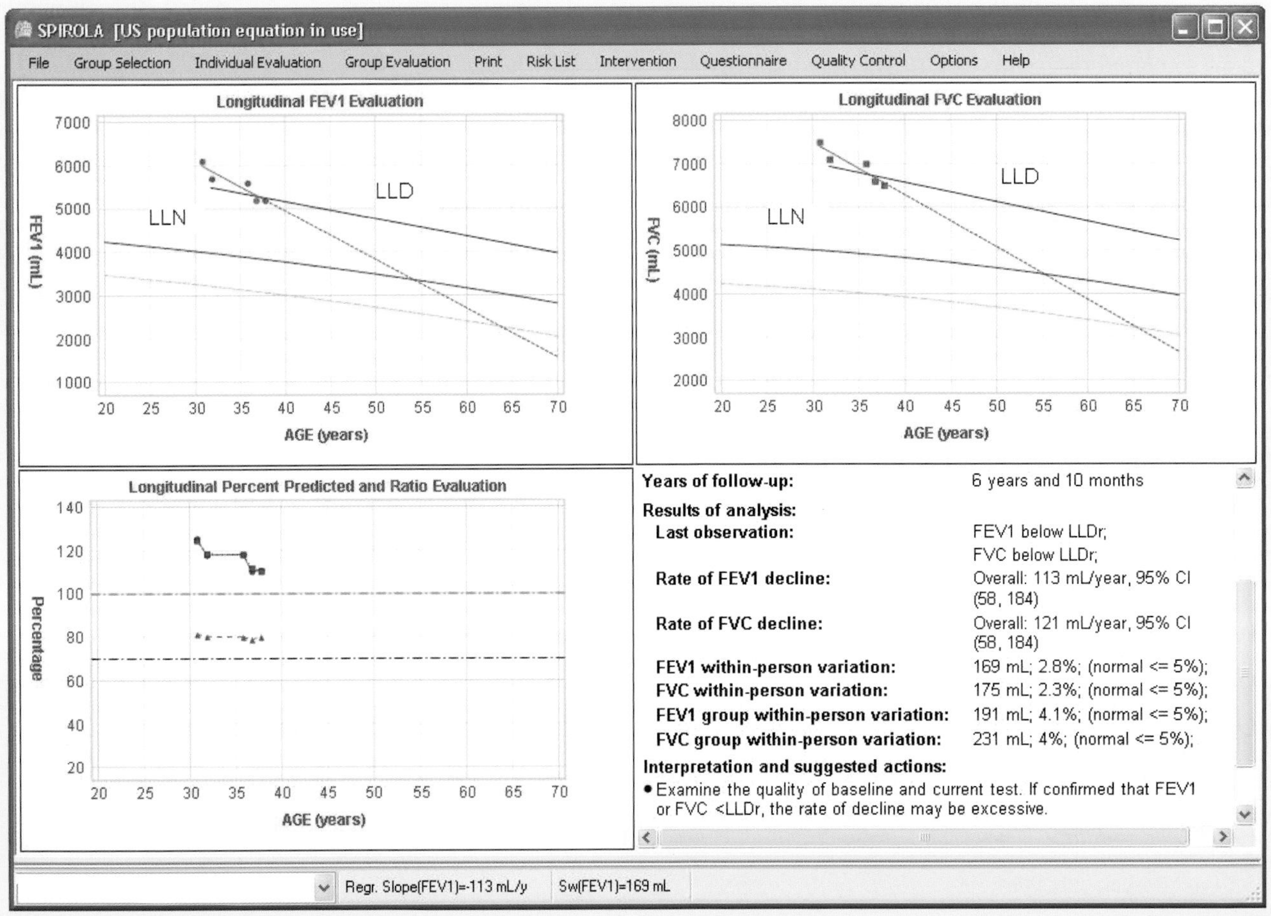

Figure 10-7. Screen capture of SPIROLA multiple charts for an individual with <8 years of follow-up. Longitudinal FEV_1, FVC, and the percentage of predicted values are plotted against age and the report summarizing findings. FEV_1 and FVC are below LLD, indicating an excessive decline. De-identified data obtained from spirometry monitoring program conducted on firefighters.
CI: confidence interval; FEV1: forced expiratory volume in 1 sec; FVC: forced vital capacity; LLD: limit of longitudinal decline; LLDr: relative limit of longitudinal decline; LLN: lower limit of normal; Regr.: regression; Sw: within-person variation; y: year
Data source: Hnizdo E, Hakobyan A, Fleming J, Beeckman-Wagner L. Periodic spirometry in occupational setting: improving quality, accuracy, and precision. *J Occup Environ Med.* 2011;53:1205–1209.

Software Environment and Data Requirement

SPIROLA runs on the PC and requires Microsoft Windows 2000/XP/Vista/Windows 7, Microsoft .NET Framework 2.0, and Microsoft Database Engine (which are Microsoft default options). The User Guide, available on the Internet[19] or from SPIROLA's Help menu, describes the installation procedure, data input, functions, and theoretical background on which the data analysis is based. The SPIROLA databases should be kept in a secured folder or in a secured shared folder, if needed.

At a minimum, SPIROLA requires the following data:

- a unique personal identifier,
- age,
- height,
- race/ethnicity,
- best FEV_1 and FVC test values, and
- date of test.

Where the spirometry system assigns quality grades from each testing session (i.e., quality grades for acceptability and repeatability), these data can be also uploaded into the SPIROLA database and analyzed by SPIROLA. Data for intervention decision-making (eg, weight, occupational exposure factors, smoking data, and questionnaire responses) can be included in the database for display in individual records. Also, a direct link can be created between a spirometer and SPIROLA.[19]

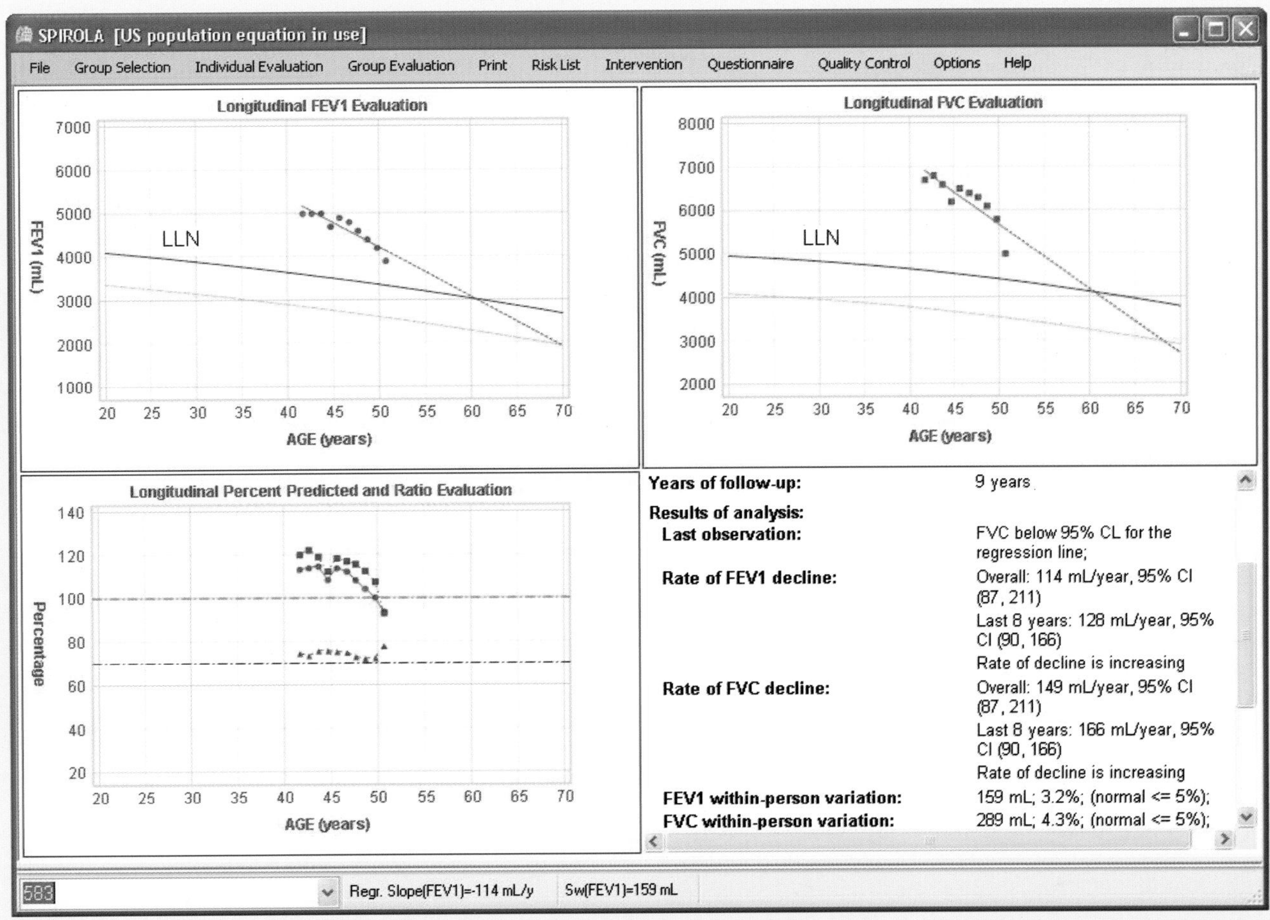

Figure 10-8. Screen capture of a SPIROLA chart shows results for an individual with >8 years of follow-up. Regression lines for FEV_1 and FVC can be projected to indicate whether the person is at risk for developing moderate airflow obstruction based on the LLN and 0.01th percentile. De-identified data obtained from spirometry monitoring program conducted on firefighters.
CI: confidence interval; CL: confidence limit; FEV1: forced expiratory volume in 1 sec; FVC: forced vital capacity; LLN: lower limit of normal; Regr.: regression; Sw: within-person variation; y: year
Data source: Hnizdo E, Hakobyan A, Fleming J, Beeckman-Wagner L. Periodic spirometry in occupational setting: improving quality, accuracy, and precision. *J Occup Environ Med.* 2011;53:1205–1209.

SPIROLA's main menu options are easy to operate and allow for a spirometry file selection, a group selection and evaluation, evaluation of an individual's data, monitoring of longitudinal spirometry data precision and tests quality scores, and automatic selection of individuals whose tests need review because of abnormal findings.

DISCUSSION

Periodic spirometry is often recommended for individuals with actual and potential exposures to respiratory hazards.[20,21] To achieve the full potential of spirometry-based medical monitoring in detecting a signal due to adverse health effects, it is necessary to maintain acceptable test quality and apply interpretive strategies that have high sensitivity and specificity in identifying individuals at risk of developing lung function impairment. Longitudinal data precision determines how soon and how reliably a "true" excessive decline can be identified (Figure 10-1).[34]

SPIROLA software was developed as a visual and analytical tool to assist healthcare professionals in addressing challenges arising from monitoring the respiratory health of individuals potentially at risk.[19] The software is intended to assist the user in assembling the information required to make medical decisions; however, it cannot be substituted for competent and informed professional judgment.

To assist in the evaluation of the practical utility of SPIROLA, managers of several ongoing spirometry-based health surveillance programs have adopted use of the software. The results from monitoring programs conducted on US workers reported here demonstrate that the information displayed by SPIROLA on longitudinal data precision can assist the healthcare professionals in determining potential sources of excess variability (eg, a change in spirometry systems and procedural errors) and recognizing when an intervention on data quality is needed and, subsequently, whether the intervention improved longitudinal data precision (Figures 10-3, 10-4, and 10-5). SPIROLA can also aid in optimizing the performance of individual technicians through the spirometry quality grades analysis (Figure 10-5). Although appropriate equipment, trained technicians, knowledgeable professional oversight, and comprehensive procedure manuals are basic components of a quality testing program,[20,21] data precision can vary over time for various reasons, and such changes may not be noticeable on individual tests.[36]

The estimate of data precision provided by the software affords additional benefits during the interpretation of longitudinal change for individuals. It facilitates determination of an appropriate limit of longitudinal decline, LLD, a criterion applied by SPIROLA software to maintain longitudinal data precision and detect early (within 8 years) excessive lung function decline. The LLD method increases flexibility to develop stringent quality control and to increase sensitivity for detecting long-term excessive decline or acute respiratory effects under different monitoring conditions.[34] The knowledge of group longitudinal data precision and data quality increases the likelihood of discerning whether an observed change in lung function is from procedural error or incipient lung disease. However, workplace or environmental factors may be responsible for increased FEV_1 and FVC variabilities by causing respiratory illness.

Because COPD is a preventable disease that usually takes many years to develop, early recognition of abnormal pulmonary function decline followed by an effective intervention is important in disease prevention.[14] The longitudinal assessment over all follow-up years based on evaluation that takes into account data variability, as done by SPIROLA, helps to improve the accuracy of recognition of the development of respiratory disease. By helping to improve longitudinal data precision, SPIROLA improves the precision of the estimated rate of decline and identification of those with a true excessive rate of decline. Furthermore, the Risk List function helps the healthcare provider to identify individuals whose spirometry results may be abnormal and who may need further evaluation; this function is especially useful in occupational settings where a large number of workers undergo spirometry monitoring.

A limitation of this work is that the long-term implications of the application of SPIROLA for disease prevention have not yet been fully evaluated in ongoing monitoring programs.

All the data presented in this chapter are from a project that has been approved by the NIOSH Human Subject Review Board.

SUMMARY

Prevention of environmental and lifestyle exposures that increase the risk of lung function impairment and disease is important because these conditions often profoundly diminish the affected individual's quality of life. These conditions are also associated with premature functional impairment and disability, early retirement from work, and increased future morbidity and mortality.

Prevention through early recognition and effective interventions directed at controlling known risk factors—including environmental, occupational, and lifestyle exposures—is possible in spirometry monitoring of at-risk populations.

SPIROLA software is designed to assist healthcare providers in managing and interpreting periodic spirometric measurements. Thus, this helps to achieve the full potential of spirometry monitoring in disease prevention and management.

Application of SPIROLA in an ongoing spirometry monitoring program has helped to identify previously unrecognized increases in longitudinal data variability from equipment and procedural problems. It also helped to demonstrate that subsequent data quality interventions resulted in improvement in spirometry quality, longitudinal data precision, and validity.[36]

By organizing and analyzing longitudinal spirometry data, SPIROLA software has helped to improve the use of periodic spirometry data in disease prevention and to improve the wellness of construction workers potentially exposed to respiratory hazards.[27]

Collection of spirometric measurements can be costly; thus, it important that the measurements are of recommended quality and that the data are effectively used for its purpose. Computerized monitoring of data quality and precision, and ongoing data analysis help to achieve the full potential of spirometry monitoring in clinical, occupational, or other settings.

REFERENCES

1. King MS, Miller R, Johnson J, et al. Bronchiolitis in soldiers with inhalational exposures in the Iraq war [abstract]. *Am J Respir Crit Care Med.* 2008;177:A885.

2. Said SI, Hamidi SA, Szema AM, Lyubsky S. Is there a common pathogenetic mechanism for pulmonary vascular remodeling and inflammation in PAH [poster board #725]? Paper presented at: American Thoracic Society 2008 International Conference; May 16–21, 2008; Toronto, Ontario, Canada.

3. Kelsall HL, Sim MR, Forbes AB, et al. Respiratory health status of Australian veterans of the 1991 Gulf War and the effects of exposure to oil fire smoke and dust storms. *Thorax.* 2004;59:897–903.

4. Korényi-Both AL, Molnár AC, Fidelus-Gort R. Al Eskan disease: Desert Storm pneumonitis. *Mil Med.* 1992;157:452–462.

5. Lange JL, Campbell KE, Brundage JF. Respiratory illnesses in relation to military assignments in the Mojave Desert: retrospective surveillance over a 10-year period. *Mil Med.* 2003;168:1039–1043.

6. Shorr AF, Scoville SL, Cersovsky SB, et al. Acute eosinophilic pneumonia among US military personnel deployed in or near Iraq. *JAMA.* 2004;292:2997–3005.

7. King MS, Eisenberg R, Newman JH, et al. Constrictive bronchiolitis in soldiers returning from Iraq and Afghanistan. *N Engl J Med.* 2011;365:222–230. [Erratum in *N Engl J Med.* 2011;365:1749.]

8. Crum-Cianflone NF. Respiratory outcomes among returning service members: data from the Millennium Cohort Study. Paper presented at: the VA/DoD Airborne Hazards Symposium; August 2012; Arlington, VA.

9. World Health Organization. *Burden of COPD.* Geneva, Switzerland: WHO; 2007.

10. Mannino DM, Reichert MM, Davis KJ. Lung function decline and outcomes in an adult population. *Am J Respir Crit Care Med.* 2006;173:985–990.

11. Beeckman LA, Wang ML, Petsonk EL, Wagner GR. Rapid declines in FEV_1 and subsequent respiratory symptoms, illnesses, and mortality in coal miners in the United States. *Am J Respir Crit Care Med.* 2001;163:633–639.

12. Sircar K, Hnizdo E, Petsonk E, Attfield M. Decline in lung function and mortality: implication for medical monitoring. *Occup Environ Med.* 2007;64:461–466.

13. Anthonisen NR, Connet JE, Enright PL, Manfreda J, and the LHS Research Group. Hospitalizations and mortality in the Lung Health Study. *Am J Respir Crit Care Med.* 2002;166:333–339.

14. Anthonisen NR, Connett JE, Murray RP. Smoking and lung function of Lung Health Study participants after 11 years. *Am J Respir Crit Care Med.* 2002;166:675–679.

15. Harber P, Tashkin DP, Simmons M, Crawford L, Hnizdo E, Connett J. Effect of occupational exposures on decline of lung function in early chronic obstructive pulmonary disease. *Am J Respir Crit Care Med.* 2007;176:994–1000.

16. Balmes J, Becklake M, Blanc P, et al. American Thoracic Society Statement: occupational contribution to the burden of airway disease. *Am J Respir Crit Care Med.* 2003;167:787–797.

17. Hnizdo E, Sullivan PA, Bang KM, Wagner G. Association between chronic obstructive pulmonary disease and employment by industry and occupation in the US population: a study of data from the Third National Health and Nutrition Examination Survey. *Am J Epidemiol.* 2002;156:738–746.

18. Weinmann S, Vollmer WM, Breen V, et al. COPD and occupational exposures: a case-control study. *J Occup Environ Med.* 2008;50:561–569.

19. Spirometry Longitudinal Data Analysis. SPIROLA software, version 3.0.1. http://www.cdc.gov/niosh/topics/spirometry/spirola-software.html. Accessed September 10, 2012.

20. Hankinson JL, Wagner GR. Medical screening using periodic spirometry for detection of chronic lung disease. *Occup Med.* 1993;8:353–361.

21. Townsend MC. Evaluating pulmonary function change over time in the occupational setting. ACOEM evidence-based statement. *J Occup Environ Med.* 2005;47:1307–1316.

22. Kreiss K, Fedan KB, Nasrullah M, et al. Longitudinal lung function declines among California flavoring manufacturing workers. *Am J Ind Med.* 2012;55:657–668.

23. Miller MR, Hankinson J, Brusasco V, et al. Standardisation of spirometry. *Eur Respir J.* 2005;26:319–338.

24. Hnizdo E, Yu L, Freyder L, Attfield M, Lefante J, Glindmeyer HW. The precision of longitudinal lung function measurements: monitoring and interpretation. *Occup Environ Med.* 2005;62:695–701.

25. Hnizdo E. The value of periodic spirometry for early recognition of long-term excessive lung function decline in individuals. *J Occup Environ Med.* 2012;54:1506–1512.

26. Wang ML, Avashia BH, Petsonk EL. Interpreting periodic lung function tests in individuals: the relationship between 1- to 5-year and long-term FEV_1 changes. *Chest.* 2006;130:493–499.

27. Hnizdo E, Berry A, Hakobyan A, Beeckman-Wagner L-A, Catlett L. Worksite wellness program for respiratory disease prevention in heavy-construction workers. *J Occup Environ Med.* 2011;53:274–281.

28. Sherrill DL, Lebowitz MD, Knudson RJ, Burrows B. Continuous longitudinal regression equations for pulmonary function measures. *Eur Respir J.* 1992;5:452–462.

29. Schlesselman JJ. Planning a longitudinal study: II. Frequency of measurement and study duration. *J Chron Dis.* 1973;26:561–570.

30. Hnizdo E, Sircar K, Glindmeyer H, Petsonk E. Longitudinal limits of normal decline in lung function in an individual. *J Occup Environ Med.* 2006;48:625–634.

31. Hnizdo E, Sircar K, Yan T, Harber P, Fleming J, Glindmeyer HW. Limits of longitudinal decline for the interpretation of annual changes in FEV_1 in individuals. *Occup Environ Med.* 2007;64:701–707.

32. Burrows B, Lebowitz MD, Camilli AE, Knudson RJ. Longitudinal changes in forced expiratory volume in one second in adults. Methodologic considerations and findings in healthy nonsmokers. *Am Rev Respir Dis.* 1986;133:974–980.

33. American Thoracic Society. Lung function testing: selection of reference values and interpretative strategies. *Am Rev Resp Dis.* 1991;144:1202–1218.

34. Hnizdo E, Glindmeyer HW, Petsonk EL. Workplace spirometry monitoring for respiratory disease prevention: a method review. *Int J Tuberc Lung Dis.* 2010;14:796–805.

35. Chaisson NF, Kreiss K, Hnizdo E, Hakobyan A, Enright PL. Evaluation of methods to determine excessive decline of forced expiratory volume in one second in workers exposed to diacetyl-containing flavorings. *J Occup Environ Med.* 2010;52:1119–1123.

36. Hnizdo E, Hakobyan A, Fleming J, Beeckman-Wagner L. Periodic spirometry in occupational setting: improving quality, accuracy, and precision. *J Occup Environ Med.* 2011;53:1205–1209.

37. Becklake MR, White N. Sources of variation in spirometric measurements. Identifying the signal and dealing with noise. *Occup Med.* 1993;8:241–264.

38. National Institute for Occupational Safety and Health. NIOSH spirometry training course. http://www.cdc.gov/niosh/topics/spirometry. Accessed April 9, 2013.

39. Enright PL, Johnson LR, Connett JE, Voelker H, Buist AS. Spirometry in the Lung Health Study. 1. Methods and quality control. *Am Rev Respir Dis.* 1991;143:1215–1223.

40. Hankinson JL, Odencrantz JR, Fedan KB. Spirometric reference values from a sample of the general US population. *Am J Respir Crit Care Med.* 1999;159:179–187.

AIRBORNE HAZARDS RELATED TO DEPLOYMENT

Section III: Follow-up Medical Care of Service Members and Veterans

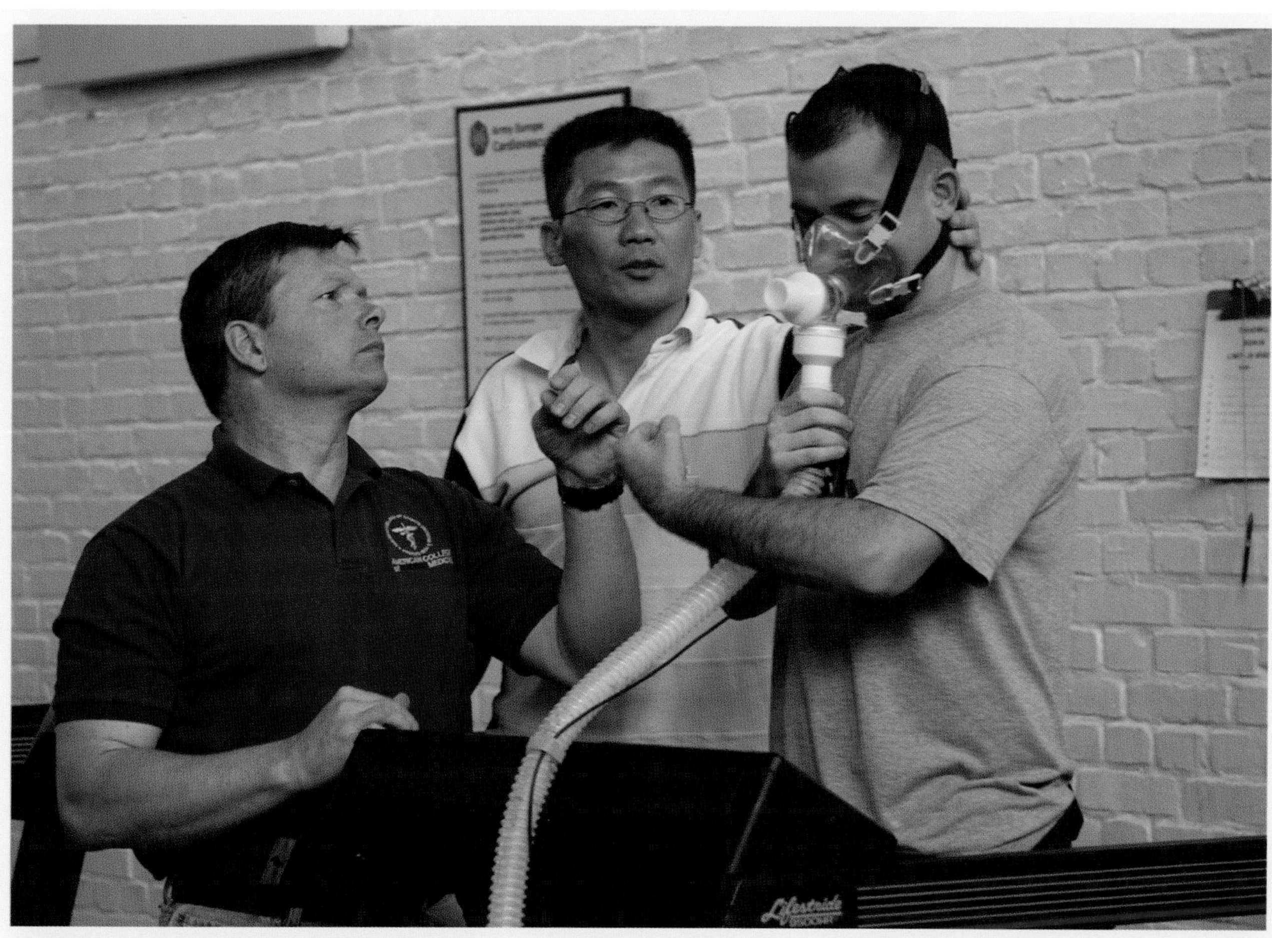

A patient receiving maximal oxygen uptake (VO_{2max}) testing.

Photograph: Courtesy of the US Army Public Health Command (Aberdeen Proving Ground, Maryland).

Chapter 11

DISCUSSION SUMMARY: BASIC DIAGNOSIS AND WORKUP OF SYMPTOMATIC INDIVIDUALS

MICHAEL J. MORRIS, MD*; CORINA NEGRESCU, MD, MPH†; DAVID G. BELL, MD‡; AND CAROLE N. TINKLEPAUGH, MD, MBA§

*Colonel (Retired), Medical Corps, US Army; Department of Defense Chair, Staff Physician, Pulmonary/Critical Care Medicine and Assistant Program Director, Internal Medicine Residency, San Antonio Military Medical Center, 3551 Roger Brooke Drive, Fort Sam Houston, Texas 78234

†Veterans Administration Chair and Medical Director, Veterans Benefits Administration, Contract Exams, US Department of Veterans Affairs, 810 Vermont Avenue, NW, Washington, DC 20420

‡Lieutenant Colonel, Medical Corps, US Army; Program Director, Pulmonary/Critical Care, San Antonio Military Medical Center, 3551 Roger Brooke Drive, Fort Sam Houston, Texas 78234

§Occupational Medicine Physician, Environmental Medicine Program, US Army Public Health Command, 5158 Blackhawk Road, Aberdeen Proving Ground, Maryland 21010-5403

INTRODUCTION

Crucial to the understanding of the potential associations between airborne hazards and deployment is an appreciation of the extent and types of respiratory symptoms and diseases related to deployment of military personnel to southwest Asia (SWA) since 2003. Although it has been reported that deployment may be associated with new-onset respiratory disease, accurate analysis of trends and rates of postdeployment respiratory diseases are dependent on identification and characterization of respiratory disease in military personnel. A primary task for the group was to review and modify a proposed diagnostic algorithm in conjunction with the referral and diagnostic recommendations at both the primary care and specialty care levels. The following six discussion questions were developed and proposed to the convened working group on the basic evaluation of postdeployment military personnel with dyspnea or undiagnosed respiratory complaints:

1. What are the essential elements of a complementary standardized questionnaire for symptomatic individuals?
2. Which elements of the diagnostic workup should be done at the primary care level?
3. Is there a need to collect/archive information apart from individual medical records? Will there be any value for the epidemiological research community when collecting and interpreting data from the electronic medical record?
4. What are the possible programmatic, policy, logistical, and feasibility issues that might arise from a standardized evaluation?
5. What other needs (outreach, education, and risk communication) for symptomatic individuals might be important for implementation?
6. Is there additional benefit from use of standardized *International Classification of Diseases* (ICD)-9 or ICD-10 codes along with a diagnostic algorithm?

PRIMARY CARE EVALUATION

Service members may complain of respiratory symptoms that include cough, shortness of breath, wheezing, and chest tightness. There are numerous reported causes of exertional dyspnea in the active duty military patient to include anemia, metabolic disorders, anxiety, cardiovascular disorders, deconditioning, and multiple pulmonary disorders (eg, airway, parenchymal, pleural, vascular, and thoracic cage diseases).[1] Whereas obstructive lung disease—such as asthma and exercise-induced bronchospasm (EIB)—is most common, consideration needs to be given for other etiologies.[2] Basic indications for evaluation of active duty are listed in Exhibit 11-1. Initial evaluation at the primary care level should document the following six items:

1. Type and length of respiratory symptoms to include dyspnea, cough, sputum production, wheezing, chest tightness, and level of decreased exercise tolerance. Specific questions should address any decrement in regular exercise or changes in fitness testing run times. Symptoms should generally be at least 3 months in length to be considered chronic in nature.
2. Relationship of onset symptoms to deployment (before, during, and after) and history of preexisting lung disease.
3. Basic exposure history to include deployment exposure, such as burn pits, dust storms, vehicle exhaust, air pollution, or other atypical exposures. Cigarette smoking should likewise be documented in terms of pack-years (which is packs per day times the number of years smoking), as well as any change in smoking habits with deployment.

EXHIBIT 11-1

INDICATIONS FOR POSTDEPLOYMENT DYSPNEA EVALUATION

- Cough, shortness of breath, wheezing, or chest tightness for >3 months duration
- New-onset or worsened pulmonary symptoms during or postdeployment
- Excessive decline compared with earlier service-specific aerobic endurance event or failure to pass the running event
- Any abnormal spirometry pattern (below the lower limit of normal)
- >15% decline in FEV_1 or FVC between pre- and postdeployment testing or >10% if new-onset respiratory symptoms are also reported, even if spirometry is within the normal range

FEV_1: forced expiratory volume in 1 sec; FVC: forced vital capacity

4. Physical examination findings should include basic vital signs, including calculation of body mass index; pulse oximetry (if available); examination of the upper airway; cardiac examination; and auscultation of lung sounds for expiratory wheezing, crackles, or inspiratory stridor.
5. Posteroanterior and lateral chest X-ray (CXR) radiograph should be obtained in all patients with new symptoms to rule out pulmonary infiltrates, masses, or pleural effusions. It is expected that most patients have a normal CXR.
6. Baseline spirometry should be obtained at initial evaluation in all patients with new symptoms. If not available locally, the individual should be referred to obtain this test. Interpretation should be provided according to the current Third National Health and Nutrition Examination Survey (NHANES III) reference values.[3] Peak flow monitoring is not an acceptable substitute measurement in place of spirometry.

SPECIALTY EVALUATION

Indications for referral for specialty evaluation (cardiology, pulmonary, or allergy) are listed in Exhibit 11-2. The threshold for referral in those postdeployment patients with persistent symptoms, but normal CXR and spirometry, should be fairly low. A chronic dyspnea evaluation should be performed according to the specialty clinic and not strictly according to a specific algorithm. Recommended studies that may be performed are listed in Exhibit 11-3. The differential for chronic dyspnea changes considerably as patients age.[4] The provided commentary from the workshop is intended to describe the possible components of the evaluation and diagnosis of individuals who present with unexplained chronic dyspnea. It is a guideline and should not be substituted for the clinical judgment of a pulmonologist or any other medical practitioner based on the results of particular studies done during an evaluation. Potential causes of respiratory symptoms in military personnel are shown in Exhibit 11-4.

EXHIBIT 11-2

INDICATIONS FOR REFERRAL FOR SPECIALTY EVALUATION

- Abnormal chest radiograph (interstitial changes, lung mass, hilar adenopathy, lung infiltrate, and pleural effusion)
- Restrictive indices on spirometry (both FEV_1 and FVC < 70%)
- Resting pulse oximetry below 95% or a decrease of 4% with ambulation during a 6-min walk test
- Need for bronchoprovocation testing to confirm asthma or exercise-induced bronchospasm
- Symptoms >3 months with no response to treatment
- Prior treatment with oral steroids, hospitalization, or endotracheal intubation
- Unexplained dyspnea, cough, and/or sputum production
- Symptomatic individuals with normal basic evaluation (spirometry and chest radiograph)

FEV_1: forced expiratory volume in 1 sec; FVC: forced vital capacity

Medical and Exposure Histories

At the specialty level, more detailed pulmonary and exposure histories should be obtained along with the complete medical history. It is expected that the relationship of respiratory symptoms to deployment and prior history of pulmonary disease be extensively documented. There are questionnaires developed by the US Army Public Health Command, such as the Exposure and Respiratory Questionnaire, that may be used as part of the evaluation. An important consideration in this specialty evaluation should be a description of the dyspnea as outlined by the 2012 American Thoracic Society. Dyspnea can be linked to specific physiological processes based on sensations of work or effort (exercising muscle), tightness (bronchoconstriction), or air hunger/unsatisfied inspiration (imbalance in efferent activation and feedback from afferent receptors).[5]

Physical examination should focus on the upper airway, and pulmonary and cardiac examinations to document evidence of seasonal allergic rhinitis, gastroesophageal reflux disease, chest wall abnormalities, and auscultation of the heart and lungs. Pulse oximetry should be tested, and readings below 95% at rest or a decrease of 4% with ambulation should prompt further evaluation. In unexplained dyspnea, it may also be helpful to obtain both a complete blood count (particularly in females) to rule out anemia and thyroid stimulating hormone to eliminate subclinical thyroid disorders. Additional laboratory studies, such as immunoglobulins or radioallergosorbent testing, will not establish a specific diagnosis but may suggest underlying allergic disorders in atopic patients.

EXHIBIT 11-3

SPECIALTY EVALUATION STUDIES

- Pulse oximetry (rest and ambulation)
- Laboratory studies (complete blood count, thyroid stimulating hormone level, immunoglobulin E level)
- Spirometry with postbronchodilator testing
- Full pulmonary function testing with lung volumes and diffusing capacity
- Impulse oscillometry
- Maximal voluntary ventilation, inspiratory/expiratory pressures
- High-resolution computed tomography of the chest
- Bronchoprovocation testing (exercise spirometry, methacholine challenge testing, mannitol testing, or eucapneic voluntary hyperventilation)
- Exercise laryngoscopy
- Cardiopulmonary exercise testing with gas analysis
- Fiberoptic bronchoscopy
- Cardiac evaluation (electrocardiogram, echocardiogram)

Chest Imaging

Chest imaging needs to be obtained in all patients presenting for a postdeployment dyspnea evaluation. In most cases, the CXR will be normal, but may be insensitive for detecting some types of parenchymal lung disease. In the evaluation of major outbreaks of environmental or occupational pulmonary disease related to metal-working, swimming pools, or indoor environments, CXRs are typically insensitive.[6] It was shown to be uniformly normal in the results of a recent postdeployment study.[7] The exact role for high-resolution computed tomography (HRCT) of the chest has yet to be determined in the deployed population and may be considered for chronic symptoms or evidence of spirometric changes with a normal CXR.

Patterns of abnormality on HRCT in diffuse lung diseases consist of linear and reticular opacities; nodules and nodular opacities; or increased lung opacification, including consolidation of the airspaces and ground glass opacity. The use of HRCT may identify mosaic attenuation during the expiratory phase that may not be identified with a standard noncontrast chest computed tomography (CT) protocol. The diseases and patterns that can lead to a specific diagnosis by means of the HRCT include bronchiectasis, emphysema, usual interstitial pneumonitis, hypersensitivity pneumonitis, pneumoconiosis, sarcoidosis, and potentially constrictive bronchiolitis (CB). In these cases, the diagnosis may be sufficiently specific to obviate tissue confirmation.[8] Because there have been case series reporting findings suggestive of CB and hypersensitivity pneumonitis in patients with otherwise normal imaging, it is reasonable to perform HRCT in symptomatic patients given the low radiation risk with a single scan. A normal HRCT without interstitial changes, airway findings, or air trapping makes the diagnosis of an occult interstitial lung disease much less likely.

Pulmonary Function Testing

As part of any initial dyspnea evaluation, spirometry (off any long-acting inhaled medications) should be repeated by the specialty clinic to confirm findings done in primary care clinics. Given the frequency of airway hyperresponsiveness (AHR) in the military population, both pre- and postbronchodilator (PBD) spirometry should be done on a routine basis, especially when the forced expiratory volume in 1 second (FEV_1)/forced vital capacity (FVC) ratio is reduced. A PBD increase in FEV_1 may indicate AHR even when:

- the FEV_1/FVC ratio is normal or slightly reduced,
- there is reduction in the midexpiratory flow, or
- FEV_1 and FVC are elevated above 90% predicted and obstruction is present based on the FEV_1/FVC ratio.[9]

Identifying obstructive indices on spirometry does not establish the diagnosis of asthma unless there is a compatible clinical history with evidence of AHR on PBD testing or reac-

EXHIBIT 11-4

COMMON CAUSES OF DYSPNEA IN MILITARY PERSONNEL

- Obstructive lung disease (asthma, exercise-induced bronchospasm, chronic obstructive pulmonary disease, or bronchiectasis)
- Chest wall deformities (eg, pectus excavatum, scoliosis, trauma)
- Interstitial lung diseases (sarcoidosis, idiopathic pulmonary fibrosis)
- Hyperventilation/anxiety disorders
- Vocal cord dysfunction and other upper airway disorders
- Diaphragmatic weakness
- Gastroesophageal reflux disease or seasonal allergic rhinitis
- Deconditioning
- Metabolic disorders (anemia, thyroid disease)
- Other chronic lung diseases

tive bronchoprovocation testing (BPT). Consideration still needs to be given for chronic obstructive pulmonary disease, bronchiectasis, or other underlying obstructive lung diseases. An integral portion of a spirometry study is careful review of the flow volume loop (FVL) to identify evidence of fixed or variable airway obstruction. However, the airway needs to be significantly obstructed to cause FVL abnormalities. For example, in patients with vocal cord dysfunction, only 25% of patients will have baseline truncation of the inspiratory FVL because of the variability of symptoms.

Full pulmonary function testing (PFT) with lung volumes and diffusing capacity of the lung for carbon monoxide (DLCO) are generally less important in younger military populations. However, in the symptomatic, postdeployment military population, the threshold should be low and considered in the following situations:

- evidence of restriction or mixed restriction/obstruction on spirometry,
- obstruction with lack of significant bronchodilator response,
- evidence of hypoxia on pulse oximetry,
- radiographic changes suggesting interstitial lung disease, and
- truncal obesity or chest wall deformities to include kyphoscoliosis or pectus excavatum.

Patients with a body mass index above 30 kg/m^2 may have mild restriction solely because of their truncal obesity. It is thought to be from both deposition of adipose tissue around the chest and abdominal adipose tissue decreasing the excursion of the diaphragm.[10]

Bronchoprovocation Testing

Unless the patient clearly has asthma on the basis of obstructive spirometry with a bronchodilator response or a definite imaging abnormality suggestive of interstitial lung disease, BPT should be performed in all military patients as part of the diagnostic evaluation. A number of techniques are currently available to determine the presence of AHR. Methacholine challenge testing (MCT) is the most widely available and is the current test of choice at most military centers. The MCT lacks specificity, but is generally sensitive for AHR. Thus, a negative test essentially rules out AHR as the underlying cause for symptoms in this population. Alternative methods include mannitol and eucapneic voluntary hyperventilation that have a similar diagnostic yield as MCT.[11] Exercise spirometry may also be considered, but is surprisingly insensitive for detecting EIB.[12] A reactive BPT in a patient with exertional dyspnea and normal spirometry is highly suggestive of EIB, but should be confirmed with a clinical response to treatment during exercise.

Other Pulmonary Function Testing

There are other pulmonary function testing modalities available that may assist in establishing a diagnosis in selected individuals.

- The maximal voluntary ventilation may be an optional study and a significantly reduced value less than 70% predicted may be a marker of underlying airway obstruction, respiratory muscle weakness, or a reduced level of fitness.[2]
- Maximal inspiratory and expiratory pressures can be done rapidly in the pulmonary function laboratory. They are most helpful when ruling out diaphragmatic dysfunction based on findings of either restrictive PFTs or an elevated hemidiaphragm on CXR.
- Impulse oscillometry is a new technique that uses sound waves to measure central and peripheral airway resistance and reactance. In those patients with normal spirometry, evidence of increased airway resistance with a reduction PBD may indicate AHR not evident on spirometry.[13]

Exercise Laryngoscopy

In the presence of normal spirometry and negative BPT, another common diagnosis in the military population is vocal cord dysfunction. Although the inspiratory FVL may indicate the presence of a variable extrathoracic obstruction, because of the intermittent nature of the condition, the FVL may be normal in the absence of symptoms. Generally, exercise is the most common trigger for vocal cord dysfunction in this population, although consideration needs to be given to other triggers that include psychogenic or irritant-related causes (gastroesophageal reflux or postnasal drip). Additionally, the appearance of the glottis and associated structures may indicate the presence of a fixed anatomical lesion or findings of pachyderma and erythema consistent with gastroesophageal reflux disease. We generally perform laryngoscopy pre- and postexercise to document differences in vocal cord motion (paradoxical adduction) and glottis appearance postexercise.[14]

Cardiopulmonary Exercise Testing

Generally, cardiopulmonary exercise testing (CPET) is reserved for those patients in whom the diagnosis is not clear despite imaging and the other kinds of testing as described previously. This is a maximum exercise test that provides expired gas analysis and measurements of both cardiac and pulmonary limitation to exercise. In an older population,

CPET may be helpful in differentiating pulmonary or cardiac limitations to exercise or the presence of deconditioning. However, for the younger military population, there is generally little cardiac disease, and the presence of most pulmonary disease can be detected by other testing. Additionally, there are no established reference values for CPET parameters in this population.[15] Despite these limitations, CPET may further provide an estimate of the patient's ability to perform maximal exercise, which is important in determining further invasive testing. It may further clarify the differential diagnosis in the following situations: where the etiology of the dyspnea is unclear, where there is coexistent cardiac and pulmonary diseases, or where the severity of dyspnea is disproportionate to other objective findings.

Fiberoptic Bronchoscopy

Fiberoptic bronchoscopy (FOB) is generally not part of the evaluation for the military population, and the workshop did not deem it to be an essential component in all patient evaluations. It is currently being utilized as a research tool in the postdeployment dyspnea studies to establish the presence of an inflammatory milieu as part of the postdeployment dyspnea syndrome. In the general population, FOB is evaluated for suspected airway lesions or lung masses, infiltrates, or the presence of interstitial changes. For the evaluation of dyspnea in the postdeployment patient, normal chest imaging obviates the need for FOB unless there is a chronic productive cough or there is a need to identify respiratory cell populations in such conditions as eosinophilic bronchitis or neutrophilic asthma. In the presence of either focal findings or diffuse interstitial changes, FOB should be the first test of choice to further evaluate the patient. Both bronchoalveolar lavage and transbronchial biopsies may provide additional information on the etiology of the underlying lung disease. FOB has a limited yield for many interstitial diseases, but is less invasive than surgical lung biopsy.

Surgical Lung Biopsy

The report of CB in redeployed soldiers in the 2011 issue of *The New England Journal of Medicine* was described as the presence of extrinsic narrowing of the luminal wall caused by subepithelial fibrosis and smooth muscle hypertrophy in membranous bronchioles in patients with otherwise normal lung pathology.[16] Typical conditions associated with the histological finding of CB include

- inhalation of a variety of gases or toxins;
- drug reactions;
- viral or mycoplasma infections;
- connective tissue disease, especially rheumatoid arthritis;
- chronic rejection in heart-lung, lung, and bone marrow transplant recipients;
- hypersensitivity reactions;
- ulcerative colitis; and
- idiopathic causes.[17]

There may be identifiable CT findings in clinical cases of CB with the presence of interstitial changes, mosaicism, and air trapping.[18] Apart from the pathological findings, CB can be a progressive clinical disorder in which patients have a continued decline in pulmonary function with continued exposure. The patients described in the King series primarily had symptoms with high levels of exertion, and the majority had normal PFT and CT findings.

Surgical lung biopsy is generally indicated to establish a specific diagnosis in the presence of identifiable changes on CT imaging. In the absence of PFT or CT changes, there is no defined indication in the medical literature for a surgical lung biopsy. It was recommended at the workshop that a comprehensive evaluation, as outlined previously, be completed first to eliminate other causes of dyspnea. This should include full PFTs with DLCO, pulse oximetry, BPT, exercise laryngoscopy, and CPET. Additionally, prior to consideration of surgical lung biopsy, a less invasive procedure—such as FOB—should be performed first. FOB allows for transbronchial biopsy of the lung parenchyma in affected areas if present and obtaining BAL samples to demonstrate the presence of inflammatory cells.

The workshop further recommended the establishment of a central joint US Department of Veterans Affairs (VA)/ US Department of Defense (DoD) board (pulmonologists, radiologists, pathologists, and cardiothoracic surgeons) to review the evaluation of any patients under consideration for surgical lung biopsy. It was further recommended that all biopsies be sent to the DoD's Joint Pathology Center for review.

Exposure Questionnaire

Every comprehensive clinical examination starts with medical history taking, to which components of occupational and environmental exposure histories should be added for evaluation of respiratory diseases related to airborne hazards exposure. For both military and civilian personnel returning from SWA, the definitions of occupational and environmental exposures have fine nuances. Exposure history, as well as personal medical history, should be accurately recorded by means of a questionnaire that is the most important research tool for collecting exposure information. Any questionnaire should be a standardized self-assessment tool by which individuals can identify, as well as characterize, their deployment environmental exposures. Individual exposures are highly variable and complex in terms of duration, location, intensity, and frequency. A questionnaire should be designed to capture this variability, but every questionnaire has limitations because of the subjectivity of the recalled information provided. Because self-reporting of past exposures involves different degrees of accuracy, relevance, and potential bias, yes/no questions should be used instead of open-ended/free text questions.

Expanded exposure history questions should also be asked and may have an important role in assessing the risk for respiratory disease.[19] These questions would refer to deployment concurrent with and/or confounding respiratory injury, infections, and nondeployment inhalation exposures related to hobbies, geographical residence, and lifestyle exposure (eg, tobacco smoke). The occupational exposure component will be represented by questions regarding workplace exposure pre- and postdeployment, deployment service branch, and specific military service job description. As a public health tool, it would also collect demographic data, such as gender, age, height, weight, marital status, race/ethnicity, and education. From the disability perspective, the questionnaire does not constitute a legal document for individual claims or compensation, but can assist public health research on deployment exposures that potentially can translate in VA-rating schedule changes that will accurately address the degrees of disability because of airborne hazards exposure and its progression in time. Several airborne hazards evaluation questionnaires have been employed for specific research studies to include the Clinical Evaluation of Respiratory Conditions and Deployment Airborne Respiratory Exposures, but none reached the level of complexity needed to comprehensively collect required airborne hazards data.

Coding

The ICD-9 codes and Current Procedural Terminology (CPT) codes are important for a multitude of practical reasons. The codes constitute the main data source for incidence and prevalence reports for respiratory conditions in service members or veterans exposed to airborne hazards. Equally important, these codes serve as information for the financial and economic analyses and disability benefits recognition that results from the incidence and/or prevalence data of these diseases. The ICD-9 codes could be the most important source by which a respiratory condition can be studied as a disease and/or public health concern, guiding researchers to where and what to look for in individual medical charts. Considering only these two useful roles of information derived from coding, it is important to have the right codes for all respiratory diseases and symptoms, and to update the diagnostic code as the disease progresses or is better characterized. Previously deployed personnel with respiratory symptoms, such as exertional dyspnea, may have multiple reasons for these symptoms to include prior disease, deconditioning, occupational exposures, or cigarette smoking.

In the veteran's or service member's medical chart, the first ICD-9 code indicating a respiratory disease, independent of its cause, can appear as a code of only one symptom or a few symptoms together, not an ICD-9 code of a definite diagnosis or condition. At this stage in the diagnosis process, to choose the correct ICD-9 code can be challenging, and too often the conditions are miscoded. The most common cases of miscoding, especially from the electronic medical records where providers are required to select a diagnosis code, are the ones of very rare diagnosis or new conditions that are not well defined. A review of ICD-9 codes for CB in the DoD electronic medical record identified that the majority (>95%) of the patients did not have this condition. From the VA disability and compensation point of view, ICD-9 codes represent fundamental information. It is important that all symptoms and conditions be well coded and documented during the military service because they constitute evidence for the condition's service connection. It is also instrumental to keep ICD-9 codes updated when the diagnosis is definitely established or the disease progresses or a condition was discovered to be miscoded. To avoid medical errors, education in good coding practices becomes a priority, with Current Procedural Terminology codes being of no less importance than the primary care evaluation algorithm, referrals, and laboratory and imaging tests, at least from a disability point of view.

The most important goal for veterans and service members, besides treatment, is to be awarded the right disability for the diseases and conditions acquired as a result of their military service. Education in good coding is needed for all providers and should be mandatory in the context that most providers hired by the VA to perform disability examinations are from outside the VA and DoD health systems and practice medicine in private offices.

Education and Risk Communication

One of the benefits of integrating the results of clinical medical practice and research studies is better educational and risk communication expertise resulting in tools to distribute a clear message to military personnel and provide services with maximum positive impact. Respiratory diseases diagnosed in redeploying service members from SWA can be considered an occupational disease, that is that they are either caused or aggravated by exposure. The top environmental exposures noted by veterans in SWA are shown in Exhibit 11-5. Primary prevention would be the major priority for airborne hazards, such as the appropriate use of respiratory protection in high exposure areas. In addition to the programs and new initiatives to better control and/or eliminate the sources of exposure (eg, efforts to eliminate open-air burn pits), improved education, increased awareness, and avoidance of exposure risks play a pivotal role in preventing or exacerbating disease.

EXHIBIT 11-5

SOUTHWEST ASIA ENVIRONMENTAL HAZARDS

- Smoke from burning trash or feces
- Sand and dust storms
- Fuels (gasoline, jet fuel, diesel)
- Depleted uranium
- Paint, solvents, other petrochemicals
- Oil well fire smoke
- Contaminated food and water
- Anthrax vaccinations

For proper awareness of the airborne hazards risk, communication tools have to be used efficiently. The awareness campaign on airborne hazards has to be at the national level, using all combined tools, such as the Internet, publications, and other print materials; public service broadcasts and videos; media relations; spokespersons; and special events (exhibitions, seminars, and special days). The VA has robust experience with the previous hot topic awareness campaigns (eg, posttraumatic stress disorder and traumatic brain injury) that did not get the message through until a coordinated and sustained media informational assault was perfected.

The awareness campaign on airborne hazards should consist of two parts. First would be a public health effort with education on prevention of environmental exposures. Second would be recognition of disease symptoms and how to quickly seek medical evaluation and treatment early after exposure. Using the physician–patient relationship, DoD and VA providers have the best opportunity to disseminate the material and offer direct education with the greatest impact. A distinctive point that is uniquely important to all communication tools is the role of smoking and additive interactions with airborne hazards.

Programmatic Issues

Numerous programmatic issues obstruct the way forward in establishing a clear and concise understanding of the problem and the relationship to airborne hazards during deployment. Survey questionnaires are often retrospective; use self-reported data; and involve different degrees of accuracy, relevance, and potential bias. Numerous limitations are acknowledged in terms of subjectivity of the recalled information, characterization of exposures, and potential biases of the individual regarding the cause of symptoms. The information gathered through questionnaires will lack the precision to link respiratory conditions to specific exposures and (for military personnel with multiple deployments) to a specific location or country, although evidence of an increase in risk exposure among persons with land-based deployments will be statistically relevant. For the moment, data collected are insufficient to determine the long-term consequences of exposure to airborne hazards (eg, rate and severity of disease progression) or the impact of other co-morbidities.[20] Miscoding of respiratory symptoms and misdiagnosing early disease will make research very difficult and laborious. There is a tendency to label most respiratory symptoms in a young, healthy cohort as asthma. From the point of view of education and risk communication, it is clear that not all military personnel will benefit from all the tools of the awareness campaign. Depending on age, gender, and cultural background, some tools will be more efficient than others. Some time will pass until an implementation and monitoring study will show a way to tailor the programs to be efficient at all levels, especially considering all demographic, cultural, and geographical factors.

SUMMARY

All individuals with postdeployment respiratory symptoms require a basic evaluation to identify common lung diseases, such as asthma. This should primarily consist of describing symptoms, relating their onset to deployment, establishing specific exposures, performing an examination, and obtaining both CXR and spirometry. Common pulmonary diseases—such as asthma, EIB, and chronic cough—may be detected. A more in-depth evaluation may be necessary in some individuals and require the expertise of specialists to provide a diagnosis. Establishing a specific diagnosis may be difficult, but given the potential for occupational lung disease in deployed military personnel, determining current limitations and future risk are important.

REFERENCES

1. Parker JM, Mikita JA, Lettieri CJ. Appendix 2: causes of dyspnea in military recruits. In: DeKoning BL, ed. *Recruit Medicine*. Washington, DC: Department of the Army, Office of The Surgeon General, Borden Institute, 2006; 575–581.

2. Morris MJ, Grbach VX, Deal LE, Boyd SY, Morgan JA, Johnson JE. Evaluation of exertional dyspnea in the active duty patient: the diagnostic approach and the utility of clinical testing. *Mil Med.* 2002;167:281–288.

3. Hankinson JL, Odencrantz JR, Fedan KB. Spirometric reference values from a sample of the general U.S. population. *Am J Respir Crit Care Med.* 1999;159:179–187.

4. Pratter MR, Curley FJ, Dubois J, Irwin RS. Cause and evaluation of chronic dyspnea in a pulmonary disease clinic. *Arch Intern Med.* 1989;149:2277–2282.

5. Parshall MB, Schwarzstein RM, Adams L, et al. An official American Thoracic Society statement: update on the mechanisms, assessment, and management of dyspnea. *Am J Respir Crit Care Med.* 2012;185:435–452.

6. Hodgson MJ, Parkinson DK, Karpf M. Chest X-rays in hypersensitivity pneumonitis: a metaanalysis of secular trend. *Am J Ind Med.* 1989;16:45–53.

7. Dodson DW, Zacher L, Lucero P, Morris M. Study of active duty military for pulmonary disease related to environmental dust exposure (STAMPEDE) [abstract]. *Am J Respir Crit Care Med.* 2011;183:A4784.

8. Worthy SA, Müller NL. Small airway diseases. *Radiol Clin North Am.* 1998;36:163–173.

9. Kotti GH, Bell DG, Matthews T, Lucero PF, Morris MJ. Correlation of airway hyper-responsiveness with obstructive spirometric indices and FEV(1) > 90% of predicted. *Respir Care.* 2012;57:565–571.

10. Sutherland TJ, Goulding A, Grant AM, et al. The effect of adiposity measured by dual-energy X-ray absorptiometry on lung function. *Eur Respir J.* 2008;32:85–91.

11. Anderson SD, Charlton B, Weiler JM, Nichols S, Spector SL, Pearlman, DS. Comparison of mannitol and methacholine to predict exercise-induced bronchoconstriction and a clinical diagnosis of asthma. *Respir Res.* 2009;10:4.

12. Eliasson AH, Phillips YY, Rajagopal KR, Howard RS. Sensitivity and specificity of bronchial provocation testing. An evaluation of four techniques in exercise-induced bronchospasm. *Chest.* 1992;102:347–355.

13. Blonshine S, Goldman MD. Optimizing performance of respiratory airflow resistance measurements. *Chest.* 2008;134:1304–1309.

14. Morris MJ, Christopher KL. Diagnostic criteria for the classification of vocal cord dysfunction. *Chest.* 2010;138:1213–1223.

15. Morris MJ, Johnson JE, Allan PF, Grbach VX. Cardiopulmonary exercise test interpretation using age-matched controls to evaluate exertional dyspnea. *Mil Med.* 2009;174:1177–1182.

16. King MS, Eisenberg R, Newman JH, et al. Constrictive bronchiolitis in soldiers returning from Iraq and Afghanistan. *N Engl J Med.* 2011;365:222–230.

17. Myers JL, Colby TV. Pathologic manifestations of bronchiolitis, constrictive bronchiolitis, cryptogenic organizing pneumonia, and diffuse panbronchiolitis. *Clin Chest Med.* 1993;14:611–622.

18. Garg K, Lynch DA, Newell JD, King TE Jr. Proliferative and constrictive bronchiolitis: classification and radiologic features. *AJR Am J Roentgenol.* 1994;162:803–808.

19. Baird CP, DeBakey S, Reid L, Hauschild VD, Petruccelli B, Abraham JH. Respiratory health status of US Army personnel potentially exposed to smoke from 2003 Al-Mishraq Sulfur Plant fire. *J Occup Environ Med.* 2012;54:717–723.

20. Abraham JH, DeBakey SF, Reid L, Zhou J, Baird CP. Does deployment to Iraq and Afghanistan affect respiratory health of US military personnel? *J Occup Environ Med.* 2012;54:740–745.

Chapter 12

ALLERGIC AIRWAY DISEASE AND DEPLOYMENT TO THE MIDDLE EAST

JENNIFER MBUTHIA, MD*; ANTHONY M. SZEMA, MD†; AND JONATHAN LI, BS‡

*Lieutenant Colonel, Medical Corps, US Army; Office of The Army Surgeon General, Defense Health Headquarters, 7700 Arlington Boulevard, Falls Church, Virginia 22042; Assistant Professor of Pediatrics, Uniformed Services University of the Health Sciences, 4301 Jones Bridge Road, Bethesda, Maryland 20814
†Assistant Professor of Medicine and Surgery, Stony Brook University School of Medicine, 101 Nicolls Road, Stony Brook, New York 11794; Chief, Allergy Section, Northport Veterans Affairs Medical Center, 79 Middleville Road, Northport, New York 11768
‡Postbaccalaureate premedical student, Stony Brook University, 101 Nicolls Road, Stony Brook, New York 11794

INTRODUCTION

Globally, allergic respiratory disorders are a growing disease burden. In 2012, the National Center for Health Statistics (Atlanta, GA) reported that, in adults aged 18 years and older, 13% had been told they had asthma, with 8% reporting they still had asthma. Seven percent of this population had been told within the prior 12 months that they had hay fever, and 4% self-reported being told that they had chronic bronchitis.[1]

A key immune mechanism in allergic diseases is the sensitization of immunoglobulin E (IgE) antibody to triggers in the environment that are not normally considered infectious pathogens, such as pollens, animal dander, food protein, or *Hymenoptera* venom. The allergic respiratory disorders included in this chapter are limited to those whose primary clinical effect is limited to the nasal and bronchial mucosa: allergic rhinitis and asthma. The presence of IgE responses to airborne environmental triggers, or aeroallergens, can be identified by means of testing methods that look for allergen-specific IgE, both in vitro and in vivo. However, a thorough symptom history is often sufficient to raise clinical suspicion for the diagnosis, and initial management often occurs at the primary care level.

ALLERGIC AIRWAY DISEASES

Allergic rhinitis is one of the most common chronic diseases in the United States and is associated with allergen exposure that causes inflammation and an immune-mediated response, leading to symptoms such as sneezing, nasal itching, rhinorrhea, and nasal congestion.[2] Rhinitis due to non–IgE-mediated responses is also common and can be present alone or as a co-morbid condition in those with allergic rhinitis. Nonallergic rhinitis is characterized by nasal symptoms that are not due to allergen-specific IgE, and testing will not show clinically significant results. Common nonallergic rhinitis diagnoses include infectious, vasomotor, drug-induced, ingestion, hormonal, and nonallergic rhinitis with eosinophilia syndrome.[2]

Asthma can also have triggers that are mediated by specific IgE; however, the spectrum of triggers leading to an asthma exacerbation is broader in nature and comprises an evolving area of research. The increasing prevalence of asthma suggests an environmental component in the development of disease, but there are also genetic patterns of asthma seen in individual patients and in families. Such patterns suggest a gene–environment interaction, further suggesting that a genetically susceptible individual, when exposed to certain environmental conditions, is likely to develop asthma.[3]

The airway of an asthmatic is hyperresponsive to triggers, demonstrating reversible and variable airflow limitations—which are also key features of asthma—and the disease can show a waxing and waning pattern of variability.[3] This variability can present a challenge in diagnosing asthma in the young adult population from which the US military recruits, particularly when there is a childhood history of a reactive airway or wheezing that also includes extended asymptomatic periods. In general, the highest rate of asthma diagnosis is made during early childhood, and new-onset asthma is not commonly diagnosed in young adults.[3] However, there is evidence in the medical literature that subjects with a diagnosis of childhood asthma can have intermittent wheezing into adulthood.[4] The risk of respiratory symptoms in young adults creates a challenge for military service due to the limitations it may place on duty performance. A retrospective review of the British Army showed that recurrence of asthma in those with previously diagnosed childhood disease was most common between the ages of 17 to 21 years.[5]

MILITARY RELEVANCE OF ALLERGIC AIRWAY DISEASE

The US military is not immune to the health problems facing the US population. Accession standards for entrance to military service are intended to protect both the potential service member, as well as the military organization. Although medical management of diagnoses such as asthma and allergic rhinitis continues to improve, and these medical conditions are not limiting in many situations faced by young adults, military service demonstrates a unique situation. Physical fitness and the ability to work in a variety of global environments and unpredictable circumstances are mandatory conditions for service members of all military occupational specialties. The military environment requires the ability to wear protective masks and gear; to live and work in a broad range of austere climate conditions and elevations; and to endure exposure to sandstorms, vehicle fumes, or smoke from nearby explosive devices or burn pits. Medical providers evaluating potential military candidates or conducting medical screenings prior to a military deployment must consider these unpredictable factors as part of their decision-making process.

Army Regulation 40-501, *Standards of Medical Fitness,*[6] details the standards regarding both accession and retention for military service. Asthma, to include a diagnosis of reactive airway disease or asthmatic bronchitis, reliably diagnosed and symptomatic after the thirteenth birthday, is considered disqualifying for entrance to military service.[6] Applicants with disqualifying medical conditions can be granted waivers for entrance to military service. A review of medical waivers considered between 1997 and 2002 showed that asthma was one of the most common conditions for which waivers were requested and granted.[7] Of the more than 3,000 applicants initially disqualified from entering military service every year because of chest or lung problems, approximately 1,500 receive waivers for a history of asthma, and 750 of those eventually enter the military. The impact of allowing these applicants with a history of asthma to enter military service may not become evident during their training and time spent in a garrison environment, but the significance of asthma increases as the environment becomes more austere.[8]

Retention standards for service members diagnosed with new-onset asthma after entering military service are determined based on the ability to perform duty, and the diagnosis does not trigger an automatic discharge. Increased bronchial responsiveness and reversible airflow obstruction must be demonstrated for asthma to be diagnosed, and a soldier with chronic asthma may still meet retention standards if the clinical condition does not prevent the soldier from otherwise performing all military training and duties.[6]

CONSIDERATIONS FOR SERVICE MEMBERS WITH ALLERGIC RHINITIS AND ASTHMA BEFORE AND DURING DEPLOYMENT

Medical Screening

Service members eligible to deploy are expected to be in good health, particularly compared with the general population. Because of the limited availability of healthcare services for chronic medical conditions in an austere environment, healthcare professionals perform medical screenings to identify chronic conditions, determine whether any such conditions are currently stable, and identify the potential impact of deployment on that stability. In some cases, an individual must receive clearance from a subspecialty provider to deploy. Due to unique circumstances and the variations in medical echelons of care in a theater of operations, medical providers familiar with military regulations, occupations, and current theater conditions should serve as the clearance authority. The US military has board-certified subspecialists in allergy/immunology, pulmonology, and otolaryngology, some of whom have deployed and provided lessons learned on the impact that deployment conditions can have on underlying allergic airway disease.

Respiratory symptoms are common in a deployed environment, even in those personnel without underlying pulmonary conditions. However, adequate baseline control in service members with a diagnosis of asthma is key because those who deploy with poor control are at increased risk of developing worsening symptoms. In a survey of service members returning from Iraq and Afghanistan, cough and allergy symptoms were the most common respiratory complaints in both asthmatic and nonasthmatic individuals. Respiratory complaints were more prevalent in those asthmatic patients with poor baseline control of symptoms.[9] These poorly controlled patients also required more frequent visits to healthcare providers and were more likely to require hospitalization or evacuation from theater.[9]

Aeroallergens and Other Exposures During Deployment

Aeroallergens are derived from a variety of sources in the environment, including pollens (tree, grass, or weed), fungal/mold spores, animal dander, and insect feces. Individuals who demonstrate sensitization to aeroallergens are commonly poly-sensitized, which can make exposure control a difficult task.[3] Additionally, seasonal and geographical variations can impact military populations who have a global presence.

Seasonal and perennial allergens observed in the United States are also found in the Middle East. Seasonal patterns of pollination are similar as well, with tree pollen peaking in the spring, grasses in the late spring and summer (except for coastal regions where year-round grass pollen is found), and weeds in the fall.[10]

A pollen study conducted in Baghdad, Iraq, concluded that most of the pollen collected was from plants that are genetically related to plants of the southeastern part of the United States and known to trigger allergic rhinitis and allergic asthma.[11]

In Kuwait, the most prevalent species of molds found in the air were similar to those in the United States to which patients may be sensitized. The predominant mold species detected was *Aspergillus,*[12] a clinically relevant species for allergic asthma patients sensitized to this mold. Based on clinical and serological testing for *Aspergillus* sensitization, patients with *Aspergillus*-sensitive asthma and allergic bronchopulmonary aspergillosis had a significantly more severe asthma, indicating the importance of this exposure and potential sensitization in atopic individuals.[13] Other mold species identified in Kuwait include *Cladosporium* and *Alternaria*, both of which have also been identified with worsening respiratory symptoms in those asthma patients sensitized to these spores.[12,14]

Individuals with and without asthma or allergic rhinitis can suffer similar symptoms from airborne irritants or airway infections, such as those commonly found during deployment in the Middle East. Fine particulate dust, sandstorms, vehicle fumes, and smoke from burn pits or exploded ordinances are all potential airway irritants, especially in those individuals with underlying asthma. During a 5-year population-based study in Kuwait, 569 days (33.6%) had dust storm events, and they were significantly associated with an increased risk of same-day asthma and respiratory admission to the hospital.[15] Sandstorms are common in Iraq and Afghanistan and have been associated with an increased risk of hospital admission for both asthma and heart disease.[16]

The underlying etiology of worsening airway symptoms following sandstorms may not be solely from irritant-induced airway inflammation. In 2011, bacterial studies were conducted on the fine topsoil particles and airborne dust particles from 19 locations in Iraq and Kuwait. The results indicated the presence of potential human pathogens, including *Mycobacterium*, *Brucella*, *Coxiella burnetii*, *Clostridium perfringens*, and *Bacillus*. *C burnetii*, the causative agent of Q fever, was confirmed and detected in additional samples by use of polymerase chain reaction, indicating a high prevalence of this organism in the analyzed samples.[17] *C burnetii* has been associated with the exacerbation of asthma in adults and should be considered on the differential for infectious agents in deployed service members with nonspecific febrile illness in conjunction with other systemic symptoms, including pneumonia.[18]

The collective impact of minerals, metals, mold, pollen, pollutants, and climate change on the exacerbation of allergic disease in the local population suggests that healthcare providers should counsel deploying soldiers with allergic rhinitis regarding relevant allergen trends, ensuring that these individuals have appropriate medications.[10]

Medications

Availability and durability of medications while deployed should be considered during the predeployment medical evaluation screenings conducted on service members and certain civilians who will be working for the Department of Defense. Attention should be focused on the expiration dates of medications, the length of deployment, and the temperature conditions that may impact medications. According to several package inserts, the upper limit of daily temperature exposure for inhalers and topical nasal steroids is between 77°F and 86°F, which is difficult to ensure for self-carried medications given the desert temperatures.[19–21]

The first-line medications for patients with either allergic rhinitis or well-controlled asthma include short-acting beta-agonists, nonsedating antihistamines, and nasal corticosteroids.[2,22] Leukotriene inhibitors are effective as prophylactic medication for exercise-induced asthma and can be an additional agent used for allergic rhinitis; however, their use for mild persistent asthma is not preferred.[22,23]

Service members who are on a daily, inhaled corticosteroid at the time of their predeployment screening should receive additional medical screening to include a pulmonary function test that assesses how well controlled they are at baseline. These individuals, according to Army Regulation 40-501 (*Standards of Medical Fitness*), should already have received a P-2 medical profile (that notes the presence of minimally significant organic defects or systemic diseases) due to the requirement for a daily controller.[6]

Allergy immunotherapy (AIT), in general, cannot be supported in an austere environment, including deployment to a relatively well-established base such as Kandahar Airfield (Afghanistan). Specific challenges include temperature restrictions during transportation (extracts should be stored at 48°C to reduce the rate of potency loss) to the final facility, and the inability to account for medical training on AIT administration, including AIT-specific issues such as recognition and management of side effects (eg, anaphylaxis), as well as documentation and dose adjustment for those with local injection site reactions.[24]

Service members who are being considered for treatment with immunomodulators (eg, Omalizumab) are likely to be ineligible to deploy. Their condition may even prove too severe to permit their retention on active duty.

POSTDEPLOYMENT CONSIDERATIONS

All service members returning from deployment to Iraq or Afghanistan are required to have at least one healthcare encounter near their time of return to complete postdeployment health assessment processing, and another visit 3 to 6 months later to complete postdeployment health reassessment processing. These mandatory encounters present opportunities for healthcare providers to identify those individuals who may have symptoms that either began or worsened during deployment and have not waned since.

The Millennium Cohort Study collected health information on a variety of topics (eg, respiratory health, smoking status, demographic information, and deployment history). Respiratory questions included self-reported asthma, emphysema, chronic bronchitis, and persistent cough. Data analyzed from the Millennium Cohort Study concluded that there was no increased prevalence of clinically significant pulmonary abnormalities 10 years after deployment.[25] However, this does not preclude the possibility that an individual with a specific exposure history or genetic predisposition could not develop a chronic respiratory condition during his/her time deployed. Clinical symptoms that are indicators that asthma is the likely diagnosis include historic symptoms, as well as those noted during current clinical presentation:

- cough, particularly worse at night;
- recurrent wheeze or difficulty breathing;
- recurrent shortness of breath;
- symptoms that worsen during exercise;
- viral infections;
- inhalant allergen exposure (animals, mold, pollen, and dust mite); and
- irritants (tobacco smoke, wood smoke, and airborne chemicals).

These symptoms should raise clinical suspicion for new-onset asthma in a patient who did not have previous symptoms.[22]

The differential for chronic respiratory complaints not responding to standard asthma therapy should include the following:

- cardiac issues;
- gastrointestinal reflux;
- pharmacological agents (eg, angiotensin-converting enzyme inhibitors);
- vocal cord dysfunction;
- chronic obstructive pulmonary disease;
- allergic bronchopulmonary aspergillosis;
- pulmonary infiltration with eosinophilia; and
- chronic infections (eg, tuberculosis).[22]

In addition to current clinical symptoms, a thorough history for redeployed service members with respiratory symptoms includes documenting detailed airborne exposure history. Although recall bias is an understood limitation, documentation of exposures while deployed may provide information for treating providers. A study that examined the pre- and postdeployment rates of inpatient and outpatient medical encounters for service members deployed to Iraq and Afghanistan found that the overall number of encounters decreased after deployment. However, there was a statistically significant increase in the encounter rates for obstructive respiratory diseases, primarily asthma or bronchitis, from the pre- to postdeployment periods for one-time deployers.[26] This study was limited by the lack of specific deployment-related exposures. Yet, in another study by Smith et al,[25] new-onset respiratory symptoms and cumulative exposure time suggest that specific exposures, rather than deployment in general, are better determinants of postdeployment respiratory conditions.

SUMMARY

Clearly, deployment to austere environments, in addition to the addressed physical requirements (eg, gear, protective masks, and unpredictable stressors), can have an adverse impact on service members. In particular, airborne irritants, allergens, and viral infections can further impact the health and capabilities of those warfighters who have an underlying predisposition to allergic airway conditions. The potential acute health effects of exposure to airborne pollutants on those with preexisting medical conditions (eg, asthma) are better studied in the near term.[27] However, efforts such as the Millennium Cohort Study demonstrate the forethought of researchers to identify long-term impacts on the respiratory health of US service members.

REFERENCES

1. Schiller JS, Lucas JW, Peregoy JA. Summary health statistics for U.S. adults: National Health Interview Survey, 2011. National Center for Health Statistics. *Vital Health Stat*. 2012;10:5–6, 22–26.

2. Wallace DV, Dykewicz MS, Bernstein DI, et al. The diagnosis and management of rhinitis: an updated practice parameter. *J Allergy Clin Immunol*. 2008;122:S1–S84.

3. Boulet L-P. Approach to adults with asthma. In: Adkinson N, Bochner B, Busse W, Holgate S, Lemanske R, Simons E, eds. *Middleton's Allergy: Principles and Practice*. 7th ed. Philadelphia, PA: Elsevier, Inc; 2009: 1346–1366.

4. Martin AJ, McLennan LA, Landau LI, Phelan PD. The natural history of childhood asthma to adult life. *Br Med J*. 1980;280:1397–1400.

5. Dickinson JG: Asthma in the Army: a retrospective study and review of the natural history of asthma and its implications for recruitment. *J R Army Med Corps*. 1988;134:65–73.

6. US Department of the Army. *Standards of Medical Fitness*. http://www.apd.army.mil/pdffiles/r40_501.pdf. Accessed August 4, 2011. Army Regulation 40-501 (Rapid Action Revision).

7. AMSARA. *Accession Medical Standards Analysis and Research Activity 2003 Annual Report*. Silver Spring, MD: Walter Reed Army Institute of Research; 2003.

8. Martin BL, Engler RJM, Nelson MR, Klote MM, With CM, Krauss MR. Asthma and its implications for military recruits. In: DeKoning BL, ed, *Recruit Medicine*. Washington, DC: Department of the Army, Office of The Surgeon General, Borden Institute; 2006: 89–108.

9. Roop SA, Niven AS, Calvin BE, Bader J, Zacher LL. The prevalence and impact of respiratory symptoms in asthmatics and non-asthmatics during deployment. *Mil Med*. 2007;172:1264–1269.

10. Waibel KH. Allergic rhinitis in the Middle East. *Mil Med*. 2005;170:1026–1028.

11. Al-Tikriti SK, Al-Salihi M, Gaillard GE. Pollen and mold survey of Baghdad, Iraq. *Ann Allergy*. 1980;45:97–99.

12. Khan ZU, Khan MA, Chandy R, Sharma PN. Aspergillus and other moulds in the air of Kuwait. *Mycopathologia*. 1999;146:25–32.

13. Maurya V, Gugnani HC, Sarma PU, Madan T, Shah A. Sensitization to Aspergillus antigens and occurrence of allergic bronchopulmonary aspergillosis in patients with asthma. *Chest*. 2005;127:1252–1259.

14. Black PN, Udy AA, Brodie SM. Sensitivity to fungal allergens is a risk factor for life-threatening asthma. *Allergy*. 2000;55:501–504.

15. Thalib L, Al-Taiar A. Dust storms and the risk of asthma admissions to hospitals in Kuwait. *Sci Total Environ*. 2012;433:347–351.

16. Bell ML, Levy JK, Lin Z. The effect of sandstorms and air pollution on cause-specific hospital admissions in Taipei, Taiwan. *Occup Environ Med*. 2008;65:104–111.

17. Leski TA, Malanoski AP, Gregory MJ, Lin B, Stenger DA. Application of a broad-range resequencing array for detection of pathogens in desert dust samples from Kuwait and Iraq. *Appl Envirol Microbiol*. 2011;77:4285–4292.

18. Okimoto N, Asaoka N, Yamato K, et al. Q fever (*Coxiella burnetii* infection) and acute exacerbation of bronchial asthma. *Intern Med*. 2005;44:79–80.

19. Proventil HFA (albuterol sulfate) [package insert]. Whitehouse Station, NJ: Schering Corporation; 2012. http://www.spfiles.com/piproventilhfa.pdf. Accessed September 12, 2013.

20. Flonase (fluticasone propionate) [package insert]. Research Triangle Park, NC: GlaxoSmithKline; 2003. us.gsk.com/products/assets/us_flonase.pdf. Accessed September 12, 2013.

21. Nasacort AQ (triamcinolone acetonide) [package insert]. Bridgewater, NJ: Sanofi-aventis U.S. LLC; 2010. products.sanofi.us/nasacort_aq/nasacortaq.pdf. Accessed September 12, 2013.

22. National Institutes of Health. Expert Panel Report 3 (EPR 3). *Guidelines for the Diagnosis and Management of Asthma*. Bethesda, MD: National Heart, Lung and Blood Institute (NHLBI), National Institutes of Health; 2007. NIH Publication No. 08-4051.

23. Weiler JM, Anderson SD, Randolph C, et al. Pathogenesis, prevalence, diagnosis, and management of exercise-induced bronchoconstriction: a practice parameter. *Ann Allergy Asthma Immunol*. 2010;105:S1–S47.

24. Cox L, Nelson H, Lockey R, et al. Allergen immunotherapy: a practice parameter third update. *J Allergy Clin Immunol*. 2011;127:S1–S55.

25. Smith B, Wong CA, Smith TC, Boyko EJ, Gacksetter GS, Ryan MAK. Newly reported respiratory symptoms and conditions among military personnel deployed to Iraq and Afghanistan: a prospective population-based study. *Am J Epidemiol*. 2009;170:1433–1442.

26. Abraham JH, DeBakey SF, Reid L, Zhou J, Baird C. Does deployment to Iraq and Afghanistan affect respiratory health of US military personnel? *J Occup Environ Med*. 2012;54:740–745.

27. The Armed Forces Health Surveillance Center, The Naval Health Research Center, and The U.S. Army Public Health Command. *Epidemiologic Studies of Health Outcomes Among Troops Deployed to Burn Pit Sites*. http://www.afhsc.mil/viewDocument?file=100604_FINAL_Burn_Pit_Epi_Studies.pdf. Accessed September 12, 2012.

Chapter 13

FOLLOW-UP MEDICAL CARE OF SERVICE MEMBERS AND VETERANS—CARDIOPULMONARY EXERCISE TESTING

WILLIAM ESCHENBACHER, MD*

Pulmonologist, Veterans Health Administration, Pulmonary/Critical Care, Cincinnati VA Medical Center, 3200 Vine Street, Cincinnati, Ohio 45220; Professor of Medicine, Division of Pulmonary and Critical Care Medicine, Department of Internal Medicine, University of Cincinnati College of Medicine, 231 Albert Sabin Way, Cincinnati, Ohio 45229

INTRODUCTION

Individuals who present with respiratory symptoms will have standard screening medical tests performed, including spirometry and chest X-ray radiographs. If further testing is indicated based on history, symptoms, and results of screening studies, this may include more complete lung function testing: lung volumes, diffusing capacity measurement, and response to the one-time use of a bronchodilator. For some individuals, even more advanced testing may be needed for complete evaluation of possible causes of respiratory symptoms, which may include bronchoprovocation challenge testing and cardiopulmonary exercise testing (CPET). CPET is the evaluation of the lungs, the heart, the circulation, and certain muscle groups under the conditions of exercise.

When a person exercises, the muscles involved in the type of exercise (eg, lower extremity musculature for running or cycling) require increased amounts of energy production by mitochondria in the muscle cells. This increased energy production depends on increased metabolism that, in turn, requires oxygen and substrates for the generation of that energy.

AEROBIC METABOLISM

If oxygen is available, this energy production is accomplished by the utilization of substrates, such as pyruvate (from glucose) through metabolic pathways of the tricarboxylic acid or Krebs cycle. For this to occur, the lungs need to take in increased quantities of oxygen from the atmosphere and transfer the oxygen to the hemoglobin of red blood cells in the circulation. The heart will then need to increase its output of blood to deliver the oxygen to the exercising muscles. As oxygen is utilized by the mitochondria within the exercising muscles, carbon dioxide is produced as a byproduct of this aerobic (with oxygen) metabolism. This extra carbon dioxide must then be transported by the heart and the circulation to the lungs where it is exhaled.

ANAEROBIC METABOLISM

In a situation where the pattern of exercise includes steadily increasing workloads for the individual, the amount of oxygen delivered to the exercising muscles may become limited or inadequate for the usual metabolic pathways for energy production (ATP [or adenosine triphosphate] formation by the Krebs cycle). At that time, energy production is shifted to a pathway that results in lactic acid production. This is known as a shift from aerobic (with oxygen) to anaerobic metabolism (without oxygen).

THE BODY'S RESPONSE TO EXERCISE

There are changes that occur within the body with exercise to supply the exercising muscles with adequate oxygen for energy production. As previously described, the lungs must be able to move more air to take in oxygen from the atmosphere and transfer that oxygen to the blood. This movement of air is measured as minute ventilation (V_E) : liters of air moved per minute. The heart then has to pump more blood to carry the oxygen to the muscles. This increased pumping ability is referred to as cardiac output in liters per minute of blood pumped by the heart to the arterial circulation. Finally, the oxygen delivered to the exercising muscles must be extracted from the blood to be used by mitochondria in the muscles. Those changes with exercise are shown in Figure 13-1.

V_E can increase from a resting value of 7 to 10 L/min to upwards of 70 to 140 L/min. Cardiac output can increase from 4 to 5 L/min at rest to 20 to 25 L/min with exercise. Extraction of oxygen in the periphery by the exercising muscles (the difference between the oxygen-carrying capacity of arterial blood and the venous blood) can increase from 5 mL of oxygen for every 100 mL of blood to 15 to 16 mL of oxygen for every 100 mL of blood. As a result of these changes, the uptake or consumption of oxygen by the body (primarily the exercising muscles) can increase from 4 mL/kg/min to 40 to 50 mL/kg/min (or even higher for some well-trained athletes). This maximal oxygen consumption (VO_{2max}) for the individual is an overall measure of the work performance or exercise capacity for that individual.

INDICATIONS FOR CARDIOPULMONARY EXERCISE TESTING

The adequate supply of oxygen to exercising muscles requires close coordination among

- the lungs (to take in oxygen),
- the heart (to pump the blood with oxygen),
- the circulation (to move oxygenated blood to the muscles), and
- the muscles themselves (to extract and use oxygen efficiently).

When a portion of this system breaks down, the delivery and utilization of oxygen by the exercising muscles are limited, and exercise or work performance for the individual is lower or worse than expected. The individual may experience this reduced or limited performance as excessive dyspnea or shortness of breath. Dyspnea with exercise that is out of proportion to what is expected for the individual may indicate decreased exercise performance and require further evaluation beyond the usual testing of the lungs and heart: pulmonary function tests, echocardiography, etc. In those instances, a CPET can be performed to help in determining the cause of dyspnea. The following are common indications for performing a CPET:

- evaluating unexplained activity-related dyspnea or exercise intolerance;
- differentiating the causes for dyspnea among the lungs, the heart, the circulation, or the exercising muscles;
- determining the impairment rating for disability; and
- monitoring the response to an intervention for a known disease or determining progression of a known disease.

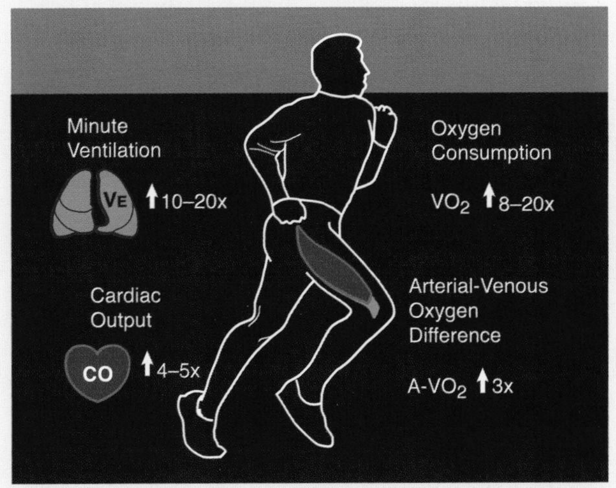

Figure 13-1. Typical changes from rest to maximal exercise.
A-VO_2: arterial-venous oxygen difference; CO: cardiac output; V_E: minute ventilation; VO_2: oxygen consumption (or oxygen uptake)

In most cases, testing is done to determine what might limit exercise performance.

TECHNICAL ASPECTS OF CARDIOPULMONARY EXERCISE TESTING: WHAT IS BEING MEASURED?

To assess contributions of the lungs, the heart, and the circulation to the delivery of oxygen to the exercising muscles, the following parameters are measured:

- V_E (tidal volume × respiratory rate) in L/min,
- oxygen uptake (VO_2) in mL/min,
- carbon dioxide production (VCO_2) in mL/min,
- heart rate in beats/min, and
- oxyhemoglobin saturation in percent.

There may also be electrocardiographic tracings obtained for heart rate and any electrocardiogram changes that may occur with exercise. Ideally, for the evaluation of the heart as the limiting factor, actual measurement of the pumping function of the heart or cardiac output itself would be important. However, this is usually not technically possible with most CPET equipment.

Other parameters that are used for interpretation of the test results are mathematical interactions of the previously described parameters:

- ventilatory equivalents: V_E/VO_2 and V_E/VCO_2; and
- lactate threshold: in a progressive test, it is the determination when there is a shift from aerobic metabolism to anaerobic metabolism.

APPLICATION OF WORKLOAD

An exercise test requires the use of an apparatus for generating a workload for the individual to perform. This is usually in the form of a treadmill or stationary bicycle.

Advantages of a treadmill include

- a more familiar form of exercise for most individuals (walking or running), and
- exercise protocols that have been designed for cardiac stress testing for the evaluation of possible cardiac ischemia.

Disadvantages of a treadmill include

- more difficult for overweight individuals;
- more motion artifact for monitoring equipment, such as oxygen saturation and electrocardiographic measurements; and
- workload achieved is not as precise from individual to individual, but in turn depends on the weight of the individual and speed/incline of the treadmill.

Cycle ergometers or stationary bicycles have the following advantages:

- more reproducible workloads from individual to individual,
- measuring devices that may work more reliably, and
- overweight individuals may be able to perform exercise more efficiently.

The disadvantage of a stationary bicycle is that many individuals may have difficulty pedaling it.

For progressive exercise testing, protocols for treadmills exist (eg, Bruce or Naughton protocols). However, these protocols may increase the workload too quickly to get a complete evaluation of work performance. For the stationary bicycle, the increase in workload can be adjusted, depending on the individual with gradual or progressive increases in wattage (work output or power), from 10 W/min to 50 W/min.

INTERPRETATION OF CARDIOPULMONARY EXERCISE TESTING RESULTS

The results of progressive CPET are interpreted by comparing the individual's performance in terms of the parameters previously described, with predicted or expected values based on normal reference values that have been established and identified in the literature.[1] As previously described, the goal of interpretation is to determine if the person appears limited (usually identified by a lower than expected VO_{2max}), wherein the limitation may be the lungs, the heart, the circulation, or the exercising muscles.

TYPICAL PATTERNS OF INTERPRETATION

Different approaches to interpretation of CPETs have been proposed in the past. These include simple algorithms based on decision points for certain measurement parameters[2] to complete textbooks that discuss the subject and propose interpretation strategies.[3] The statement by the American Thoracic Society/American College of Chest Physicians contains the following regarding interpretation approaches:

- There is no consensus on any one approach.
- Algorithms based on a single key measurement and conceptual framework may be helpful in differential diagnosis, but are limited by excessive reliance on that single measurement.
- An integrative approach that emphasizes the interrelationships, trending phenomena, and patterns of key variable responses in a clinical setting framework is recommended.
- Typical patterns of interpretation results include the following:
  - normal response to CPET,
  - deconditioning or obesity,
  - ventilatory or pulmonary limitation,
  - cardiac limitation.
  - persistent hyperventilation, and
  - chronotropic incompetence (including use of a medication such as a beta-blocker).

Because this test is similar to other testing done in the clinical setting where maximal effort is required for most representative results for that individual, there may be times when suboptimal efforts may make interpretation difficult.

SUMMARY

Evaluation of an individual who presents with respiratory symptoms can involve lung function testing to determine the presence of a respiratory illness or disease. In some instances, the results of this testing (spirometry, lung volumes, and diffusing capacity) may not reveal the cause for the symptoms endorsed by the individual, including the symptom of activity-related dyspnea. Also, if the individual appears to have a reduced exercise performance based on a standard exercise protocol (eg, the Army standard 2-mile run that must be completed in a certain time based on age of the individual), then further testing may be indicated, including performance of CPET. Results of such a test can indicate reduced exercise performance and, in many instances, the cause or causes for that reduced exercise performance.

REFERENCES

1. American Thoracic Society / American College of Chest Physicians. ATS / ACCP Statement on Cardiopulmonary Exercise Testing. *Am J Respir Crit Care Med.* 2003;167:211–277.

2. Eschenbacher WL, Mannina A. An algorithm for the interpretation of cardiopulmonary exercise tests. *Chest.* 1990;97:263–267.

3. Wasserman K, Hansen JE, Sue DY, Stringer WW, Whipp BJ. *Principles of Exercise Testing and Interpretation: Including Pathophysiology and Clinical Applications.* Baltimore, MD: Lippincott Williams & Wilkins; 2005.

Chapter 14

VALUE OF LUNG BIOPSY IN WORKUP OF SYMPTOMATIC INDIVIDUALS

ROBERT MILLER, MD*

*Associate Professor of Medicine, Vanderbilt University School of Medicine, Division of Allergy, Pulmonary, and Critical Care Medicine, 6134 Medical Center East, Nashville, Tennessee 37232-8288

INTRODUCTION

More than 2 million US service members have been deployed to the Middle East since 2001, including Operation Enduring Freedom (OEF) beginning in 2001 and Operation Iraqi Freedom (OIF) beginning in 2003. Service members participating in both conflicts experienced a variety of inhalational exposures. Some exposures, such as dust storms, were related to climate and location. Other inhalational exposures were associated with mission-oriented settings, including battlefield smoke, burning solid waste, burning oil, diesel exhaust, etc. There were still other exposures that were unique to specific countries, regions, and events. These unique exposures may have been limited in duration and scope, but frequently impacted large numbers of service members.

Inhalational exposures associated with service in Iraq and Afghanistan have received a lot of attention because of the number of troops involved and the high incidence of respiratory complaints linked to service. Reports of respiratory symptoms were common among service members deployed to Operation Desert Storm in the 1990s and more recently in soldiers returning from Iraq and Afghanistan. Epidemiological studies in the United States, England, and Australia have documented an increased incidence of respiratory disorders in soldiers who served in the Middle East versus soldiers deployed elsewhere. A 2009 study of 46,000 military personnel described increased respiratory symptoms among service members functioning in inland settings versus shore environments.[1–4]

Deployments to Iraq and Afghanistan have been associated with a spectrum of respiratory complaints, including

- cough,
- bronchitis,
- shortness of breath,
- asthma,[1,2,5–8]
- eosinophilic pneumonia,[9] and
- small airway disease.[10]

Many soldiers became symptomatic during deployment. However, a larger number became symptomatic following deployment.[2,10]

Surveys of soldiers returning from OEF/OIF estimate that 69% of personnel reported respiratory symptoms associated with deployment.[7] Based on the *International Classification of Diseases, Ninth Revision, Clinical Modification* coding, Abraham et al[11] showed that a large number of these cases may be from obstructive lung disease (asthma and bronchitis). Their methods relied on coding and did not require supportive data, such as pulmonary function testing (PFT), X-ray films, or exercise testing that may offer more specific definition of the disorders. The Millennium Cohort Study (MCS) surveyed 46,000 soldiers and found an increased incidence of respiratory symptoms among soldiers who had been deployed versus those who had not been deployed. However, the differences that investigators initially noted between deployed versus nondeployed soldiers within the MCS could not be explained by an increased incidence of asthma, bronchitis, or emphysema.[4] The MCS findings suggest that there may be other respiratory disorders contributing to the high incidence of respiratory complaints.

Clearly, there is a high incidence of respiratory disorders associated with Middle East deployment. Although many individuals returning from service in the Middle East have respiratory disorders that meet criteria for specific diagnoses, a significant number of service members returning with symptoms have been more difficult to characterize.

THE MISHRAQ SULFUR MINE FIRE

Approximately 20,000 soldiers from the 101st Airborne (Fort Campbell, KY) were deployed to Northern Iraq as part of OIF in early 2003. In July 2003, the Mishraq Sulfur Mine—located 25 km northeast of Camp Q West and 50 km south of Mosul Airfield—caught fire. Most of the Fort Campbell soldiers resided in the vicinity of the fire.

Extinguishing the Mishraq Sulfur Mine fire presented risks to both civilians and military personnel. The fire burned for 1 month and reportedly released 21 million pounds of sulfur dioxide (SO_2) a day.[12] Sulfur fires, like the Mishraq fire, release both hydrogen sulfide (H_2S) and SO_2. H_2S is a noxious gas with an odor compared to rotten eggs; it causes neuromuscular weakness and, in severe cases, respiratory failure. The effects of H_2S are believed to be reversible once exposure to H_2S has ended. SO_2 has an odor compared to burning matches and is a potent pulmonary toxin. It is associated with upper airway irritation, irritant asthma, and constrictive bronchiolitis (CB).[13]

The US Army collected a limited number of random air samples during the fire. More than 50% of the 32 samples were above the Army's maximal standard of 13 parts per million (ppm). Some of the concentrations were as high as 120 parts per million.[14]

The health effects of SO_2 exposure can manifest at the time of exposure or long afterward. Acute effects include airway irritation, cough, bronchoconstriction, and wheezing. Asthmatics are particularly sensitive to SO_2. Chronic effects of SO_2 exposure include reactive airways dysfunction syndrome, chronic obstructive pulmonary disease, CB, and increased frequencies of acute asthma exacerbations.[10,15]

Most of the soldiers deployed with the 101st Airborne in early 2003 returned in early 2004. Many deployers returned to Fort Campbell complaining of increased dyspnea on exertion and an inability to complete their 2-mile runs within regulation time. Standard pulmonary evaluations at Fort Campbell's Blanchfield Army Community Hospital failed to reveal a specific cause for the soldier's exercise limitations.

CONSTRICTIVE BRONCHIOLITIS

Fort Campbell's Blanchfield Army Community Hospital began referring patients with exercise limitations to Vanderbilt University Medical Center in 2004. Vanderbilt providers were aware of the increase in respiratory complaints associated with Operation Desert Storm in 2001[1,2,5] and reports of eosinophilic pneumonia associated with OIF in 2003 to 2004.[9] Patients referred to Vanderbilt, however, did not seem to have asthma and did not fit the pattern of eosinophilic pneumonia.

Vanderbilt and Blanchfield providers created a protocol to evaluate soldiers returning with unexplained shortness of breath. The protocols included chest X-ray radiographs, high-resolution computerized tomography (HRCT), full PFT, and cardiopulmonary exercise testing (CPET). For most patients, these studies were normal or near normal and did not identify the cause for their exercise limitation.

Approximately one-half of the soldiers referred underwent thoracoscopic lung biopsy to better understand the cause for their limitation. Performing surgical lung biopsy in the setting of normal chest imaging, normal PFT, and CPET is unusual. However, at the time of deployment, the majority of the soldiers exhibited high levels of physical fitness, and, on return, these deployers were incapable of completing a 2-mile run within regulation time. Exercise limitations persisted, and service members were declared nondeployable and were facing discharge without a compensable diagnosis.

Lung biopsies appeared to provide an explanation for the soldiers' exercise limitations. In the majority of cases, the small airways had features of CB. Several of the biopsies had other small airway and/or parenchymal abnormalities, including respiratory bronchiolitis, respiratory bronchiolitis with interstitial lung disease, nonspecific small airway scarring, and sarcoidosis (Table 14-1).

The pathological characteristics of CB consist of extrinsic narrowing of the luminal wall from subepithelial fibrin or smooth-muscle deposition in membranous bronchioles. In most cases, the remaining portions of the lung parenchyma appear normal. All soldiers diagnosed with CB met this case definition, but individual variations were noted. There were varying degrees of smooth muscle versus fibrin deposition. Most, but not all, biopsies had accompanying arteriopathy. Many biopsies had associated inflammation noted as inflammatory luminal granulation, bronchial-associated lymphoid tissue, or respiratory bronchiolitis. Almost all cases had peribronchial pigment deposition, the composition of which is currently being investigated (Figure 14-1).

TABLE 14-1

HISTOPATHOLOGY OF 65 SERVICE MEMBERS UNDERGOING SURGICAL LUNG BIOPSY AT VANDERBILT UNIVERSITY MEDICAL CENTER BETWEEN 2005–2012

No.	Pathological Diagnosis
52	Constrictive bronchiolitis
4	Respiratory bronchiolitis
2	Respiratory bronchiolitis with interstitial lung disease
2	Hypersensitivity pneumonitis
3	Sarcoidosis
2	Other

Note: Between 2004–2010, 80 soldiers were evaluated with unexplained shortness of breath; 49 of them were referred for video-assisted thoracoscopic surgery. The majority of them met the criteria for constrictive bronchiolitis. Although all of the diagnoses are consistent with inhalational causes, the focus is on those soldiers who were diagnosed with constrictive bronchiolitis.

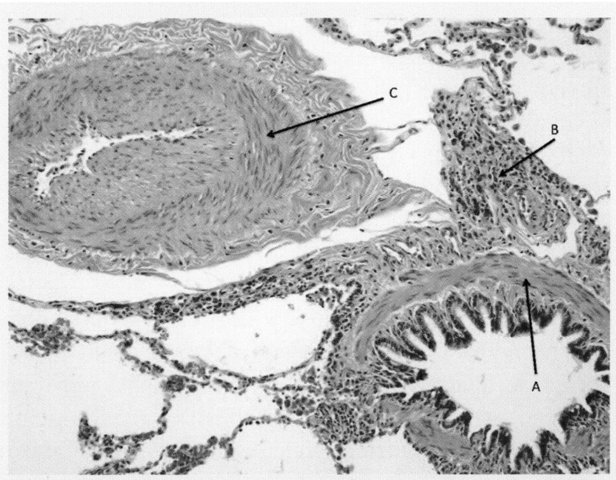

Figure 14-1. Peribronchial pigment deposition. (**A**) Intraluminal deposition of fibrin and smooth muscle resulting in airway narrowing. (**B**) Peribronchial pigment deposition. (**C**) Arteriopathy associated with bronchiolar changes.

The initial suspicion was that the sulfur mine fire was the only cause for constrictive bronchiolitis. Over time, however, more soldiers presented with exercise limitations who had not been exposed to the Mishraq Sulfur Mine fire. Twenty-five percent of the original 38 soldiers with CB had only the usual exposures and were not exposed to the sulfur fire. Vanderbilt investigators have now biopsied 65 soldiers, with 52 having CB. More than 50% of those examined had the usual exposures associated with deployment and no exposure to the sulfur mine fire.[10]

The diagnosis of CB did not lead to significant changes in therapy, but did provide an explanation for symptoms. More importantly, soldiers diagnosed with the disorder were able to receive disability benefits that would not have been available without biopsy. Soldiers who have unexplained exercise limitation and who do not undergo biopsy typically do not receive a rating for their disorder unless another label such as asthma is assigned.

Surgical biopsies of the lung have always been controversial. The controversy for returning service members and their providers involves doing biopsies for those with symptoms who happen to have normal preoperative studies. The procedure is invasive and is associated with a small, but real, risk of complications. There is always a question of how a positive biopsy will affect clinical management or benefit the patient. Clinicians often wonder if there is enough of a benefit to justify the risk. They will also consider the possibility of less invasive approaches for either diagnosis or to direct therapy.

Fort Campbell and Vanderbilt providers felt that biopsies were appropriate and in the best interest of the soldiers. Biopsies provided an explanation for the patients' exercise limitations. Biopsies also confirmed inhalational injury and helped characterize a disorder that had not been previously described in service members. Biopsy results did not usually affect treatment as there are no known treatment options for patients with constrictive bronchiolitis. Many soldiers were spared treatment with potentially high-risk therapy, such as systemic corticosteroids that are not effective in this disorder.

At some point, it may be possible to identify this disorder without a biopsy. An example is the use of surgical lung biopsies for interstitial lung disease. Lung biopsies for interstitial lung disease are less common than they were in the past. Noninvasive studies, including better serological studies and recognizable patterns on HRCT, have allowed clinicians to identify disorders such as idiopathic pulmonary fibrosis without biopsy. For now, however, the only way for soldiers to obtain appropriate compensation for this war-related injury is histological confirmation.

CLINICAL PRESENTATIONS

Soldiers serving in Iraq and Afghanistan appear to experience a wide spectrum of respiratory symptoms. Service members deployed to Operation Desert Storm had a higher incidence of respiratory complaints and asthma-like symptoms[1–4] that manifested more frequently in postdeployment settings.[2,10] Service members in both OEF and OIF commonly complained of cough upon arrival in the Middle East.[11] There have been reports of acute respiratory failure from eosinophilic pneumonia,[9] as well as an increased incidence of asthma among OEF/OIF deployers.[8]

All of the soldiers diagnosed with CB had exercise limitations, and most of them also had cough or chest tightness. Unexplained exercise limitations and, specifically, an inability to complete a 2-mile run within regulation time strongly correlated with the presence of CB (in the absence of other explanations for such limitations).

Service members typically became symptomatic postdeployment, with a unique association to restarting their training regimens. Two of the Vanderbilt patients diagnosed with CB, however, developed acute respiratory distress during deployment and later ended up with exercise and PFT impairments more severe than other patients.

EVALUATIONS

Providers caring for soldiers with shortness of breath or other respiratory symptoms postdeployment should obtain a formal occupational exposure history for each deployment. Most patients will need standard chest X-ray radiographs and full PFT. Methacholine challenge may be helpful in screening for asthma, but was usually negative for patients diagnosed with CB.[10]

CPET appears to be a less-sensitive screening tool for small airways disease. Patients with CB appear to have mean levels of maximal oxygen consumption and anaerobic thresholds at lower limits of normal; however, many CB patients are clearly within normal range (maximal oxygen consumption: 80% of the predicted value; anaerobic threshold: 40% of the predicted maximal oxygen consumption). PFT and CPET measurements in this cohort were lower than those reported for soldiers who had not been deployed (Tables 14-2 and 14-3).[16,17] CPET will be difficult to use as a diagnostic screen until better baseline data exist for CPET studies of healthy soldiers who have never been deployed. CPET may be valuable to monitor for progression in those diagnosed

TABLE 14-2

PULMONARY FUNCTION TESTING IN THE INITIAL 38 SOLDIERS DIAGNOSED WITH CONSTRICTIVE BRONCHIOLITIS*

	Comparison Group[1,2]	Patient†	*p* Value
FEV_1 (%pred)	99.1 ± 9.2	86.7 ± 13.3	<0.001
FVC (%pred)	101.6 ± 10.7	90.3 ± 13.2	<0.001
FEV_1/FVC (%)	97.4 ± 5.0	79.1 ± 7.6	<0.001
TLC (%pred)	99.6 ± 12.0	96.1 ± 15.5	0.230
DLCO (%pred)	90.6 ± 12.6	73.4 ± 15.4	<0.001

* Not matched for age and body mass index.
† Only one of our patients had pulmonary function testing prior to deployment.
DLCO: diffusing capacity of the lungs for carbon monoxide; FEV_1: forced expiratory volume in 1 second; FVC: forced vital capacity; pred: predicted; TLC: total lung capacity
Data sources: (1) Morris MJ, Grbach VX, Deal LE, Boyd SY, Morgan JA, Johnson JE. Evaluation of exertional dyspnea in the active duty patient: the diagnostic approach and the utility of clinical testing. *Mil Med.* 2002;167:281–288. (2) Still JM, Morris MJ, Johnson JE, Allan PF, Grbach VX. Cardiopulmonary exercise test interpretation using age-matched controls to evaluate exertional dyspnea. *Mil Med.* 2009;174:1177–1182.

TABLE 14-3

CARDIOPULMONARY EXERCISE TESTING IN THE INITIAL 38 SOLDIERS DIAGNOSED WITH CONSTRICTIVE BRONCHIOLITIS*

	Comparison Group[1,2]	Patient	*p* Value
VO_{2max} (%pred)	105.4 ± 14.3	85.1 ± 15.2	<0.001
VATS (%VO_{2max})	78.2 ± 15.3	45.0 ± 9.5	<0.001
Max HR (%pred)	95.2 ± 5.7	87.2 ± 9.5	<0.001
RR (breaths/min)	44.5 ± 6.7	34.2 ± 7.7	<0.001
V_E/VCO_2 (%pred)	31.9 ± 4.0	28.3 ± 3.5	<0.001

*Not matched for age and body mass index.
Max HR: maximal heart rate; pred: predicted; RR: respiratory rate; VATS: video-assisted thoracoscopic surgery; V_E: minute ventilation; VCO_2: carbon dioxide production; VO_{2max}: maximal oxygen consumption
Data sources: (1) Morris MJ, Grbach VX, Deal LE, Boyd SY, Morgan JA, Johnson JE. Evaluation of exertional dyspnea in the active duty patient: the diagnostic approach and the utility of clinical testing. *Mil Med.* 2002;167:281–288. (2) Still JM, Morris MJ, Johnson JE, Allan PF, Grbach VX. Cardiopulmonary exercise test interpretation using age-matched controls to evaluate exertional dyspnea. *Mil Med.* 2009;174:1177–1182.

with CB or suspected of having CB.

When standard PFT and chest X-ray radiographs fail to yield a diagnosis or to help guide therapy, additional testing should include HRCT. The HRCT test was usually normal or near-normal in patients who were ultimately diagnosed with CB. However, HRCT did show changes with other diagnoses, such as hypersensitivity pneumonitis, sarcoidosis, and bronchiectasis.[10]

Some clinicians have recommended screening all soldiers with unexplained respiratory problems for vocal cord dysfunction (VCD).[18,19] Although this may be a simple maneuver, the cohort with CB did not have symptoms typical for VCD (eg, wheezing, stridor, or throat clearing). Patients evaluated at Vanderbilt did not have any upper airway symptoms to suggest VCD. Vanderbilt patients had CB, a diagnosis that seemed to explain their respiratory complaints.

WHY NONINVASIVE STUDIES FAIL TO DETECT CONSTRICTIVE BRONCHIOLITIS

Noninvasive studies, such as PFT, CPET, and HRCT do not appear to provide adequate screening for CB in soldiers following deployment. Many reasons for this have been considered. The small airways of the lungs represent the largest cross-sectional area of the tracheobronchial tree. As a result, symptoms may not occur until a large cross-section has been affected.[20–22]

Those soldiers diagnosed with CB were highly trained, elite athletes prior to becoming symptomatic. Most patients presented because they could no longer exercise at high capacity. The PFT and CPET were within normal limits for most patients diagnosed with CB. The question became this: Were CB patients' PFT/CPET results lower than what they would have been prior to deployment? Only one of the soldiers had predeployment PFT, and his predeployment study appeared to be much better than his PFTs prior to biopsy. The possibility exists that this cohort suffered significant loss of function, but still tested in a range of normal. This possibility was supported when the Vanderbilt cohort was compared with historical controls.[16,17] An analogous cohort would include firefighters who worked at the World Trade Center site in 2011 to 2012. Each firefighter had annual spirometry prior to the World Trade Center attacks. Mean forced expiratory volume in 1 second measurements several months after working at the World Trade Center site were 439 cc lower than pre-September 2011 studies.[23]

Vanderbilt biopsies showed that 64% (95% confidence interval, 57.6–71 on nonparametric bootstrap analysis) of the small airways were affected in the 38 soldiers diagnosed with CB.[10] Findings of CB appear to be correlated with a reduced exercise capacity, but not severe changes in PFT and CPET; these disparities need to be examined. Could CB possibly be associated with exercise-induced air-trapping not evident at rest? Pathology examination shows significant arteriopathy associated with small airway changes. Is pulmonary hypertension with exertion a possibility? Both of these prospects need to be considered as we evaluate this population.

Clearly, CB is one of the conditions contributing to a rising incidence of respiratory disorders following deployment. The relative contribution of CB to the rising incidence of respiratory complaints has not been quantified because as many clinicians fail to consider the disorder. The fact that CB requires surgical biopsy for diagnosis has hampered efforts to identify the association between CB and deployment-related respiratory complaints. Experts from a number of fields agree that exposures in Iraq and Afghanistan place deployers at risk for respiratory symptoms and disease. Evaluations of deployed populations would be easier if we had both pre- and postdeployment data from service members.

LONG-TERM FOLLOW-UP

The majority of service members diagnosed with CB left military service with a disability rating or retirement. A few continued to serve in noncombat capacities, and others continued to serve with further exposure to Middle East environments. Those who have followed up at Vanderbilt complain of persistent exercise limitations and, in some cases, progressive exercise limitations. Most service members have gained weight from being more sedentary and not being able to exercise. Follow-up chest X-ray radiographs, HRCT, and PFTs have been performed on several of those diagnosed with CB and have generally remained stable. Many service members undergoing follow-up CPET have demonstrated reduced exercise capacities compatible with deconditioning, but also consistent with disease progression. The US Department of Veterans Affairs has recognized CB as being associated with service in the Middle East. They will inherit the responsibility for following this population over time and monitoring disease progression.

RECOMMENDATIONS

In February 2010, a working group of pulmonologists, occupational and preventive specialists, industrial hygienists and exposure scientists, the US Department of Defense, and the Department of Veterans Affairs convened at National Jewish Health (Denver, CO) to discuss inhalational exposures and the risk of respiratory disease associated with deployment to the Middle East.[24] This group recommended

- pre- and postdeployment respiratory questionnaires, as well as pre- and postdeployment spirometry;
- formal pulmonary evaluations for soldiers experiencing persistent cough, shortness of breath, or an unexplained drop in physical readiness testing; and
- surgical lung biopsies, when appropriate.

SUMMARY

Respiratory symptoms and a number of respiratory disorders have been linked to service in the Middle East. Some service members become symptomatic during deployment, but many will become symptomatic only after returning home. Disorders such as asthma may be easy to diagnose with PFT and may respond to standard treatment. Some patient complaints may be nonspecific in nature and appropriate to follow or treat empirically. Disorders affecting small airways may be more difficult to diagnose and even more disabling. Providers need to be aware that there is a group of patients who served in the Middle East who may have advanced airways disease in the absence of normal noninvasive testing. Individuals with this presentation should be evaluated by providers with expertise in the area of interstitial lung disease or postdeployment respiratory disorders. Lung biopsies may be necessary to complete the evaluation of some individuals presenting with unexplained shortness of breath.

REFERENCES

1. Haley RW, Kurt TL. Self-reported exposure to neurotoxic chemical combinations in the Gulf War: a cross-sectional epidemiologic study. *JAMA.* 1997;277:231–237.

2. Coker WJ, Bhatt BM, Blatchley NF, Graham JT. Clinical findings for the first 1000 Gulf war veterans in the Ministry of Defence's Medical Assessment Programme. *BMJ.* 1999;318:290.

3. Kelsall HL, Sim MR, Forbes AB, et al. Respiratory health status of Australian veterans of the 1991 Gulf War and the effects of exposure to oil fire smoke and dust storms *Thorax.* 2004;59:897–903.

4. Smith B, Wong CA, Smith TC, et al. Newly reported respiratory symptoms and conditions among military personnel deployed to Iraq and Afghanistan: a prospective population-based study. *Am J Epidemiol.* 2009;170:1433–1442.

5. Petruccelli BP, Goldenbaum M, Scott B, et al. Health effects of the 1991 Kuwait oil fires: a survey of US Army troops. *J Occup Environ Med.* 1999;41:433–439.

6. Roop SA, Niven AS, Calvin BE, et al. The prevalence and impact of respiratory symptoms in asthmatics and nonasthmatics during deployment. *Mil Med.* 2007;172:1264–1269.

7. Sanders JW, Putnam SD, Frankart C, et al. Impact of illness and non-combat injury during Operations Iraqi Freedom and Enduring Freedom (Afghanistan). *Am J Trop Med Hyg.* 2005;73:713–719.

8. Szema AM, Peters MC, Weissinger KM, et al. New-onset asthma among soldiers serving in Iraq and Afghanistan. *Allergy Asthma Proc.* 2010;31:67–71.

9. Shorr A, Scoville S, Cersovsky S, et al. Acute eosinophilic pneumonia among US military personnel deployed in or near Iraq. *JAMA.* 2004;292:2997–3005.

10. King MS, Eisenberg R, Newman JH, et al. Constrictive bronchiolitis in soldiers returning from Iraq and Afghanistan. *N Engl J Med.* 2011;365:222–230.

11. Abraham JH, DeBakey SF, Reid L, Zhou J, Baird CP. Does deployment to Iraq and Afghanistan affect respiratory health of US military personnel? *J Occup Environ Med.* 2012;54:740–745.

12. Defend America. US Department of Defense News About the War on Terrorism. http://www.defendamerica.mil/iraq/update/june2003/iu063003.html. Accessed September 17, 2013.

13. Charan NB, Myers CG, Lakshminarayan S, Spencer TM. Pulmonary injuries associated with acute sulfur dioxide inhalation. *Am Rev Respir Dis.* 1979;119:555–560.

14. Department of the Army, Headquarters, 61st Medical Detachment (Sanitation). *Executive Summary: Sulfur Mine Fire, Mishraq Sulfur State Company, Objective Cheetah.* Washington, DC: DOA; July 8–14, 2003.

15. The National Academies. *Health Effects of Project Shad Chemical Agent: Sulfur Dioxide [CAS 7446-09-5].* Silver Spring, MD: The Center for Research Information, Inc; 2004.

16. Morris MJ, Grbach VX, Deal LE, Boyd SY, Morgan JA, Johnson JE. Evaluation of exertional dyspnea in the active duty patient: the diagnostic approach and the utility of clinical testing. *Mil Med.* 2002;167:281–288.

17. Still JM, Morris MJ, Johnson JE, Allan PF, Grbach VX. Cardiopulmonary exercise test interpretation using age-matched controls to evaluate exertional dyspnea. *Mil Med.* 2009;174:1177–1182.

18. King M, Newman J, Miller R. Constrictive bronchiolitis in soldiers. *N Engl J Med.* 2011;365:1743–1744.

19. Chang AB, Masel JP, Masters B. Post-infectious bronchiolitis obliterans: clinical, radiological and pulmonary function sequelae. *Pediatr Radiol.* 1998;28:23–29.

20. Devakonda A, Raoof S, Sung A, Travis WD, Naidich D. Bronchiolar disorders: a clinical-radiological diagnostic algorithm. *Chest.* 2010;137:938–951.

21. Visscher DW, Myers JL. Bronchiolitis: the pathologist's perspective. *Proc Am Thorac Soc.* 2006;3:41–47.

22. Schwarz MI, King TE. *Interstitial Lung Disease.* 4th ed. Hamilton, Ontario, Canada: B. C. Decker; 2003: 796.

23. Aldrich TK, Gustave J, Hall CB, et al. Lung function in rescue workers at the World Trade Center after 7 years. *N Engl J Med.* 2010;362:1263–1272.

24. Rose C, Abraham J, Harkins D, et al. Overview and recommendations for medical screening and diagnostic evaluation for post-deployment lung disease in returning US warfighters. *J Occup Environ Med.* 2012;54:1–6.

Chapter 15

THE PROBLEMS WITH CONSTRICTIVE BRONCHIOLITIS: HISTOPATHOLOGICAL AND RADIOLOGICAL PERSPECTIVES

MICHAEL R. LEWIN-SMITH, MB, BS*; MICHAEL J. MORRIS, MD†; JEFFREY R. GALVIN, MD‡; RUSSELL A. HARLEY, MD§; AND TERI J. FRANKS, MD§

*Senior Environmental Pathologist, The Joint Pathology Center, Joint Task Force National Capital Region Medical, 606 Stephen Sitter Avenue, Silver Spring, MD 20910-1290

†Colonel (Retired), Medical Corps, US Army; Department of Defense Chair, Staff Physician, Pulmonary/Critical Care Medicine and Assistant Program Director, Internal Medicine Residency, San Antonio Military Medical Center, 3551 Roger Brooke Drive, Fort Sam Houston, Texas 78234

‡Professor, Departments of Diagnostic Radiology, Thoracic Imaging, and Internal Medicine, Pulmonary/Critical Care Medicine, University of Maryland School of Medicine, 685 West Baltimore Street, Baltimore, MD 21201

§Senior Pulmonary and Mediastinal Pathologist, The Joint Pathology Center, Joint Task Force National Capital Region Medical, 606 Stephen Sitter Avenue, Silver Spring, MD 20910-1290

INTRODUCTION

Much of the focus of pulmonary health issues following deployment of US service members to Iraq and Afghanistan has centered on the diagnosis of constrictive bronchiolitis (CB). This is largely because of the article published in 2011 by King et al[1] that reported that 38 of 49 soldiers who underwent lung biopsy had "changes that were diagnostic of constrictive bronchiolitis." Of those 38 soldiers, 28 (74%) reported a history of exposure to sulfur fires in 2003, for which CB could be an expected sequela. However, in 10 of 38 soldiers (26%), the exposure leading to the development of CB was less clear, although dust storms, burn pits, exposure to human waste, and combat smoke were reported exposures for between 33 of 38 (87%) and 17 of 38 (45%). Twenty-five of the 38 soldiers (66%) were reported to have been lifetime nonsmokers.[1] This chapter provides background information concerning CB, highlighting some of the problems associated with this histopathological diagnosis. The information is presented to place the histopathological diagnosis of CB in context so that it may be neither overemphasized nor underemphasized as an entity associated with the clinical picture of postdeployment respiratory illnesses among US military service members.

HISTOPATHOLOGICAL CLASSIFICATION OF NONNEOPLASTIC LUNG DISEASE

Nonneoplastic lung diseases are generally classified histopathologically by light microscopic observations made from formalin-fixed, paraffin-embedded, routinely stained 3- to 5-µm-thick lung tissue sections mounted on glass slides. Each slide from an open lung biopsy may contain as much as a 2 × 3 cm (essentially two-dimensional) sample that provides a limited, but high (microscopic)-resolution picture of the lung, compared with the virtual three-dimensional images of the entire thorax provided by radiological imaging. Histopathological diagnosis is optimized by correlation with clinical and laboratory data and radiological imaging studies, such as high-resolution computed tomography (HRCT).

Additional tests that can be performed on lung biopsy specimens include histochemical special stains, for example, for the detection of infectious microorganisms; immunohistochemical tests, primarily for immunophenotyping of tumors and viral infections; molecular studies; and, in certain circumstances, chemical analytical studies, such as infrared microspectroscopy and scanning electron microscopy with energy dispersive X-ray analysis. Transmission electron microscopy routinely uses different fixation than formalin, but also has diagnostic utility in rare situations (eg, evaluation of ciliary dyskinesia). Light microscopic evaluation includes addressing the following questions:

- Is the specimen adequate?
- What part(s) of the lung is (are) involved?
- What type of process is present?
- Can the duration of the process be determined?
- How is the process distributed anatomically and chronologically?
- Can additional tests performed on the tissue specimen confirm the cause of the process?

Is the Specimen Adequate?

Clinicians wish to establish a diagnosis quickly and with minimal risk of harm to the patient. Therefore, they strive to perform the least invasive procedure and obtain the smallest amount of tissue that will allow them to attain their diagnostic goals. Unfortunately, the least invasive procedures, primarily transbronchial and percutaneous needle biopsies, rarely obtain a sufficient amount of tissue for the evaluation of nonneoplastic lung diseases, such as CB. In the case of CB, this outcome is primarily because of the patchy distribution of the histopathological lesions within the lungs.[2,3] Therefore, more invasive techniques, such as open lung biopsy or video-assisted thoracoscopic surgery biopsy, are usually required.

What Part(s) of the Lung Is (Are) Involved?

The key task for the pathologist is to determine distribution of disease, which, in nonneoplastic lung disease, frequently requires correlation of chest imaging studies with histopathology. Upper versus lower lobe and central versus peripheral zone distribution of disease in the lung are readily assessed with chest CT (computed tomography). Chest CT is also valuable for determining distribution of abnormalities in the secondary lobule of the lung for correlation with histology. Identifying, histologically, whether a process is distributed specifically to anatomical sites within the secondary lobule (eg, the bronchioles) is critical to understanding the route of injury. The anatomical sites, or compartments, within the secondary lobule include the airways and their paired pulmonary arteries in the centrilobular bronchovascular bundles; the alveolar parenchyma; the veins in the pleura and interlobular septa; and the lymphatics in the bronchovascular bundles, pleura, and interlobular septa.

What Type of Process Is Present?

In nonneoplastic lung disease, this question specifically addresses

- whether there is fibrosis and how it is distributed;
- whether an inflammatory cell infiltrate is present and what constituent cell types are present; and
- whether there are diagnostic/pathognomonic findings, such as asbestos bodies, viral cytopathic effects, or aspirated foreign materials.

Can the Duration of the Process Be Determined?

Pathologists use clues such as the composition of inflammatory cell infiltrates and the presence of fibrosis to determine, in general terms, whether a disease process is acute (of recent onset), subacute (longer onset), or chronic (longstanding). CB is a disease that is usually diagnosed histopathologically after fibrous tissue has been deposited in the walls of bronchioles in a circumferential manner, constricting and obliterating the bronchiolar lumen. Because this process develops over time, it is therefore generally considered to be a chronic process.

How Is the Process Distributed Anatomically and Chronologically?

After the site and duration of a disease process have been determined, ascertaining whether these facets are heterogenous or homogeneous among biopsies from different lung lobes—or even within the same open lung biopsy—can be diagnostically important. For example, a single episode of exposure to an infectious microorganism or toxic fumes may result in lesions of the same type, location, and age, whereas repeated episodes of aspiration pneumonia may show a variety of lesions of different ages.

Can Additional Tests Performed on the Tissue Specimen Confirm the Cause of the Process?

In the field of infectious diseases, there are histochemical stains that can rapidly confirm the presence of fungal, bacterial, and mycobacterial infections, although they cannot speciate microorganisms as a microbiological culture can. Immunohistochemical stains, such as those for cytomegalovirus, can be performed on sections from a biopsy specimen to specifically identify the presence of a microorganism. Histochemical stains, such as Masson's trichrome stain, are useful in highlighting collagen deposition in areas of fibrosis and can be helpful in recognizing the pattern of fibrosis typical of CB. Elastin stains are particularly useful in diagnosing CB because they help to identify residual bronchiolar elastic tissue encircling fibrous scar tissue and to highlight the presence of pulmonary arteries without adjacent patent bronchioles.[4] CB is a pattern of histopathological change that has been associated with a variety of distinctly different causes and clinical scenarios. There is no single specific stain or test for CB, and establishing the diagnosis typically requires examination of several tissue sections from biopsies from more than one lung lobe. In addition, in most cases, the underlying cause of CB is not identified by routine tests that can be performed on the formalin-fixed, paraffin-embedded lung tissue, but rather are determined by correlation with patients' clinical and occupational histories, laboratory findings, and radiological findings.

WHAT IS THE REPERTOIRE OF HISTOLOGICAL RESPONSES OF HUMAN LUNG TISSUE?

The human lung has a limited repertoire of responses to injury. In nonneoplastic lung disease injury, the response is most commonly expressed as variable amounts of fibrosis and inflammatory cell infiltrates. Responses that are more specific, such as sarcoidosis and the granulomas (seen secondary to infection), can help narrow the etiological differential diagnosis. Pathognomonic tissue reactions do occur and are often diagnosed because of the presence of identifiable objects within the lesions of interest (eg, asbestos bodies associated with airway and alveolar wall fibrosis or cytomegalovirus cytopathic changes). Conversely, findings such as asbestos bodies, in the absence of histopathological lesions, are evidence of exposure, but not necessarily of disease causation.

Similarly, both carbon and silicate deposits are common findings in lung tissue from adult, urban-dwelling patients, but the presence of deposits alone does not establish a silicate-related lung disease.

Patterns of lung injury in nonneoplastic lung disease are generally not specific for a single etiology and may be associated with a wide spectrum of both inhalational and noninhalational clinical settings. For example, CB is most commonly seen in lung and bone marrow transplant recipients where it is regarded to be a manifestation of chronic rejection in the former and graft-versus-host disease in the latter.[4] In most of these instances, the histopathology alone does not indicate which of these possible causes is responsible for the pathological changes seen. It is usually only by correlating the histopathology with clinical, laboratory, and radiological data (and exposure histories where appropriate) that a likely cause can be identified.

It has also been well documented that single materials are capable of eliciting different patterns of histopathological response in lung tissue; inhaled silica (silicon dioxide) is a good example. Fibrotic nodules appearing after prolonged exposure to crystalline silica are seen in silicosis, but a histopathological picture of pulmonary alveolar proteinosis associated with acute silicosis can also develop, usually after heavy exposure to small silica particles over a short time period.[4]

HOW DO PARTICLE SIZE AND COMPOSITION AFFECT THE DISTRIBUTION OF INHALED MATERIALS?

The part of the lung involved is influenced by particle characteristics, including size. In general, particles >10 µm in greatest dimension usually deposit in the upper aerodigestive tract and large airways where they are removed by the mucociliary escalator. In this case, there may be no histopathological response visible on the lung biopsy. Particles 1 to 3 µm in size are small enough to reach respiratory bronchioles and alveoli where they may deposit.[5]

Solubility is among the factors that influence whether irritant gases affect upper/larger airways or peripheral airspaces. Sulfur dioxide, for example, is an irritant gas that is readily soluble in the aqueous milieu of the upper airways, causing inflammatory or corrosive structural changes. Nitrogen oxides, however, are relatively insoluble and tend to injure respiratory bronchioles and alveoli.[5]

WHAT IS CONSTRICTIVE BRONCHIOLITIS?

There is a problem of inconsistency in the terminology that has been used to describe the histopathological lesion referred to as CB. A clear understanding of what is meant by this pathological term is central to much of the debate surrounding respiratory illnesses among previously deployed military service members.

The term bronchiolitis denotes inflammatory injury to the small airways which, by definition, lack cartilage and submucosal glands and have an internal diameter of <2 mm. However, bronchiolitis is often confusing because it encompasses a group of clinically, etiologically, and pathologically divergent lesions.[6] Bronchiolar disorders have historically been difficult to classify; clinical, pathological, and radiological schemes have all been offered. However, classification into primary bronchiolar disorders (eg, CB), interstitial lung diseases with a prominent bronchiolar involvement (eg, hypersensitivity pneumonitis), and bronchiolar involvement in large airway diseases (eg, chronic bronchitis) highlights the necessity of assessing the distribution of disease both radiologically and histologically so that involvement of parts of the lungs other than the small airways is not overlooked, thus resulting in an erroneous diagnosis.[6]

CB is a pattern of injury rather than a specific disease entity and is characterized histologically by circumferential submucosal deposition of fibrous tissue that leads to extrinsic, concentric compression of the airway rather than filling the airway lumen, which may result in obliteration of the bronchiolar lumen.[3,7] Obliteration of the bronchiolar lumen has led some authors to use the term "constrictive bronchiolitis obliterans,"[4] and has led clinicians to use "bronchiolitis obliterans" or "obliterative bronchiolitis" for the same diagnosis.[2] This terminology may be confused with the more common condition of cryptogenic organizing pneumonia (COP), formerly termed bronchiolitis obliterans organizing pneumonia. COP differs from CB in its clinical course, radiological appearance, histological findings, treatment, and more favorable prognosis. In contrast to CB, COP demonstrates plugs of granulation tissue most commonly distributed in airspaces and, to a lesser degree, in the lumens of small airways. Additionally, CB is considered to be a diffuse progressive process resistant to medical treatment, whereas COP is most often patchy and bilateral in distribution and typically responds to steroid therapy.[8]

In practice, mixed histopathological features may be present, and the confidence with which a pathologist can make a diagnosis of CB is influenced by other features that may be present in the biopsy. Peribronchiolar fibrosis and chronic inflammation are not specific findings because they have been noted in many settings; in particular, they are common findings in cigarette smokers[9] and are seen in a minority of cases of chronic pulmonary aspiration.[10]

Pathological diagnosis of CB is generally made when CB is recognized as a predominant pattern rather than merely as a focal feature within other histopathological processes. Pathological changes may be subtle, and, as previously noted, CB can be patchy in distribution. Sampling issues may also lead to underdiagnosis.

CB is a histopathological pattern of injury rather than an etiologically specific diagnosis. The rate at which CB lesions will progress to the point of becoming symptomatic will vary among individuals and among different etiologies. However, the process is progressive and considered to be irreversible.

WHAT ARE THE KNOWN ASSOCIATIONS OF CONSTRICTIVE BRONCHIOLITIS?

Although CB is a relatively rare pulmonary diagnosis, it has been associated with the following:

- organ transplant recipients (bone marrow, heart-lung, and lung);
- autoimmune disease (rheumatoid arthritis, eosinophilic fasciitis, systemic lupus erythematosus, psoriatic arthritis, pemphigus vulgaris, and ulcerative colitis);
- postinfections, mainly in childhood (viral and mycoplasmal);
- inhaled or ingested toxins (nitrous oxides, sulfur dioxide, sulfur mustard, ammonia, chlorine, phosgene, and *Sauropus androgynus*);
- drugs (penicillamine and lomustine);
- peripheral carcinoids/neuroendocrine cell hyperplasia; and
- occupations (microwave popcorn manufacturers and possibly fiberglass workers).

Some cases are idiopathic/cryptogenic.[3,8,11–13]

WHAT ARE THE LIMITS OF HISTOPATHOLOGY?

Intra- and interobserver variabilities have been documented for many histopathological diagnoses, and even among experts in specific fields, the rate at which universal diagnostic agreement can be attained is in some instances surprisingly low.[14,15] A study of open lung biopsies for the histological classification of patients with clinical cryptogenic fibrosing alveolitis documented a kappa value of 0.49 between two expert lung pathologists.[16] We are not aware of large studies examining intra- and interobserver variabilities among lung pathologists examining open lung biopsies for the diagnosis of CB. One study reporting poor agreement in the presence of CB in transplant recipients between two lung pathologists was published in 2005, but was based on transbronchial biopsies that are generally considered to be suboptimal specimens for diagnosing CB.[17]

In addition to specimen adequacy, there are (as previously noted) sampling issues that may prevent the recognition of CB. As with histopathology specimens in general, the preservation, fixation, and staining of tissue sections can influence the diagnostic yield.

Even in situations where there is well-documented exposure (ie, to diacetyl in popcorn workers and sulfur mustard exposure during the Iran-Iraq War), expert pulmonary pathologists have made the diagnosis of CB in only approximately 50% of cases or less in open lung biopsies.[18,19] This outcome may be partially explained by a lack of classic morphological findings, but it is also influenced by the presence of other processes that may either obscure or serve as alternative explanations for bronchiolar fibrosis and inflammation.

WHAT IS THE ROLE OF RADIOLOGY?

The utility of functional imaging is based on the seminal work by Hogg et al,[20] demonstrating that small airways with an internal diameter of <2 mm contributed <25% of total airflow resistance.[21] Damage to these peripheral, noncartilagenous airways can be substantial and yet can remain undetected by standard pulmonary function tests because of the relatively high resistance to airflow normally presented by the central bronchi.

Typical findings of CB on HRCT cross-sectional imaging include large airway thickening and multilobular regions of decreased lung attenuation.[6,22,23] This lobular pattern of alternating high and low attenuation has been termed either "mosaic attenuation" or "mosaic perfusion" (Figure 15-1). The extent of decreased lung attenuation on expiratory HRCT, obtained with the patient at residual volume, has the strongest correlation with physiological tests of small airway function.[23] Mosaic attenuation on expiratory CT is a consistent finding in patients with both dyspnea and a clinical diagnosis of CB. A substantial minority of these patients (approximately 15%) will not demonstrate obstruction on the pulmonary function test.[24] As such, screening with expiratory HRCT provides the most sensitive and easily obtained objective indicator of small airway disease.[6]

A number of areas related to the accuracy of expiratory HRCT will require further clarification. It is important to confirm that a normal expiratory HRCT precludes the diagnosis of CB. Although highly sensitive to the presence of small airway dysfunction, the exact correlation between findings of expiratory mosaic attenuation on imaging and pathological specimens is unknown because the majority of patients who carry the clinical diagnosis of CB are not subjected to open lung biopsy.[6] It is also important to recognize that minimal change of lobular mosaic attenuation can be identified in apparently normal individuals.[25,26]

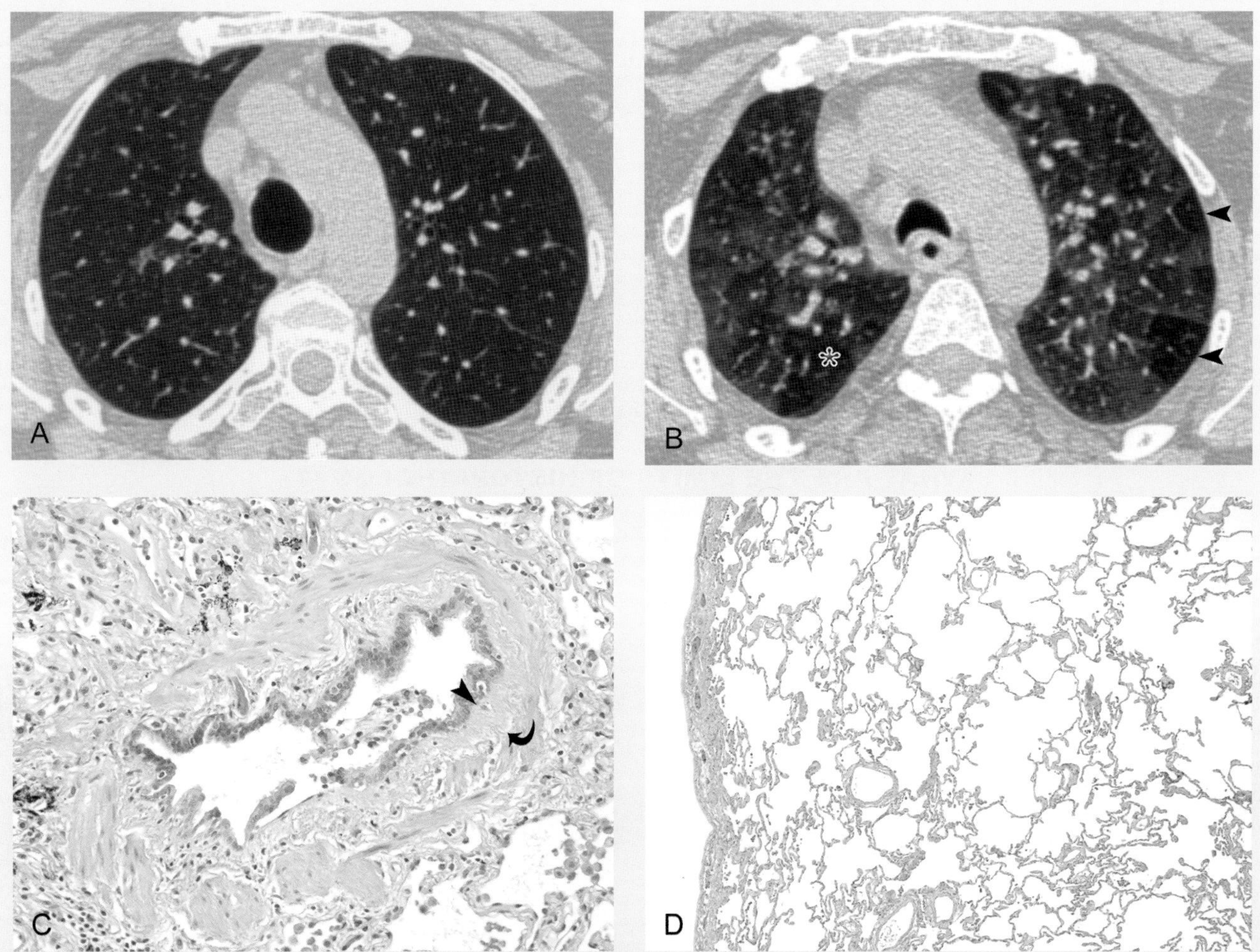

Figure 15-1. Mosaic attenuation. This 38-year-old female with dyspnea on exertion and normal pulmonary functions demonstrates normal lung parenchyma on this axial high-resolution computed tomographic image (**A**) acquired through the upper lobes at full inspiration. The expiratory phase image (**B**) at the same level demonstrates multiple, lobular (*arrowheads*), and larger (*asterisk*) regions of low attenuation consistent with air-trapping. In the same patient, the open lung biopsy demonstrates a prominent layer of fibrous tissue (**C**) between the bronchiolar epithelium (*arrowhead*) and the smooth muscle layer (*curved arrow*); normally, the bronchiolar epithelium rests directly on the smooth muscle layer. Airway fibrosis in constrictive bronchiolitis is typically present in a background of essentially normal lung parenchyma (**D**).

WHAT OTHER INFLUENCES IMPACT THE DIAGNOSIS OF CONSTRICTIVE BRONCHIOLITIS?

In as much as the timing of biopsy is influenced by clinical suspicion of CB, documentation of exposure history is likely to influence the rate at which CB is detected pathologically. The deployment history of military patients, occupational history, and inclusion in groups exposed to known hazards—such as the 2003 Mishraq Sulfur Mine fire—are factors that may lead to greater clinical suspicion of CB and, if supported by additional findings, greater likelihood of lung biopsy.

In the study by King et al,[1] reduced performance in physical fitness tests was a principal presenting feature of the patients studied. In a relatively young military population that includes individuals who have undergone medical screening upon joining the military and who are more physically fit than age- and gender-matched members of the general US population, one might expect to see the "healthy warrior effect." This phenomenon is considered to confer lower incidences of many medical conditions on the active duty military population than the general US population. Military personnel may also be reluctant to present with respiratory symptoms for fear of being prevented from remaining in their current military occupational specialty.

The impact of cigarette smoking on the interpretation of lung biopsies cannot be overemphasized. The US military still includes a relatively high number of tobacco smokers, with more smoking reported among the deployed.[27–29] The group of patients reported by King et al[1] to have CB had a relatively high reported proportion of lifelong nonsmokers for a previously deployed US military population.

Another issue that influences assessment of pulmonary function is body mass index. The diagnosis of overweight/obesity tripled in the active component of the US armed forces between 1998 to 2010.[30] Reduced performance in respiratory function testing has been associated with increases in body mass index and age.[31] Age is inevitably a factor not only in the histopathological diagnosis of CB, but also in clinical assessment parameters.

The impacts of other clinical findings are also likely to influence the ability of pathologists to diagnose CB. In particular, gastrointestinal reflux disease can lead to CB through aspiration of gastric contents and has been particularly associated with postlung transplant bronchiolitis obliterans syndrome.[32] Upper airway lesions, including laryngeal dysfunction, may also lead to aspiration and fibrosis.

SUMMARY

CB is a pattern of histopathological findings that have been associated with a wide variety of clinical scenarios. A rare diagnosis associated with specific inhaled toxic exposures, CB is not likely to be present in a large population of deployed veterans, but is possible in subgroups (eg, specific units or occupational groups). The histopathological diagnosis of CB should be reserved for cases with recognizable and broadly accepted pathological features to retain the utility of this diagnosis and preclude overdiagnosing CB as a focal finding in the presence of other lung pathology. Clinically, in the absence of objective findings, such as changes in pulmonary function tests and abnormal expiratory phase HRCT, it is difficult to classify patients as candidates for invasive open lung biopsies as the next step in their diagnostic evaluation. In the large military population with prior deployment histories to Iraq and Afghanistan, it is likely that a spectrum of pulmonary pathology will arise, as with any large population followed over time. However, CB described in a small cohort with a large proportion of patients who reported to have been exposed to the 2003 Mishraq Sulfur Mine fire is not likely to comprise such a large proportion of the pulmonary disease burden of the entire deployed military cohort. Although it is important for pathologists to recognize CB, it is equally important that they do not underdiagnose other (treatable) conditions among active duty military service members and retirees who were previously deployed to Iraq and Afghanistan.

REFERENCES

1. King MS, Eisenberg R, Newman JH, et al. Constrictive bronchiolitis in soldiers returning from Iraq and Afghanistan. *N Engl J Med*. 2011;365:22–30.

2. Epler GR. Diagnosis and treatment of constrictive bronchiolitis. *F1000 Med Rep*. 2010;2:ii, 32.

3. Schlesinger C, Meyer CA, Veeraraghavan S, Koss MN. Constrictive (obliterative) bronchiolitis: diagnosis, etiology, and a critical review of the literature. *Ann Diagn Pathol*. 1998;2:321–334.

4. Katzenstein A-LA. *Katzenstein and Askin's Surgical Pathology of Non-neoplastic Lung Disease; Major Problems in Pathology*. 4th ed. Philadelphia, PA: Saunders Elsevier; 2006: 459–461.

5. Ziskind MM. Occupational pulmonary disease. *CIBA Clin Symp*. 1978;30:1–32.

6. Ryu JH, Myers JL, Swensen SJ. Bronchiolar disorders. *Am J Respir Crit Care Med*. 2003;168:1277–1292.

7. Myers JL, Colby TV. Pathologic manifestations of bronchiolitis, constrictive bronchiolitis, cryptogenic organizing pneumonia, and diffuse panbronchiolitis. *Clin Chest Med*. 1993;14:611–622.

8. Visscher DW, Myers JL. Bronchiolitis: the pathologist's perspective. *Proc Am Thorac Soc*. 2006;3:41–47.

9. Adesina AM, Vallyathan V, McQuillen EN, et al. Bronchiolar inflammation and fibrosis associated with smoking. A morphologic cross-sectional population analysis. *Am Rev Respir Dis*. 1991;143:144–149.

10. Mukhopadhyay S, Katzenstein AL. Pulmonary disease due to aspiration of food and other particulate matter: a clinicopathologic study of 59 cases diagnosed on biopsy or resection specimens. *Am J Surg Pathol.* 2007;31:752–759.

11. Kreiss K, Gomaa A, Kullman G, et al. Clinical bronchiolitis obliterans in workers at a microwave-popcorn plant. *N Engl J Med.* 2002;347:330–338.

12. Rowell M, Kehe K, Balszuweit F, Thiermann H. The chronic effects of sulfur mustard exposure. *Toxicology.* 2009;263:9–11.

13. Cullinan P, McGavin CR, Kreiss K, et al. Obliterative bronchiolitis in fiberglass workers: a new occupational disease? *Occup Environ Med.* 2013;70:357–359.

14. Rosai J. Borderline epithelial lesions of the breast. *Am J Surg Pathol.* 1991;15:209–221.

15. Jain RK, Mehta R, Dimitrov R, et al. Atypical ductal hyperplasia: interobserver and intraobserver variability. *Mod Pathol.* 2011;24:917–923.

16. Nicholson AG, Colby TV, du Bois RM, Hansell DM, Wells AU. The prognostic significance of the histologic pattern of interstitial pneumonia in patients presenting with the clinical entity of cryptogenic fibrosing alveolitis. *Am J Respir Crit Care Med.* 2000;162:2213–2217.

17. Stephenson A, Flint J, English J, et al. Interpretation of transbronchial lung biopsies from lung transplant recipients: inter- and intraobserver agreement. *Can Respir J.* 2005;12:75–77.

18. Akpinar-Elci M, Travis WD, Lynch DA, Kreiss K. Bronchiolitis obliterans syndrome in popcorn production plant workers. *Eur Respir J.* 2004;24:298–302.

19. Ghanei M, Tazelaar HD, Chilosi M, et al. An international collaborative pathology study of surgical lung biopsies from mustard gas-exposed patients. *Respir Med.* 2008;102:825–830.

20. Hogg JC, Macklem PT, Thurlbeck WM. Site and nature of airway obstruction in chronic obstructive lung disease. *N Engl J Med.* 1968;278:1355–1360.

21. Macklem PT. The physiology of small airways. *Am J Respir Crit Care Med.* 1998;157(5 Pt 2):S181–S183.

22. Desai SR, Hansell DM. Small airways disease: expiratory computed tomography comes of age. *Clin Radiol.* 1997;52:332–337.

23. Hansell DM, Rubens MB, Padley SP, Wells AU. Obliterative bronchiolitis: individual CT signs of small airways disease and functional correlation. *Radiology.* 1997;203:721–726.

24. Parambil JG, Yi ES, Ryu JH. Obstructive bronchiolar disease identified by CT in the non-transplant population: analysis of 29 consecutive cases. *Respirology.* 2008;14:443–448.

25. Stern EJ, Webb WR. Dynamic imaging of lung morphology with ultrafast high-resolution computed tomography. *J Thoracic Imaging.* 1993;8:273–282.

26. Webb WR, Stern EJ, Kanth N, Gamsu G. Dynamic pulmonary CT: findings in healthy adult men. *Radiology.* 1993;186:117–124.

27. Ornelas S, Benne PD, Rosenkranz RR. Tobacco use at Fort Riley: a study of the prevalence of tobacco use among active duty soldiers assigned to Fort Riley, Kansas. *Mil Med.* 2012;177:780–785.

28. Smith B, Ryan MA, Wingard DL, et al. Cigarette smoking and military deployment: a prospective evaluation. *Am J Prev Med.* 2008;35:539–546.

29. Talcott GW, Cigrang J, Sherrill-Mittleman D, et al. Tobacco use during military deployment. *Nicotine Tob Res.* 2013;15:1348–1354.

30. US Armed Forces Health Surveillance Center. Diagnosis of overweight / obesity, active component, U.S. Armed Forces, 1998–2010. *MSMR*. 2011;18:7–11.

31. Thyagarajan B, Jacobs DR Jr, Apostol GG, et al. Longitudinal association of body mass index with lung function: the CARDIA study. *Respir Res*. 2008;9:31.

32. Morehead RS. Gastro-oesophageal reflux disease and non-asthma lung disease. *Eur Respir Rev*. 2009;18:233–243.

Chapter 16

MILITARY PERSONNEL WITH POSTDEPLOYMENT DYSPNEA: CHRONIC LUNG DISEASE AND THE ROLE OF SURGICAL LUNG BIOPSY

MICHAEL J. MORRIS, MD*; AND DANIEL E. BANKS, MD†

*Colonel (Retired), Medical Corps, US Army; Department of Defense Chair, Staff Physician, Pulmonary/Critical Care Medicine and Assistant Program Director, Internal Medicine Residency, San Antonio Military Medical Center, 3551 Roger Brooke Drive, Fort Sam Houston, Texas 78234

†Lieutenant Colonel, Medical Corps, US Army; Professor, Department of Medicine, Uniformed Services University for the Health Sciences, 4301 Jones Bridge Road, Bethesda, Maryland 20814; Director and Editor in Chief, Borden Institute, 2478 Stanley Road, Fort Sam Houston, Texas 78234; Staff Physician, Department of Medicine, Brooke Army Medical Center, 3551 Roger Brooke Drive, Fort Sam Houston, Texas 78234

INTRODUCTION

Deployment of military personnel to Iraq and Afghanistan in support of Operation Iraqi Freedom (OIF) and Operation Enduring Freedom has resulted in unique medical challenges due to the sustained length of combat operations with multiple deployments and the hostile desert environment. Although traumatic brain injury, posttraumatic stress disorder, and traumatic amputations have come to the forefront of military medical efforts, other medical challenges remain. Environmental sampling by the US Army Public Health Command (Aberdeen Proving Ground, MD) has established that ambient particulate matter (PM) levels from this region are elevated mainly from sandstorms and geological dusts. However, other factors (eg, fumes from burn pits, urban air pollution, and vehicle exhaust)—as well as the increased rate of cigarette smoking—remain respiratory hazards to deployed personnel.[1]

The joint US Department of Veterans Affairs (VA) and the US Department of Defense (DoD) Airborne Hazards Symposium held in 2012 in Arlington, VA, specifically addressed the potential relationship between airborne hazards and lung disease in deployed military personnel. This conference was organized as a response to numerous concerns raised in publications such as the 2011 report by the Institute of Medicine, *Long-Term Health Consequences of Exposure to Burn Pits in Iraq and Afghanistan*, that states, "Service in Iraq or Afghanistan might be associated with long-term health effects, particularly in highly exposed and/or susceptible populations, mainly because of high concentrations of particulate matter."[2] The report determined that there is "limited/suggestive evidence of an association between exposure to combustion products and reduced pulmonary function in these populations."[2] Two primary issues were at the forefront of the discussion during the conference:

1. Is there an identifiable link between deployment and the development of lung disease in general and, in particular, chronic lung diseases such as constrictive bronchiolitis (CB) as described by King et al[3]?
2. What type of clinical evaluation should be performed on military personnel returning from deployment with respiratory symptoms, but whose pulmonary function testing (PFT) results are normal and radiographic findings are unremarkable?

This chapter addresses the diagnosis of CB and other lung diseases associated with deployment to southwest Asia (SWA) as currently described in the medical literature. Furthermore, it focuses on the published recommendations concerning the evaluation of radiographic findings in symptomatic patients and the current indications for surgical lung biopsy.

LUNG DISEASE AND DEPLOYED MILITARY PERSONNEL

There is a minimal amount of published data associating deployment to SWA with chronic lung disease. Specifically, there is a lack of both cross-sectional and longitudinal studies on diagnosed lung disease. Although the survey data of deployed personnel during Operation Desert Storm (often referred to as the First Gulf War) and OIF/Operation Enduring Freedom demonstrated an increase in reported respiratory symptoms, no longitudinal data have documented an associated increase in chronic lung disease.[4] Likewise, additional epidemiological studies have not shown an increase in defined chronic lung disease from these conflicts.[5] A well-described cluster of deployment-related acute eosinophilic pneumonia cases in military personnel were initially reported during the early years of OIF. Eighteen cases of acute eosinophilic pneumonia were diagnosed among 183,000 military personnel deployed in or near Iraq in 2004.[6] Continued data collection from Landstuhl Regional Medical Center in Germany now shows 44 diagnosed cases, with an average bronchoalveolar lavage (BAL) eosinophilia of 36.8% ± 20.9%. Ninety-three percent of the patients were smokers, and 65% required mechanical ventilation.[7]

The primary respiratory concern for military personnel in general is asthma. However, very limited data exist on the effects of deployment on asthma. A survey of Army personnel deployed to SWA identified 5% with a previous diagnosis of asthma.[8] In this group, both asthmatics and nonasthmatics reported a similar increase in respiratory symptoms during deployment. A retrospective review of VA medical records based on diagnostic codes with limited PFT data noted higher rates of asthma (6.6% vs 4.3%, $p < 0.05$) in deployed military compared with nondeployed personnel.[9] A more in-depth DoD review of asthmatics undergoing a formal medical "fitness-for-duty" evaluation could not establish a definitive relationship between deployment and the diagnosis of asthma. DoD investigators reviewed 400 patient records, and the diagnosis of asthma had been objectively confirmed in 78% of the patients either by spirometry or bronchoprovocation testing. Only 25% of asthmatic individuals were diagnosed postdeployment, and no differences in spirometry or asthma severity were noted based on deployment history.[10]

Preliminary data on interstitial lung disease (ILD) diagnoses collected by military researchers showed a low overall number of cases (1.5% of military patients evaluated in Army pulmonary clinics) and were primarily attributable to sarcoidosis (53%). Fifty percent of sarcoidosis cases occurred in never-deployed personnel, and no differences in disease stage or severity were noted when comparing a pre- and postdeployment diagnosis of sarcoidosis.[11] Further collection of data to identify the prevalence of pulmonary disease in military personnel and veterans is under way in a variety of studies being conducted by DoD researchers.

CONSTRICTIVE BRONCHIOLITIS

CB, also referred to as "bronchiolitis obliterans," has been associated with numerous identified causes and is recognized to occur in various clinical settings. Clinically, it may be attributable to transplantation, medical causes, and inhalation injury. Foremost, CB is well recognized as a common complication of lung transplantation (occurring in up to 60% of patients) and is less frequently associated with bone marrow or stem cell transplantation (approximately 10%). Other noninhalational causes include postinfectious inflammatory responses (*Mycoplasma pneumoniae*, adenovirus, and influenza), drug reactions (gold, penicillamine), connective tissue disorders (rheumatoid arthritis and scleroderma), and other miscellaneous disorders (ulcerative colitis, Stevens-Johnson syndrome, neuroendocrine cell hyperplasia, and paraneoplastic pemphigus).[12]

The disorder may also be idiopathic and has been only occasionally reported as cryptogenic "adult" bronchiolitis. An initial case series from 1993 first described four nonsmoking females with chronic cough and dyspnea without any features clinically consistent with known pulmonary diseases. Three of these patients had increased bronchovascular markings on the chest X-ray radiograph (CXR). A reduced diffusing capacity and obstructive defects were identified in three patients. All were diagnosed with CB by open lung biopsy.[13] Further descriptions of cryptogenic CB have noted typical imaging features of mild hyperinflation on CXR. PFT may demonstrate obstruction, increased lung volumes, airflow limitation, lack of response to bronchodilators, and reduction in diffusing capacity of the lung for carbon monoxide (DLCO).[14]

CB may also be the result of inhalation injury and has been described in association with a variety of toxic fumes, irritant gas, mineral dust, organic dust, or volatile flavoring agent exposures.[13] Toxic fume exposures that typically cause CB include sulfur dioxide, ammonia, chlorine, methylisocyanate, or fire smoke. Inhalation of nitrogen dioxide (as in Silo-Fillers' disease) or sulfur dioxide is the classic example of a three-stage illness following toxic fume exposure. Immediately postexposure, there may be burning of the mucous membranes (eyes and throat) with minimal respiratory symptoms noted. An asymptomatic latent period of a few hours may be followed by the development of acute respiratory distress syndrome. If the patient survives, there will be a second latent period followed by the development of bronchiolitis obliterans with obstructive pneumonia (in the case of nitrogen dioxide) or CB (after sulfur dioxide exposure).[13] Other detailed reports have implicated diacetyl exposure from butter flavoring in microwave popcorn workers,[15,16] mustard gas exposure during the Iran-Iraq war,[17–19] and dust from the World Trade Center (WTC) collapse[20] as causes of CB. In East Asian countries, oral toxin-related CB has been linked to consumption of the leafy vegetable *Sauropus androgynous* used for weight control.[21,22]

Radiographic Findings

As described in multiple studies, the routine CXR is generally of minimal value in CB because often, chest imaging may either be normal or show a mild degree of hyperinflation. Typical high-resolution computed tomography (HRCT) findings in patients with CB show increased bronchiolar wall thickening and expiratory air trapping. This is recognized as the classic "mosaic pattern," an alternating pattern of increased and decreased density of the pulmonary lobules. The most striking HRCT feature is the finding of lobular or segmental areas of decreased lung attenuation, interpreted as air trapping with oligemia associated with narrowing of pulmonary vessels.[23] Bronchiectasis and bronchiolectasis are late findings in more severe disease. A composite computed tomography (CT) score may be useful for early detection in lung transplant patients. This score correlates with a decreasing forced expiratory volume at 1 second (FEV_1) and includes bronchiectasis, mucus plugging, airway wall thickening, consolidation, mosaic pattern during inspiration, and air trapping during expiration.[24]

The use of HRCT to detect CB has been studied extensively because it may provide earlier detection of disease. Breatnach and Kerr[25] first described the CXR findings in 13 known CB patients. The researchers reported what would become recognized as the characteristic CXR appearance of diminished midzone to lower zone vasculature and mild hyperinflation in seven patients. Padley et al[26] characterized the appearances of 18 patients with CB on HRCT (biopsy confirmed in six) and correlated these findings to PFT results. Sixteen of 18 performed PFTs with a mean FEV_1 of 41% predicted, a mean residual volume (RV) of 165% predicted, and an average FEV_1/forced vital capacity (FVC) of 61.6%

predicted. There was no significant correlation between the extent of HRCT abnormalities and the static lung volumes or impairment in gas diffusion. The most common abnormalities were patchy areas of decreased parenchymal attenuation ($n = 15$), subsegmental ($n = 12$) and segmental ($n = 6$) bronchial dilatation, and centrilobular branching structures ($n = 5$).

Studies by Leung et al[27] and Worthy et al[28] showed that air trapping on expiratory scans was both sensitive (80%–91%) and specific (80%–94%) in diagnosing bronchiolitis obliterans in lung transplant recipients. The role of HRCT in the early diagnosis of CB is less clear. Lee et al[29] correlated thin-section CT findings with biopsy results in 28 patients following lung transplant, 7 of whom had pathological features of CB. Using an air trapping score >3 (based on a maximum score of 4 for >75% involvement), the sensitivity of expiratory CT was 74%, specificity was 67%, and accuracy was 71%.

Pathological Findings of Constrictive Bronchiolitis

A detailed discussion of the pathological features of CB is provided in Chapter 15 (The Problems With Constrictive Bronchiolitis: Histopathological and Radiological Perspectives). In brief, the pathological features of CB include the following:

- peribronchiolar fibrotic process that surrounds, rather than fills, the lumen;
- submucosal collagenous fibrosis with progressive concentric narrowing associated with luminal distortion;
- fibrosing bronchiolitis that preferentially involves membranous bronchioles and is characterized by fibrosis of the stroma (the muscle layer may be hypertrophic in early lesions, atrophic in late stages, and replaced by fibrotic tissue at the end stage); and
- concentric narrowing or obliteration of the airway lumen due to submucosal lesions occurring in the membranous bronchioles and sparing the distal respiratory bronchioles.

Clinical Syndromes of Constrictive Bronchiolitis

The largest case series (29 patients) of nontransplant and noninhalational CB was published in 2008.[30] The mean age was 54 years, and 69% of the patients were females. All presented primarily with dyspnea and/or cough, and only 14% reported a smoking history. Identified causes in 20 patients (69%) included

- rheumatoid arthritis,
- hypersensitivity pneumonitis,
- multiple carcinoid tumorlets,
- Sjögren's syndrome,
- paraneoplastic pemphigus,
- inflammatory bowel disease, and
- Swyer–James syndrome.

An underlying cause was not identified in nine patients (31%) and was considered to be cryptogenic CB. CXRs were normal in 28% of the patients. Hyperinflation was the primary abnormality seen in an additional 55% of patients. HRCT showed mosaic perfusion and air trapping in all patients, whereas bronchiectasis was noted in an additional 21 patients. PFTs were abnormal in all patients, and 86% of patients had an obstructive defect (exceptions were those patients with hypersensitivity pneumonitis and extreme obesity). Mean PFT values included

- FEV_1 (% predicted) = 42 ± 16,
- FVC (% predicted) = 60 ± 14,
- FEV_1/FVC = 0.55 ± 0.15,
- total lung capacity (% predicted) = 104 ± 19,
- RV (% predicted) = 176 ± 65, and
- DLCO (% predicted) = 79 ± 21.

Another series presented 19 biopsy-proven CB patients with varying clinical presentations.[31] Of those, 11 demonstrated airflow limitation, 1 had a restrictive pattern, 1 had a mixed pattern, 2 had isolated gas trapping, and 4 had normal spirometry. Mild-to-moderate bronchiolar inflammation in the subepithelial layers, the adventitial layer, or both, was invariably present in all patients. HRCT performed in 10 patients revealed inspiratory (50%) and expiratory air trapping (100%), ground-glass opacities (70%), bronchial wall thickening (50%), bronchiectasis (20%), and centrilobular nodules (20%). Interestingly, six patients had a prior clinical diagnosis of asthma with progressive deterioration of lung function prior to the diagnosis of CB. One patient died, 4 patients eventually underwent lung transplantation, and 6 additional patients responded to antiinflammatory therapy. Follow-up clinical evaluations were not available in the remaining patients.

In popcorn workers with diacetyl exposure, nine patients were described in detail by Akpinar-Elci et al.[16] after the initial report was published in 2002. All workers had respiratory complaints of cough, dyspnea, wheezing, myalgia, and fatigue. Eight of the nine patients underwent HRCT. All showed marked bronchial wall thickening and mosaic attenuation with air trapping on expiratory imaging. Mild cylindrical bronchiectasis was seen in five cases, and mild upper lobe volume loss and subpleural nodularity suggestive of fibrosis were seen in three cases. Initial spirometry noted impairment with FEV_1 ranging from 14.0% to 66.8%

predicted, FVC of 24% to 84% predicted, and FEV_1/FVC of 23% to 75%. Thoracoscopic lung biopsy was performed and was consistent with CB in two of three cases. After leaving employment, there was stabilization of lung function among the patients, although five patients were on lung transplantation waiting lists. An additional report describing the screening of 175 workers employed in a diacetyl production plant located in The Netherlands showed three cases consistent with CB among the process operators with highest exposure.[32] All cases had moderate-to-severe airways obstruction with hyperinflation with air trapping on HRCT. A video-assisted thoracoscopic lung biopsy was performed in one case. Some histological sections showed emphysema and chronic bronchiolitis, reflecting nonspecific small airway disease but no sign of CB.

Studies of Iranian soldiers exposed to mustard gas in the 1980 to 1988 Iran-Iraq war reported ILDs (including CB) in patients with chronic respiratory complaints.[18–20] Of 15 patients who underwent surgical lung biopsy, 6 had severe and 9 had mild exposure to mustard gas 20 years earlier. Thirteen patients had normal spirometry, 1 had obstruction, and 1 had mild restriction. Six patients in the mild exposure group and 3 in the severe exposure group showed evidence of >25% air trapping on chest HRCT. Pathological findings varied; 33% of the patients (both mild and severe exposure) had definitive findings of CB and various other types of bronchiolar injury.

Each of these case series provides insight on the unique and clinically distinct spectrum of disease associated with the diagnosis of CB. Etiologies for CB range from various inflammatory diseases to inhalational causes, as seen in diacetyl and mustard gas exposures. In many cases, the etiology remains undetermined.

Deployed Military Personnel and Constrictive Bronchiolitis

In 2011, King et al[3] reported the outcomes of evaluations addressing the respiratory symptoms of 80 military personnel who had returned from Iraq and Afghanistan with dyspnea on exertion. Patients comprising this case series had varied deployment exposures. Self-reported inhalational exposures included the 2003 Mishraq Sulfur Mine fire, dust storms, burn pits, combat smoke, and human waste. Forty-nine of the patients underwent surgical lung biopsy. No members of the nonbiopsied group (0/31) and 36/49 (73%) in the biopsied group reported exposure to the 2003 Mishraq Sulfur Mine fire. A pathological diagnosis of CB was made in 38 (78%) of the biopsied patients. Evaluation consisted of complete lung function testing (results of postbronchodilator testing were not reported) and HRCT in this group, whereas cardiopulmonary exercise testing was completed in 30/38 (79%) soldiers diagnosed with CB. The methacholine challenge test was performed in 12/38 (32%) patients. Additional diagnostic testing, such as flexible laryngoscopy or bronchoscopy, was not reported. Spirometry was normal in the majority of patients diagnosed with CB because 16% had evidence of obstruction or restriction. Full PFTs revealed that half of the patients had a reduction in DLCO (mean value of 73.4 ± 15.4), but the reported mean total lung capacity (96.1 ± 15.5) did not reflect hyperinflation; mean RV values were not reported. Chest radiography was normal in 37/38 patients. HRCT showed mild air trapping in 16%, but the diffuse radiographic pattern of mosaicism was not described in any patients. The pathological diagnoses of the lung biopsy specimens were made by two clinical pathologists. The authors associated these findings with inhalational exposures during deployment.

An epidemiological study conducted by the US Army Public Health Command found no increase in the number of postdeployment medical encounters among military personnel exposed to the 2003 Mishraq Sulfur Mine fire, compared with unexposed personnel: "This exploratory analysis did not show a definite link between sulfur fire exposure in Iraq and either chronic or recurring respiratory diseases."[33] The report did not address any specific reported illness, but only reported whether there were an excess number of respiratory complaints related to acute exposures. An important issue not addressed was the long-term outcome of these soldiers. According to the previously cited report, the majority of soldiers had symptoms with high levels of exercise only. No outcome data was provided that would identify whether these soldiers had a progressive clinical course. Follow-up questionnaire information is only available for 43% of them. It is important to know the severity and chronicity of their illness as a baseline, and to undertake further longitudinal evaluation to determine if there was a progressive worsening of symptoms, a decline in exercise tolerance or lung physiological indices, or a response to specific therapies.

Does the pathological finding of CB on the surgical lung biopsy equate with the clinical syndrome of CB or bronchiolitis obliterans in these patients? We summarized the clinical, physiological, and radiological data from manuscripts describing patients with non–transplant-related CB and contrasted this information with the findings in the King et al[3] article (Table 16-1).[34] Manuscripts that addressed the clinical features and outcomes of CB in transplant patients were excluded because confounding issues (eg, graft-versus-host response or infections in the immunosuppressed host) occur with frequency and mask the features of CB. At 23.5%, smoking was less prevalent in the historical CB population as compared with the rate of 34.2% in the soldiers. PFT data show that the presence of nonreversible obstruction (89.2%) is consistent with a diagnosis of CB, yet the patients from King et al[3] were rarely obstructed (5.3%). Although a normal CXR can be identified in CB cases (53.2%), 97.4% of the soldiers had normal CXR imaging in the King study.

TABLE 16-1

CLINICAL FEATURES OF REPORTS OF CONSTRICTIVE BRONCHIOLITIS

Author	*N*	Smoking History	Etiology	Spirometry	Reduced DLCO	Normal CXR	Normal HRCT	Open Lung Biopsy
Turton et al, 1981 Breatnach and Kerr, 1982	13	0/13	RA–6 Cryptogenic–7	Obst–10/10	5/10	4/13	NR	0/10
Kraft et al, 1993	4	0/4	Idiopathic	Obst–3/4 Norm–1/4	3/4	1/4	1/3	4/4
Padley et al, 1993	18	NR	Various	Obst–16/16	NR	NR	0/18	2/18
Lai et al, 1996	23	0/23	*Sauropus* leaves	Obst–23/23	6/17	23/23	0/23	4/23
Yang et al, 1997	24	NR	*Sauropus* leaves	Obst–24/24	21/24	NR	0/24	4/24
Markopoulou et al, 2002	19	9/19	Various	Obst–11/17 Rest–1/17 Mixed–1/17 Norm–4/17	3/19	NR	0/10	19/19
Akpinar-Elci et al, 2004	9	6/9	Diacetyl	Obst–9/9	2/7	5/9	0/8	1/3
Van Rooy et al, 2007	3	1/3	Diacetyl	Obst–3/3	1/3	NR	0/3	1/3
Parambil et al, 2008	29	4/9	Various	Obst–25/28 Rest–3/28 Norm–1/28	1/1	8/28	0/29	5/29
Ghanei et al, 2007	5	0/5	Mustard gas	Norm–5/5	NR	NR	0/5	5/5
King et al, 2011	38	13/38 (34.2%)	Sulfur 74%	Obst–2/38 (5.3%) Rest–2/38 (5.3%) Mixed–1/38 (2.6%) Norm–33/38 (87%)	23/38 (60.5%)	37/38 (97.4%)	31/38 (81.6%)	38/38 (100%)
TOTAL	**147**	**20/85 (23.5%)**	—	**Obst–124/139 (89.2%) Norm–11 (7.9%) Rest–4 (2.9%) Mixed–1 (0.7%)**	**42/85 (49.4%)**	**41/77 (53.2%)**	**1/123 (0.8%)**	**45/128 (35.2%)**

CXR: chest X-ray radiography; DLCO: diffusing capacity of the lung for carbon monoxide; HRCT: high-resolution computed tomography; Norm: normal; NR: not reported; Obst: obstructive; RA: rheumatoid arthritis; Rest: restrictive

Data sources: Akpinar-Elci M, Travis WD, Lynch DA, Kreiss K. Bronchiolitis obliterans syndrome in popcorn production plant workers. *Eur Respir J.* 2004;24:298–302. Breatnach R, Kerr I. The radiology of cryptogenic obliterative bronchiolitis. *Clin Radiol.* 1982;33:657–661. Ghanei M, Tazelaar HD, Harandi AA, Peyman M, Akbari HMH, Aslani J. Clinical differentiation between resistant asthma and chronic bronchiolitis: testing a practical approach. *Iran J Allergy Asthma Immunol.* 2007;6:207–214. King MS, Eisenberg R, Newman JH, et al. Constrictive bronchiolitis in soldiers returning from Iraq and Afghanistan. *N Engl J Med.* 2011;365:222–230. Kraft M, Mortenson RL, Colby TV, Newman L, Waldron JA Jr, King TE Jr. Cryptogenic constrictive bronchiolitis, a clinicopathologic study. *Am Rev Respir Dis.* 1993;148(4 Pt 1):1093–1101. Lai R-S, Chiang AA, Wu M-T, et al. Outbreak of bronchiolitis obliterans associated with consumption of *Sauropus androgynus* in Taiwan. *Lancet.* 1996;348:83–85. Markopoulou KD, Cool CD, Elliot TL, et al. Obliterative bronchiolitis: varying presentations and clinicopathological correlation. *Eur Respir J.* 2002;19:20–30. Padley SP, Adler BD, Hansell DM, Muller NL. Bronchiolitis obliterans: high resolution CT findings and correlation with pulmonary function tests. *Clin Radiol.* 1993;47:236–240. Parambil JG, Yi ES, Ryu JH. Obstructive bronchiolar disease identified by CT in the non-transplant population: analysis of 29 consecutive cases. *Respirology.* 2008;14:443–448. Turton CW, Williams G, Green M. Cryptogenic obliterative bronchiolitis in adults. *Thorax.* 1981;36:805–810. van Rooy FGBG, Rooyackers JM, Prokop M, Houba R, Smit LAM, Heederik DJJ. Bronchiolitis obliterans syndrome in chemical workers producing diacetyl for food flavorings. *Am J Respir Crit Care Med.* 2007;176:498–504. Yang CF, Wu MT, Chiang AA, et al. Correlation of high-resolution CT and pulmonary function in bronchiolitis obliterans: a study based on 24 patients associated with consumption of *Sauropus androgynus*. *AJR Am J Roentgenol.* 1997;168:1045–1050.

The greatest difference demonstrated is the lack of HRCT findings. While <1% of patients from the combined CB series had a normal HRCT, 81.6% of the biopsied soldiers had normal HRCT findings without evidence of the reported abnormalities typically found in CB (ie, diffuse air trapping, nodular pattern, or mosaicism). Finally, in the combined group of CB cases, surgical lung biopsy was only considered necessary to verify the diagnosis in 35.2% of patients. In the majority of cases, the diagnosis of CB was made based on the clinical presentation, the basis of known exposure, significant nonreversible obstruction, and typical findings on HRCT imaging.

Indications for Surgical Lung Biopsy

A controversial issue from the 2011 King et al[3] case series was the routine use of surgical lung biopsy in the evaluation of soldiers with postdeployment dyspnea. Although the soldiers reported a decline in exercise tolerance, the amount of decline did not correlate with objective measures of reduced lung function, such as PFT or imaging findings. Although the DLCO was mildly reduced in 50% of the study cohort, none of the soldiers had diffuse parenchymal changes on CT imaging. Mild air trapping may be identified in normal subjects and is a nonspecific finding on CT imaging.[35] Pulmonologists have not advocated a surgical approach in patients with unexplained dyspnea in the absence of CT findings suggestive of parenchymal changes or solely with minimal abnormalities in lung function. There are potential risks with surgical lung biopsy to include general anesthesia, bleeding, infection, chronic thoracic pain, and persistent pneumothorax.[36]

Numerous studies on the utility of surgical lung biopsy in the diagnosis of ILD have been published. Aside from lung transplant patients, CB has been only infrequently reported.[37–40] As noted previously, most patients with CB have both of the abnormal imaging features associated with physiological impairment.[31,32] HRCT has been increasingly included in the investigation of unknown lung disease, particularly when ILD is suspected. Compared with lung parenchymal resolution gained from the CXR and routine CT scan images, HRCT has the ability to identify the features of the lung interstitium. HRCT is most helpful in recognizing ILD and, in certain cases, HRCT may provide a definitive diagnosis. In a study comparing HRCT and pathology in 58 ILD patients, the correct diagnosis was reached by the radiologist in 64% of cases.[39] Alternatively, if a surgical procedure is needed, HRCT helps identify the most appropriate site for a lung biopsy.

Characteristic HRCT findings in patients with idiopathic pulmonary fibrosis (IPF) may obviate the need for lung biopsy in certain patients.[41] Orens et al[42] assessed the sensitivity of HRCT in diagnosing IPF and in determining the degree of physiological abnormalities in those with IPF, but with a negative HRCT. Of the 25 patients with biopsy-proven IPF, three patients (12%) had a normal HRCT result. Based on composite scoring, their disease was less severe, but they still had moderate reduction in spirometry and lung volumes with a normal DLCO. Physiological testing was determined to be more sensitive than HRCT in detecting mild disease in this patient cohort.

The American Thoracic Society and the British Thoracic Society have published guidelines on the role of transbronchial lung biopsy (TBLB) and BAL in the evaluation of clinically suspected ILD. The American Thoracic Society guideline reports that

- the BAL cellular analysis may be a useful adjunct in patients who lack a typical usual interstitial pneumonia pattern on HRCT;
- an inflammatory cellular pattern may narrow the differential diagnosis, although patterns are nonspecific; and
- BAL cellular analysis is insufficient to establish a specific diagnosis.[43]

The British Thoracic Society guidelines on BAL and TBLB make similar statements (with the exception of suspected IPF) and emphasize the timing of the procedure before initiation of treatment, the usefulness of the procedure in identifying suspected infection or malignancy, and the recognition that TBLB is the initial procedure of choice in those patients likely to have ILD in which small samples may be diagnostic, particularly if the disease has a tendency for bronchocentric involvement.[43] There is little question, however, that TBLB has a lower diagnostic yield than does open lung biopsy (59% vs 94%) in the investigation of the etiology of ILD. This procedure may not be indicated in particular cases where diagnostic accuracy is needed for specific treatment options.[44]

No published data exist on the pathological findings in patients with dyspnea who have undergone surgical lung biopsy in the absence of PFT or imaging abnormalities. Three large studies have been conducted on patients with unexplained dyspnea. In these reports, the use of lung biopsy is very limited. The first study by Pratter et al[45] reviewed the utility of diagnostic studies in 85 patients (mean age: 52 years) with chronic dyspnea (2.9 years). The variety of diagnosed disorders included asthma (29%), ILD (14%), chronic obstructive pulmonary disease (14%), cardiomyopathy (10%), upper airway causes (8%), and numerous other etiologies (25%). Most patients underwent bronchoprovocation testing, and only two had a surgical lung biopsy. A subsequent study by DePaso et al[46] evaluated 72 patients with chronic dyspnea unexplained by history, physical examination, chest roentgenogram, and spirometry. Pulmonary disease was identified in 36%, with the majority having asthma and only two having ILD. The most common causes were cardiac disease (19%), hyperventilation (14%), and "unexplained" (19%). The most recent study, specifically performed on 105 military personnel with exertional dyspnea, demonstrated a different spectrum of disease.[33] This study had a corresponding control group (n = 69), and all patients underwent a standardized evaluation. Airways obstruction (exercise-induced bronchospasm, asthma, bronchitis, and emphysema) was by far the most frequent explanation for dyspnea (52%). Of the remainder, 10% had vocal cord dysfunction, 14% had other disorders, and 24% had no discernible etiology despite comprehensive testing. With the exception of two patients diagnosed with sarcoidosis, lung biopsy (bronchoscopic or surgical) was not indicated.

A recent study published by Doyle et al[47] provides a reasonable perspective on the proposed evaluation for subclinical lung disease. They evaluated smokers and patients at risk for developing pulmonary fibrosis (to include familial pulmonary fibrosis) and rheumatoid arthritis. In these patients with clinically suspected ILD or others with incidentally noted interstitial lung abnormalities found on HRCT, the risk for progression is unclear. Their algorithm outlined the evaluation process and suggested that, in the absence of symptoms or physiological impairment on full PFTs, patients can be followed periodically for progression of HRCT findings, symptoms, or physiological changes on PFTs prior to a formal ILD evaluation. The authors emphasized that a primary step after a nondiagnostic HRCT is the utilization of BAL cellular analysis to narrow the differential diagnosis before proceeding with surgical lung biopsy.

EVALUATION OF WORLD TRADE CENTER RESPONDERS

The evaluation of firefighters, police, and other persons exposed to the airborne hazards associated with the 2001 WTC collapse is an excellent example of repeated inhalation exposures of particulate matter exposure in a defined population. Numerous studies have been published as part of the systematic evaluation of respiratory complaints made after exposure to the WTC dusts. A spectrum of pulmonary diseases has been diagnosed that reflects chronic inflammation of the lung with associated airflow obstruction. These diseases include irritant-induced asthma, chronic bronchitis, aggravated preexisting asthma or chronic obstructive pulmonary disease, and bronchiolitis. To a lesser extent, chronic rhinosinusitis, upper airway disease, and gastroesophageal reflux were noted in this population, with uncommon reports of ILD (eg, sarcoidosis or interstitial pulmonary fibrosis).[48] Evaluation of WTC dust demonstrated predominantly coarse particles (955) with high alkalinity (pH of 9.0–11.0). The high alkalinity of this dust produced bronchial hyperreactivity, persistent cough, and increased risk of asthma.[49]

Increased symptoms were commonly reported in heavily exposed areas. New-onset respiratory symptoms were described by 55.8% of area residents (survey of 2,812 persons) in an exposed area, compared with 20.1% in the control area. Persistent symptoms were identified in 26.4% of residents in the exposed area versus 7.5% in the control areas, but no differences in screening spirometry were detected.[50]

Examinations of 9,442 responders from 2002 to 2004 identified 69% who experienced new or worsened respiratory symptoms while performing work at the WTC site.[51] Pulmonary function analysis of symptomatic individuals was notable for a variety of findings. Results from the WTC Worker and Volunteer Medical Screening Program identified 61% with new-onset respiratory symptoms that persisted after the WTC attacks. Twenty-eight percent of all tested individuals had abnormal spirometry; FVC was below the 95th percentile in 21%, and obstruction was present in 5%. The rate of abnormal spirometry was 27% among nonsmokers (compared with 13% in the general US population), and the prevalence of low FVC among nonsmokers (20%) was fivefold greater than the US population. Respiratory symptoms and spirometry abnormalities were significantly associated with early arrival at the WTC site.

Longitudinal studies showed a reduction in adjusted average FEV_1 in WTC-exposed workers for the year following exposure, and the decrement correlated with intensity of exposure and the presence of respiratory symptoms.[52] Spirometry in nearly 13,000 fire department workers showed a reduction in FEV_1 (affecting 13% of firefighters and 22% of the emergency medical services personnel), with little recovery over the 6-year follow-up period.[53] In an early study of 179 workers, hyperreactivity was increased 6.8 times for those highly exposed, compared with those moderately exposed, and it persisted beyond 6 months in 55% of workers with airway hyperreactivity.[54]

Evidence for other lung diseases is relatively uncommon despite the extensive follow-up care these patients received. Pathological evidence consistent with new-onset sarcoidosis was found in 26 patients. Thirteen patients were identified during the first year after the initial WTC disaster, and the remaining 13 patients were identified over the next 4 years. In this cohort, a high percentage (69%) had airway hyperreactivity not previously seen in sarcoidosis patients from this area.[55] There is a single case report of a patient with granulomatous pneumonitis who developed cough and dyspnea 3 weeks postexposure with diffuse miliary nodularity on imaging and lung biopsy showing diffuse, noncaseating granulomatous nodules and large quantities of silicates by electron microscopy.[56] A single case of acute eosinophilic pneumonia was reported in a firefighter with 70% eosinophilia on BAL.[57] Only one patient was reported to have CB identified by surgical lung biopsy. Despite the lack of radiographic findings and a normal HRCT, he demonstrated chronic unresponsive respiratory symptoms and a 50% reduction in FVC.[21] In this case, the patient's progressive respiratory decline was unresponsive to corticosteroid therapy, but did improve following chronic azithromycin therapy.[58]

Overall, surgical lung biopsy in this large symptomatic population was a relatively rare procedure for interstitial changes or unexplained pulmonary disease. Wu et al[59] reported on seven WTC responders with severe respiratory impairment or unexplained radiological findings. Histopathology showed ILD consistent with small airways disease, bronchiolocentric parenchymal disease, and nonnecrotizing granulomas. Tissue analysis for minerals showed variable amounts of substances, including silicates, asbestos, calcium compounds, shards of glass, and carbon nanotubes.[59] Similar findings were noted in a study of 12 patients who underwent surgical lung biopsy for suspected ILD or abnormal PFTs (predominantly restrictive with normal imaging).[60] Findings included interstitial fibrosis, emphysematous change, and small airway abnormalities. All cases had particles within macrophages containing silica, aluminum silicates, titanium dioxide, talc, and metals.

SUMMARY

The clinical approach to the deployed military patient with unexplained respiratory complaints should be comprehensive. Based on limited data, the association between deployment in Iraq or Afghanistan and the development of chronic lung disease is not well defined at this time. Patients with postdeployment respiratory symptoms should receive a comprehensive, noninvasive evaluation that includes a detailed history of inhalational exposures, examination, complete PFTs, CXR, HRCT, and routine testing to eliminate asthma as the causative etiology. Bronchoscopy with BAL and TBLB (if indicated) may provide additional information for evidence of inflammatory or infectious etiologies. For most deployed military personnel with unexplained dyspnea, close observation with interval imaging and PFTs can determine any progressive nature to their underlying symptoms. Invasive testing, such as surgical lung biopsy, should be reserved for only those patients with significant PFT or imaging abnormalities who have shown no improvement over time. As noted by Ryu[61] in his 2006 review of bronchiolar disease, the finding of "bronchiolitis" on lung biopsy may either be a major finding or a minor component of the underlying disorder and not relevant to the final diagnosis. The clinician must determine the relevance of this finding with clinical, radiological, and physiological findings.

REFERENCES

1. Weese CB, Abraham JH. Potential health implications associated with particulate matter exposure in deployed settings in southwest Asia. *Inhal Toxicol*. 2009;21:291–296.

2. Institute of Medicine of the National Academies. *Long-Term Health Consequences of Exposure to Burn Pits in Iraq and Afghanistan*. Washington, DC: The National Academies Press; 2011: 1–9, 31–44, 117–129.

3. King MS, Eisenberg R, Newman JH, et al. Constrictive bronchiolitis in soldiers returning from Iraq and Afghanistan. *N Engl J Med*. 2011;365:222–230.

4. Smith B, Wong CA, Smith TC, Boyko EJ, Gackstetter G, Ryan MAK. Newly reported respiratory symptoms and conditions among military personnel deployed to Iraq and Afghanistan: a prospective population-based study. *Am J Epidemiol*. 2009;170:1433–1442.

5. Abraham JH, DeBakey SF, Reid L, Zhou J, Baird CP. Does deployment to Iraq and Afghanistan affect respiratory health of US military personnel? *J Occup Environ Med*. 2012;54:740–745.

6. Shorr AF, Scoville SL, Cersovsky SB, et al. Acute eosinophilic pneumonia among US military personnel deployed in or near Iraq. *JAMA*. 2004;292:2997–3005.

7. Sine C, Allan P, Haynes R, et al. Case series of 44 patients with idiopathic acute eosinophilic pneumonia in the deployed military setting [abstract]. *Chest*. 2011;140:675A.

8. Roop SA, Niven AS, Calvin BE, Bader J, Zacher LL. The prevalence and impact of respiratory symptoms in asthmatics and non-asthmatics during deployment. *Mil Med*. 2007;172:1264–1269.

9. Szema AM, Peters MC, Weissinger KM, Gagliano CA, Chen JJ. New-onset asthma among soldiers serving in Iraq and Afghanistan. *Allergy Asthma Proc.* 2010;31:67–71.

10. Delvecchio, S, Zacher L, Morris M. Correlation of asthma with deployment in active duty military personnel [abstract]. *Chest.* 2010;138:145A.

11. Rawlins F, Morris M. Pulmonary evaluation of active duty military personnel for deployment-related respiratory symptoms [abstract]. *Chest.* 2012;142:749A.

12. Epler GR. Constrictive bronchiolitis obliterans: the fibrotic airway disorder. *Expert Rev Respir Med.* 2007;1:139–147.

13. Kraft M, Mortenson RL, Colby TV, Newman L, Waldron JA Jr, King TE Jr. Cryptogenic constrictive bronchiolitis, a clinicopathologic study. *Am Rev Respir Dis.* 1993;148(4 Pt 1):1093–1101.

14. King TE Jr. Miscellaneous causes of bronchiolitis: inhalational, infectious, drug-induced, and idiopathic. *Semin Respir Crit Care Med.* 2003;24:567–576.

15. Kreiss K, Gomaa A, Kullman G, et al. Clinical bronchiolitis obliterans in workers at a microwave-popcorn plant. *N Engl J Med.* 2002;347:330–338.

16. Akpinar-Elci M, Travis WD, Lynch DA, Kreiss K. Bronchiolitis obliterans syndrome in popcorn production plant workers. *Eur Respir J.* 2004;24:298–302.

17. Ghanei M, Harandi AA. Long term consequences from exposure to sulfur mustard: a review. *Inhal Toxicol.* 2007;19:451–456.

18. Ghanei M, Tazelaar HD, Chilosi M, et al. An international collaborative pathologic study of surgical lung biopsies from mustard gas-exposed patients. *Respir Med.* 2008;102:825–830.

19. Ghanei M, Tazelaar HD, Harandi AA, Peyman M, Akbari HMH, Aslani J. Clinical differentiation between resistant asthma and chronic bronchiolitis: testing a practical approach. *Iran J Allergy Asthma Immunol.* 2007;6:207–214.

20. Mann JM, Sha KK, Kline G, Breuer FU, Miller A. World Trade Center dyspnea: bronchiolitis obliterans with functional improvement: a case report. *Am J Ind Med.* 2005;48:225–229.

21. Lai R-S, Chiang AA, Wu M-T, et al. Outbreak of bronchiolitis obliterans associated with consumption of *Sauropus androgynus* in Taiwan. *Lancet.* 1996;348:83–85.

22. Yang CF, Wu MT, Chiang AA, et al. Correlation of high-resolution CT and pulmonary function in bronchiolitis obliterans: a study based on 24 patients associated with consumption of *Sauropus androgynus. AJR Am J Roentgenol.* 1997;168:1045–1050.

23. Garg K, Lynch DA, Newell JD, King TE Jr. Proliferative and constrictive bronchiolitis: classification and radiologic features. *AJR Am J Roentgenol.* 1994;162:803–808.

24. de Jong PA, Dodd JD, Coxson, HO, et al. Bronchiolitis obliterans following lung transplantation: early detection using computed tomographic scanning. *Thorax.* 2006;61:799–804.

25. Breatnach R, Kerr I. The radiology of cryptogenic obliterative bronchiolitis. *Clin Radiol.* 1982;33:657–661.

26. Padley SP, Adler BD, Hansell DM, Muller NL. Bronchiolitis obliterans: high resolution CT findings and correlation with pulmonary function tests. *Clin Radiol.* 1993;47:236–240.

27. Leung AN, Fisher K, Valentine V, et al. Bronchiolitis obliterans after lung transplantation: detection using expiratory HRCT. *Chest.* 1998;113:365–370.

28. Worthy SA, Park CS, Kim JS, Muller NL. Bronchiolitis obliterans after lung transplantation: high resolution CT findings in 15 patients. *AJR Am J Roentgenol.* 1997;169:673–677.

29. Lee ES, Gotway MB, Reddy GP, Golden JA, Keith FM, Webb WR. Early bronchiolitis obliterans following lung transplantation: accuracy of expiratory thin-section CT for diagnosis. *Radiology*. 2000;216:472–477.

30. Parambil JG, Yi ES, Ryu JH. Obstructive bronchiolar disease identified by CT in the non-transplant population: analysis of 29 consecutive cases. *Respirology*. 2008;14:443–448.

31. Markopoulou KD, Cool CD, Elliot TL, et al. Obliterative bronchiolitis: varying presentations and clinicopathological correlation. *Eur Respir J*. 2002;19:20–30.

32. van Rooy FGBG, Rooyackers JM, Prokop M, Houba R, Smit LAM, Heederik DJJ. Bronchiolitis obliterans syndrome in chemical workers producing diacetyl for food flavorings. *Am J Respir Crit Care Med*. 2007;176:498–504.

33. Baird CP, DeBakey S, Reid L, Hauschild VD, Petruccelli B, Abraham JH. Respiratory health status of US Army personnel potentially exposed to smoke from 2003 Al-Mishraq Sulfur Plant fire. *J Occup Environ Med*. 2012;54:717–723.

34. Turton CW, Williams G, Green M. Cryptogenic obliterative bronchiolitis in adults. *Thorax*. 1981;36:805–810.

35. Tanaka N, Matsumoto T, Miura G, et al. Air trapping at CT: high prevalence in asymptomatic subjects with normal pulmonary function. *Radiology*. 2003;227:776–785.

36. Zhang D, Liu Y. Surgical lung biopsies in 418 patients with suspected interstitial lung disease in China. *Intern Med*. 2010;49:1097–1102.

37. Sigurdsson MI, Isaksson HJ, Gudmundsson G, Gudbjartsson T. Diagnostic surgical lung biopsies for suspected interstitial lung diseases: a retrospective study. *Ann Thorac Surg*. 2009;88:227–232.

38. Ayed AK. Video-assisted thoracoscopic lung biopsy in the diagnosis of diffuse interstitial lung disease. A prospective study. *J Cardiovasc Surg*. 2003;44:115–118.

39. Fibla JJ, Molins L, Blanco A, et al. Video-assisted thoracoscopic lung biopsy in the diagnosis of interstitial lung disease: a prospective, multi-center study in 224 patients. *Arch Bronconeumol*. 2012;48:81–85.

40. Swensen SJ, Aughenbaugh GL, Myers JL. Diffuse lung disease: diagnostic accuracy of CT in patients undergoing surgical biopsy of the lung. *Radiology*. 1997;205:229–234.

41. Meyer KC, Raghu G, Baughman RP, Brown KK, Costabel U, du Bois RM. An official American Thoracic Society clinical practice guideline: the clinical utility of bronchoalveolar lavage cellular analysis in interstitial lung disease. *Am J Respir Crit Care Med*. 2012;185:1004–1014.

42. Orens JB, Kazerooni EA, Martinez FJ, et al. The sensitivity of high-resolution CT in detecting idiopathic pulmonary fibrosis proved by open lung biopsy. A prospective study. *Chest*. 1995;108:109–115.

43. Bradley B, Branley HM, Egan JJ, et al. Interstitial lung disease guideline: the British Thoracic Society in collaboration with the Thoracic Society of Australia and New Zealand and the Irish Thoracic Society. *Thorax*. 2008;63(suppl 5):v1–v58.

44. Rizzato G. The role of thoracic surgery in diagnosing interstitial lung disease. *Curr Opin Pulm Med*. 1999;5:284–286.

45. Pratter MR, Curley FJ, Dubois J, Irwin RS. Cause and evaluation of chronic dyspnea in a pulmonary disease clinic. *Arch Intern Med*. 1989;149:2277–2282.

46. DePaso WJ, Winterbauer RH, Lusk JA, Dreis DF, Springmeyer SC. Chronic dyspnea unexplained by history, physical examination, chest roentgenogram, and spirometry. Analysis of a seven-year experience. *Chest*. 1991;100:1293–1299.

47. Doyle TJ, Hunninghake GM, Rosas IO. Subclinical interstitial lung disease: why you should care. *Am J Respir Crit Care Med*. 2012;185:1147–1153.

48. Guidotti TL, Prezant D, de la Hoz RE, Miller A. The evolving spectrum of pulmonary disease in responders to the World Trade Center tragedy. *Am J Ind Med*. 2011;54:649–660.

49. Landrigan PJ, Lloy PJ, Thurston G, et al. Health and environmental consequence of the World Trade Center disaster. *Environ Health Perspect*. 2004;112:731–739.

50. Reibman J, Lin S, Hwang SA, et al. The World Trade Center residents' respiratory health study: new-onset respiratory symptoms and pulmonary function. *Environ Health Perspect*. 2005;113:406–411.

51. Herbert R, Moline J, Skloot G, et al. The World Trade Center disaster and the health of workers: five-year assessment of a unique medical screening program. *Environ Health Perspect.* 2006;114:1853–1858.

52. Banauch GI, Hall C, Weiden M, et al. Pulmonary function after exposure to the World Trade Center collapse in the New York City Fire Department. *Am J Respir Crit Care Med*. 2006;174:312–319.

53. Aldrich TK, Gustave J, Hall CB, et al. Lung function in rescue workers at the World Trade Center after 7 years. *N Engl J Med*. 2010;362:1263–1272.

54. Banauch GI, Alleyne D, Sanchez R, et al. Persistent hyperreactivity and reactive airway dysfunction at the World Trade Center. *Am J Respir Crit Care Med*. 2003;168:54–62.

55. Izbicki G, Chavko R, Banauch GI, et al. World Trade Center "sarcoid-like" granulomatous pulmonary disease in New York City Fire Department rescue workers. *Chest*. 2007;13:1414–1423.

56. Safirstein BH, Klukowicz A, Miller R, Teirstein A. Granulomatous pneumonitis following exposure to World Trade Center collapse. *Chest*. 2003;123:301–304.

57. Rom WN, Weiden M, Garcia R, et al. Acute eosinophilic pneumonia in a New York City firefighter exposed to World Trade Center dust. *Am J Respir Crit Care Med*. 2002;166:797–800.

58. Gerhardt SG, McDyer JF, Girgis RE, Conte JV, Yang SC, Orens JB. Maintenance azithromycin therapy for bronchiolitis obliterans syndrome: results of a pilot study. *Am J Respir Crit Care Med*. 2003;168:121–125.

59. Wu M, Gordon RE, Herbert R, et al. Case report: lung disease in World Trade Center responders exposed to dust and smoke: carbon nanotubes found in the lungs of World Trade Center patients and dust samples. *Environ Health Perspect.* 2010;118:499–504.

60. Caplan-Shaw CE, Yee H, Rogers L, et al. Lung pathologic findings in a local residential and working community exposed to World Trade Center dust, gas, and fumes. *J Occup Environ Med*. 2011;53:981–991.

61. Ryu JH. Classification and approach to bronchiolar diseases. *Curr Opin Pulm Med*. 2006;12:145–151.

Chapter 17

EVALUATING THE EFFECTS OF AIRBORNE HAZARDS: A CLINICAL PERSPECTIVE FROM THE WAR RELATED ILLNESS AND INJURY STUDY CENTER

MICHAEL J. FALVO, PhD*; RONALD F. TEICHMAN, MD, MPH†; and DREW A. HELMER, MD, MS‡

*Research Physiologist, War Related Illness and Injury Study Center, Veterans Affairs New Jersey Health Care System, 385 Tremont Avenue, East Orange, New Jersey 07018; Assistant Professor, Rutgers University–New Jersey Medical School, 185 South Orange Avenue, Newark, New Jersey 07103

†Occupational and Environmental Medicine Specialist, War Related Illness and Injury Study Center, Veterans Affairs New Jersey Health Care System, 385 Tremont Avenue, East Orange, New Jersey 07018; Teichman Occupational Health Associates, 4 Forest Drive, West Orange, New Jersey 07052

‡Director, War Related Illness and Injury Study Center, Veterans Affairs New Jersey Health Care System, 385 Tremont Avenue, East Orange, New Jersey 07018; Associate Professor, Rutgers University–New Jersey Medical School, 185 South Orange Avenue, Newark, New Jersey 07103

INTRODUCTION

Brief Overview of the War Related Illness and Injury Study Center

The War Related Illness and Injury Study Center (WRIISC) of the US Veterans Health Administration (VHA) was founded by Congressional Mandate in 2001 in the context of continued concerns about the etiology, pathophysiology, and prognosis of Gulf War illnesses. Two WRIISCs were initially established, with a third created in 2007. With a mission to promote research, education, clinical care, and risk communication related to deployment health issues, the WRIISC focuses on difficult-to-diagnose conditions in veterans of the US armed forces and their possible link to deployment-related experiences. Based in the VHA's Office of Public Health, the WRIISCs have an explicit role in surveillance of the population health of deployed veterans. The VHA providers throughout the country refer patients with difficult-to-diagnose conditions to one of the three WRIISCs located in

- East Orange, NJ;
- Palo Alto, CA; and
- Washington, DC.

Each center offers a similar multiday, comprehensive, multidisciplinary evaluation of exposure and health concerns, as well as previous workups. The WRIISC works with patients to create a roadmap for moving forward with the referring team of providers. Through prospective, active review of clinical activity, the WRIISC program identifies novel exposure concerns and health conditions for further investigation.

Airborne Hazards Experience of the War Related Illness and Injury Study Center

One of the most frequent exposure concerns reported by Gulf War veterans seen at the WRIISCs in New Jersey and Washington, DC, was smoke from burning oil wells.[1] These concerns were explicitly addressed by New Jersey WRIISC clinicians in a comprehensive, lifetime exposure assessment for every patient with additional diagnostic evaluation recommended on a case-by-case basis. In 2004, New Jersey WRIISC clinicians began evaluating veterans deployed to Operation Enduring Freedom/Operation Iraqi Freedom (OEF/OIF) and gaining clinical experience with their health and exposure concerns. By January 2006, New Jersey WRIISC experience with the first 56 OEF/OIF veterans evaluated indicated that air quality was one of the most common exposure concerns. Ear, nose, and throat symptoms were among the most prevalent, although the small sample size precluded the detection of a definitive association between these two observations.[2] Review of a larger sample of New Jersey WRIISC patients (n = 469) from 2006 to 2010 indicated that approximately 90% of veterans evaluated at the New Jersey WRIISC reported exposure to airborne hazards, including smoke from burn pits, sand/dust, and general air pollution. The same proportion reported somewhat or greater concern about these exposures. This was the most prevalent exposure concern in this clinical population.[3]

Given the near universality of concern about airborne hazards during deployment to OEF/OIF, the clinical team developed an approach to addressing both concern about the exposure and symptoms reported that might be associated with airborne hazards exposure.

CLINICAL EVALUATION

Clinical Approach to Airborne Hazards at the War Related Illness and Injury Study Center

The comprehensive clinical evaluation for all patients seen at the WRIISC was designed to assess as many organ systems, symptoms, and health concerns as possible during the 1- to 3-day stay in East Orange, NJ. This included an extensive set of intake questions—some as formal, validated questionnaires (such as the Patient Health Questionnaire-15) and others developed by WRIISC staff to ascertain responses specific to postdeployment veterans. In 2006, a newly revised self-report exposure measure created by one of the authors (R.F.T.) was added to the set of questions. This measure allowed veterans to indicate whether they believe themselves to have been exposed and whether they were concerned about the exposure. Further details of this measure and analysis of responses have already been published.[3] Veterans' responses to all questions in the intake packet are electronically scanned or manually entered into an electronic database through which WRIISC investigators may access under an approved protocol.

Each veteran seen at the WRIISC was given a thorough history and physical examination by either a primary care physician with an interest in postdeployment health issues or a nurse practitioner with additional specialized training in conducting these examinations. In addition, each veteran was given a neuropsychological screening battery and a psychological interview, as well as an evaluation by a social worker. An occupational medicine physician conducted an in-person exposure evaluation with each veteran. This involved taking a lifelong exposure history, conducting an in-depth discussion of exposures during military service and deployment, and executing a discussion of all postmilitary exposures. Each exposure was explored with the veteran in regard to location, duration, intensity, and frequency of exposure; a strong emphasis was placed on eliciting a temporal correlation between exposure and the onset or worsening of health symptoms. All provider notes from this comprehensive evaluation are entered into the US Department of Veterans Affairs (VA) Computerized Patient Record System.

Sometime in late 2009, the WRIISC clinical staff noted that the portion of OEF/OIF veterans reporting respiratory symptoms was increasing. At the same time, review of these veterans' pulmonary function testing (PFT) conducted at their home VA Medical Centers revealed values within normal range, defined as forced expiratory volume in 1 second (FEV_1) and forced vital capacity, both equal to or above 80% of predicted (see section below for further discussion of this definition of "normal"). Several reports were published in 2009 and 2010 that proposed a correlation between OEF/OIF veterans' deployment airborne exposures and their respiratory symptoms.[4–6] Personal communications between one of the authors (R.F.T.) and several colleagues, both with the Department of Defense and the VA, indicated that there were veterans evaluated with normal PFTs who revealed significant bronchodilator response when tested.

In September 2011, an agreement was established with the Pulmonary Function Laboratory at the East Orange VA Medical Center and the WRIISC to enable each veteran (with or without respiratory symptoms) seen at the WRIISC to have a comprehensive PFT performed during their brief visit. This testing would include diffusion capacity and spirometric testing without and then subsequent to the administration of a bronchodilator medication. The remainder of this chapter discusses these preliminary findings of the first 20 consecutive WRIISC OEF/OIF veterans to undergo this testing. The PFT was performed as part of the clinical surveillance mission of the WRIISC and therefore did not require institutional review board approval. However, retrospective analysis of these data has received local institutional review board approval.

Clinical Observations of 20 Operation Enduring Freedom/Operation Iraqi Freedom Veterans

We reviewed retrospectively medical records and intake questionnaire packets from OEF/OIF veterans who underwent clinical evaluations at the New Jersey WRIISC. Chest roentgenograms were already being obtained on all veterans seen who had not had this test within 1 to 2 years of their visit to the WRIISC. Overall, these roentgenograms were unremarkable. We selected the first 20 consecutive veterans who completed PFT as part of their comprehensive clinical evaluation—a process that started at the New Jersey WRIISC in the fall of 2011.

For the purposes of characterizing our clinical sample, we extracted key demographic variables, medical histories, and symptom reports from both the veterans' medical records and intake questionnaire packet responses. These data are presented individually for each veteran in Table 17-1. Variables were computed as follows:

- *Mental Health Diagnosis*—Provider diagnosis of posttraumatic stress disorder, panic disorder, and/or depression.
- *Respiratory Symptoms in Top Three*—Each veteran self-reports his/her top three symptoms of concern. For example, these may include widespread pain, balance or dizziness, and/or shortness of breath or coughing. These top three symptoms are part of the intake packet and often represent reasons why the veteran is seeking evaluation at the WRIISC.
- *Smoking Status*—Veterans were categorized as never, current, or past (>100 cigarettes/cigars/pipes in lifetime) smokers.
- *Lower Respiratory Symptoms*—Symptoms include coughing, bronchitis, wheezing, and/or dyspnea.
- *Upper Respiratory Symptoms*—Symptoms include sinusitis and/or rhinitis.
- *Abnormal Radiological Findings*—Abnormalities reported in the medical record may include abnormal findings on chest X-ray, computed tomography, and/or magnetic resonance imaging.

Summary of Findings From Clinical Evaluation and Questionnaires

Our sample is predominantly young (40.4 ± 12.2 years), male (85%), white non-Hispanic (85%), and overweight/obese (with a body mass index of 31.02 ± 4.9). Most are Army veterans (80%), and 75% served in OIF. Three veterans had served in conflicts prior to 2001 (Persian Gulf, Kosovo, and Vietnam), and five veterans had served in OEF.

Mental health diagnoses were observed in all but five of these veterans, and 30% (6 of 20) were current smokers. Respiratory symptoms of lower (75%) and upper (55%) airways were present in most veterans; however, only 6 of 20 veterans (30%) listed respiratory symptoms in their top three symptom concerns. Four veterans had abnormal lung radiological findings.

All but two veterans endorsed exposure to airborne hazards during their exposure evaluation with an occupational medicine physician. Exposure medical notes were further reviewed in these 18 veterans to determine the frequency of *specific* airborne hazards concerns that were grouped into the following five categories:

TABLE 17-1

DATA ABSTRACTED FROM THE COMPUTERIZED MEDICAL RECORD AND WRIISC DATABASE

ID	Age	Gender	BMI	Mental Health Diagnosis	Respiratory Symptoms	Smoking Status in Top 3	Lower Respiratory Symptoms	Upper Respiratory Symptoms	Abnormal Radiological Findings
1	43	Female	25.23	Y	N	Current	Y	Y	N
2	42	Male	34.78	N	Y	Never	Y	Y	N
3	33	Male	27.73	Y	N	Past	Y	Y	N
4	64	Male	31.39	Y	Y	Past	Y	N	Y
5	29	Female	24.18	Y	N	Past	Y	N	Y
6	43	Male	32.56	Y	Y	Never	N	Y	N
7	51	Male	41.14	Y	N	Current	N	Y	Y
8	23	Male	33.64	Y	N	Current	N	N	N
9	64	Male	37.67	Y	Y	Never	Y	Y	N
10	56	Male	24.33	Y	Y	Never	Y	Y	Y
11	44	Male	29.49	N	N	Never	Y	N	Y
12	26	Male	29.35	Y	N	Current	Y	Y	N
13	26	Female	29.16	N	N	Never	Y	Y	N
14	41	Male	37.67	Y	N	Never	Y	N	N
15	38	Male	30.44	N	N	Never	N	N	N
16	29	Male	22.57	Y	N	Current	Y	Y	N
17	47	Male	35.05	Y	N	Past	N	N	N
18	25	Male	29.63	Y	N	Never	Y	N	N
19	38	Male	33.98	Y	N	Current	Y	N	N
20	46	Male	30.48	N	Y	Past	Y	Y	N

BMI: body mass index; DoD: Department of Defense; ID: identification; N: no; WRIISC: War Related Illness and Injury Study Center; VA: Veterans Affairs; Y: yes
Data source: VA/DoD Airborne Hazards Symposium, Arlington, Virginia, August 2012.

1. smoke from burning trash,
2. sand and/or dust,
3. regional air pollution,
4. fuels and/or chemicals, and
5. other (eg, cigarette smoke, mold, and asbestos).

The frequencies of specific airborne hazards concerns are shown in Figure 17-1. Note that the most common exposure was exposure to sandstorms and/or airborne dust (80%).

Pulmonary Function Testing

The PFTs were conducted by a Registered Respiratory Therapist in the Department of Pulmonary and Critical Care Medicine at the VA New Jersey Health Care System (East Orange, NJ). Lung volumes and flows were obtained according to standardized guidelines[7] via body box and pneumotach, respectively. PFTs were performed in the morning in a fasted state by all veterans. Predicted values for our laboratory are based on the reference equations listed in Table 17-2.

Data are presented individually for each veteran in Table 17-3 and expressed as a percentage of their predicted values.

Summary of Findings From Pulmonary Function Testing

We used the simplified algorithm provided by the American Thoracic Society and the European Respiratory Society (see Pelligrino et al,[7] Figure 2) to assess lung function in

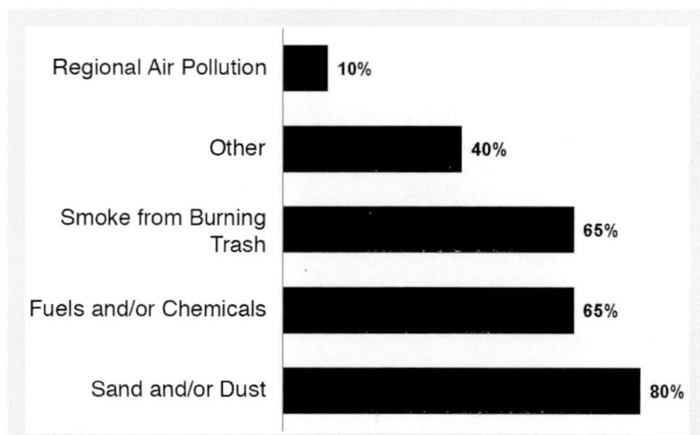

Figure 17-1. Frequency of specific airborne hazards exposure in 18 veterans. "Other" refers to cigarette smoke, mold, and asbestos.

this sample. Using these classic patterns, we observed four veterans with abnormal patterns (patient no. 4 = restriction; patient nos. 16, 17, and 20 = obstruction). Therefore, the majority of the sample performed within normal ranges. However, there was a considerable range in our measured variables, with some veterans producing values close to the lower limit of normal (LLN). For example, one in four veterans had FEV_1 values that were lower than the LLN. Means and standard deviations for each of these variables are provided in Table 17-4.

SUMMARY

Prior work from the New Jersey WRIISC has shown that veterans of Afghanistan and Iraq are concerned about their deployment-related exposures,[2,3] and these concerns are associated with their somatic symptom burden.[3] This concern seems justified because prior reports have indicated that the deployment environment of OEF/OIF contains high levels of particulate matter that exceed environmental, occupational, and military exposure guidelines.[6,8] In fact, exposure to these particulates—especially those that are combustion-derived—may induce pulmonary inflammation that is associated with the pathogenesis and exacerbation of airway diseases.[9,10] The military population also warrants additional attention given the physically active nature of their service which, like exercise, necessitates an increase in pulmonary ventilation and diffusion capacity. Therefore, if service members are physically active in a location with high-ambient particulate matter, the lung concentration of inhaled particulates will increase. This has been demonstrated experimentally because the total amount of particulate matter deposited in the lungs is 4.5-fold higher during exercise than at rest, thereby making deposition of particles a function of minute ventilation.[11] This significant increase in particle deposition during exercise may also be related to a greater increase in oral rather than nasal breathing as the intensity of physical activity increases, thereby bypassing protective filtering functions of the nasopharyngeal region. These experimental data may support the reports of new-onset respiratory conditions in OEF/OIF veterans[4,12,13] and reports of exercise intolerance.[14]

Several features of the military environment are favorable for the development of respiratory illnesses that include close living quarters, unique stressors, and barracks with closed ventilation systems. Therefore, respiratory infections during deployment to OEF/OIF have been commonly reported. Thus, the incidence of self-reported respiratory illness has been estimated between 40% to 70% during deployment to Afghanistan or Iraq.[12,13] Although these rates have appeared to decline from the early stages of the conflict (ie, 69% vs 40%), the question remains whether respiratory symptoms persist postdeployment, and whether these symptoms and illnesses precede the development of respiratory disease. Few experimental studies are available to determine whether exposure to airborne hazards during deployment negatively impacts lung function postdeployment. To this end, the WRIISC has introduced standardized pulmonary evaluations for all veterans who participate in our clinical evaluation. Herein, we present our preliminary findings from the first 20 consecutive OEF/OIF veterans who performed PFTs as part of their evaluation.

The overwhelming majority of OEF/OIF veterans clinically evaluated at the WRIISC endorsed exposure to airborne hazards during their deployment (90%), as well as lower airway respiratory symptoms (75%), such as coughing, wheezing, and shortness of breath. It remains unclear whether symptoms are attributable to these exposures; however, it is concerning that symptoms are maintained several years following their deployment to OEF/OIF (5.4 ± 2.6 years = date of WRIISC visit − date of separation). Despite the frequency of symptoms, only 30% of our sample indicated respiratory symptoms as one of their top three reasons for coming to the WRIISC.

TABLE 17-2

REFERENCE EQUATIONS FOR PULMONARY FUNCTION TESTING

Pulmonary Function Testing Variables	Reference Equations
Lung volumes	
Total lung capacity	Crapo, 1982
Vital capacity	Crapo, 1981
Forced residual capacity	Boren and Korey, 1966
Residual volume	Boren and Korey, 1966
Spirometry	
Forced vital capacity	Crapo, 1981
Forced expiratory volume in 1 second	Morris, 1985
Forced expiratory flow between 25%–75% of vital capacity (FMEF 25%–75%)	Crapo, 1981

FMEF: forced midexpiratory flow

Data sources: Crapo RO, Morris AH, Clayton PD, Nixon CR. Lung volumes in healthy nonsmoking Adults. *Bull Eur Physiopathol Respir.* 1982;18:419–425. Crapo RO, Morris AH, Gardner RM. Reference spirometric values using techniques and equipment that meet ATS recommendations. *Am Rev Respir Dis.* 1981;123:659–664. Boren HG, Kory RC, Syner JC. The Veterans Administration Army Cooperative Study of Pulmonary Function. II. The lung volume and its subdivisions in normal men. *Am J Med.* 1966;41:96–114. Morris J, Temple W. Spirometric "lung age" estimation for motivating smoking cessation. *Prev Med.* 1985;14:655–662.

TABLE 17-3

LUNG VOLUME AND SPIROMETRY DATA

ID	TLC (%)	VC (%)	FRC (%)	RV (%)	FVC (%)	FEV_1 (%)	FMEF (25%–75%)	FEV_1/FVC
1	106.54	125.61	129.04	61.58	125.61	111.22	83.92	0.73
2	85.74	86.72	95.13	75.38	86.72	80.69	65.42	0.76
3	95.23	102.00	120.85	63.16	97.41	98.56	99.95	0.84
4	64.91	51.84	50.86	89.02	50.71	56.81	100.23	0.86
5	91.28	97.66	75.00	67.86	97.66	99.39	108.25	0.87
6	81.45	78.79	103.75	81.22	78.79	72.39	54.25	0.75
7	93.23	103.28	82.42	64.25	99.78	100.00	105.05	0.81
8	73.26	95.12	93.09	75.63	95.12	90.67	82.69	0.79
9	75.78	89.02	87.65	48.48	89.02	94.83	136.78	0.84
10	90.93	102.15	169.42	62.61	102.15	91.52	59.15	0.70
11	92.24	92.01	93.47	85.51	92.01	93.50	104.48	0.81
12	81.17	87.84	108.36	48.62	85.64	78.56	62.70	0.75
13	99.13	100.87	114.22	93.91	100.87	88.56	63.33	0.78
14	99.72	107.66	110.39	69.50	107.66	103.32	96.26	0.78
15	87.86	86.93	101.37	82.09	86.93	85.62	81.67	0.80
16	106.82	110.37	198.04	80.92	110.37	83.18	47.66	0.62
17	25.80	108.92	128.96	128.00	107.22	88.71	54.01	0.67
18	85.05	88.43	78.35	62.07	87.74	80.50	69.39	0.76
19	86.49	94.01	83.51	58.21	94.01	91.69	90.72	0.79
20	96.55	108.75	98.55	59.62	108.15	69.63	27.67	0.52

FEV_1: forced expiratory volume in 1 second; FMEF: forced midexpiratory flow; FRC: forced residual capacity; FVC: forced vital capacity; ID: identification; %: percent of predicted value; RV: residual volume; TLC: total lung capacity; VC: vital capacity

Lung volume and spirometry data were primarily normal, with the exception of four veterans who demonstrated obstructive patterns. In addition, approximately 25% of our sample had FEV_1 values that were lower than the LLN. Given the absence of prior PFT data (ie, predeployment or pre-WRIISC visit), our assessment provides only a snapshot of lung function. Serial PFTs would afford a better assessment of lung function over time and that may facilitate a better understanding of whether deployment-related exposures and/or smoking may affect lung function.

To address the limitations of single timepoint spirometry and lung volume testing, the New Jersey WRIISC has implemented and is considering additional testing, such as reversibility testing with a bronchodilator, lung-diffusing capacity, and cardiopulmonary exercise testing. These additional tests may provide a more comprehensive evaluation of integrated lung function, and we hope to make these data available to the community in the near future. We also want to highlight that data presented herein are mostly descriptive and preliminary in nature. Therefore, one should exercise caution in extrapolating these data until further cases are evaluated and more detailed studies are performed.

There are several key issues that warrant attention from the clinical and research communities. First, the challenges of assessing exposures during deployment are substantial,[15] and previous research has demonstrated the difficulties regarding misclassifying exposures for determining associations between potential exposures and adverse health outcomes.[16] At the WRIISC, detailed exposure histories are conducted by occupational medicine physicians with veterans. There is widespread agreement that these histories are subject to recall bias, and the population of veterans seen at the WRIISC is subject to (self-) selection bias. Because

TABLE 17-4

AVERAGE VALUES FOR SELECTED PULMONARY FUNCTION TESTING VARIABLES

PFT Variables	Mean ± SD
TLC	86.0% ± 17.7%
VC	95.9% ± 15.1%
FRC	106.1% ± 32.9%
RV	72.9% ± 18.2%
FVC	95.2% ± 15.1%
FEV_1	88.0% ± 12.7%
FMEF (25%–75%)	79.7% ± 26.1%

FEV_1: forced expiratory volume in 1 second; FMEF: forced midexpiratory flow; FRC: forced residual capacity; FVC: forced vital capacity; PFT: pulmonary function testing; RV: residual volume; SD: standard deviation; TLC: total lung capacity; VC: vital capacity a one-on-one interview is not feasible for all veterans, we must develop appropriate metrics through which to quantify exposure. Second, we currently lack a well-accepted clinical protocol on how to approach the OEF/OIF veteran who may present with respiratory symptoms or limitations. Our approach must have a favorable risk-to-benefit ratio and provide appropriate sensitivity to improve the differential diagnosis. Lastly, we emphasize that the extent and severity of deployment-related lung injury remain unclear. Therefore, additional studies are greatly needed to better understand the scope of this problem, if any, and how best to treat affected veterans.

REFERENCES

1. Lincoln AE, Helmer DA, Schneiderman AI, et al. The war-related illness and injury study centers: a resource for deployment-related health concerns. *Mil Med.* 2006;171:577–585.

2. Helmer DA, Rossignol M, Blatt M, Agarwal R, Teichman R, Lange G. Health and exposure concerns of veterans deployed to Iraq and Afghanistan. *J Occup Environ Med.* 2007;49:475–480.

3. McAndrew LM, Teichman RF, Osinubi OY, Jasien JV, Quigley KS. Environmental exposure and health of Operation Enduring Freedom/Operation Iraqi Freedom veterans. *J Occup Environ Med.* 2012;54:665–669.

4. Smith B, Wong CA, Smith TC, Boyko EJ, Gackstetter GD. Newly reported respiratory symptoms and conditions among military personnel deployed to Iraq and Afghanistan: a prospective population-based study. *Am J Epidemiol.* 2009;170:1433–1442.

5. Szema AM, Peters MC, Weissinger KM, Gagliano CA, Chen JJ. New-onset asthma among soldiers serving in Iraq and Afghanistan. *Allergy Asthma Proc.* 2010;31:67–71.

6. Weese CB, Abraham JH. Potential health implications associated with particulate matter exposure in deployed settings in southwest Asia. *Inhal Toxicol.* 2009;21:291–296.

7. Pellegrino R, Viegi G, Brusasco V, et al. Interpretative strategies for lung function tests. *Eur Respir J.* 2005;26:948–968.

8. Morris MJ, Zacher LL, Jackson DA. Investigating the respiratory health of deployed military personnel. *Mil Med.* 2011;176:1157–1161.

9. Li N, Hao M, Phalen RF, Hinds WC, Nel AE. Particulate air pollutants and asthma. A paradigm for the role of oxidative stress in PM-induced adverse health effects. *Clin Immunol.* 2003;109:250–265.

10. Tao F, Gonzalez-Flecha B, Kobzik L. Reactive oxygen species in pulmonary inflammation by ambient particulates. *Free Radic Biol Med.* 2003;35:327–340.

11. Daigle CC, Chalupa DC, Gibb FR, et al. Ultrafine particle deposition in humans during rest and exercise. *Inhal Toxicol.* 2003;15:539–552.

12. Sanders JW, Putnam SD, Frankart C, et al. Impact of illness and non-combat injury during Operations Iraqi Freedom and Enduring Freedom (Afghanistan). *Am J Trop Med Hyg.* 2005;73:713–719.

13. Soltis BW, Sanders JW, Putnam SD, Tribble DR, Riddle MS. Self reported incidence and morbidity of acute respiratory illness among deployed U.S. military in Iraq and Afghanistan. *PLoS One.* 2009;4:e6177.

14. King MS, Eisenberg R, Newman JH, et al. Constrictive bronchiolitis in soldiers returning from Iraq and Afghanistan. *N Engl J Med.* 2011;365:222–230.

15. Glass DC, Sim MR. The challenges of exposure assessment in health studies of Gulf War veterans. *Philos Trans R Soc Lond B Biol Sci.* 2006;361:627–637.

16. Checkoway H, Savitz DA, Heyer NJ. Assessing the effects of nondifferential misclassification of exposures in occupational studies. *Appl Occup Environ Hyg.* 1991;6:528–533.

Chapter 18

EXPERIENCE WITH EMERGING LUNG DISEASES FROM THE NATIONAL INSTITUTE FOR OCCUPATIONAL SAFETY AND HEALTH

KATHLEEN KREISS, MD*

**Field Studies Branch Chief, Division of Respiratory Disease Studies, National Institute for Occupational Safety and Health, Centers for Disease Control and Prevention, Mailstop H-2800, 1095 Willowdale Road, Morgantown, West Virginia 26505*

INTRODUCTION

Surveillance of respiratory health or environmental conditions that impact health is efficient only when the nature of health outcomes and their causes are known. Surveillance does not establish causes. Rather, the purpose of surveillance is to follow trends over time as a means of evaluating public health interventions.[1] Interventions are often difficult to justify until specific respiratory conditions and their causes are understood. Some research studies have documented increases in respiratory symptoms and diagnoses in military personnel who have deployed to Iraq and Afghanistan,[2–4] but diagnoses and their causes remain the subject of considerable controversy,[5-6] precluding systematic preventive measures and even appropriate surveillance.

Lessons learned are from characterizing emerging occupational diseases or novel occupational efforts in new service-associated challenges, such as soldiers with constrictive bronchiolitis,[7] undiagnosed respiratory symptoms, and suspected environmental contributors. Illustrative examples of emerging diseases and causes investigated by the National Institute for Occupational Safety and Health (NIOSH) are listed in Exhibit 18-1. Like public health personnel and clinical providers in the military and Veterans Affairs facing their current challenges, NIOSH investigators could not look up answers in textbooks when these emerging problems were presented to them. Rather, some were new diseases altogether, such as chemical-associated bladder neuropathy and flock worker's lung. Others were rare or familiar diseases surfacing in an unanticipated setting, such as flavoring-related constrictive bronchiolitis and asthma related to indoor dampness. Efforts to intervene frequently failed because NIOSH knowledge had to be extended and refined, sometimes triggering experimental laboratory science to establish biological plausibility, as in control of beryllium sensitization in beryllium-exposed workers. Controversy is inevitable when previously unsuspected diseases or causes surface, because no common consensus exists regarding these phenomena among the many disciplines and institutions with stakes in the answers. Only multidisciplinary research regarding health in relation to environmental conditions will solve these challenges. Pertinent disciplines include clinical medicine, epidemiology, environmental science, and statistics. Interventions, which are often necessary to confirm cause, require military leaders, engineers, and public health personnel, among others.

This chapter illustrates several lessons from NIOSH work on emerging occupational diseases and novel causes of traditional lung diseases. It then briefly outlines the implications for surveillance and tools to identify three types of lung disease that affect service members who have deployed to southwest Asia.

LESSONS FOR APPROACHING NEW CAUSES AND NEW DISEASES

The lessons on emerging issues, distilled from investigations in occupational health practice and public health, do not apply equally to the three major respiratory health concerns discussed at the August 2012 Airborne Hazards Symposium: (1) constrictive bronchiolitis, (2) asthma, and (3) chronic obstructive pulmonary disease (COPD). However, a systematic approach to unknowns is invaluable before committing to surveillance prematurely, and confusion about cause exists for all three diseases. Consensus is often necessary to support preventive intervention and to assess benefits related to service-associated disability. These lessons include the importance of

- verifying pathology/diagnosis when cases are reported,
- interviewing patients,
- being wary of textbook descriptions,
- reviewing known etiologies,
- exploring exposure surrogates,
- generating hypotheses for epidemiological studies, and
- assessing the effectiveness of interventions.

These are steps to creating the knowledge base that will underlie consensus building regarding the allegations that service in southwest Asia has impaired respiratory health in US service persons.

EXHIBIT 18-1

EXAMPLES OF EMERGING ISSUES ILLUSTRATING LESSONS FOR SUCCESSFUL INVESTIGATION

- Flavoring-related bronchiolitis obliterans
- Bladder neuropathy related to the catalyst dimethylaminopropionitrile
- Dampness-related asthma
- Nylon flock worker's lung
- Lifeguard lung
- Beryllium sensitization via skin exposure

Verify Pathology/Diagnosis When Cases Are Reported

Environmental insults to the respiratory system may affect the larynx, the large airways, the small airways (bronchioli), the alveoli, or a combination of these compartments. Symptoms of chest illness are nonspecific and cannot differentiate among compartments reliably. For example, wheezing may have its origin in vocal cord adduction, asthma, bronchiolitis, and emphysema—all of which reflect damage at different levels of the respiratory tract. Additional information is usually necessary for differential diagnosis, such as age of the patient, onset and time course, cigarette smoking history, reversibility of symptoms, whether exacerbations exist, physiological measurements, and pathology. For example, to differentiate asthma from other respiratory diseases with common symptom presentations requires demonstration of reversible airflow limitation by spirometry in serial clinic visits, with a bronchodilator, or a test of airways hyperreactivity with methacholine or mannitol. Without distinguishing between asthma and other respiratory diseases, the investigator may misclassify the disease outcome, making it less likely that associations with environmental conditions can be demonstrated. An example of potential misdiagnosis is respiratory symptom data from a Veterans Affairs hospital, in which specific diagnostic tests *for* asthma (eg, methacholine challenge) were unavailable, and diagnosis was required on the form requesting spirometry to evaluate the diagnosis.[8]

An example of the need to verify diagnosis is the recognition of microwave popcorn-associated constrictive bronchiolitis. Several cases of severe respiratory illness had occurred over 8 years among workers who had manufactured microwave popcorn in a small plant in rural Missouri. In 2000, eight former workers were recognized as having constrictive bronchiolitis, a rare disease that is usually the late sequel of massive overexposure to irritant gases.[9] Misdiagnoses of more common diseases (eg, asthma, bronchitis, and COPD) were the norm in these cases.[10] Clinicians and public health investigators had no inkling about cause. The only way to establish that a new cause of occupational constrictive bronchiolitis existed was to epidemiologically evaluate the current workforce. The investigation documented that current workers had a 3.3-fold excess of obstructive spirometric abnormalities, that exposure to the flavoring chemical diacetyl (2,3-butanedione) was associated with abnormality in an exposure-dependent manner, and that exposed rodents had respiratory epithelial necrosis.[10]

Verifying the pathological diagnosis is particularly important for exploring constrictive bronchiolitis. Controversy about this unsuspected diagnosis in US soldiers serving in Iraq and Afghanistan dates from 2008[11,12] and is finally being resolved by an independent pathology panel. If the pathology is confirmed that this rare disease exists in a number of soldiers who served in Iraq and Afghanistan, exploration of cause will be required, regardless of whether case-patients had fixed airways obstruction, high-resolution computerized tomography (HRCT) findings of mosaic attenuation, or expected clinical course. The absence of some of the classic characteristics of constrictive bronchiolitis has been used to question the diagnosis, but the pathology findings are the gold standard in this instance. Discovery of new causes of constrictive bronchiolitis or attribution of case-patients to known causes must follow this first step.

Interview Patients

The cases of constrictive bronchiolitis diagnosed at Vanderbilt University (Nashville, TN) puzzled military pulmonologists because they largely had normal pulmonary functions and radiology studies.[7,11] When patients have symptoms that do not "make sense" in light of conventional medical practice, it is especially important to obtain their health and exposure histories in an open-ended fashion (ie, interview patients to obtain their insights). Standardized questionnaires are limited for emerging issues because they only work when you know what to ask, and they may not be appropriate for new patterns of disease, such as indolent onset of constrictive bronchiolitis.

A chemically induced bladder neuropathy illustrates this lesson.[13] Nine workers from a factory manufacturing foam automobile seats came to an emergency room together saying that they could not urinate. However, they all produced urine specimens, which appeared to contradict their chief complaint. Each individual worker had consulted his or her physician without resolution of urinary symptoms, but they knew that most of their co-workers had developed the same chronic symptoms in the same time course. Their clinicians had never heard of a chemical that caused patients to complain that they could drink a six-pack of beer and feel no need to void. Some workers had undergone surgery for prostatic obstruction without resolution of urinary symptoms. The county health department had investigated and reported that the restrooms were sanitary. Interviewing these sentinel nine patients led to clues about both the diagnosis and the potential causes. The investigators could only devise a questionnaire to collect systematic information from the workforce after interviewing them and their managers. An investigation of the current workforce showed that half of the workers in the facility had developed abnormalities of urination beginning shortly after a new catalyst was introduced, and incident cases paralleled the volume of its use (Figure 18-1). Workers had bladder neuropathy following introduction of dimethylaminopropionitrile, a chemical catalyst that had been used as a grouting agent for decades outdoors in construction without recognition of a sensorimotor neuropathy of the bladder. When the catalyst was removed from production, new cases immediately fell to zero.

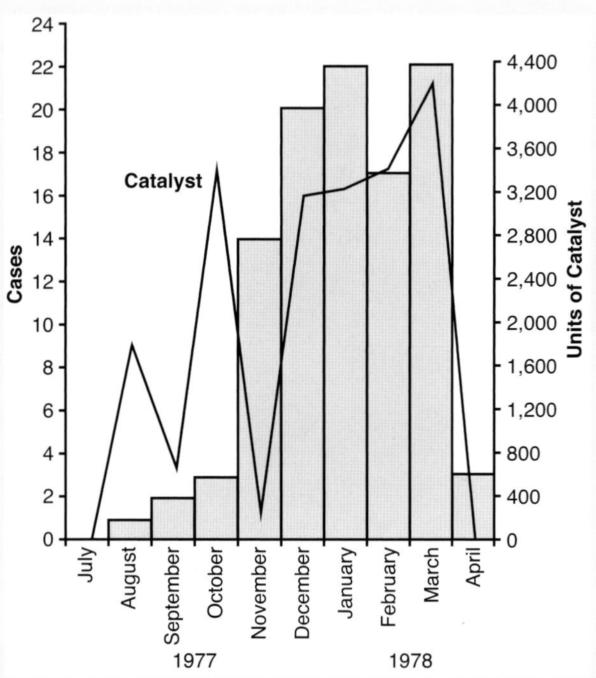

Figure 18-1. Number of incident cases of urinary symptoms and dimethylaminopropionitrile catalyst used by month during bladder neuropathy outbreak in automobile seat manufacturing plant.[13]
Data source: Kreiss K, Wegman DH, Niles CA, Siroky MB, Krane RJ, Feldman RG. Neurological dysfunction of the bladder in workers exposed to dimethylaminopropionitrile. *JAMA*. 1980;243:741–745.

The 38 Vanderbilt-diagnosed soldiers with pathological constrictive bronchiolitis were not systematically queried, but this was to be expected for an emerging condition that was likely recognized as a potential "outbreak" only after a number of similar cases had come to thoracoscopic biopsy. A challenge in this outbreak was the confusion about military versus Veterans Affairs jurisdiction to follow up these soldiers after they left the Army, which has delayed the ability to learn as much as possible from those affected. Among the 38 patients, 28 reported having been exposed to smoke from a sulfur mine fire near Mosul. Their probable chemical exposures include sulfur dioxide and hydrogen sulfide, both known causes of bronchiolitis.[14,15] In the instance of new-onset respiratory symptoms in soldiers deploying to southwest Asia, case-patients can

- report the circumstances of their recognizing new dyspnea on exertion and any associated symptoms;
- communicate whether co-workers had similar symptoms;
- reveal work assignments and exposures preceding or concurrent with the symptoms;
- describe progression or stabilization in relation to deployment dates; and
- report suspected causes.

Be Wary of Textbook Descriptions

Emerging issues are not described in textbooks, and prudence requires careful consideration of the basis of textbook knowledge. This is particularly evident for occupational constrictive bronchiolitis. Those individuals writing textbooks convey knowledge from case reports with recognized causes. In individual cases, the clue to cause has been acute pulmonary edema from an overwhelming accidental exposure; such cases seemingly recover and then develop fixed obstruction weeks or months later. The drama of acute presentation in previously healthy farmers or workers makes it easy to identify the cause of constrictive bronchiolitis, even though it is a rare condition. Without a dramatic acute event, persons with constrictive bronchiolitis would not be diagnosed or would be considered to have an idiopathic lung disease.

In flavoring-related constrictive bronchiolitis, there were no accidental high exposures, and yet 25% of plant workers had abnormal spirometry, many without chest symptoms.[10] They reported no work-aggravated chest symptoms and had no idea that they had work-related disease. The clue to a common etiology was the cluster of eight former workers with severe fixed obstruction, half on lung transplant lists, among a small workforce. Only epidemiological investigation in several microwave popcorn plants established the cause to be diacetyl. Diacetyl is an alpha diketone used in artificial butter flavorings. This example of chemical exposure-related constrictive bronchiolitis may be similar to the military case series of soldiers in Iraq with indolent development of dyspnea that subsequently precluded their meeting military requirements for exercise performance. Without an acute overexposure resulting in clinical contact for acute symptoms, only epidemiological investigation can resolve confusion about contributing exposures. In the example of diacetyl-related constrictive bronchiolitis, the cluster of severe lung disease in former workers motivated epidemiological investigation of current workers whose distribution of abnormal lung functions was related to current and estimated past exposures to flavoring ingredients of microwave popcorn production.

Textbook knowledge of constrictive bronchiolitis from inhaled toxins is largely based on case reports; it is not informed by population-based research on those at risk of indolent constrictive bronchiolitis. Only within the last decade has investigation of flavoring-exposed populations and population-based case series allowed characterization of the broader spectrum of findings in constrictive bronchiolitis. These recent findings contradict and thus must extend the classic descriptions of occupational constrictive bronchiolitis. Specifically, biopsy-confirmed cases do not always have fixed airways obstruction, expiratory mosaic attenuation on HRCT scans, or relentlessly progressive disease.[7,16,17] These three characteristics, detailed in the following paragraphs, are no longer required for diagnosis.

The spectrum of spirometric findings in biopsy-confirmed constrictive bronchiolitis now includes normal pulmonary function and spirometric restriction, as well as fixed obstruction and mixed obstruction and restriction (as described in textbooks). In a consecutive clinical case series, Markopoulou and co-authors[17] described 19 cases: 4 had normal spirometry, 2 had isolated gas trapping, 1 had restriction, 1 had mixed obstruction and restriction, and the remaining 11 had airflow obstruction. Similarly, among 7 biopsied mustard gas cases from the Iraq-Iran war with constrictive bronchiolitis, Ghanei and co-workers[16] showed that all had normal spirometry; of 4 additional cases with chronic cellular bronchiolitis on biopsy after mustard gas exposure, 2 had normal spirometry, 1 had restrictive abnormalities, and 1 had obstructive abnormalities. Distribution of spirometric findings among 38 US soldiers in Iraq and Afghanistan with biopsy-documented constrictive bronchiolitis included 32 with normal spirometry, 3 with restriction, 2 with obstruction, and 1 with mixed obstruction and restriction.[7] This last case series was unusual in that invasive workups were conducted to describe unexplained decreases in exercise performance. All of these case series reflect the limitations of spirometry (and a textbook requirement for fixed obstruction in constrictive bronchiolitis) in identifying bronchiolar abnormalities.[18]

In NIOSH work on flavoring-related lung disease starting in 2000, researchers concentrated on fixed obstructive spirometric abnormalities because they were guided by textbook descriptions, and their efforts preceded the publications just cited. In the sentinel microwave popcorn plant investigation, researchers found nearly equal numbers of current workers with spirometric obstruction, restriction, and mixed obstruction and restriction.[10] NIOSH investigators classified those with mixed abnormalities with the obstructed because it was assumed that air trapping explained the restrictive component. With the advent of publications on biopsy-confirmed constrictive bronchiolitis, researchers have reexamined the spectrum of spirometric abnormalities in the many flavoring-exposed worker populations now studied.[19] Distribution of spirometric abnormalities in many flavoring-exposed worker populations parallels that of the sentinel microwave popcorn plant. In addition, we found one flavoring manufacturing plant in which 28% of the workers had abnormal spirometric restriction; those workers in jobs or areas with higher potential for flavorings exposure had a 5.8-fold risk of excessive decline in forced expiratory volume in 1 second (FEV_1) during employment, compared to workers with lower potential for flavorings exposure.[20] In retrospect, we underestimated the burden of disease associated with flavoring chemical exposure by concentrating on obstructive and mixed spirometric abnormalities. In addition, we neglected the excesses of exertional dyspnea in flavoring-exposed workers in microwave popcorn and flavoring manufacturing industries because we had not recognized the insensitivity of spirometry abnormalities in biopsy-documented constrictive bronchiolitis. The insensitivity of spirometry was demonstrated in a study of 34,000 Iranians who developed respiratory complications of sulfur mustard gassing in the 1980s: 57.5% had normal pulmonary function testing, 37.0% had mild impairment, 4.5% had moderate impairment, and 1.0% had severe pulmonary function testing impairment, primarily obstructive but occasionally mixed and purely restrictive in pattern.[21,22]

Radiographic diagnostic tests, the second classic criterion for constrictive bronchiolitis, are also insensitive for identifying bronchiolar abnormalities, as reflected in the biopsy-documented case series described previously. In the consecutive clinical case series, air trapping reflecting mosaic attenuation was found in only 5 of 10 cases.[17] Similarly, Ghanei and co-workers[16] showed that biopsy-confirmed cases in Iran did not all have HRCT abnormalities. In US soldiers with southwest Asia experience, 25 of 37 (68%) had normal HRCT scans, and 6 (16%) had mild air trapping.[7] Similarly, in flavoring worker surveillance in California, only 4 of 7 cases with moderate-to- severe obstruction had abnormal HRCTs consistent with constrictive bronchiolitis.[23] Our conclusion is that workers and soldiers with unexplained dyspnea and normal radiological studies and physiology may require thoracoscopic biopsies for a diagnosis.

The third presumed characteristic of constrictive bronchiolitis, unrelenting progression, has its origin in the experience of persons who have undergone lung or bone marrow transplant. This common source of posttransplant demise is thought to reflect an immune-mediated phenomenon. In contrast, we have found that the natural history of flavoring-related constrictive bronchiolitis is quite different. Even the sentinel former worker cases of constrictive bronchiolitis in 2000 and 2003 appeared to have stabilized in their physiological impairment with the cessation of exposure,[24] and none of them have received lung transplants to date to our knowledge. Similarly, an incident case of flavoring-related lung disease during the eight cross-sectional surveys of the sentinel microwave popcorn plant had much slower deterioration in FEV_1 2 years after he left employment (Figure 18-2).

As factory exposures were brought under control, excessive lung function declines normalized for the aggregate population with spirometry over all eight surveys (Figure 18-3).[25,26] Thus, there is good reason to suspect that

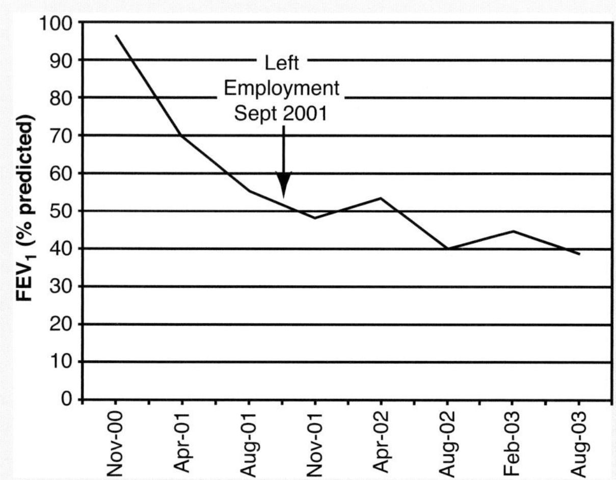

Figure 18-2. Serial forced expiratory volume in 1 second (FEV_1) by month of employment of incident case of fixed obstruction in microwave popcorn plant. *Arrow* indicates cessation of employment.

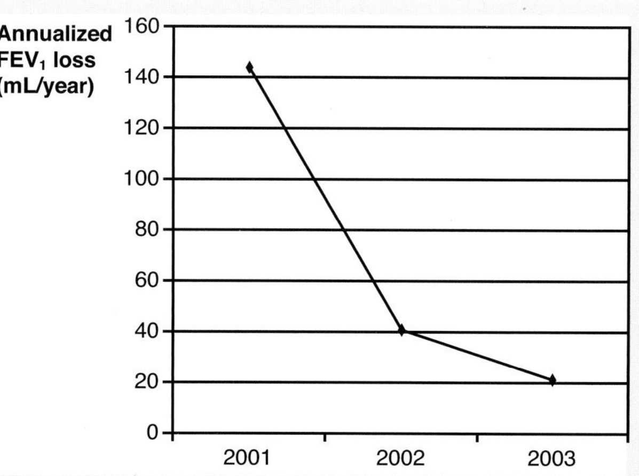

Figure 18-3. Annualized decline in forced expiratory volume in 1 second (FEV_1) by year of follow-up in sentinel microwave popcorn plant, November 2000–August 2003 for participants in all eight cross-sectional studies.

exposure-related indolent evolution of constrictive bronchiolitis does not progress after exposure ceases, and this may be true for the US soldiers in Iraq and Afghanistan who were diagnosed postdeployment. Even for constrictive bronchiolitis from an acute overwhelming exposure, long-term follow-up shows that disease can be stable.[14,21,27–29] In the case of follow-up studies of patients gassed with chlorine from transportation accidents, the absence of progressive disease from 2 to 6 years postexposure has been taken as lack of evidence of chronic effects, even when excessive declines in pulmonary functions were evident in the first 2 years postexposure and did not improve.[30]

In summary, classic characteristics of constrictive bronchiolitis in textbooks are incomplete. Without findings from population-based epidemiology and biopsy-documented case series, conclusions about the extent of disease, its characteristics, and its causes may be inaccurate.

Review Known Etiologies

In approaching unidentified causes of respiratory disease, exploration of known or suspected causes is the first step. Because environmental sampling is never available for unsuspected causes, the known causes may suggest exposure surrogates that can be explored in epidemiological studies. In turn, exposure surrogates that are associated with increased incidence or prevalence of health outcomes can form the basis of intervention studies. Effectiveness of interventions in interrupting adverse health outcomes in longitudinal surveillance can form evidence that the causal hypotheses were correct.

For constrictive bronchiolitis, known etiologies based on case reports of acute injury followed by delayed fixed obstruction include nitrogen dioxide, sulfur dioxide, the halogens, ammonia, methyl isocyanate, hydrogen sulfide, and sulfur mustard (see Table 18-1[14–18,21,26–29,31–58]). All of these are gases, with the exception of sulfur mustard aerosols.

Gases are also associated with constrictive bronchiolitis without recognition of acute injury (see Table 18-1). Many of these causes of insidious disease required epidemiological investigation to substantiate cause or assembly of case series in particular industrial settings. The best studied is diacetyl, a constituent of artificial butter flavoring, with cases and risk associated with microwave popcorn production, manufacturing of flavorings, and diacetyl manufacture.[26] With substitution of other alpha diketones for diacetyl (2,3-butanedione) in flavoring manufacture, experimental laboratory work documents that compounds with similar structure, such as 2,3-pentanedione, have similar epithelial toxicity in rodents and are likely no safer.[59]

Chemicals associated with reinforced plastic resins used in fiberglass boat building likely include a cause of constrictive bronchiolitis, and this may be styrene. Diagnoses of constrictive bronchiolitis were made in five boat builders in four fiberglass boatyards; in a worker building fiberglass water towers using similar chemicals; and in someone who burned Styrofoam insulation indoors, liberating styrene gas.[55,60] Another fiberglass boat builder was diagnosed on clinical grounds with hypersensitivity pneumonitis.[61] Two mortality studies of workers exposed to styrene in boat building document excess deaths from "other chronic obstructive disease" (not emphysema, bronchitis, or asthma) in short tenure workers with high exposure.[62,63] This pattern is consistent with a short latency, exposure-related, severe

TABLE 18-1

KNOWN OR SUSPECTED CAUSES OF CONSTRICTIVE BRONCHIOLITIS BY GASEOUS OR PARTICULATE FORM AND COURSE OF INJURY

Gaseous or Particulate Form and Course of Injury	Illustrative Setting	References
Irritant Gases Causing Acute Injury		
Nitrogen dioxide	Explosive detonation, silage decomposition, nitric acid use, nitrocellulose fires, welding gases	Lowry & Schuman, 1956 Grayson, 1956 Becklake et al, 1957 Darke & Warrack, 1958 Milne, 1969 Ramirez & Dowell, 1971 Horvath et al, 1978 Yockey et al, 1980 Zwemer et al, 1992
Sulfur dioxide	Paper mill bleaching, sulfur mine fire	Woodford et al, 1979 Charan et al, 1979
Thionyl chloride	Lithium batteries	Konichezky et al, 1993
Chlorine	Transportation spill	Jones et al, 1986 Seaton, 2008
	Industrial accident	Chester et al, 1977
Bromine and compounds	Flavoring research and development	Kraut & Lilis, 1988
Ammonia	Chemical industry; refrigerant	Kass et al, 1972 Monforte et al, 2003
Methyl isocyanate	Bhopal pesticide manufacture leak	Weill, 1987 Cullinan et al, 1997 Mishra et al, 2009
Polymethylene polyphenol isocyanate	Plastics factory maintenance	Markopoulou et al, 2002
Hydrogen sulfide	Crude oil, natural gas, manure pits, toilets	Arnold et al, 1985 Parra et al, 1991 Richardson 1995 Doujaiji & Al-Tawfiq, 2010
Sulfur mustard	Chemical war gassing (with aerosol)	Thomason et al, 2003 Ghanei & Harandi, 2007 Ghanei et al, 2008 Weinberger et al, 2011 Tang & Loke, 2012
Dimethyl disulfide		Seaton, 2008
Hydrochloric acid		Seaton, 2008
Irritant Gases Causing Subacute Injury		
Diacetyl and other alpha diketones	Microwave popcorn, flavoring, and diacetyl manufacture	Kreiss, 2007
Oxides of nitrogen	Silo filling	Zwemer et al, 1992 Ramirez & Dowell, 1971

(**Table 18-1** *continues*)

Table 18-1 *continued*

Possible Particulate Causes		
Smoke inhalation	Plastics factory fire	Seggev et al, 1983
	Synthetic materials in house fire	Tasaka et al, 1995
	Styrofoam combustion	Janigan et al, 1997
	Photography processing fire (ammonia, nitrogen dioxide)	Markopoulou et al, 2002
Overheated cooking oil fumes	Commercial cooking	Simpson et al, 1985
Fly ash	Incineration of coal and oil; particulate (may have adsorbed toxic gases)	Boswell & McCunney, 1995
Dusts and combustion products	World Trade Center collapse	Mann et al, 2005
Food production dusts	Animal feed manufacture (could have been flavorings)	Spain et al, 1995
Powder of chlorine-liberating disinfectant	Cleaning	Seaton, 2008

Data sources: Arnold IM, Dufresne RM, Alleyne BC, Stuart PJ. Health implication of occupational exposures to hydrogen sulfide. *J Occup Med.* 1985;27:373–376. Becklake MR, Goldman HI, Bosman AR, Freed CC. The long-term effects of exposure to nitrous fumes. *Am Rev Tuberc.* 1957;76:398–409. Boswell RT, McCunney RJ. Bronchiolitis obliterans from exposure to incinerator fly ash. *J Occup Environ Med.* 1995;37:850–855. Charan NB, Myers CG, Lakshminarayan S, Spencer TM. Pulmonary injuries associated with acute sulfur dioxide inhalation. *Am Rev Respir Dis.* 1979;119:555–560. Chester EH, Kaimal J, Payne CB, Kohn PM. Pulmonary injury following exposure to chlorine gas. Possible beneficial effects of steroid treatment. *Chest.* 1977;72:247–250. Cullinan P, Acquilla S, Dhara VR. Respiratory morbidity 10 years after the Union Carbide gas leak at Bhopal: a cross sectional survey. The International Medical Commission on Bhopal. *Br Med J.* 1997;314:338–342. Darke CS, Warrack AJ. Bronchiolitis from nitrous fumes. *Thorax.* 1958;13:327–333. Doujaiji B, Al-Tawfiq JA. Hydrogen sulfide exposure in an adult male. *Ann Saudi Med.* 2010;30:76–80. Ghanei M, Harandi AA. Long term consequences from exposure to sulfur mustard: a review. *Inhal Toxicol.* 2007;19:451–456. Ghanei M, Tazelaar HD, Chilosi M, et al. An international collaborative pathologic study of surgical lung biopsies from mustard gas-exposed patients. *Respir Med.* 2008;102:825–830. Grayson RR. Silage gas poisoning: nitrogen dioxide pneumonia, a new disease in agricultural workers. *Ann Intern Med.* 1956;45:393–408. Horvath EP, doPico GA, Barbee RA, Dickie HA. Nitrogen dioxide-induced pulmonary disease: five new cases and a review of the literature. *J Occup Med.* 1978;20:103–110. Janigan DT, Kilp T, Michael R, McCleave JJ. Bronchiolitis obliterans in a man who used his wood-burning stove to burn synthetic construction materials. *Can Med Assoc J.* 1997;156:1171–1173. Jones RN, Hughes JM, Glindmeyer H, Weill H. Lung function after acute chlorine exposure. *Am Rev Respir Dis.* 1986;134:1190–1195. Kass I, Zamel N, Dobry CA, Holzer M. Bronchiectasis following ammonia burns of the respiratory tract. A review of two cases. *Chest.* 1972;62:282–285. Konichezky S, Schattner A, Ezri T, Bokenboim P, Geva D. Thionyl-chloride-induced lung injury and bronchiolitis obliterans. *Chest.* 1993;104:971–973. Kraut A, Lilis R. Chemical pneumonitis due to exposure to bromine compounds. *Chest.* 1988;94:208–210. Kreiss K. Flavoring-related bronchiolitis obliterans. *Curr Opin Allergy Clin Immunol.* 2007;7:162–167. Lowry T, Schuman LM. Silo-filler's disease; a syndrome caused by nitrogen dioxide. *JAMA.* 1956;162:153–160. Mann JM, Sha KK, Kline G, Breuer FU, Miller A. World Trade Center dyspnea: bronchiolitis obliterans with functional improvement: a case report. *Am J Ind Med.* 2005;48:225–229. Markopoulou KD, Cool CD, Elliot TL, et al. Obliterative bronchiolitis: varying presentations and clinicopathological correlation. *Eur Respir J.* 2002;19:20–30. Milne JE. Nitrogen dioxide inhalation and bronchiolitis obliterans. A review of the literature and report of a case. *J Occup Med.* 1969;11:538–547. Mishra PK, Samarth RM, Pathak N, Jain SK, Banerjee S, Maudar KK. Bhopal gas tragedy: review of clinical and experimental findings after 25 years. *Int J Occup Med Environ Health.* 2009;22:193–202. Monforte V, Roman A, Gavalda J, et al. Nebulized amphotericin B concentration and distribution in the respiratory tract of lung-transplanted patients. *Transplantation.* 2003;75:1571–1574. Parra O, Monso E, Gallego M, Morera J. Inhalation of hydrogen sulphide: a case of subacute manifestations and long term sequelae. *Br J Ind Med.* 1991;48:286–287. Ramirez J, Dowell AR. Silo-filler's disease: nitrogen dioxide-induced lung injury. Long-term follow-up and review of the literature. *Ann Intern Med.* 1971;74:569–576. Richardson DB. Respiratory effects of chronic hydrogen sulfide exposure. *Am J Med.* 1995;28:99–108. Seaton A. Bronchiolar disease. In: Seaton A, Seaton D, Leitch AG, eds, *Crofton and Douglas's Respiratory Disease*, 5th ed. London, UK: Wiley Inc; 2008: 829–838. Chapter 29. Seggev JS, Mason UG 3rd, Worthen S, Stanford RE, Fernandez E. Bronchiolitis obliterans: report of three cases with detailed physiologic studies. *Chest.* 1983;83:169–174. Simpson FG, Belfield PW, Cooke NJ. Chronic airflow limitation after inhalation of overheated cooking oil fumes. *Postgrad Med J.* 1985;61:1001–1002. Spain BA, Cummings O, Garcia JG. Bronchiolitis obliterans in an animal feed worker. *Am J Ind Med.* 1995;28:437–443. Tang FR, Loke WK. Sulfur mustard and respiratory diseases. *Crit Rev Toxicol.* 2012;42:688–702. Tasaka S, Kanazawa M, Mori M, et al. Long-term course of bronchiectasis and bronchiolitis obliterans as late complication of smoke inhalation. *Respiration.* 1995;62:40–42. Thomason JW, Rice TW, Milstone AP. Bronchiolitis obliterans in a survivor of a chemical weapons attack. *JAMA.* 2003;290:598–599. Weill H. Disaster at Bhopal: the accident, early findings and respiratory health outlook in those injured. *Bull Eur Physiopathol Respir.* 1987;23:587–590. Weinberger B, Laskin JD, Sunil V, Sinko PJ, Heck DE, Laskin DL. Sulfur mustard-induced pulmonary injury: therapeutic approaches to mitigating toxicity. *Pulm Pharmacol Ther.* 2011;24:92–99. Woodford DM, Coutu RE, Gaensler EA. Obstructive lung disease from acute sulfur dioxide exposure. *Respiration.* 1979;38:238–245. Yockey CC, Eden BM, Byrd RB. The McConnell missile accident: clinical spectrum of nitrogen dioxide exposure. *JAMA.* 1980;244:1221–1223. Zwemer FL Jr, Pratt DS, May JJ. Silo filler's disease in New York State. *Am Rev Respir Dis.* 1992;146:650–653. (**Note:** References 14–18, 21, 26–29, and 31–58 are cited herein.)

respiratory disease in which those affected leave employment. Epidemiological studies in the plastic-reinforced fiberglass industry are needed to refine the causal hypotheses by looking at exposure–response relations.

Finally, causes of acute injury (eg, nitrogen oxides) have also been reported to result in constrictive bronchiolitis in workers who did not seek medical attention for acute illness following causative exposures.[36,38,40,41] Such workers presented with fixed obstruction weeks after exposure without recognized acute injury, as happens with indolent constrictive bronchiolitis in flavoring-exposed workers.

There is much poorer evidence for particulate etiologies for constrictive bronchiolitis. Case reports exist for smoke inhalation, overheated cooking oil fumes, fly ash inhalation, World Trade Center exposures, a plastics factory fire, and an animal feed worker (see Table 18-1). Interestingly, cases involving animal feed manufacture,[58] overheated cooking oil fumes,[56] and bromine compounds[41] occurred in settings with likely artificial flavorings exposure before diacetyl was recognized as causing constrictive bronchiolitis. It is difficult to separate particulate and gaseous exposures in situations involving combustion effluents. It is uncertain whether aerosols and particulates, independent of their combination with or source of toxic gases, are capable of eliciting a constrictive bronchiolitis response.[29,57,58]

Thus, the existing literature documents a multitude of associations of gas exposures and perhaps a few particulate exposures with constrictive bronchiolitis. Some of these exposures almost certainly existed in Iraq and Afghanistan. Exposures to burning plastics, burning batteries, burning Styrofoam, and nonspecific combustion products were surely episodic from burn pits. The possibility of nitrogen dioxide exposures from explosions might also need exploration, whether in the setting of improvised explosive devices or conventional fire fights. The oil field fires in Iraq and Kuwait may have been a source of hydrogen sulfide exposures. In all of these cases, episodic or single exposure may have been sufficient to result in epithelial cell injury in the distal airway with subacute evolution of constrictive bronchiolitis.

Attributing incident cases of asthma and COPD among service members is usually limited to known etiologies. These diseases are common in any population, unlike constrictive bronchiolitis that is a rare disease with an extremely low background rate. The usual way to find *new* occupational causes of asthma and COPD is to study new cases clustered in time and space in relation to exposure–response relationships. This is unlikely to be possible in a military situation.

Explore Exposure Surrogates

When no measurements of suspected causal agents are available, nearly always the case in the setting of an unexpected health outcome, markers or surrogates of exposure may be suggested by case-patient interviews and knowledge of deployment conditions in which known causes might be present. In industry, process-related risks and work practices are sometimes clues to exposures that may be associated with illness. Associations of health outcomes with such surrogates of exposure can guide further investigations and interventions. Sometimes exposure measurements are impossible to obtain or useless because they are not biologically relevant.

An example of this situation was an investigation of a pathologically unique new disease, lymphocytic bronchiolitis and peribronchiolitis with lymphoid hyperplasia, dubbed "flock worker's lung." Several cases of this interstitial pneumonitis occurred in four plants in the nylon flock industry in which long filaments of nylon were cut into short fibers and impacted onto adhesive-covered cloth to make a velvet upholstery for automobile seats.[64–66] The nylon fibers were too large to be respirable, and no one suspected a respirable dust in the plants. In searching for a cause, we found an unexpected respirable dust from milling the cut flock. Fibrils generated in the cutting of nylon into fibers were broken off in milling (Figure 18-4).[67] This respirable dust melted at the precise melting point of nylon, suggesting that it was nylon particulate, for which no analytic method existed.

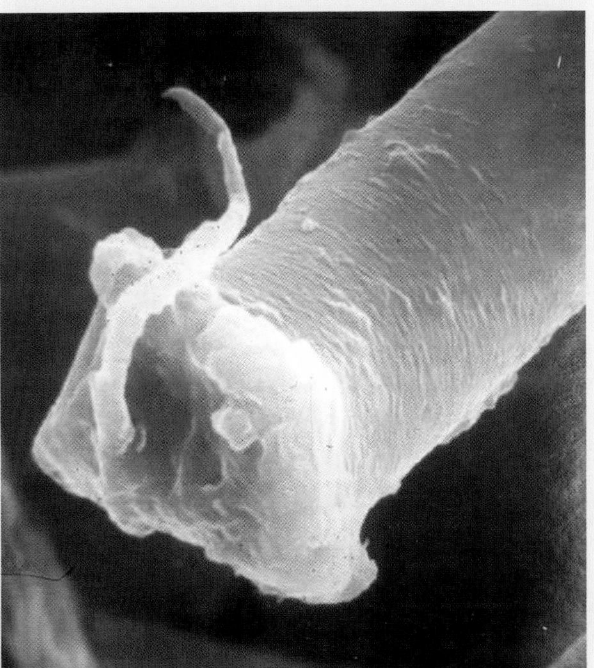

Figure 18-4. Scanning photomicrograph of nylon flock fiber with fibril on cut end that can be dislodged to form a respirable dust associated with flock worker's lung.
Data source: Burkhart J, Piacitelli C, Schwegler-Berry D, Jones W. Environmental study of nylon flocking process. *J Toxicol Environ Health.* 1999;57:1–23.

Exhausting the milling procedure removed the respirable particulate in the plant. Animal studies demonstrated that respirable nylon particulate from the plant was toxic on intratracheal instillation.

For another emerging issue—damp indoor spaces in relation to asthma and hypersensitivity pneumonitis—bioaerosol measurements do not correlate with health risk; but, observational indices of dampness, mold, and mold odor do. These observational indices are a marker of presumed causal microbial constituents in water-damaged indoor environments, in which the epidemiological evidence is overwhelming that there are health risks.[68] We do not use bioaerosol measurements to recommend remediation of the source of water incursion, nor do we recommend clearance air sampling after remediation.[69]

Generate Hypotheses for Epidemiological Studies

Pathologically confirmed cases of constrictive bronchiolitis or another unexpected lung disease are an opportunity to extend our knowledge for the sake of intervention. Opportunities for exposure to known causes can be explored using surrogates of possible exposure. For potential causes requiring intervention, focusing on personal susceptibility or predeployment exposures are diversions, sometimes motivated by attempts to deny occupational risk factors and responsibility for prevention. Personal risk factors and predeployment exposures are only important in the differential diagnosis of individual cases in a clinical setting. In the epidemiology of risk factors, personal factors are usually irrelevant because persons do not sort into particular military categories of exposure by their genetics, hobbies, or prior exposure experience.

Hypothesis generation arises from exposure surrogate clues from "sentinel cases" regarding deployment processes, times, locations, and the case-patients' own ideas about risky situations. These clues should be winnowed to a reasonable number by in-depth study of known etiologies and surrogates for these potential exposures. In southwest Asia, possible exposure surrogates are the sulfur mine fire with sulfur dioxide and hydrogen sulfide ambient exposures; burn pits with many potential exposures to causes of constrictive bronchiolitis, including battery and Styrofoam combustion products; explosions with possible exposure to nitrogen dioxide; and oil fires with possible hydrogen sulfide exposures.

To identify likely candidate exposure risk factors for intervention, appropriate epidemiological designs are important for efficiency and feasibility. For rare diseases, such as constrictive bronchiolitis, case-control studies are efficient, and cross-sectional designs are not. Surveillance is not the mechanism for finding epidemiological associations, but is a way of monitoring trends in response to interventions.

Assess Effectiveness of Intervention

Knowing specific chemical or particulate cause is not required to intervene to prevent future workers or service personnel from being affected. It may be enough to find "process-related" risk, in which potential causal exposures can be lowered with engineering controls, changes in work practices, and/or personal protective equipment.

An illustrative example is flavoring-related lung disease in microwave popcorn manufacture. From the eight sentinel cases in former workers, we knew that the mixing room conferred high risk because half of these severe case-patients had been mixers, despite each shift having only one mixer.[9] The engineering recommendation was to isolate the mixing room from the packaging line so that the source of the potential cause did not contaminate the work spaces of the larger number of microwave production workers. Because microfine salt dumped into an auger in the mixing room billowed dust into the room, our industrial hygienists initially recommended particulate respirators, as had an earlier generation of NIOSH industrial hygienists investigating constrictive bronchiolitis in a company adding liquid flavors to powders for the baking industry.[70] In both of these investigations, the initial counsel for intervention was inappropriate and would have been ineffective because constrictive bronchiolitis is usually related to gases and would require organic vapor protection. Luckily, in the microwave popcorn investigation, the hypothesis that volatile flavoring exposure was the cause, rather than salt dust, surfaced quickly from the multidisciplinary team. In later microwave popcorn plant investigations, we found that some plants used encapsulated flavors that required a combination of particulate and organic vapor respiratory protection until engineering controls were put into place. In an emerging issue, evaluation of intervention is critical and can substantiate the likelihood of having found the cause.

A problem with epidemiology is that associations between exposure surrogates and health outcomes may not be causal. Granted, Sir Austin Bradford Hill gave the criteria for interpreting associations as causal, including strength of association, consistency of findings by different investigators, appropriate temporal relations between exposure and outcome, biological plausibility, and exposure–response relationships.[71] In the microwave popcorn industry with diacetyl exposure, it was years before the criteria had been met for interpreting associations as causal, and the seriousness of the health effect dictated intervention before there was proven cause.[72]

Sometimes effective interventions cement our understanding of cause. For the emerging issues listed in Exhibit 18-1, several encompassed examples of successful interventions. In the bladder neuropathy outbreak, new cases disappeared with removal of the catalyst dimethylaminopropionitrile (see Figure 18-1).[13] In the sentinel popcorn plant, control of diacetyl exposure resulted in average annualized FEV_1 declines falling from 144 to 40 to 22 mL/yr over a 3-year follow up period (see Figure 18-3).[25,26] In a damp building with cross-sectional evaluations before and after remediation of water infiltration, new asthma cases with building-related symptoms were prevented.[73] Surveillance is an effective tool to study intervention. If interventions result in lower incidence, that finding contributes to causal criteria for associations.

If interventions fail, it generally means that the cause has not been found or that the controls have been inadequate. For example, in another damp building, incomplete remediation did not lower a seven-fold excess incidence of building-related asthma since occupancy after remediation.[74,75] For emerging occupational lung diseases, unsuccessful interventions are a stimulus to learn more to prevent them. Reexamination of hypotheses and other intervention strategies are required.

An example of a failed intervention occurred in NIOSH work in the beryllium industry. Beryllium sensitization is a precondition for developing beryllium disease, a granulomatous interstitial disease. A 10% prevalence of sensitization was found in beryllium workers who had worked at least a year.[76] The company invested millions of dollars in lowering beryllium air concentrations. On a repeat cross-sectional survey, a 10% prevalence of beryllium sensitization was found in new workers regardless of tenure.[77] The intervention had failed. The company then decided that the only thing they had not considered was protecting workers' skin from beryllium exposure. Only after developing a comprehensive program that included keeping beryllium off the skin did sensitization prevalence fall in each of the three production facilities of this company.[78–80] The company did not need scientific proof of skin as a route of beryllium sensitization to institute this intervention. It was a matter of economic survival. As in the military situation with unexpected respiratory disease in southwest Asia, solving the problem with interventions is more important than developing proof of causation.

Another example of a failed intervention involved a leisure swimming pool with many water spray features. A lifeguard developed granulomatous lung disease with work-related symptoms and an abnormal chest X-ray.[81] Symptomatic co-workers were also found to have abnormal biopsies consistent with hypersensitivity pneumonitis, despite having normal chest X-rays. With systematic public health investigation, 33 lifeguards had abnormal biopsies (an attack rate of 27% of pool-exposed employees). The pool was closed for ventilation improvements, but within 3 months of the pool reopening, 65% of the lifeguards had developed work-related chest symptoms. The only abnormal industrial hygiene measurement was elevated endotoxin levels in air, particularly when the spray water features were on.

The pool was closed again, the chlorination system was replaced with ozonation, and corroded water circuits were replaced. This time the outbreak was beat. The cause could not be found, but the problem had been solved. In retrospect, it might have been wise to perform a culture for environmental mycobacteria, which was subsequently implicated in hypersensitivity pneumonitis in hot tubs, therapy pools, and machinists exposed to contaminated metal working fluids.[82] Targeted surveillance allowed a second solution to be evaluated as successful.

IMPLICATIONS FOR EMERGING CAUSES OF LUNG DISEASES

Approaches to Constrictive Bronchiolitis

Recent investigations of biopsy-documented constrictive bronchiolitis in survivors of mustard gassing in the Iraq-Iran war and in a sequential clinical case series document that spirometric results range from normal to obstructive, restrictive, and mixed abnormalities. In this disease, FEV_1 is not an indicator of severity of impairment, unlike in COPD. The spectrum of abnormalities in flavoring-exposed populations is also diverse, and NIOSH investigations of constrictive bronchiolitis ignored the many workers with similar flavoring exposures who had exertional dyspnea without obstructive abnormalities. NIOSH investigators are currently trying to rectify this oversight in their further studies of flavoring-related constrictive bronchiolitis. Spirometry and radiological imaging are both insensitive for bronchiolar pathology. In US service members with unexplained dyspnea after conventional noninvasive clinical evaluations, only open biopsies will make or exclude the diagnosis of constrictive bronchiolitis. Without looking for this disease systematically, the military and the Department of Veterans Affairs will not know the extent of the problem and will not have a rigorous case series with which to conduct epidemiological studies of possible causes, such as burn pit effluents, the sulfur mine fire, or nitrogen oxides from exploded ordinance. An efficient design for furthering understanding of associations would be case-control studies, guided by hypotheses based on known causes and surrogates of potential exposure to known or unsuspected causes. Trying to reconstruct historical exposures is usually impossible for individual cases or even groups with similar exposure levels, but surrogates of exposure may be illuminating. The focus of some at the 2012 Airborne Hazards Symposium on individual exposure measurements being necessary to prove cause is an unrealistic distraction that ignores the potential contribution of epidemiological study.

Interventions for known causes of constrictive bronchiolitis should be implemented as quickly as possible, with efforts to evaluate effectiveness in preventing new cases. Because little is known about exposure–response relationships for chemicals causing constrictive bronchiolitis, lowered exposure measurements by themselves will not be sufficient evidence of intervention effectiveness. Furthermore, concentrations of particulate exposures may not be relevant to this health outcome, and future assessment of gaseous exposures may be of more utility. Surveillance of clinical outcomes, rather than environmental surveillance, is the means of evaluating intervention effectiveness, but depends on adequate symptom and clinical abnormality data.

Approaches to Asthma

In studies presented at the August 2012 Airborne Hazards Symposium, objective measures of lung function have not always been available to validate the reports of new-onset asthma or asthma exacerbation in Gulf War veterans. Normal spirometry does not exclude the diagnosis of asthma in which airflow limitation is episodic. When spirometry is normal, tests of airways hyperreactivity are needed. Physician misdiagnosis of asthma is common in the setting limited to history taking and stethoscopic examination. Serial spirometry is also not helpful usually, because asthmatic persons typically have normal spirometry between attacks of asthma. Case definitions should include airways hyperreactivity and not spirometry alone, unless abnormalities respond to the bronchodilator, documenting reversibility of airflow limitation.

Although allergic occupational asthma has a latency period to development after exposure begins, symptoms of occupational asthma and asthma exacerbation (in the case of preexisting asthma) occur during or within about 12 hours of the implicated exposure. Similarly, asthma caused by irritant exposures has onset in close temporal sequence to exposure. Asthma symptoms do not have **onset** weeks after the postexposure period. Thus, incident asthma cases lend themselves to hypothesis generation about causal exposures that can be addressed in case-control or cohort studies.

Allergic occupational asthma of many causes is curable if identified early in its course, and implicated exposures cease. When asthma becomes severe, steroid-dependent, and prolonged in duration, the prognosis switches to permanent asthma with many nonspecific triggers. For this reason, early identification of service members with incident asthma and removal from further exposure are critical to their long-term respiratory health. In meta-analyses of population-based asthma studies, about 21% of current asthma is attributable to indoor dampness,[83] and housing during deployment may warrant consideration.

Approaches to Chronic Obstructive Pulmonary Disease

COPD, unlike asthma, can be diagnosed with spirometry demonstrating obstruction that is not fully reversible with bronchodilators. However, even in smokers, airflow limitation below the lower limits of normal is not usually demonstrated until the fifth decade of age.[84] COPD is a long latency respiratory outcome that results from accelerated decline

TABLE 18-2

ODDS RATIOS FOR MEASURED AIRWAYS OBSTRUCTION BY INDUSTRY OR OCCUPATION IN THE US WORKING POPULATION FROM 1988 TO 1994 (EXCLUDING THOSE REPORTING PHYSICIAN-DIAGNOSED CURRENT ASTHMA)*

Industry & Occupation	Odds Ratio
Industry	
Rubber, plastics, and leather manufacturing	**2.5**
Utilities[†]	2.4
Office building services	2.4
Textile mill products manufacturing	**2.2**
US armed forces[‡]	**2.2**
Food products manufacturing	**2.1**
Occupation	
Freight, stock, and material handlers	**2.2**
US armed forces[§]	**2.0**
Vehicle mechanics	2.0
Records processing and distribution clerks[¥]	1.8

*Adjusted for age, race/ethnicity, smoking status, pack-years of cigarette smoking, body mass index, education, and socioeconomic status. **Bold font** indicates that 95% confidence intervals exclude 1.0 in comparison to office workers which is both an industry and an occupation.

[†]Among never-smokers, odds ratio in this industry was 27.2 (confidence interval = 3.6–214).

[‡]Among never-smokers, odds ratio in this industry was 4.4 (confidence interval = 0.9–20).

[§]Among never-smokers reporting armed forces employment, odds ratio was 4.1 (confidence interval = 0.9–19.4).

[¥]Among never-smokers reporting records processing and distribution clerk employment, odds ratio was 2.9 (confidence interval = 1.1–7.6).

Adapted from: Hnizdo E, Sullivan PA, Bang KM, Wagner G. Association between chronic obstructive pulmonary disease and employment by industry and occupation in the US population: a study of data from the Third National Health and Nutrition Examination Survey. *Am J Epidemiol.* 2002;156:738–746.

of FEV_1, year after year, until abnormal airflow limitation manifests. In smokers, excessive annual decline usually disappears with the cessation of smoking, but recovery of lost reserves does not usually occur. Few service members are in the age range in which smokers have abnormal obstructive spirometry. This is the one health outcome that merits predeployment and postdeployment spirometry to identify excessive declines of FEV_1 within the normal range of lung function in service members who may go on to develop clinical COPD. This group with excessive declines should be targeted for smoking cessation efforts and attention to occupational exposures related to COPD.

Population-based studies suggest that occupational exposures account for 26% to 53% of COPD in nonsmokers,[85] and the nonsmoking group of soldiers would be the easiest in which to study likely military causes of obstructive lung disease. In smokers, the attributable risks of smoking and occupational exposures are at least additive. Before the advent of widespread cigarette smoking, there was clear recognition of the risk of chronic airways disease with dusty trades, and there is now good evidence for airways disease among workers exposed to silica, coal mine dusts, and asbestos, independent of pneumoconioses and smoking. In population-based community surveys in many countries, being exposed to vapors, gas, dust, or fumes at work in the longest-held job has been associated with poorer or abnormal pulmonary function comparable in size of effect to cigarette smoking. With respect to specific agents associated with occupational COPD, there is ample evidence of the hazards of cadmium for emphysema, vanadium (as in oil field fires) for bronchitis, and welding gas and fume exposures for airways obstruction.[85]

In addition to well-established causes of occupational COPD, the third National Health and Nutrition Survey data demonstrated industries and occupations with an excess of measured airways obstruction, adjusted for cigarette smoking, where causative exposures remain to be explained (Table 18-2).[86] Among these is the armed forces category, and these data—collected from a general population sample in 1988 to 1994—largely precede the conflicts in southwest Asia. The excess respiratory outcomes among veterans are likely a long-standing risk of military service independent of ambient dust storms in Iraq and Afghanistan. To begin to prevent the substantial burden of COPD in veterans, research and intervention on exposures during military service, apart from smoking, are prudent.

LIMITATIONS OF OUR TOOLS

Looking for causes of health outcomes with our limited surveillance tools may be insufficient, akin to looking for lost keys at night under a lamppost because light is available. Questionnaires can give us symptoms of constrictive bronchiolitis and asthma, but are less useful for identifying subclinical evolving COPD in the military age group. In addition, symptoms alone are nonspecific for differentiating among lung diseases. In constrictive bronchiolitis, even dyspnea may be insensitive for spirometric abnormality, as demonstrated in microwave popcorn manufacture in which one-quarter of workers with abnormal spirometry had no chest symptoms.[10] In public health surveillance of the flavoring industry, half of those with spirometric obstruction reported no chest symptoms.[23]

Questionnaires for exposure classification need different approaches for the health outcomes of constrictive bronchiolitis, asthma, and COPD. These health outcomes have different time courses of pertinent exposure and different known exposure types. Particulate exposures are more important for COPD and asthma, and gaseous exposures are likely more important for constrictive bronchiolitis.

Serial spirometry is useful for subclinical COPD to identify excessive declines in FEV_1. Spirometry alone is not useful for identifying asthmatics because they have intermittent airflow obstruction. Instead, case definitions for epidemiological studies of deployment-associated asthma should measure airway hyperreactivity in the absence of bronchodilator response to spirometry. Finally, spirometry is insensitive for constrictive bronchiolitis because case-patients can have normal, obstructive, restrictive, or mixed patterns.

Our questionnaire tools for symptoms, exposures, and spirometry must each be tailored for specific respiratory disease outcomes. Even then, their interpretation is limited, particularly for constrictive bronchiolitis because we do not have good clinical tests for bronchiolar disease apart from open lung biopsy.

SUMMARY

The reason to better understand exposures associated with health outcomes is to intervene, both to prevent US service members from having exposures and to improve prognosis of those who have developed health conditions in relation to exposure. The role of surveillance is the repeated assessment of health outcomes in a population to assess trends, and there is no reason to repeatedly assess health outcomes unless interventions are undertaken. Surveillance is not a substitute for understanding military respiratory hazards with targeted hypothesis-driven research.

Longitudinal surveillance is premature when unexpected health outcomes occur. Such health outcomes need to be acknowledged as unknowns and restated as hypotheses about plausible causes to facilitate research regarding causes and interventions. Targeted epidemiological research studies should test hypotheses about plausible causes of specific health outcomes. Past exposures that were not measured cannot be known, and this is particularly true of the uncharacterized gases that may have caused constrictive bronchiolitis, the bioaerosols in damp indoor spaces that may induce asthma, or the various occupational exposures that will eventually lead to COPD. Indices of exposure can be as simple as deployment in specific locations and dates or information about participation in exposure-generating processes gathered by questionnaires. For constrictive bronchiolitis arising in an indolent way, report of severity of exposures may not be helpful at all because respiratory epithelial toxins may not induce irritant symptoms, even in those with spirometric abnormality. For incident asthma, however, symptoms would have arisen during pertinent exposures in deployment.

Prevention of respiratory diseases in service members requires research efforts to assess causality and to evaluate the effectiveness of interventions so that fighting strength can be preserved. These efforts should take precedence over determination of compensation eligibility for service-related health outcomes. In clinical occupational medicine practice, a high level of evidence about proof of cause in the workers' compensation system is needed. The military cannot afford to risk the health of its troops, even if causal associations have not yet been demonstrated. The occurrence of pathological and objective disease requires attempts at intervention.

Acknowledgments

Findings and conclusions in this chapter are those of the author and do not necessarily represent those of the National Institute for Occupational Safety and Health (NIOSH) and the Centers for Disease Control and Prevention. The author has no financial relationship with a commercial entity that has an interest in the subject of this paper and wrote this chapter during the course of NIOSH employment.

The author thanks LCDR Anna-Binney McCague, MD, and CDR Rachel Bailey, DO, MPH, US Public Health Service (NIOSH in Morgantown, WV) for providing helpful comments on this chapter.

REFERENCES

1. Baker EL, Matte TP. Surveillance of occupational illness and injury. In: Halperin W, Baker EL, eds. *Public Health Surveillance*. New York, NY: Van Nostrand Reinhold; 1992: 178–194.

2. Smith B, Wong CA, Smith TC, Boyko EJ, Gacksetter GS, Ryan MAK. Newly reported respiratory symptoms and conditions among military personnel deployed to Iraq and Afghanistan: a prospective population-based study. *Am J Epidemiol*. 2009;170:1433–1442.

3. Baird CP, DeBakey S, Reid L, Hauschild VD, Petruccelli B, Abraham JH. Respiratory health status of US Army personnel potentially exposed to smoke from 2003 Al-Mishraq Sulfur Plant fire. *J Occup Environ Med*. 2012;54:717–723.

4. Szema AM, Peters MC, Weissinger KM, Gagliano CA, Chen JJ. New-onset asthma among soldiers serving in Iraq and Afghanistan. *Allergy Asthma Proc*. 2010;31:67–71.

5. Morris MJ, Zacher LL, Jackson DA. Investigating the respiratory health of deployed military personnel. *Mil Med*. 2011;176:1157–1161.

6. Abraham JH, DeBakey SF, Reid L, Zhou J, Baird C. Does deployment to Iraq and Afghanistan affect respiratory health of US military personnel? *J Occup Environ Med*. 2012;54:740–745.

7. King MS, Eisenberg R, Newman JH, et al. Constrictive bronchiolitis in soldiers returning from Iraq and Afghanistan. *N Engl J Med*. 2011;365:222–230.

8. Szema AM, Salihi W, Savary K, Chen JJ. Respiratory symptoms necessitating spirometry among soldiers with Iraq/Afghanistan war lung injury. *J Occup Environ Med*. 2011;53:961–965.

9. Centers for Disease Control and Prevention. Fixed obstructive lung disease in workers at a microwave popcorn factory—Missouri, 2000–2002. *MMWR Morb Mortal Wkly Rep*. 2002;51:345–347.

10. Kreiss K, Gomaa A, Kullman G, et al. Clinical bronchiolitis obliterans in workers at a microwave-popcorn plant. *N Engl J Med*. 2002;347:330–338.

11. Morris MJ, Zacher LL. Constrictive bronchiolitis in soldiers [letter]. *N Engl J Med*. 2011;365:1743–1745.

12. Zacher LL, Browning R, Bisnett T, Bennion JR, Postlewaite RC, Baird CP. Clarifications from representatives of the Department of Defense regarding the article "Recommendations for medical screening and diagnostic evaluation for postdeployment lung disease in returning US warfighters." *J Occup Environ Med*. 2012;54:760–761.

13. Kreiss K, Wegman DH, Niles CA, Siroky MB, Krane RJ, Feldman RG. Neurological dysfunction of the bladder in workers exposed to dimethylaminopropionitrile. *JAMA*. 1980;243:741–745.

14. Woodford DM, Coutu RE, Gaensler EA. Obstructive lung disease from acute sulfur dioxide exposure. *Respiration*. 1979;38:238–245.

15. Doujaiji B, Al-Tawfiq JA. Hydrogen sulfide exposure in an adult male. *Ann Saudi Med*. 2010;30:76–80.

16. Ghanei M, Tazelaar HD, Chilosi M, et al. An international collaborative pathologic study of surgical lung biopsies from mustard gas-exposed patients. *Respir Med*. 2008;102:825–830.

17. Markopoulou KD, Cool CD, Elliot TL, et al. Obliterative bronchiolitis: varying presentations and clinicopathological correlation. *Eur Respir J*. 2002;19:20–30.

18. Seaton A. Bronchiolar disease. In: Seaton A, Seaton D, Leitch AG, eds, *Crofton and Douglas's Respiratory Disease*, 5th ed. London, UK: Wiley Inc; 2008: 829–838. Chapter 29.

19. Kreiss K. Respiratory disease among flavoring-exposed workers in food and flavoring manufacture. *Clin Pulm Med*. 2012;19:165–173.

20. Kreiss K. Work-related spirometric restriction in flavoring manufacturing workers. *Am J Ind Med*. 2014;57:129–137.

21. Ghanei M, Harandi AA. Long term consequences from exposure to sulfur mustard: a review. *Inhal Toxicol*. 2007;19:451–456.

22. Saber H, Saburi A, Ghanei M. Clinical and paraclinical guidelines for management of sulfur mustard induced bronchiolitis obliterans; from bench to bedside. *Inhal Toxicol*. 2012;24:900–906.

23. Kim TJ, Materna BL, Prudhomme JC, et al. Industry-wide medical surveillance of California flavor manufacturing workers: cross-sectional results. *Am J Ind Med*. 2010;53:857–865.

24. Akpinar-Elci M, Travis WD, Lynch DA, Kreiss K. Bronchiolitis obliterans syndrome in popcorn production plant workers. *Eur Respir J*. 2004;24:298–302.

25. Kanwal R, Kullman G, Fedan KB, Kreiss K. Occupational lung disease risk and exposures to butter-flavoring chemicals after implementation of controls at a microwave popcorn plant. *Public Health Rep*. 2011;126:480–494.

26. Kreiss K. Flavoring-related bronchiolitis obliterans. *Curr Opin Allergy Clin Immunol*. 2007;7:162–167.

27. Horvath EP, doPico GA, Barbee RA, Dickie HA. Nitrogen dioxide-induced pulmonary disease: five new cases and a review of the literature. *J Occup Med*. 1978;20:103–110.

28. Chester EH, Kaimal J, Payne CB, Kohn PM. Pulmonary injury following exposure to chlorine gas. Possible beneficial effects of steroid treatment. *Chest*. 1977;72:247–250.

29. Mann JM, Sha KK, Kline G, Breuer FU, Miller A. World Trade Center dyspnea: bronchiolitis obliterans with functional improvement: a case report. *Am J Ind Med*. 2005;48:225–229.

30. Jones RN, Hughes JM, Glindmeyer H, Weill H. Lung function after acute chlorine exposure. *Am Rev Respir Dis*. 1986;134:1190–1195.

31. Lowry T, Schuman LM. Silo-filler's disease; a syndrome caused by nitrogen dioxide. *JAMA*. 1956;162:153–160.

32. Grayson RR. Silage gas poisoning: nitrogen dioxide pneumonia, a new disease in agricultural workers. *Ann Intern Med*. 1956;45:393–408.

33. Becklake MR, Goldman HI, Bosman AR, Freed CC. The long-term effects of exposure to nitrous fumes. *Am Rev Tuberc*. 1957;76:398–409.

34. Darke CS, Warrack AJ. Bronchiolitis from nitrous fumes. *Thorax*. 1958;13:327–333.

35. Milne JE. Nitrogen dioxide inhalation and bronchiolitis obliterans. A review of the literature and report of a case. *J Occup Med*. 1969;11:538–547.

36. Ramirez J, Dowell AR. Silo-filler's disease: nitrogen dioxide-induced lung injury. Long-term follow-up and review of the literature. *Ann Intern Med*. 1971;74:569–576.

37. Yockey CC, Eden BM, Byrd RB. The McConnell missile accident: clinical spectrum of nitrogen dioxide exposure. *JAMA*. 1980;244:1221–1223.

38. Zwemer FL Jr, Pratt DS, May JJ. Silo filler's disease in New York State. *Am Rev Respir Dis*. 1992;146:650–653.

39. Charan NB, Myers CG, Lakshminarayan S, Spencer TM. Pulmonary injuries associated with acute sulfur dioxide inhalation. *Am Rev Respir Dis*. 1979;119:555–560.

40. Konichezky S, Schattner A, Ezri T, Bokenboim P, Geva D. Thionyl-chloride-induced lung injury and bronchiolitis obliterans. *Chest*. 1993;104:971–973.

41. Kraut A, Lilis R. Chemical pneumonitis due to exposure to bromine compounds. *Chest*. 1988;94:208–210.

42. Kass I, Zamel N, Dobry CA, Holzer M. Bronchiectasis following ammonia burns of the respiratory tract. A review of two cases. *Chest*. 1972;62:282–285.

43. Monforte V, Roman A, Gavalda J, et al. Nebulized amphotericin B concentration and distribution in the respiratory tract of lung-transplanted patients. *Transplantation*. 2003;75:1571–1574.

44. Weill H. Disaster at Bhopal: the accident, early findings and respiratory health outlook in those injured. *Bull Eur Physiopathol Respir*. 1987;23:587–590.

45. Cullinan P, Acquilla S, Dhara VR. Respiratory morbidity 10 years after the Union Carbide gas leak at Bhopal: a cross sectional survey. The International Medical Commission on Bhopal. *Br Med J*. 1997;314:338–342.

46. Mishra PK, Samarth RM, Pathak N, Jain SK, Banerjee S, Maudar KK. Bhopal gas tragedy: review of clinical and experimental findings after 25 years. *Int J Occup Med Environ Health*. 2009;22:193–202.

47. Arnold IM, Dufresne RM, Alleyne BC, Stuart PJ. Health implication of occupational exposures to hydrogen sulfide. *J Occup Med*. 1985;27:373–376.

48. Parra O, Monso E, Gallego M, Morera J. Inhalation of hydrogen sulphide: a case of subacute manifestations and long term sequelae. *Br J Ind Med*. 1991;48:286–287.

49. Richardson DB. Respiratory effects of chronic hydrogen sulfide exposure. *Am J Med*. 1995;28:99–108.

50. Thomason JW, Rice TW, Milstone AP. Bronchiolitis obliterans in a survivor of a chemical weapons attack. *JAMA*. 2003;290:598–599.

51. Weinberger B, Laskin JD, Sunil V, Sinko PJ, Heck DE, Laskin DL. Sulfur mustard-induced pulmonary injury: therapeutic approaches to mitigating toxicity. *Pulm Pharmacol Ther*. 2011;24:92–99.

52. Tang FR, Loke WK. Sulfur mustard and respiratory diseases. *Crit Rev Toxicol*. 2012;42:688–702.

53. Seggev JS, Mason UG 3rd, Worthen S, Stanford RE, Fernandez E. Bronchiolitis obliterans: report of three cases with detailed physiologic studies. *Chest*. 1983;83:169–174.

54. Tasaka S, Kanazawa M, Mori M, et al. Long-term course of bronchiectasis and bronchiolitis obliterans as late complication of smoke inhalation. *Respiration*. 1995;62:40–42.

55. Janigan DT, Kilp T, Michael R, McCleave JJ. Bronchiolitis obliterans in a man who used his wood-burning stove to burn synthetic construction materials. *Can Med Assoc J*. 1997;156:1171–1173.

56. Simpson FG, Belfield PW, Cooke NJ. Chronic airflow limitation after inhalation of overheated cooking oil fumes. *Postgrad Med J*. 1985;61:1001–1002.

57. Boswell RT, McCunney RJ. Bronchiolitis obliterans from exposure to incinerator fly ash. *J Occup Environ Med*. 1995;37:850–855.

58. Spain BA, Cummings O, Garcia JG. Bronchiolitis obliterans in an animal feed worker. *Am J Ind Med*. 1995;28:437–443.

59. Morgan DL, Jokinen MP, Price HC, Gwinn WM, Palmer SM, Flake GP. Bronchial and bronchiolar fibrosis in rats exposed to 2,3-pentanedione vapors: implications for bronchiolitis obliterans in humans. *Toxicol Pathol*. 2012;40:448–465.

60. Cullinan P, McGavin CR, Kreiss K, et al. Obliterative bronchiolitis in fiberglass workers: a new occupational disease? *Occup Environ Med*. 2013;70:357–359.

61. Volkman KK, Merrick JG, Zacharisen MC. Yacht-maker's lung: a case of hypersensitivity pneumonitis in yacht manufacturing. *Wisc Med J*. 2006;105:47–50.

62. Wong O, Trent LS, Whorton MD. An updated cohort mortality study of workers exposed to styrene in the reinforced plastics and composites industry. *Occup Environ Med*. 1994;51:386–396.

63. Ruder AM, Ward EM, Dong M, Okun AH, Davis-King K. Mortality patterns among workers exposed to styrene in the reinforced plastic boatbuilding industry: an update. *Am J Ind Med*. 2004;45:165–176.

64. Lougheed MD, Roos JO, Waddell WR, Munt PW. Desquamative interstitial pneumonitis and diffuse alveolar damage in textile workers. Potential role of mycotoxins. *Chest*. 1995;108:1196–1200.

65. Washko RM, Day B, Parker JE, Castellan RM, Kreiss K. Epidemiologic investigation of respiratory morbidity at a nylon flock plant. *Am J Ind Med*. 2000;38:628–638.

66. Daroowalla F, Wang ML, Piacitelli C, Attfield MD, Kreiss K. Flock workers' exposures and respiratory symptoms in five plants. *Am J Ind Med*. 2005;47:144–152.

67. Burkhart J, Piacitelli C, Schwegler-Berry D, Jones W. Environmental study of nylon flocking process. *J Toxicol Environ Health*. 1999;57:1–23.

68. Mendell MJ, Mirer AG, Cheung K, Tong M, Douwes J. Respiratory and allergic health effects of dampness, mold, and dampness-related agents: a review of the epidemiologic evidence. *Environ Health Perspect*. 2011;119:748–756.

69. National Institute for Occupational Safety and Health. *Alert: Preventing Occupational Respiratory Disease from Exposures Caused by Dampness in Office Buildings, Schools, and Other Nonindustrial Buildings*. Morgantown, WV: US Department of Health and Human Services, US Public Health Service, Centers for Disease Control and Prevention, National Institute for Occupational Safety and Health; 2012. NIOSH publication no. 2013-102.

70. National Institute for Occupational Safety and Health. *Health Hazard Evaluation and Technical Assistance Report: International Bakers Services, Inc., South Bend, Indiana*. Cincinnati, OH: US Department of Health and Human Services, US Public Health Service, Centers for Disease Control and Prevention, National Institute for Occupational Safety and Health; 1986. NIOSH publication no. 85-171-1710.

71. Hill AB. The environment and disease: association or causation? *Proc R Soc Med*. 1965;58:295–300.

72. Kreiss K. Occupational bronchiolitis obliterans masquerading as COPD. *Am J Respir Crit Care Med*. 2007;176:427–429.

73. Jarvis JQ, Morey PR. Allergic respiratory disease and fungal remediation on a building in a subtropical climate. *Appl Occup Environ Hyg*. 2001;16:380–388.

74. Cox-Ganser JM, White SK, Jones R, et al. Respiratory morbidity in office workers in a water-damaged building. *Environ Health Perspect*. 2005;113:485–490.

75. Iossifova Y, Cox-Ganser JM, Park JH, White SK, Kreiss K. Lack of respiratory improvement following remediation of a water-damaged office building. *Am J Ind Med*. 2011;54:269–277.

76. Kreiss K, Mroz MM, Newman LS, Martyny J, Zhen B. Machining risk of beryllium disease and sensitization with median exposures below 2 micrograms/m^3. *Am J Ind Med*. 1996;30:16–25.

77. Henneberger PK, Cumro D, Deubner DD, Kent MS, McCawley M, Kreiss K. Beryllium sensitization and disease among long-term and short-term workers in a beryllium ceramics plant. *Int Arch Occup Environ Health*. 2001;74:167–176.

78. Cummings KJ, Deubner DC, Day GA, et al. Enhanced preventive programme at a beryllium oxide ceramics facility reduces beryllium sensitisation among new workers. *Occup Environ Med*. 2007;64:134–140.

79. Bailey RL, Thomas CA, Deubner DC, Kent MS, Kreiss K, Schuler CR. Evaluation of a preventive program to reduce sensitization at a beryllium metal, oxide and alloy production plant. *J Occup Environ Med*. 2010;52:505–512.

80. Thomas CA, Bailey RL, Kent MS, Deubner DC, Kreiss K, Schuler CR. Efficacy of a program to prevent beryllium sensitization among new employees at a copper-beryllium alloy processing facility. *Public Health Rep*. 2009;124(suppl 1):112–124.

81. Rose CS, Martyny JW, Newman LS, et al. "Lifeguard lung": endemic granulomatous pneumonitis in an indoor swimming pool. *Am J Public Health*. 1998;88:1795–1800.

82. Kreiss K, Cox-Ganser J. Metalworking fluid-associated hypersensitivity pneumonitis: a workshop summary. *Am J Ind Med*. 1997;32:423–432.

83. Mudarri D, Fisk WJ. Public health and economic impact of dampness and mold. *Indoor Air*. 2007;17:226–235.

84. Hnizdo E, Glindmeyer HW, Petsonk EL, Enright P, Buist AS. Case definitions for chronic obstructive pulmonary disease. *COPD*. 2006;3:95–100.

85. Blanc PD, Hnizdo E, Kreiss K, Toren Kjell. Chronic obstructive airway disease due to occupational exposure. In: Bernstein IL, Chan-Yeung M, Bernstein DL, eds. *Asthma in the Workplace*. 4th ed. Boca Raton FL: CRC Press; 2013: 375–391.

86. Hnizdo E, Sullivan PA, Bang KM, Wagner G. Association between chronic obstructive pulmonary disease and employment by industry and occupation in the US population: a study of data from the Third National Health and Nutrition Examination Survey. *Am J Epidemiol*. 2002;156:738–746.

Chapter 19

FOLLOW-UP MEDICAL CARE OF SERVICE MEMBERS AND VETERANS: CASE REPORTS—USUAL AND UNUSUAL

MICHAEL R. LEWIN-SMITH, MB*; RUSSELL A. HARLEY, MD†; JEFFREY R. GALVIN, MD‡; AND TERI J. FRANKS, MD†

*Senior Environmental Pathologist, The Joint Pathology Center, Joint Task Force National Capital Region Medical, 606 Stephen Sitter Avenue, Silver Spring, Maryland 20910-1290

†Senior Pulmonary and Mediastinal Pathologist, The Joint Pathology Center, Joint Task Force National Capital Region Medical, 606 Stephen Sitter Avenue, Silver Spring, Maryland 20910-1290

‡Professor, Departments of Diagnostic Radiology, Thoracic Imaging, and Internal Medicine, Pulmonary/Critical Care Medicine, University of Maryland School of Medicine, 685 West Baltimore Street, Baltimore, Maryland 21201

INTRODUCTION

Two case reports are presented from the perspective of pulmonary and environmental pathologists who have reviewed many pulmonary pathology specimens from US service members deployed to Iraq and Afghanistan. Pulmonary pathology specimens from these service members were sent for expert second opinion review to the former Armed Forces Institute of Pathology (AFIP) and to the current Joint Pathology Center (JPC), Departments of Pulmonary and Mediastinal Pathology. The two cases selected are examples of nonneoplastic pulmonary histopathology that illustrate a breadth of diagnoses seen in biopsies from US military personnel previously deployed to the Iraq theater.

CASE 1

In 2009, a 29-year-old male—active duty, enlisted, US Air Force military service member—presented with fever, chills, productive cough, night sweats, anorexia, myalgia, and general malaise. He gave a history of having cleaned out an unoccupied dusty apartment 1 week prior to the onset of symptoms. The patient's social history included tobacco use, smoking one-quarter to one-half pack of cigarettes per day for a total of 2¼ to 4½ pack-years, but stopping with the onset of his current illness. He reported mild alcohol use, but denied high-risk behavior or the use of illicit substances. His occupational history included working in the communications field repairing computers and electrical systems. He reported having worked in buildings under construction and in disrepair in Iraq. His deployment history included deployments to Iraq in 2004 and to Kuwait in 2007.

His past medical history included sickle cell trait and minor traumas, but nothing else of note. He had no known allergies to medications. The patient was treated with antibiotics, but was seen in the emergency room 1 week after initial presentation, with no improvement in his symptoms. A chest radiograph was obtained in which multiple pulmonary nodules were seen. The patient had a normal chest radiograph in 2007. Computed tomography (CT) of the thorax was performed, which revealed numerous blood vessel-associated consolidative nodules involving all five lung lobes. The majority of the nodules measured between 1.5 and 2.5 cm. Multiple air bronchograms were also noted (Figure 19-1). The radiological impression from this study was of multifocal consolidative nodules, and the differential diagnosis proffered included infection, lymphoma, organizing pneumonia, and sarcoidosis.

He was admitted to the hospital and underwent a bronchoscopy in which his airways were noted to have a "cobblestone" appearance suggestive of a sarcoid or a fungal infection. Cultures were taken, and no growth was reported. An endobronchial biopsy was also performed that showed acute and chronic inflammation, but no granulomas were seen. Bronchoalveolar lavage (BAL) revealed a lymphocytosis, and both the bronchoalveolar lavage and sputum were negative for acid-fast bacilli by examination of smears and polymerase chain reaction. A fine-needle aspiration cytology specimen was obtained from lymph nodes that were reported as showing a reactive process. No granulomas or malignancy were seen. The patient was treated with antibiotics and voriconazole,

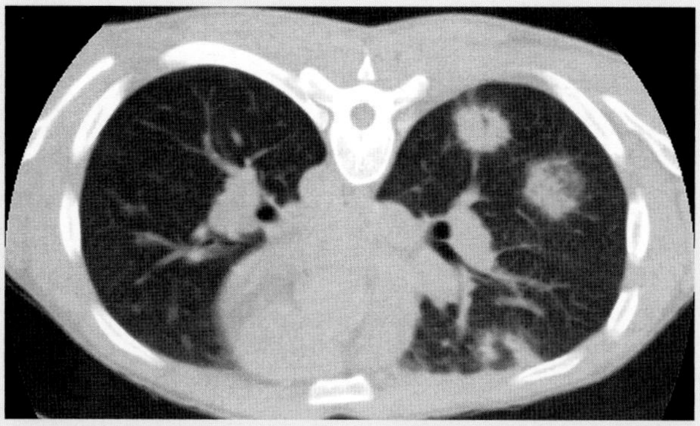

Figure 19-1. Case 1. Axial chest computed tomography scan acquired in the prone position demonstrates multiple pulmonary nodules.

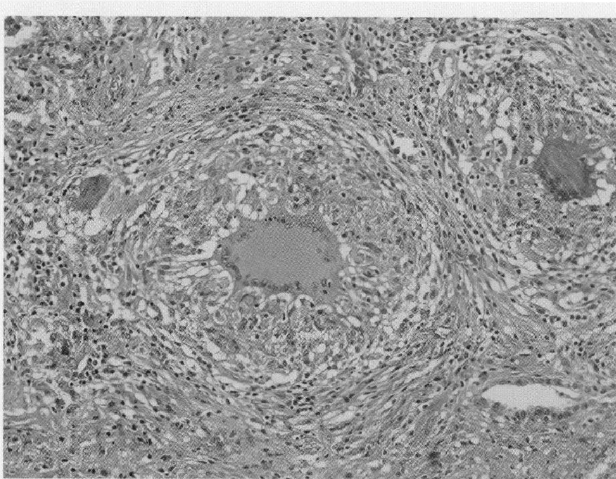

Figure 19-2. Case 1. Lung wedge biopsy showing non-necrotizing granulomas. (Hematoxylin & eosin stain; original magnification 20×.)

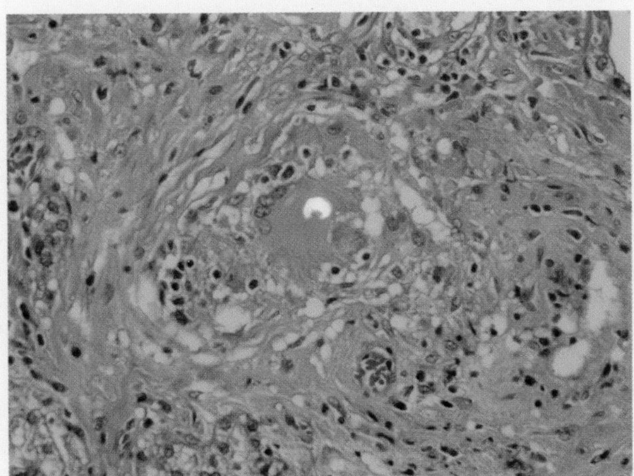

Figure 19-3. Case 1. Lung-wedge biopsy showing a multinucleated giant cell containing a birefringent cup-shaped particle of calcium oxalate. (Hematoxylin & eosin, photographed under polarized light; original magnification 40×.)

but failed to improve. He continued to have anorexia, malaise, night sweats, nosebleeds, and back pain. A CT-guided lung biopsy was performed, but was reported as nondiagnostic. A video-assisted thoracoscopic surgery (VATS) biopsy was obtained from the lung after marking with methylene blue. Additional *negative* or normal study results reported at this time included

- serological tests for histoplasma and *Coccidioides* antibodies,
- immunoglobulin E,
- quantitative immunoglobulins,
- myeloperoxidase antibody,
- proteinase antibody,
- human immunodeficiency virus, and
- *Legionella* urine antigen.

Positive laboratory findings included

- antinuclear antibody titer of 1:160 with a speckled pattern,
- double-stranded deoxyribonucleic acid antibody of 30 IU/mL (normal: 0–24 IU/mL),
- C-reactive protein of 10 mg/dL,
- erythrocyte sedimentation rate of 66 mm/h, and
- complement factor 4 of 40 mg/dL (high normal).

A rheumatology consult was arranged to rule out an autoimmune process.

After the VATS biopsy and the results of fungal stains, which were negative, the patient was treated with high-dose intravenous steroids followed by oral prednisone. His clinical status showed significant improvement. Clinically

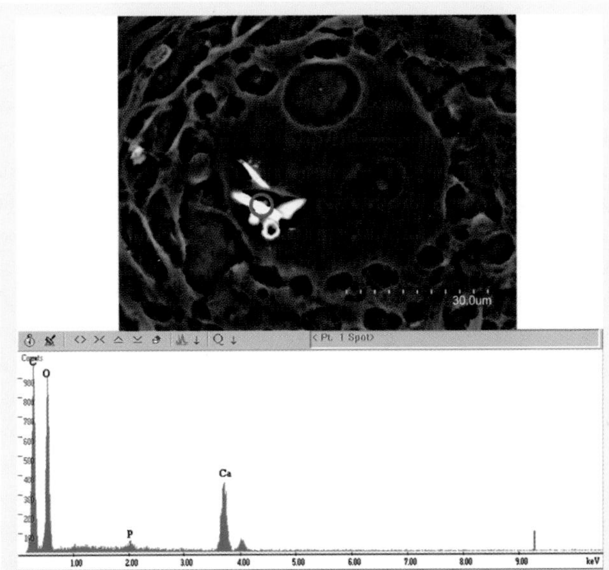

Figure 19-4. Case 1. Scanning electron microscopic image of a multinucleated giant cell containing calcium oxalate crystals and energy dispersive X-ray analysis (*red circle*), demonstrating the presence of carbon (C), oxygen (O), calcium (Ca), and a small phosphorus (P) peak.

and radiologically, the patient's illness was considered to be consistent with sarcoidosis, but particulate matter noted in the VATS biopsy material was not considered to be

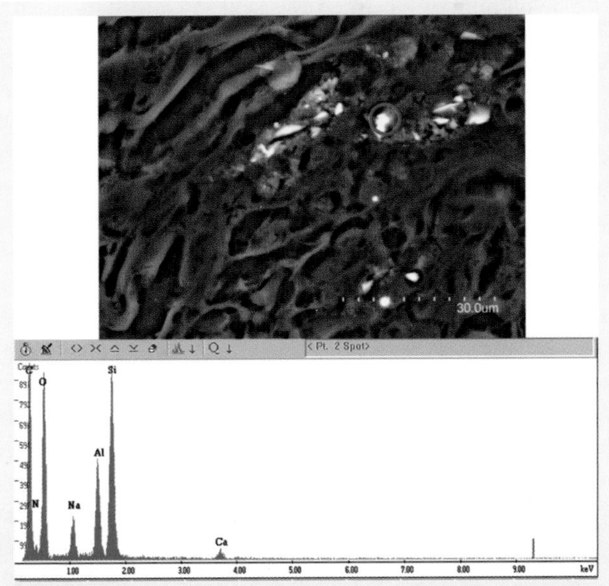

Figure 19-5. Case 1. Scanning electron microscopic image of a small birefringent particle consistent with a silicate and energy dispersive X-ray analysis (*red circle*), demonstrating the presence of carbon (C), nitrogen (N), oxygen (O), sodium (Na), aluminum (Al), silicon (Si), and calcium (Ca).

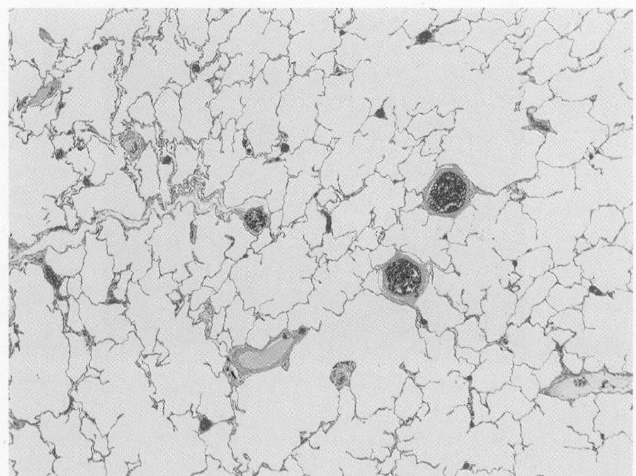

Figure 19-6. Case 2. Lung wedge biopsy showing an area of emphysematous change. (Hematoxylin & eosin; original magnification 2×.)

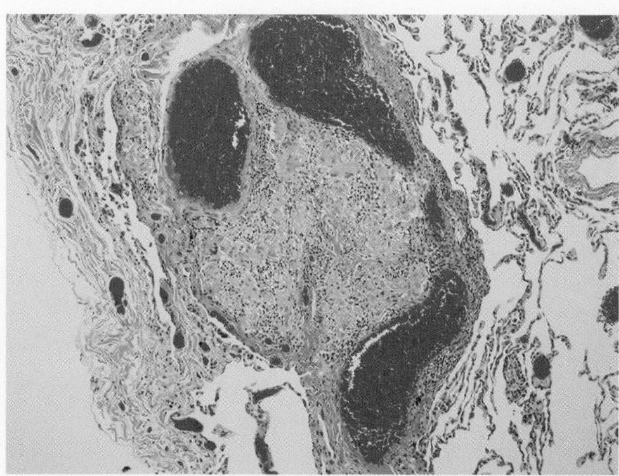

Figure 19-7. Case 2. Lung-wedge biopsy showing poorly formed granulomas adjacent to blood vessels. (Hematoxylin & eosin; original magnification 10×.)

classically consistent with sarcoidosis. Consideration was given to performing a lymphocyte proliferation assay, but the patient's history was not thought to be consistent with significant beryllium exposure. The contributing pathologist's diagnosis of the two wedge biopsies obtained from the VATS procedure was of noncaseating granulomatous inflammation with polarizable foreign material detected within granulomas and within giant cells. Special stains for fungi and mycobacteria were negative.

The pathology specimen was sent in consultation with the AFIP to rule out pneumoconiosis because of the birefringent material seen, with beryllium, aluminum, or talc being considered. The AFIP diagnosis rendered was nonnecrotizing and rare necrotizing granulomas. Birefringent material located in giant cells was characterized as calcium oxalate by scanning electron microscopy with energy dispersive X-ray analysis (SEM-EDXA) and infrared spectroscopy. This material was considered to be endogenous in origin (not a "foreign body"). Smaller rod-shaped birefringent particles containing silicon, oxygen, magnesium, and aluminum consistent with silicates were also detected. Rare particles consistent with silica and possibly talc (a magnesium silicate) were also identified (Figures 19-2 to 19-5). Inductively coupled plasma mass spectroscopy was

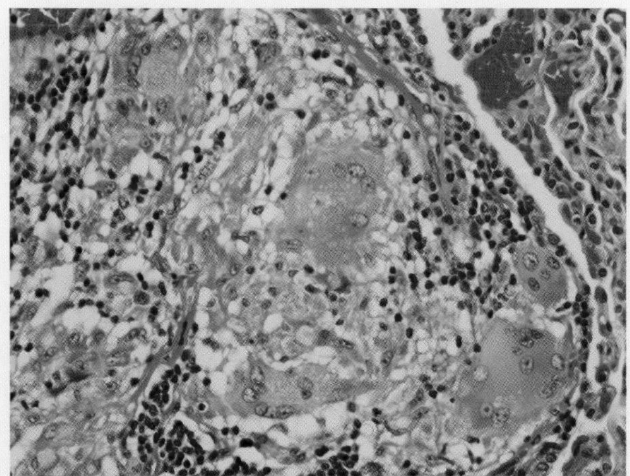

Figure 19-8. Case 2. Lung-wedge biopsy higher magnification from Figure 19-7 showing a poorly formed granuloma with an endogenous asteroid body in a multinucleated giant cell. No "foreign bodies" are seen. (Hematoxylin & eosin; original magnification 40×.)

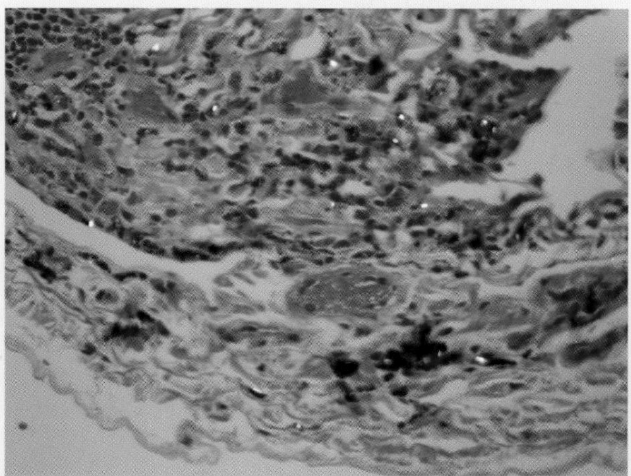

Figure 19-9. Case 2. Lung wedge biopsy showing a subpleural pigment deposit containing black carbon and birefringent silicate particles. (Hematoxylin & eosin, photographed under partially polarized light; original magnification 40×.)

also performed on the formalin-fixed lung tissue, but no abnormalities were detected. A possible small increase in nickel was reported.

Limited follow-up information was available, but the patient responded to steroid treatment with tapering doses of prednisone. The rheumatology consult included noting that the patient had a family history of lupus, but he was felt to have sarcoidosis responding to treatment with tapering steroids. The immunology studies were reviewed and thought to be nonspecific abnormal findings.

CASE 2

In 2011, a 42-year-old male—active duty, enlisted US Army service member—presented with pulmonary follow-up after being noted as hypoxemic on air evacuation from the Iraqi theater for musculoskeletal injuries. The patient's social history included tobacco use and smoking 1 to 1½ packs of cigarettes per day for a total of 25-pack years. He reported rarely consuming alcohol. The patient's occupational history included working as a combat medic, and his deployment history included deployments to Iraq in 2004, 2005, and 2007, and deployments to Kuwait and Iraq in 2009 to 2010.

Low oxygen saturation was confirmed on polysomnography as mild (88%–92% range), and after titrated continuous positive airway pressure lying flat from nocturnal oximetry. Spirometry revealed mild obstruction. Other normal or negative studies included a methacholine challenge, diffusing capacity of the lung for carbon monoxide, high-resolution CT scan, and shunt study. The patient's medications included chronic opioid use for musculoskeletal injuries. His past medical history included posttraumatic stress disorder, psoriasis, and obstructive sleep apnea. His body mass index was 30.

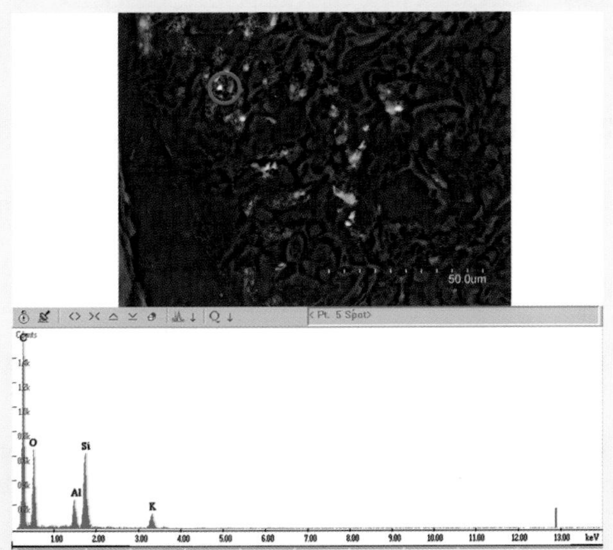

Figure 19-10. Case 2. Scanning electron microscopic image of a particle-rich area of lung, and energy dispersive X-ray analysis data showing the presence of carbon (C), oxygen (O), aluminum (Al), silicon (Si), and potassium (K) at the point indicated by the *red circle.*

Deployment-related exposures to benzene and beryllium were included in his record.

The patient underwent a VATS lung biopsy to rule out interstitial lung disease, with the sole abnormality being low arterial oxygen tension (to the low 70 mm Hg) on multiple arterial blood gases.

The contributing pathologist's diagnosis was nonnecrotizing granulomatous inflammation and emphysematous changes. The case was sent in consultation with the JPC and the contributor favoring a diagnosis of sarcoidosis. The JPC diagnosis was microgranulomatous pneumonitis. The JPC pathologist noted that the granulomas were not as well-formed as usual for sarcoidosis. He favored hypersensitivity pneumonitis, but the granulomas were located in lymphatics adjacent to small vessels, and there was minimal lymphocytic infiltration. No constrictive bronchiolitis and no nonspecific interstitial pneumonia were seen (Figures 19-6 to 19-8).

Scanning electron microscopy with energy dispersive X-ray analysis was performed on the biopsy, and particle counting was performed on particle-rich and particle-poor fields. In the richest deposit, 103 particles were counted (in a 1.5K magnification field). Twenty-seven particles had an area of $<0.25\ \mu m^2$. All but five particles contained silicon. Of these, three particles contained titanium and oxygen. Most (>90%) were aluminum silicates (Figures 19-9 to 19-12). Rare silica particles (with higher silicon content) were identified. In a particle-poor area, all of the particles had an area of $>0.39\ \mu m^2$. Few contained silicon. Most contained oxygen, iron, aluminum, and some titanium.

Follow-up information was available for this patient. His blood beryllium level was normal, and his lymphocyte stimulation test was negative. The patient's pulmonary function testing stabilized with an improved PaO_2 of 88 mm Hg. He reported no exposure history to suggest a potential etiology for hypersensitivity pneumonitis. In particular, he reported no contact with birds or other animals (except a cat), no hot tub use, and so forth. The patient still experienced dyspnea with exertion that "he felt was slightly worse," but he had none at rest. The patient had obstructive sleep apnea and continued to use continuous positive airway pressure unchanged. He was noted as having mild polycythemia persisting after reported smoking cessation and resolving hypoxia. Etiology was uncertain, and a hematology oncology consultation was performed that favored a respiratory hypoxic etiology.

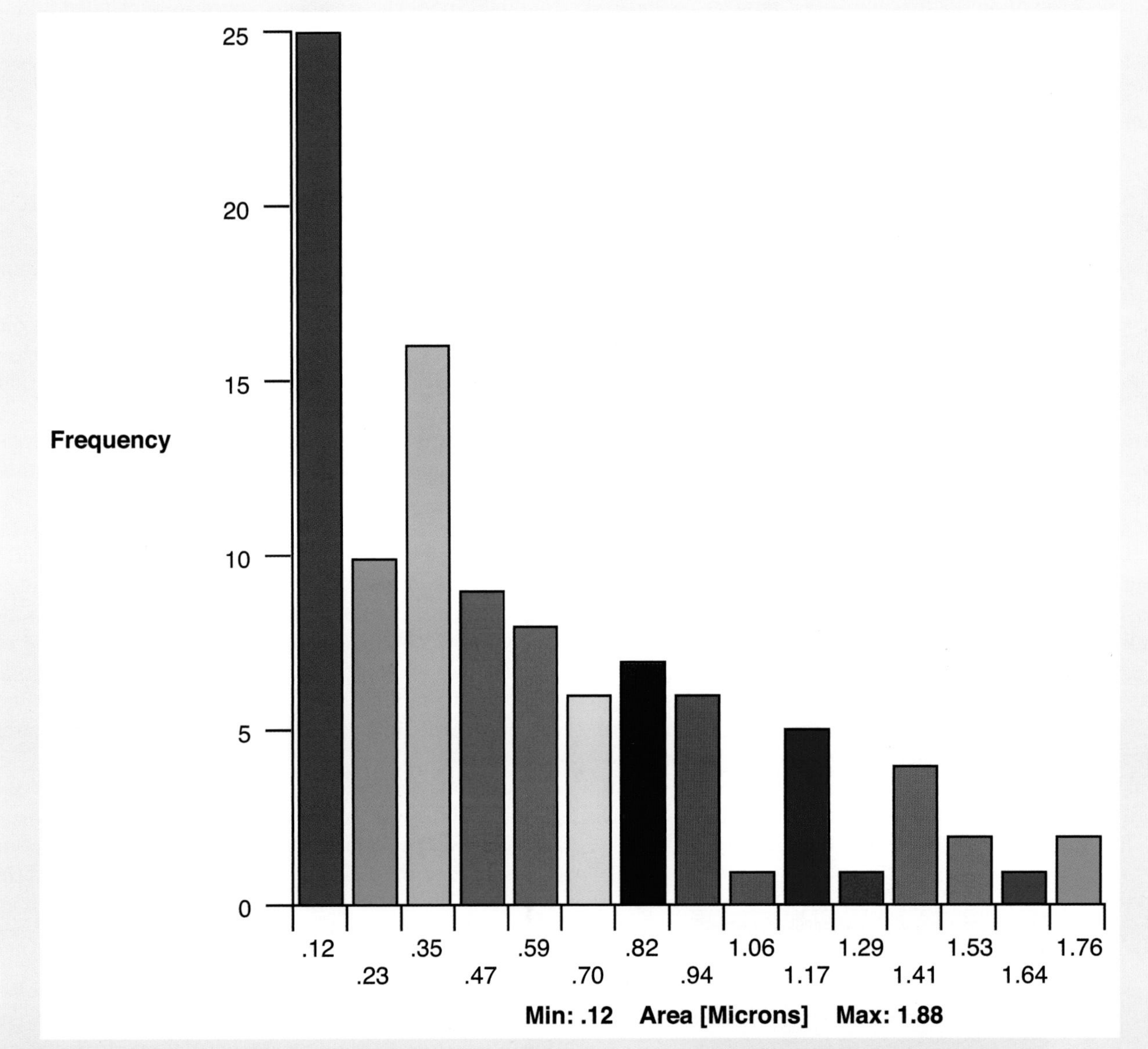

Figure 19-11. Case 2. Particle size (area) distribution histogram for a particle-rich area of the lung biopsy. Max: maximum; Min: minimum

SUMMARY

Since the start of the wars in Iraq and Afghanistan, several hundred cases have been reviewed by the Departments of Pulmonary and Mediastinal Pathology, Environmental Pathology, and Radiologic Pathology at the AFIP and the JPC, from US military personnel previously deployed to Iraq and Afghanistan. There is a breadth of histopathological diagnoses in this population. Two of these cases with nonneoplastic histopathology have been described in this chapter. The working/clinical diagnosis for case 1 was sarcoidosis. In case 2—involving a patient with a more complicated clinical picture—hypersensitivity pneumonitis was considered, but was not supported by the available clinical information. Because a certain number of respiratory illnesses occur in any population, their presence in previously deployed military personnel is not of itself an unexpected finding. What is difficult to determine is what proportion of lung injury in the previously deployed military population can be specifically attributed to exposures encountered during deployment.

The human lung has a limited repertoire of responses to inhaled materials, which are categorized by histopathologists into various patterns based on light microscopy. Although there are a few notable exceptions, broadly speaking these categories are not pathognomonic for exposure to a single specific environmental agent. Indeed, there are also examples

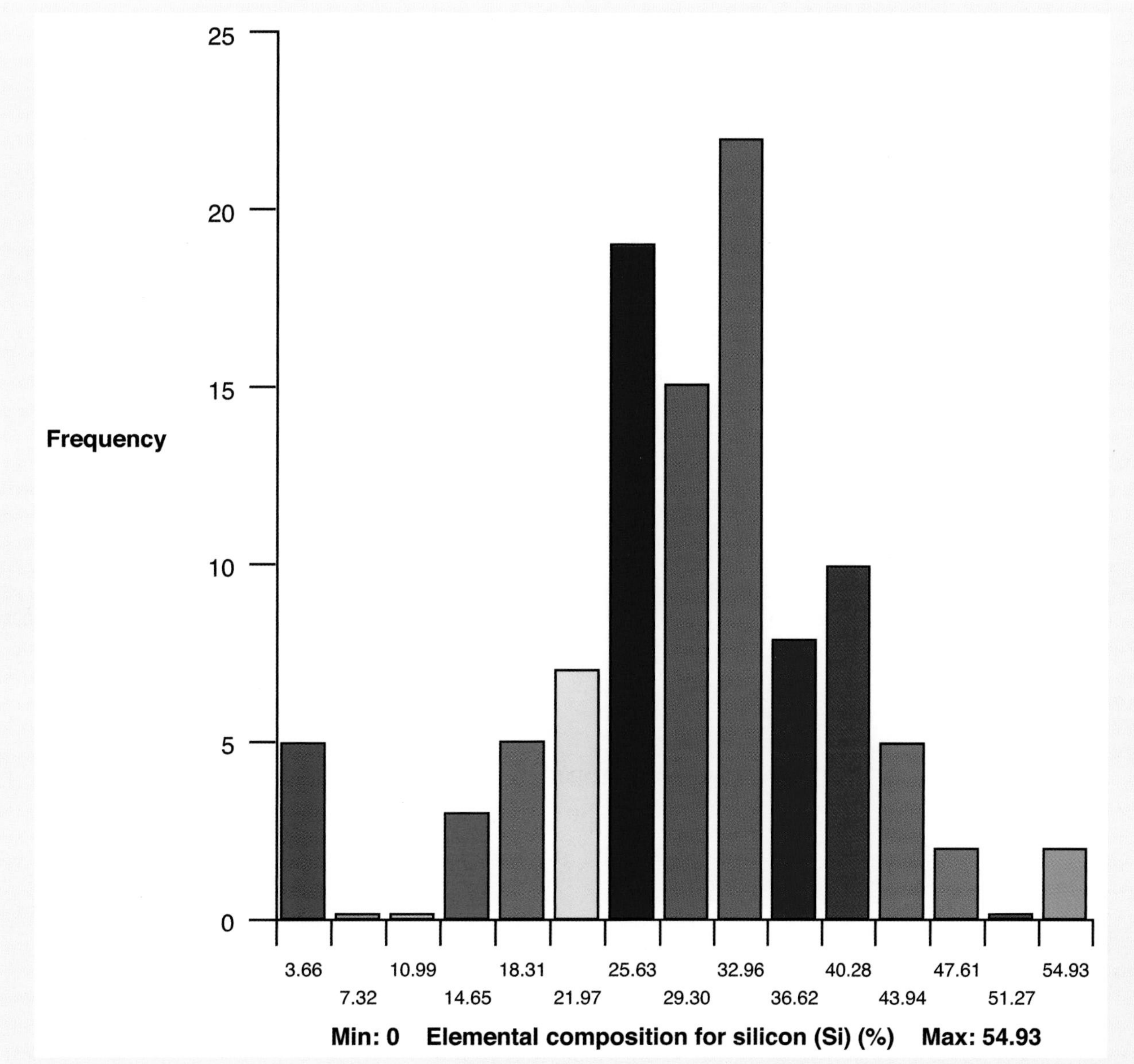

Figure 19-12. Case 2. Histogram of the same particles as seen in Figure 19-11 sorted by silicon content. A small number of particles containing the most silicon may represent silica.
Max: maximum; Min: minimum

of single environmental agents giving rise to more than one histopathological pattern. The histopathological assessment is often only part of reaching a specific diagnosis, coupled with clinical, laboratory, and radiological findings. In this assessment, factors such as occupational history, cigarette smoking, and body mass index are known to have a significant impact in many cases and should not be ignored. In each case, a link to a specific etiology is sought. Although the question of etiology is straightforward, a confident determination of etiology is frequently elusive.

Acknowledgments

The authors acknowledge the assistance of Albin Moroz and Tain-Lin Huang who provided database support and obtained Defense Manpower Data Center confirmation of deployment status. Florabel G. Mullick, MD, ScD, Former Director of the Armed Forces Institute of Pathology and Chair of the Department of Environmental and Infectious Disease Sciences, supported the creation of registries for pathology specimens from Iraq and Afghanistan veterans. We also thank Colonel Thomas Baker, MD, US Army MC, Director, The Joint Pathology Center, for his support in continuing registries focused on the histopathology of US military service members deployed to Iraq and Afghanistan.

THERE ARE NO REFERENCES IN THIS CHAPTER

Chapter 20

VETERANS AFFAIRS SYMPOSIUM: CASE REPORTS

MICHAEL J. MORRIS, MD*

*Colonel (Retired), Medical Corps, US Army; Department of Defense Chair, Staff Physician, Pulmonary/Critical Care Medicine and Assistant Program Director, Internal Medicine Residency, San Antonio Military Medical Center, 3551 Roger Brooke Drive, Fort Sam Houston, Texas 78234

INTRODUCTION

The inhaled airborne hazards related to southwest Asia deployment have resulted in higher rates of respiratory symptoms and potentially unique manifestations of respiratory disease. While the extent and chronicity of lung disease has not been delineated for deployed military personnel, common diseases such as asthma and less common etiologies should be considered. This chapter reviews several unusual manifestations of lung disease in two cases and describes the difficulties associated with establishing specific diagnoses in these symptomatic military personnel.

CASE 1

In November 2009, a 39-year-old active duty male initially presented to the Pulmonary Clinic at Brooke Army Medical Center (Fort Sam Houston, TX) with symptoms of progressive dyspnea. The soldier had previously deployed to Iraq for 12 months (from 2005 to 2006) as a helicopter door gunner. He denied any pulmonary symptoms during deployment and upon return was able to pass the semiannual Army Physical Fitness Test. Because of the onset of nystagmus from a medullary central nervous system lesion, he was unable to perform any regular exercise for the following 2 years. After gradual resolution of neurological symptoms, he noted the onset of progressive exertional dyspnea. He denied any rest symptoms, cough, or sputum production in association with his exertional symptoms. The patient had a previous 4-pack-year tobacco history, but quit in 1996. His past medical history included post-traumatic stress disorder, anxiety disorder, and sleep disturbances. Physical examination was unremarkable, with body mass index unchanged at 28 to 29. Pulmonary and cardiac examinations were normal.

The initial chest X-ray radiograph was unremarkable, with no consolidations or infiltrates. Initial spirometry demonstrated a mixed obstructive/restrictive pattern with a forced vital capacity (FVC) of 3.98 L (64% predicted), a forced expiratory volume in 1 second (FEV_1) of 2.79 L (57% predicted), and a normal FEV_1/FVC ratio with a 7% increase in postbronchodilator FEV_1. The inspiratory flow volume loop was likewise noted as partially truncated during baseline spirometry. Full pulmonary function testing (PFT) demonstrated a total lung capacity of 7.04 L (86% predicted), with a residual volume of 2.46 L (116% predicted) and a diffusing capacity of the lung for carbon monoxide at 27.1 mL/mm Hg/min (61% predicted). Further evaluation included methacholine challenge testing, which was stopped after the initial dose because of a 37% decrease in FVC and a 42% decrease in FEV_1.

The patient was referred to speech therapy and had a normal laryngoscopic examination with no evidence of gastroesophageal reflux disease. He had normal vocal cord appearance and motion. The patient underwent cardiopulmonary exercise testing and worked out for 9 minutes using a cycle ergometer. His exercise capacity was normal with a maximal oxygen consumption of 93% predicted, an anaerobic threshold of 65% maximal oxygen consumption, and no cardiac or respiratory limitation to exercise. Computed tomography (CT) imaging of the chest revealed mild ground-glass opacities at medial-to-posterior lung bases on selected high-resolution supine inspiratory and prone expiratory images with mild reticular prominence. Flexible fiberoptic bronchoscopy was normal, with negative cultures and cytology. There was no acute or chronic inflammation in the transbronchial biopsies.

Because of the persistent findings on CT imaging, the patient was referred for surgical lung biopsy where right upper lobe, middle lobe, and lower lobe samples were obtained. Tissue specimens were sent to the Armed Forces Institute of Pathology (Washington, DC; closed in September 2011). Scanning electron microscopy revealed specimens of mild, focal, nonspecific interstitial pneumonia with possible hypersensitivity pneumonitis; mild peribronchiolar fibrosis and emphysema; and mild anthracosilicotic deposits with occasional small, colorless, birefringent particles containing silicon. Further testing of the transbronchial biopsy specimens with scanning electron microscopy with energy dispersive X-ray analysis identified both gold and Teflon (E I DuPont de Nemours and Company, Wilmington, DE) particles. Based on previously described findings, there was no distinct etiology for the patient's symptoms. However, possible diagnoses included the following:

- mixed obstructive/restrictive PFTs with no clear demonstration of airway hyperreactivity,
- possible upper airway involvement, and
- deconditioning contributing to symptoms of mild interstitial lung disease.

The role of silicates and other metals to interstitial findings is unclear.

CASE 2

In November 2011, a 30-year-old active duty male was referred for abnormal imaging to the Pulmonary Clinic at Brooke Army Medical Center. The soldier was previously deployed to Iraq for 15 months in 2008 to 2009 to perform vehicle recovery. He specifically described ongoing exposure to burning vehicles from improvised explosive devices. He developed a nocturnal cough while still deployed, but was not evaluated or treated in theater. Postdeployment treatment included an inhaled corticosteroid/long-acting beta-agonist combination that did not relieve his cough symptoms. He developed both progressive exertional dyspnea and chronic cough, but denied any rest symptoms or productive sputum. The patient was an active smoker with a 6-pack-year history at the time of initial evaluation, but later quit. Past medical history was only notable for a chronic back injury and left ear deafness. Physical examination was notable for a body mass index of 32 and oxygen saturation of 97%. Cardiac and pulmonary examinations were normal. Initial spirometry revealed an FVC of 4.62 L (84% predicted), an FEV_1 of 3.61 L (81% predicted), an FEV_1/FVC of 78%, and a 7% increase in postbronchodilator FEV_1. Full PFTs demonstrated a total lung capacity of 5.48 L (77% predicted), with a residual volume of 0.70 L (40% predicted) and a diffusing capacity of the lung for carbon monoxide at 26.8 mL/mm Hg/min (65% predicted).

These findings were consistent with a mild restrictive defect. Given the mild decrease in the FEV_1/FVC ratio, mannitol challenge testing was performed, and the patient completed a maximum dose of 160 mg, with only a 1% decrease in FEV_1 (normal bronchial responsiveness). Chest X-ray radiograph demonstrated nonspecific linear opacities in the left lower lung, and CT of the chest identified a wedge-shaped opacity within the left lower lobe with subjacent pleural thickening likely related to rounded atelectasis. Because of this finding on chest CT, he underwent diagnostic fiberoptic bronchoscopy. Bronchoalveolar lavage was negative for bacterial or fungal infection, and cytology was noninflammatory. Transbronchial biopsies demonstrated focal acute inflammation with a suggestion of organization, but were otherwise nondiagnostic. Based on these findings and stable dyspnea symptoms, he opted for repeat imaging, and repeat CT performed in March 2012 showed no interval change. The patient's chronic dyspnea was thought to be deployment-related and multifactorial in etiology because of the following:

- left lower lobe rounded atelectasis,
- chronic pleural thickening with pleurisy,
- mild restrictive lung disease, and
- limited exercise from chronic back pain.

SUMMARY

These case reports highlight the complexity of lung disease found in deployed military personnel and the need for an extensive evaluation by specialists to discern the various contributing factors for their symptoms. It has been well established that deployment to southwest Asia is associated with increased respiratory symptoms and the possibility of chronic lung disease.[1,2] Potential hazards may include suspended particulate matter from geological dusts, proximity to burn pit smoke, vehicle exhaust emissions, industrial air pollution, and specific exposure incidents.[3] Other factors that may play a role in these complaints include increased rates of cigarette smoking, multiple deployments, and higher rates of posttraumatic stress disorder and traumatic brain injury affecting a significant number of military personnel. Although a specific diagnosis may not be established, a complete evaluation can establish the severity of symptoms and underlying lung disease.

REFERENCES

1. Morris MJ, Zacher LL, Jackson DA. Investigating the respiratory health of deployed military personnel. *Mil Med.* 2011;176;1157–1161.

2. Smith B, Wong CA, Smith TC, Boyko EJ, Gacksetter GS, Ryan MAK. Newly reported respiratory symptoms and conditions among military personnel deployed to Iraq and Afghanistan: a prospective population-based study. *Am J Epidemiol.* 2009;170:1433–1442.

3. Weese CB, Abraham JH. Potential health implications associated with particulate matter exposure in deployed settings in Southwest Asia. *Inhal Toxicol.* 2009;21:291–296.

Chapter 21

DENVER VETERANS AFFAIRS MEDICAL CENTER EXPERIENCE WITH POSTDEPLOYMENT DYSPNEA CASE REPORTS

CAROLYN H. WELSH, MD*; AND YORK E. MILLER, MD†

*Professor, Department of Medicine, Division of Pulmonary Sciences and Critical Care Medicine, University of Colorado Denver School of Medicine, Anschutz Medical Campus, 12700 East 19th Avenue, Aurora, Colorado 80045; Staff Physician and Sleep Program Director, Denver Veterans Affairs Medical Center, Eastern Colorado Health Care System, 1055 Clermont Street, Denver, Colorado 80220

†Thomas L. Petty Chair of Lung Research Professor, Department of Medicine, Division of Pulmonary Sciences and Critical Care Medicine, University of Colorado School of Medicine, Anschutz Medical Campus, 12700 East 19th Avenue, Aurora, Colorado 80045; Staff Physician and Chest Clinic Director, Denver Veterans Affairs Medical Center, Eastern Colorado Health Care System, 1055 Clermont Street, Denver, Colorado 80220

INTRODUCTION

Patients without symptoms prior to deployment to southwest Asia have experienced respiratory symptoms, exercise difficulty, and even impaired ability to perform basic activities of daily living after return from one or more tours of duty. A larger number of soldiers deployed to Iraq and Afghanistan are reported to have respiratory symptoms compared with soldiers deployed to other locations (14.5% vs 1.8%).[1] One series of exposed individuals reports respiratory symptoms and findings of constrictive bronchiolitis.[2] Of note, not all of these persons have a history of tobacco smoking. Although the majority of people returning stateside experience no respiratory impairment, there are a growing number of instances in which chronic, otherwise unexplained shortness of breath and cough accompany a significant alteration in exercise capacity and ability to carry out activities of daily living. Two illustrative cases are presented herein with findings that, after diagnostic workup, were not attributable to asthma or chronic obstructive pulmonary disease and showed persistence of findings on serial assessments.

CASE 1

A 36-year-old man presented in 2010 with dyspnea on exertion and productive cough. His symptoms began in 2002 while he was deployed to Bagram Airfield in Afghanistan. At that time, he had wheezing and the onset of dark, sometimes black sputum. He was told that he had smoking-related lung disease although he never smoked. While in Tikrit, Iraq, for 12 months during 2005 to 2006, he experienced dyspnea on exertion and could barely run 1½ to 2 miles. He would become lightheaded and stopped running so he would not pass out. His run time increased to 17 minutes for a 2-mile run. He lived ¼ mile from pits where trash was burned and was assigned to work in demining operations. At this time, there was an uncapped oil well burning 1 mile out of town. From 2007 to 2008, he was again in Afghanistan for 12 months. He worked in an old Russian crematorium and had contact with human remains. He also had direct contact with asbestos-wrapped pipes. Over these three separate deployments, his symptoms resolved, but never normalized with stateside return.

In his permanent residence, there were no birds, hot tub, or water damage in his home. He was a clerical worker. After his third return stateside, his running distance had decreased markedly.

On examination, he was a well-groomed man without use of accessory muscles to breathe. Pulse was elevated at 113, and blood pressure was 138/98 mm Hg. His body mass index was borderline high at 26.3. He had no lymphadenopathy and no adventitious breath sounds. On cardiac examination, there was no jugular venous distention, and heart sounds were normal without murmurs. Abdominal examination was normal, and extremities were without edema. Pulse oximetry showed 94% saturation at rest, normal at an altitude of 5,280 feet. While

TABLE 21-1

CASE 1: PULMONARY FUNCTION TESTING

	June 2010	May 2011	July 2012
FVC (L)	4.13 (84%)	4.03 (73%)	3.89 (70%)
FEV_1 (L)	3.63 (89%)	3.53 (80%)	3.22(73%)
FEV_1/FVC ratio	0.88	0.88	0.83
TGV (L)	1.79 (50%)	1.89 (53%)	2.01 (56%)
RV (L)	1.13 (62%)	1.39 (74%)	1.43 (76%)
TLC (L)	5.25 (74%)	5.46 (76%)	5.40 (75%)
DLCO/VA (mL/min/mm Hg)	112%	129%	121
Bronchodilator response	No	No	13%

DLCO/VA: diffusing capacity of the lung for carbon monoxide corrected for alveolar volume; FEV_1: forced expiratory volume in 1 second; FVC: forced vital capacity; RV: residual volume; TGV: thoracic gas volume performed by plethysmography; TLC: total lung capacity
Note: Serial pulmonary function testing. Percentages are percent predicted for gender, ethnicity, weight, and height.

running, his oxygen saturations dropped to 82%. Serial pulmonary function is shown in Table 21-1. There was a mild restrictive process without improvement over a 2-year interval.

Transthoracic echocardiograph was normal, and chest X-ray film was normal. Thoracic computed tomography scans in 2010 and 2011 showed no interstitial lung changes, airspace opacity, or mosaicism. On polysomnography, the apnea hypopnea index was mildly elevated at 6.

Lung biopsy showed nonspecific changes of hyperinflation, with mild patchy bronchiolar and peribronchiolar chronic inflammation and minimal focal cellular bronchiolitis. There was mild patchy peribronchiolar mixed dust and anthracotic pigment with pigmented macrophages in airspaces (Figure 21-1).

For his airway symptoms, he had been treated with inhaled corticosteroids, prednisone, sodium mycophenolate, and azithromycin with minimal response in dyspnea or exercise distance. He is currently using a budesonide/formoterol inhaler and azithromycin three times weekly. He notes continued dyspnea and hypoxemia when he exercises.

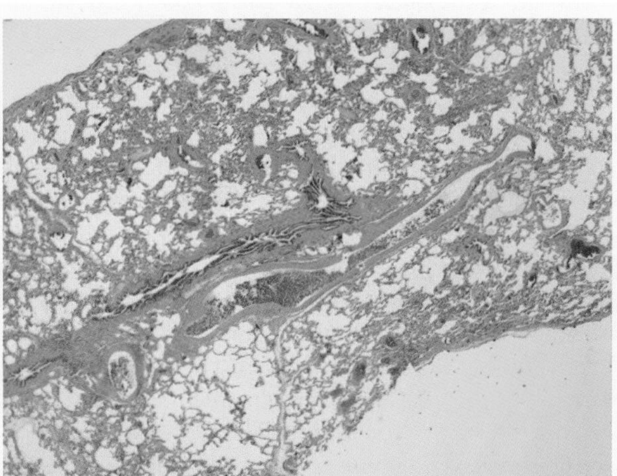

Figure 21-1. Representative areas of peribronchiolar inflammation and mild cellular bronchiolitis from lung biopsy. Hematoxylin and eosin stain, Case 1.

CASE 2

A 37-year-old man presented with pulmonary evaluation in early 2011. He noted shortness of breath while putting on socks, showering, and walking 25 feet. He was no longer able to perform his job driving a truck for a scrapyard because of coughing and shortness of breath. His wife described the onset of his trouble breathing in 2007, 4 years prior to presentation. He was short of breath when he laid flat; therefore, he slept in a recliner.

He coughed when he was supine and then regurgitated. He noted sharp anterior chest pain when he inspired. Seven years previously, he could run 2 miles in 15 minutes. He smoked briefly at age 14 for less than 1 year and has been a nonsmoker since that time.

He was deployed to Tikrit, Iraq, for 4 months in 2003. He had a second deployment of 12 months starting November 2005 in Baqubah, Iraq. During this time, he lived 2 miles

TABLE 21-2

CASE 2: PULMONARY FUNCTION TESTING

	April 2011	June 2011	April 2012
FVC (L)	4.58 (71%)	4.50 (70%)	3.29 (51%)
FEV_1 (L)	3.40 (66%)	3.63 (71%)	2.80 (50%)
Ratio FEV_1/FVC	0.74	0.81	0.85
TGV (L)	2.69 (64%)	3.43 (82%)	2.49 (59%)
RV (L)	1.54 (73%)	3.26 (155%)	2.21 (104%)
TLC (L)	7.36 (90%)	5.20 (64%)	6.29 (77%)
DLCO/VA (mL/min/mm Hg)	98%	—	108%
Bronchodilator response	33%	—	17%
MIP/MEP		44%/30%	

DLCO/VA: diffusing capacity of the lung for carbon monoxide corrected for alveolar volume; FEV_1: forced expiratory volume in 1 second; FVC: forced vital capacity; MEP: maximum expiratory pressure; MIP: maximum inspiratory pressure; RV: residual volume; TGV: thoracic gas volume performed by plethysmography; TLC: total lung capacity

Note: Serial pulmonary function testing. Percentages are percent predicted for gender, ethnicity, weight, and height. Dashes indicate that no test was performed and that data are not available.

downwind of the burn pits. He had nightly pesticide mist exposure. He took two platoons worth of trash to the burn pits every day, and these were often downwind. He worked on wash detail. During deployment, there were frequent dust storms.

On examination, blood pressure was 119/64 mm Hg, pulse was 62, and body mass index was 32. He was not using accessory muscles to breathe and had no rash. He had no lymphadenopathy or jugular venous distention. There was good air movement with mild inspiratory crackles at the bases that cleared with coughing. He had a shallow breathing pattern. Cardiac examination showed a normal S1, S2 and no murmurs or gallops. He had no pedal edema. Oxygen saturation was normal (96% on room air at rest, 95% with exertion). Serial pulmonary function is shown in Table 21-2. He had intermittent airflow limitation with a bronchodilator response and hyperinflation. He also had low thoracic gas volume, a restrictive finding that had not resolved over a 1-year interval.

The computed tomography scan of the thorax showed no consolidation, nor any abnormal findings (including ground-glass attenuation, interlobular septal thickening, subpleural reticular abnormalities, diffuse parenchymal nodularity, significant bronchiectasis, or evidence of pulmonary fibrosis).

Extensive diagnostic workup included lack of diaphragmatic paresis on sniff test and normal vocal cord movement with no vocal cord dysfunction on laryngoscopy. In addition, he had a normal apnea hypopnea index on an in-laboratory sleep study. His 6-minute walk test at 3 L/min with resting oxygen saturation was 94%, with a heart rate of 102 beats/min. Posttest oxygen saturation was 97%, and heart rate was 99 beats/min. The Borg Dyspnea Scale score was 4 (somewhat heavy), with a walking distance of only 500 feet in 6 minutes on 3 L/min of oxygen (using a cane).

Lung biopsy showed hyperinflated lung parenchyma. There was a subacute bronchiolocentric process characterized by chronic inflammation with occasional poorly formed granulomas and scattered giant cells. Changes appeared to be more prominent in lower and middle lobe sections (Figure 21-2). No fibrosis, constrictive bronchiolitis, or polarizable material was seen, and the pathologist's conclusion was inflammation that appeared most compatible with a process of subacute hypersensitivity pneumonitis.

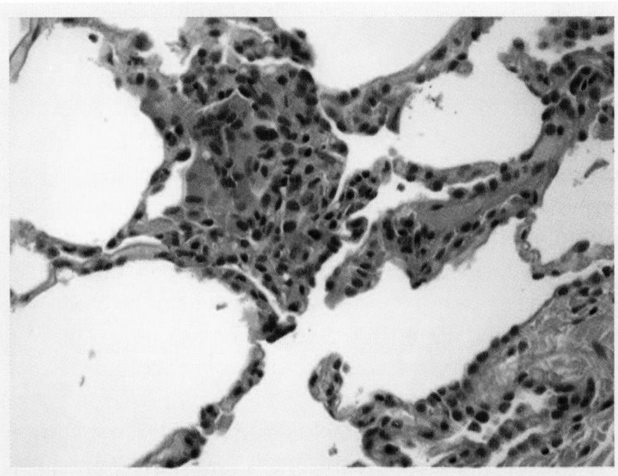

Figure 21-2. High power view of chronic inflammation area. Poorly formed giant cells were noted in other areas of the lung biopsy specimen. Hematoxylin and eosin stain, Case 2.

His treatment included inhaled mometasone, formoterol, and albuterol as needed up to 8 times daily. Tiotropium had been subsequently added. He received two courses of high-dose prednisone tapering over 2 weeks. Despite this, he had progressive worsening of symptoms such that he could no longer function in his job.

SERIES OF BIOPSIES

In our practice group, there have been more than 40 patients referred for persistent airway symptoms after deployment to southwest Asia. Of these, eight patients underwent thoracoscopic lung biopsies after careful review of their unexplained symptoms. All cases are discussed in a multidisciplinary conference with imaging, surgery, and pulmonology input prior to referral for this procedure.

Although the symptoms and time course for these patients were not classic for asthma, most were tried on bronchodilator therapy without clinical response prior to referral for biopsy. Specimens of these eight patients were reviewed by a pathologist with expertise in pulmonary pathology. Findings include comments on hyperinflation for five of the eight specimens. Assessments include the following:

- sarcoid,
- perivascular nonnecrotizing granulomas,
- constrictive bronchiolitis,
- multiple chemodectomas,
- focal cellular bronchiolitis,
- patchy lymphocytic respiratory bronchiolitis, and
- two cases with bronchocentric granulomas.

None of the specimens showed normal lung tissue.

SUMMARY

These are two illustrative cases of unanticipated dyspnea and respiratory symptoms after deployment to southwest Asia. Findings are not fully explained by a diagnosis of asthma or chronic obstructive pulmonary disease, although Case 2 has had intermittent hyperinflation and clear bronchodilator responses on two occasions. Neither patient has smoked tobacco for more than a minimal exposure. Both of these cases have experienced a dramatic drop in their functional activity and have not improved over time. Pathological findings include abnormalities in the bronchiolar and bronchial regions of the specimens, and radiographic abnormalities are not evident. Pulmonary function shows restrictive features for Case 1 and intermittent obstruction with a low thoracic gas volume, also a restrictive finding, in Case 2. Symptoms and findings in Case 2 have progressed long after his time of deployment, and both men have experienced life-altering symptoms.

This chapter notes findings for two persons and is not a comprehensive assessment of persons deployed to Afghanistan and Iraq. It does, however, illustrate that for some people there is a persistent process other than asthma with restrictive features on physiology for which treatment is unclear and prognosis not defined. Fortunately, the majority of persons do not experience such symptoms after deployment; however, referrals are common enough to warrant concern. That these pulmonary abnormalities in exposed persons do not affect the majority of those exposed is parallel to the symptom incidence in other exposures causing bronchial and interstitial diseases (eg, beryllium workers). In one series of chronic beryllium disease, only 4% of exposed workers develop clinical disease.[3] Further assessment of risk, exposures, and natural history as outlined in the working group document is warranted.[4]

REFERENCES

1. Szema AM, Salihi W, Savary K, Chen JJ. Respiratory symptoms necessitating spirometry among soldiers with Iraq/Afghanistan war lung injury. *J Occup Environ Med*. 2011;53:961–965.

2. King MS, Eisenberg R, Newman JH, et al. Constrictive bronchiolitis in soldiers returning from Iraq and Afghanistan. *N Engl J Med*. 2011;365:222–230.

3. Schuler CR, Kent MS, Deubner DC, et al. Process-related risk of beryllium sensitization and disease in a copper-beryllium alloy facility. *Am J Ind Med*. 2005;47:195–205.

4. Rose C, Abraham J, Harkins D, et al. Overview and recommendations for medical screening and diagnostic evaluation for postdeployment lung disease in returning US warfighters. *J Occup Environ Med*. 2012;54:746–751.

Chapter 22

DISCUSSION SUMMARY: METHODOLOGICAL CONSIDERATIONS TO DESIGN A PULMONARY CASE SERIES AND A NATIONAL, BROAD-BASED REGISTRY FOR VETERANS OF OPERATION IRAQI FREEDOM AND OPERATION ENDURING FREEDOM

KELLEY ANN BRIX, MD, MPH*; AND STELLA E. HINES, MD, MSPH†

*Deputy Director for the Defense Medical Research and Development Program, Office of the Assistant Secretary of Defense for Health Affairs, Force Health Protection and Readiness Defense Health Headquarters, 7700 Arlington Boulevard, Suite 5101, Falls Church, Virginia 22042-5101

†Assistant Professor, University of Maryland School of Medicine, Department of Medicine Occupational Health Program and Division of Pulmonary & Critical Care Medicine, Baltimore Veterans Affairs Medical Center, 11 South Paca Street, Suite 200, Baltimore, Maryland 21201

INTRODUCTION

In Iraq and Afghanistan, concentrations of air contaminants, such as combustion products and particulate matter, are frequently much higher than they are in the United States. The US Department of Defense (DoD) has evaluated air pollution at several locations in theater and performed risk assessments of the potential long-term health effects.[1,2] In 2010, the DoD published the proceedings of a symposium co-sponsored by the Armed Forces Health Surveillance Center and the Uniformed Services University of the Health Sciences titled Assessing Potentially Hazardous Environmental Exposures Among Military Populations.[3] The symposium focused on airborne hazards, including environmental monitoring and medical surveillance.[4–6] Several other recent studies have focused on air pollution in theater, including a comprehensive Institute of Medicine (IOM) study potential health effects of burn pit emissions.[1,2,7–9] The long-term health effects of air pollution in theater are uncertain; therefore, epidemiological, clinical, and laboratory research studies are underway.

Individual cases have been reported of service members and veterans who developed various pulmonary diseases after returning from deployment to Operation Iraqi Freedom (OIF) and Operation Enduring Freedom (OEF). However, no controlled epidemiological studies have followed up these individual cases to determine if there were linkages between them, such as living at the same military base in theater or belonging to the same military unit or military occupational specialty. The rates of chronic pulmonary diseases in deployed service members have been compared with the rates in nondeployed service members in a number of controlled, population-based studies. To date, the evidence is inconclusive.[7,8,10–15] Controlled epidemiological studies of pulmonary diseases in OIF/OEF veterans and nondeployed veterans are continuing.

In response to case reports of pulmonary diseases, the Department of Veterans Affairs (VA) and the DoD have recently discussed the possible establishment of a pulmonary disease registry for veterans of OIF and OEF. During the Joint VA/DoD Airborne Hazards Symposium in August 2012, one work group discussed the scientific issues that need to be considered to develop a registry; this chapter summarizes that discussion. The purpose of this chapter is to describe issues related to development of two possible types of medical data collection: (1) a case series that is targeted to specific pulmonary diseases and (2) a national, broad-based registry related to deployment to OIF and OEF.

During the past few years, Congress introduced multiple bills that would require the VA to establish a burn pit registry. This potential requirement for a new VA registry was discussed during the August 2012 symposium. In January 2013, President Obama signed legislation that requires the VA to establish a registry. The provisions of this law are outlined in the section on National, Broad-based Registry Related to Operation Iraqi Freedom and Operation Enduring Freedom.[16]

CASE SERIES THAT ARE TARGETED TO SPECIFIC PULMONARY DISEASES

Existing Case Series of Pulmonary Diseases in Veterans of Operation Iraqi Freedom and Operation Enduring Freedom

This section reviews the small case series that has been published or presented during the August 2012 Airborne Hazards symposium, followed by a summary of the work group discussion during that symposium. This discussion focused on the general methodological issues related to the development of a pulmonary case series.

DoD and VA physicians at different locations have identified individual cases of OIF/OEF veterans who developed pulmonary diseases after returning home. During the August 2012 symposium, several physicians presented clinical case summaries of patients who had pulmonary diseases and who had served in Iraq or Afghanistan. Each of these cases demonstrated divergent pulmonary pathology. These individual cases raised more questions than they answered related to the types of environmental exposures or other risk factors that they experienced in OIF or OEF, which may or may not have contributed to the etiology of their diseases. Currently, there is no coordinated process in the DoD and the VA to collect data on these patients and to provide long-term follow-up, if warranted.

Physicians at Vanderbilt University (Nashville, TN) evaluated 80 soldiers who had deployed to Iraq or Afghanistan and who were referred for an evaluation of dyspnea on exertion.[17] Some of the soldiers reported exposure to the large fire at a sulfur mine in Iraq in 2003; however, others did not report any specific exposures.[14] These 80 soldiers received a variety of diagnoses, including asthma, bronchitis, sarcoidosis, and several other pulmonary diseases.[17] Of the 49 soldiers who underwent surgical lung biopsy, 38 were diagnosed with constrictive bronchiolitis.

Methodological concerns have been raised about this case series.[7,18] Questions have been raised whether the diagnoses of constrictive bronchiolitis were actually correct, because the majority of cases lacked evidence of airway obstruction on pulmonary function tests, which has traditionally been a diagnostic feature of this disease. In addition, the majority of these cases (75%) did not demonstrate findings of mosaic air trapping or centrilobular nodularity on high-resolution chest computed tomography, both of which are features that are seen in constrictive bronchiolitis. Concerns have also been raised about the lack of blinding of the pathologists in this study, which could have led to bias. Results of this case series cannot be used to draw conclusions on the etiology (causes) of the individual cases. To address the methodological concerns, the DoD recently funded scientists at National Jewish Health (Denver, CO) to provide an independent pathological review of the Vanderbilt cases.[9] This pathological review will be blinded; it will include the development of a morphometric diagnostic tool for small airways diseases, such as constrictive bronchiolitis, and it will include characterization of particles associated with the lesions.

Physicians at Brooke Army Medical Center (BAMC) in San Antonio, TX, are conducting a series of studies that are systematic clinical evaluations of active duty soldiers with pulmonary symptoms.[7,9] To date, this group has evaluated approximately 100 soldiers. The first study—titled Study of Active-Duty Military for Pulmonary Disease Related to Environmental Dust Exposure (STAMPEDE)—was presented during the August 2012 symposium.[19] The purpose of the study was to evaluate 50 active duty soldiers for evidence of lung disease. These soldiers had returned from OIF/OEF in the past 6 months and had developed new-onset pulmonary symptoms. Of the 50 cases, 12 received a diagnosis of asthma and 7 received other diagnoses. There was no evidence of constrictive bronchiolitis or interstitial lung disease in any of the 50 cases. No pulmonary diagnosis was made in 31 of the cases after a comprehensive workup. No surgical lung biopsies were required as part of STAMPEDE. Patients did undergo transbronchial lung biopsies through bronchoscopy if interstitial changes were seen on chest computed tomography. The overall conclusion was that most cases had a normal evaluation. This series of studies of systematic clinical evaluations of active duty soldiers is continuing at BAMC.[7,9]

The three VA War-Related Illness and Injury Study Centers (WRIISCs)—located in East Orange, NJ, Palo Alto, CA, and Washington, DC—evaluate veterans who have pulmonary symptoms.[8] For example, the East Orange Veterans Affairs Medical Center (VAMC) evaluated 35 veterans during 2012. These evaluations included cardiopulmonary exercise testing. The Baltimore VAMC has similarly performed thorough evaluations of OIF/OEF veterans who have had pulmonary symptoms since January 2012.

In general, medical evaluation methods used in these small case series have been too disparate to permit combined analyses from different sites. The DoD and VA could build on the foundation of separate case series to establish a shared, systematically collected case series of OIF/OEF veterans who have developed pulmonary diseases. The DoD and VA could develop this as a consortium for sharing information on pulmonary cases among military treatment facilities (MTFs) and VAMCs. The consortium could consist of a network of DoD and VA sites that would report to a central coordinating site.

During the August 2012 symposium, the work group discussed the potential utility of a coordinated, shared case series. The purpose of the case series would have to be carefully defined during its development to align expectations with the purpose. If a mechanism to pool similar cases from MTFs and VAMCs nationally could be established, this mechanism could yield a larger collection of cases and more useful data that could be used to identify commonalities among the cases. This could help generate hypotheses related to possible risk factors for the development of pulmonary diseases, which are related to military service or not. The case data would be used optimally as part of a case-control study. The remainder of this section describes the general methodological considerations needed to design a pulmonary case series, and it also summarizes the work group's discussion during the 2012 symposium.

Identification of Pulmonary Cases for a Shared Case Series

Eligibility criteria for the pulmonary case series could be defined by the new onset of a specific disease after returning from deployment (eg, constrictive bronchiolitis or interstitial lung disease) or by the new onset of symptoms (eg, dyspnea on exertion). A case series based on medically validated diseases would be much more specific; therefore, it would have greater scientific utility. Patients who have been described to date were diagnosed with a wide variety of diseases. Thus, it is premature to limit the shared case series to a single diagnosis (eg, constrictive bronchiolitis). The eligibility criteria could also include a threshold level of disability. Disability would be defined on the basis of pulmonary functional abnormalities or pathological diagnoses and not on receiving compensation benefits. These criteria would exclude a veteran who has mild symptoms that do not cause abnormalities in objective tests. Progression of the disease severity over time should also be considered.

Surgical lung biopsies would not be required to include patients in this case series. Many pulmonary diagnoses can be made with confidence without biopsy, particularly when the risk of undergoing an invasive procedure outweighs the benefits gained by a pathological diagnosis. However, biopsy is the gold standard for certain nonneoplastic lung diseases, and neoplastic diagnoses require pathology specimens. If biopsy results were available for some cases, pathological results would be useful to include in a case series because they provide the most accurate data. Lung biopsy specimens can be preserved, reviewed, and used in future research.

The DoD and VA maintain electronic databases that include medical records of millions of service members and veterans. These databases could be mined to identify OIF/OEF veterans who have pulmonary diseases. A targeted approach could focus on the electronic medical records of the MTF and VAMC that evaluate a large number of pulmonary patients. These hospitals evaluate the highest proportion of patients who are difficult to diagnose, regardless of severity of disease. These hospitals also treat the most severe cases.

Coordination of a Pulmonary Disease Consortium, Including Standardized Data Collection

The DoD and VA could develop one or two central coordinating centers to collect data from the MTF and VAMC that participate in the consortium. The coordinating centers would collect periodic reports from these sites and analyze the data for patterns and trends. The coordinating centers would provide feedback on these periodic analyses to the participating sites. The three military services have pulmonary consultants who could serve as consortium coordinators for their services. The VA has a national Director of Pulmonary Medicine who could coordinate consortium activities for the VA.

To develop a shared case series, the DoD and VA would need to develop and adopt a standardized medical evaluation that would be consistently recorded to ensure comparability of results between sites. Standardized evaluations would include a thorough diagnostic algorithm. Evaluations would also require the development of standardized forms for the data entry of medical history, occupational and military histories, physical examination, and a minimal set of diagnostic tests. The minimal set of diagnostic tests could include chest X-ray films and pulmonary function tests that could be performed at all of the participating sites. At a minimum, the pulmonary function tests should include pre- and post-bronchodilator spirometry to identify mild airflow obstruction.[20–24] Medical evaluations and data reporting would need to be standardized across the participating sites. Even minor differences could prevent easy integration of the data from different sites that would lead to substantial challenges in data analysis. Central coordinating centers would collect, maintain, and analyze the results of patient evaluations.

A standardized set of questions would be needed for the occupational and military histories to combine computerized data from many patients. These questions could address common airborne hazards in theater (eg, exposure to burn pits), high concentrations of particulate matter due to sand storms, and other exposures (eg, the large sulfur fire in Iraq in 2003).[14] Questions could also address the frequency, duration, and intensity of these exposures. The DoD has collected environmental samples from many locations in theater, and data are archived at the US Army Public Health Command at Aberdeen Proving Ground, MD. DoD environmental monitoring data could be requested for specific locations in theater to compare with the occupational histories of specific patients. In a small case series, environmental monitoring data could be retrieved and used to validate self-reported exposures on the questionnaires.

Environmental monitoring data would likely be available for only a small minority of cases. In most cases, only the self-reported exposure history will be available. A more scientific exposure assessment of past exposures would not be necessary to diagnose most pulmonary diseases or to provide treatment and follow-up care. Usually, clinical care does not depend on whether the causative factor was past exposure to burn pit smoke, sandstorms, or cigarette smoking. If the exposure is continuing, identification of the environmental factors contributing to a disease is necessary as part of management and treatment, because the ongoing exposure could lead to prolongation or exacerbation of the disease.

Current capability and funding for ongoing data management must be considered before deciding on the location of the central data repositories. The coordinating centers must have an ongoing public health mission that includes information systems specialists, biostatisticians, and epidemiologists who work on health databases. The US Army Public Health Command would be a logical location for the DoD coordinating center. This Command collects data on an ongoing basis to maintain several large databases that include information from all three services. The Armed Forces Health Surveillance Center in Silver Spring, MD, would be an alternate location for the DoD coordinating center. This center has access to the great majority of health databases in the DoD, and it performs ongoing health surveillance studies.

The VA coordinating center could be located at the VA Office of Public Health in Washington, DC. This office performs environmental epidemiology studies and currently coordinates the Agent Orange and Gulf War registries. Alternatively, one of the three WRIISCs could serve as the VA coordinating center, depending on the funding mechanism that would establish the consortium. One of these centers could have an advantage, because it receives funding to perform clinical care and research. The database manager for this program could be located adjacent to clinicians, which would facilitate ongoing communications.

Longitudinal Follow-up of a Pulmonary Case Series

Patients who have advanced or diagnostically perplexing pulmonary diseases should be referred to a pulmonary specialist at the local MTF or VAMC. The pulmonary specialist would be responsible for identifying potential patients to be included in the shared case series and would be the local point of contact for the consortium. If the patient's illness is still too difficult to diagnose, or is not responding to conventional treatment, the patient could be referred to a higher level DoD or VA referral center for further evaluation, such as the BAMC or one of the WRIISCs.

Patients who have pulmonary diseases should be followed over time and reevaluated, including after the transition of care from the DoD to VA due to separation from the military. Providers at the MTF and VAMC should plan the clinical hand-off of individual patients to ensure continuity of care and to prevent loss to follow-up, similar to the hand-off for OIF/OEF veterans who have traumatic brain injuries. Planning for a shared case series should incorporate the need for seamless transition of individual patients between DoD and VA care.

Long-term follow-up would ensure the continuity of care of individual patients, as well as illuminate the natural history of the diseases. A case series could provide useful longitudinal information, if it was designed to capture clinical follow-up data. To date, physicians who assessed the small case series have evaluated their cases at only one point in time; they have not followed the cases over time to describe the longitudinal course of the diseases. This means that DoD and VA clinicians who care for these patients have no information on the prognosis of the diseases, or if there are exposure-related conditions that could lead to unique patterns of disease progression.

By periodically evaluating trends in the case series population, investigators could elucidate the natural progression of deployment-related diseases. For example, longitudinal data analysis could address questions on the stability or progression of pulmonary function, chest imaging, or severity of disability. Some of these conditions may be rare and without widely accepted standards regarding appropriate treatment (eg, constrictive bronchiolitis). Therefore, comparisons between varying medical therapies in similar patients could foster understanding of the prognosis and the appropriate medical treatments for deployment-related diseases. The consortium could provide feedback to the participating sites on these issues of progression of the diseases and responses to treatments that could lead to improvements in clinical care.

Utility of a Shared Pulmonary Case Series

Longitudinal follow-up of pulmonary cases would enable the development of a systematic, thorough description of the cases, and it would define the natural history of the diseases. The results of a shared case series could have clinical utility to inform VA and DoD physicians who care for OIF/OEF veterans. For example, the results could be used to develop guidelines for the use of specific diagnostic tests or specific treatments for veterans who have particular respiratory diseases. Results could be published as an internal DoD or VA report and in the open medical literature.

Results of the medical evaluations could be compiled to generate hypotheses, based on patterns of disease or patterns of exposure. If patterns could be detected, improvements in treatment or prevention could possibly be developed.[24] It should be emphasized that a pulmonary case series would have multiple limitations regarding causality or association. Results could not be used to determine the etiology or pathophysiology of the diseases in individual cases. In addition, diseases that are diagnosed in individual cases could not be generalized to the entire deployed population, and no estimate of the rates of diseases could be determined.[25] However, if the cases were used as the basis of a case-control study, the association of potential risk factors with disease outcomes could be ascertained.

NATIONAL, BROAD-BASED REGISTRY RELATED TO OPERATION IRAQI FREEDOM AND OPERATION ENDURING FREEDOM

Existing Department of Veterans Affairs Registries Related to Deployments and the Congressional Requirement for a New Veterans Affairs Burn Pit Registry

This section describes the existing VA registries, followed by a summary of the work group discussion during the August 2012 symposium. This discussion focuses on the general methodological issues related to the development of a broad-based VA registry.

The VA has multiple registries related to specific deployments and environmental exposures, including Agent Orange, Gulf War, depleted uranium, and ionizing radiation. The VA has maintained an Agent Orange Registry for Vietnam veterans since 1978.[26] As of mid-2012, more than 561,000 veterans had received an Agent Orange examination. Approximately 4,000 veterans per month were enrolling in the Agent Orange registry as of 2012.[26] The VA has maintained a Gulf War Registry since 1992.[26] Veterans of the 1990–1991 Gulf War and OIF are eligible to enroll in the Gulf War Registry. As of mid-2012, more than 126,000 veterans had received a Gulf War examination. From 1994 to 2002, the DoD had a similar registry for active duty service members who had deployed to the 1990–1991 Gulf War.[25]

The VA's Agent Orange and Gulf War registries are voluntary (ie, any veteran who deployed can enroll). Veterans can enroll for a medical evaluation for any type of disease, even if they are asymptomatic. Approximately 10% of the veterans who enrolled in the DoD Gulf War Registry were asymptomatic.[25] The VA Agent Orange and Gulf War registries include similar elements:

- an exposure history,
- a medical history,
- a physical examination, and
- laboratory tests, if indicated.

The exposure history relies solely on the veteran's recall and is not verified with military records. In fact, some veterans in the Agent Orange Registry were never in Vietnam.[26] These registry examinations do not provide a substitute for a VA Compensation and Pension Examination; that is, these examinations are not the first step in an application for VA disability compensation. This is confusing to some veterans.

Results of these examinations are entered into specific Agent Orange and Gulf War databases, respectively. The registry forms are paper-based, and they require data entry of multiple pages that is burdensome for the clinical staff. Registry data are not integrated with the general VA outpatient database. Data quality and usability of the databases are limited. For multiple reasons, there has been very little analysis of the data in the Agent Orange Registry, despite data collection since 1978.[26]

DoD and VA scientists performed an exhaustive analysis of the data in the DoD and VA Gulf War registries in 2002.[25] They combined the DoD and VA data on more than 100,000 patients and published a comprehensive surveillance report. This included approximately 14% of the total population of 697,000 Gulf War veterans. They concluded there was substantial clinical information in the registries that was useful to DoD and VA physicians who cared for Gulf War veterans. However, extrapolations could not be made from the registry data to the health status of the entire population of Gulf War veterans because of the substantial selection bias. Multiple research studies have demonstrated that Gulf War veterans who enrolled in the registries were sicker than Gulf War veterans who did not enroll.[25] In general, the registry data could not be used for epidemiological research.

The Disabled American Veterans (DAV), a veterans service organization, developed a burn pits registry for veterans to enroll in if they have health concerns that they believe are related to burn pit exposure. The DAV speaker at the August 2012 symposium said that 591 veterans had registered on the DAV website. They reported diseases in many organ systems, including 80 veterans who reported that they developed cancer within a few years of exposure to burn pits in theater.

During the past few years, Congress introduced multiple bills that would require the VA to establish a burn pit registry. In January 2013, President Obama signed legislation that requires the VA to establish a registry.[16] Public Law 112-260, Section 201, requires the VA to establish an "open burn pit registry for eligible individuals who may have been exposed to toxic airborne chemicals and fumes caused by open burn pits."[16(p6)] The law defines eligibility as having deployed in support of a contingency operation while serving in the military, on or after September 2001, and being based at a location where an open burn pit was used. The law does not require verification of an individual's location with military records or substantiation of exposure to burn pits. Burn pits were used at most bases in Iraq and Afghanistan; therefore, most deployed service members were located at bases with burn pits. VA implementation of the law is likely to translate into enrollment of any veteran who was deployed to OIF or OEF and who wants to volunteer for the registry.

The VA must establish this registry within 1 year of enactment of the law. The VA is also required to include information in the registry that would enable the VA to "ascertain and monitor the health effects of the exposure" in veterans that were "caused by open burn pits."[16(p6)] This would likely require periodic analyses of data on medical diagnoses of veterans enrolled in the registry.

In January 2013, the VA started planning for this mandated burn pits registry for OIF/OEF veterans. This chapter summarizes the work group discussion during the August 2012 symposium, which focused on the methods used to develop registries in general. This chapter does not address the VA's plans for the Congressionally mandated registry, which were just beginning to be formulated.

Enrollment Criteria for a National, Broad-based Registry Related to Operation Iraqi Freedom and Operation Enduring Freedom

During the August 2012 symposium, one work group discussed issues related to developing a national registry for OIF/OEF veterans. The work group recommended that veterans could enroll in this type of broad-based national registry, regardless of their disease status. The only requirement for enrollment would be verification that the veteran was deployed. The VA already has access to the military personnel database of veterans who were deployed to OIF and OEF. The VA uses this type of open enrollment in its Agent Orange and Gulf War registries.

A broad-based registry would not be limited to individuals who have pulmonary diseases. Many veterans, who have other types of diseases, believe their health problems are from exposure to burn pits. The registry would also include asymptomatic veterans who are concerned about their exposures. Burn pits were used in most large bases in theater; therefore, the great majority of veterans perceive they were exposed to burn pit emissions.[8] Many veterans are concerned about the long-term health effects of these exposures, even if an environmental scientist objectively evaluated the air concentrations at specific locations and developed a risk assessment that concluded levels that were not hazardous.[1]

Enrollment in the registry could provide improved access to the VA medical care system. The VA currently provides free medical care to OIF/OEF veterans for 5 years after they separate from the military. Enrollment in the registry would be useful to provide access to veterans who are separated from the military more than 5 years. Veterans would not need service connection for a disability to enroll in the registry.

Coordination of a Broad-based Registry, Including Standardized Data Collection

Centralized data collection would be necessary for a broad-based national VA registry for OIF/OEF veterans. Data from the patients' medical evaluations, as documented in electronic medical records, would need to be collected and archived centrally. This centralized coordination center could also perform periodic analyses of the aggregated data to detect patterns of veterans' concerns and medical diagnoses. The most likely location for this coordination center would be the VA Office of Public Health in Washington, DC.

To develop a national, broad-based registry, the VA would need to develop and adopt a standardized medical evaluation that could be consistently recorded to ensure comparability of results among the VAMCs nationwide. This would include the development of standardized forms for the data entry of medical history, occupational and military histories, physical examination, and a minimal set of diagnostic tests. If the registry was limited to lung diseases, the medical history could be focused and the minimal set of laboratory tests could include chest X-ray films and pulmonary function tests. If the registry included patients who had diseases in any organ system, a much broader medical history and a larger number of diagnostic tests would be needed.

A standardized set of questions would be needed for the occupational and military histories to combine computerized data from many patients. This could include questions on common airborne hazards in theater, such as exposure to burn pits, high concentrations of particulate matter due to sand storms, and other exposures. The occupational and military histories would reflect the patients' perceptions of their environmental exposures. Therefore, the utility of these histories would be limited, and they could not be used to determine the etiology of disease.

In 2011, the IOM published a comprehensive review of the potential health effects of exposure to burn pits in theater.[1] The IOM concluded that there was limited or suggestive evidence of an association between exposure to combustion products and decreases in pulmonary function tests. This conclusion was based on studies of industrial workers and not on military populations exposed to burn pits. The IOM concluded that there was inadequate evidence to determine if there was an association between exposure to combustion products and several other diseases. Based on IOM conclusions, pulmonary function testing would be the only scientifically justified laboratory test to include in a standardized medical evaluation.

Instead of developing a tailored medical evaluation for registry participants, the VA might choose to use the standard electronic medical records for outpatient clinic visits and hospitalizations. The names, demographics, and exposure histories of veterans who enrolled in the registry could be matched with the VA outpatient and inpatient databases. This would pull in the results of medical evaluations that were performed during routine clinical care. This approach would provide the advantage of integrating the registry data with the VA's electronic medical record systems. It would reduce the need for data entry of paper forms. It would also improve the incorporation of registry procedures into the normal clinical work flow compared with a separate stand-alone system for registry examinations.[26] However, this approach would lead to more incomplete or missing diagnostic data and less consistency in the methods of medical evaluations. This would lead to substantial challenges if analyses of aggregated diagnostic data were conducted.

Initial Small-Scale Initiative to Prepare for the Development of a National Registry

A small-scale pilot project at a few VAMCs would be very useful before the VA launches a national registry for OIF/OEF veterans. This initiative could gauge the possible interest of veterans who wanted to enroll in a registry. It could also estimate the number of veterans who would enroll and assess the types of questions, symptoms, and diseases they would have. In 2013, the VA considered use of a pilot project to refine the website and processes for its Congressionally mandated burn pits registry.

A small-scale pilot project would be useful to refine the standardized medical evaluation based on the types of diseases seen. It would also be useful to refine the information technology systems needed for the electronic reporting of medical evaluations and centralized data collection. The pilot project results would also be useful to design training for clinicians who care for OIF/OEF veterans. The VA has training programs for healthcare providers. A program outlining the purpose and methods of the registry could be developed prior to the national launch.

A pilot project would also provide useful information on the types of outreach and communications the VA should perform when it launches a national registry. The VA should include information on its website describing the purpose of the registry and how to register. Younger veterans have an affinity for social media; therefore, the VA should consider using social media to publicize the registry. Veterans service organizations should be involved in planning the outreach efforts for the launch of the national registry.

Utility of a National, Broad-based Registry for Veterans of Operation Iraqi Freedom and Operation Enduring Freedom

A registry could provide value to OIF/OEF veterans; however, the registry would have limited value for scientific analyses. Results of a voluntary registry for OIF/OEF veterans would not be useful for epidemiological research to determine the strength of association or causality. Veterans who would enroll in a registry would likely represent the most severe end of the disease spectrum. Therefore, considerable selection bias would be likely in the group of veterans who enroll. The VA has performed population-based studies that demonstrated that veterans who seek VA medical care have higher rates and severity of disease, higher rates of disability, higher rates of unemployment, and lower incomes, compared with veterans who do not seek VA care.[6] Healthy OIF/OEF veterans who are not concerned about their exposures would be much less likely to enroll in the registry. This selection bias was demonstrated in analyses of veterans who enrolled in the Gulf War Registry.[25] This means the types of diseases that are diagnosed in veterans enrolled in the registry could not be generalized to the entire population of 2.6 million veterans who have deployed to OIF and OEF. In addition, no estimate of the rates of diseases could be determined.

The registry results could not be used to determine the etiology of diseases. The registry would contain self-reported exposure data from a self-selected group of veterans that would lead to recall bias and selection bias. A registry would have some utility in hypothesis generation for design of future controlled studies. A population-based epidemiological study would be required to determine if there was a relationship between exposure to burn pits and the subsequent development of pulmonary diseases or other diseases. Appropriate population-based studies that address this issue are ongoing, including the Millennium Cohort Study and other longitudinal studies. These research studies use environmental data to classify individuals into more accurate exposure categories, and they use valid medical diagnoses and smoking histories to control for confounding factors.[9–13]

Although a voluntary registry for OIF/OEF veterans would have substantial scientific limitations, it could fulfill other needs. Veterans have benefited from previous VA registries in multiple ways.[25,26] A registry evaluation could provide OIF/OEF veterans with an opportunity to receive a high-quality medical evaluation and to address their health concerns. Informed healthcare providers could provide veterans with answers to their questions about long-term health effects related to deployments. Enrolling in such a registry would provide OIF/OEF veterans with a variety of benefits, including the following:

- Information about VA medical care and benefits for which they are eligible.
- Improved access to VA medical care without the need to establish a service connection for a disability. The VA would need to make it clear that a registry evaluation would not be a substitute for a Compensation and Pension Examination (ie, enrolling in the registry would not be the first step in applying for disability compensation).
- Recognition and validation from the VA that it takes veterans health conditions and exposure concerns seriously.
- The opportunity to provide feedback to the VA during their evaluations. In turn, the VA would gain insight on the veterans' perceptions and concerns. This would enable the VA to target its health education messages, which would be the highest priority to veterans in future VA communication efforts.
- Placement on an automatic mailing list. Veterans who enroll in the Agent Orange and Gulf War registries are placed on a mailing list and automatically receive periodic newsletters tailored to their concerns.[26] The VA could improve its communication with OIF/OEF veterans by establishing a similar mailing list and sending newsletters (via mail or email) highlighting issues of particular concern to OIF/OEF veterans.

The health surveillance data derived from the registry for OIF/OEF veterans should be shared with physicians and other healthcare providers on a periodic basis. These could be VA, DoD, and private healthcare providers. Results should be published as an internal report for VA clinicians and in the open medical literature. A summary of the results should be written in plain English and published on a VA website to communicate with veterans, active duty service members, family members, and Congress.

SUMMARY

This chapter described methodological issues related to development of two possible types of medical data collection: (1) a case series that is targeted to specific pulmonary diseases; and (2) a national, broad-based registry related to OIF and OEF deployment.

Individual cases of service members and veterans who developed various pulmonary diseases after returning from deployment to OIF and OEF have been reported. DoD and VA scientists have already developed multiple, small case series at different locations. The DoD and VA could build on this small case series foundation to establish a shared, systematically collected case series of OIF/OEF veterans. This would require collaboration to develop a standardized medical evaluation of OIF/OEF veterans that would provide data that are comparable and could be combined. The DoD and VA could develop this as a consortium for sharing information on pulmonary cases among multiple medical centers. Patients who have pulmonary diseases should be followed over time and reevaluated, including after the transition of care from the DoD to the VA after military separation. The DoD and the VA could establish one or two coordinating centers that would collect, archive, and analyze the data. Combining data from multiple sites could yield adequate numbers of cases to analyze for patterns of pathology, disease progression, and possible risk factors during military service.

The VA maintains multiple, national registries related to specific deployments, including the Agent Orange and Gulf War registries. In January 2013, Congress mandated that the VA establish a registry for OIF/OEF veterans related to burn pit exposure. This chapter described general methodological issues related to the development of a broad-based registry, focusing on the discussion during the August 2012 symposium. The work group recommended that veterans could enroll in this type of broad-based registry regardless of their disease status. The only requirement for enrollment would be verification that the veteran was deployed. The registry would not be limited to individuals who have pulmonary diseases, because many veterans who have other types of diseases believe their health problems are from burn pit exposure. The VA would need to develop and adopt a standardized medical evaluation that would be recorded consistently to ensure comparability of results among the VAMCs nationally. Instead of developing a tailored medical evaluation for the registry, the VA might choose to use the standard electronic medical records for outpatient clinic visits and hospitalizations. The names of veterans who enrolled in the registry could be matched with the VA outpatient and inpatient databases to pull in the results of medical examinations from routine clinical care. A voluntary registry could provide value to OIF/OEF veterans; however, it would have substantial scientific limitations. It would not be useful for epidemiological research to determine the strength of association or causality. In contrast, a registry could fulfill the multiple needs of veterans. Participating in the registry could provide OIF/OEF veterans with an opportunity to receive a high-quality medical evaluation and address their health concerns. In addition, the registry could inform veterans about VA medical care and benefits for which they are eligible and be used to develop an OIF/OEF veterans' mailing list for future VA communications.

REFERENCES

1. Institute of Medicine of the National Academies. *Long-Term Health Consequences of Exposure to Burn Pits in Iraq and Afghanistan.* Washington, DC: National Academies Press; 2011: 1–9, 31–44, 117–129.

2. National Research Council. *Review of the Department of Defense Enhanced Particulate Matter Surveillance Program Report.* Washington, DC: National Academies Press; 2010: 10–11, 51–56.

3. Defraites RF, Richards EE. Assessing potentially hazardous environmental exposures among military populations. *Mil Med.* 2011;176(suppl 7):1–112.

4. Martin NJ, Richards EE, Kirkpatrick JS. Exposure science in U.S. military operations: a review. *Mil Med.* 2011;176(suppl 7):77–83.

5. Baird C. The basis for and uses of environmental sampling to assess health risk in deployed settings. *Mil Med.* 2011;176(suppl 7):84–90.

6. Brix K, O'Donnell FL. Panel 1: medical surveillance prior to, during, and following potential environmental exposures. *Mil Med.* 2011;176(suppl 7):91–96.

7. Morris MJ, Zacher LL, Jackson DA. Investigating the respiratory health of deployed military personnel. *Mil Med.* 2011;176:1157–1161.

8. Teichman R. Exposures of concern to veterans returning from Afghanistan and Iraq. *J Occup Environ Med.* 2012;54:677–681.

9. Jackson DA. Research studies: overview and future direction. In: Harkins DK, ed. *Airborne Hazards Related to Deployment.* Washington, DC: Department of the Army, Office of The Surgeon General, Borden Institute; 2014. Chap 27.

10. Armed Forces Health Surveillance Center. *Epidemiological Studies of Health Outcomes Among Troops Deployed to Burn Pit Sites,* Silver Spring, MD: the Naval Health Research Center and the U.S. Army Public Health Command (Provisional); May 2010.

11. Smith B, Wong CA, Smith TC, Boyko EJ, Gackstetter GD, Ryan MAK. Newly reported respiratory symptoms and conditions among military personnel deployed to Iraq and Afghanistan: a prospective population-based study. *Am J Epidemiol.* 2009;170:1433–1442.

12. Smith B, Wong CA, Boyko EJ, et al. The effects of exposure to documented open-air burn pits on respiratory health among deployers of the Millennium Cohort Study. *J Occup Environ Med.* 2012;54:708–716.

13. Abraham JH, DeBakey SF, Reid L, Zhou J, Baird CP. Does deployment to Iraq and Afghanistan affect respiratory health of US military personnel? *J Occup Environ Med.* 2012;54:740–-745.

14. Baird CP, DeBakey S, Reid L, Hauschild VD, Petruccelli B, Abraham JH. Respiratory health status of US Army personnel potentially exposed to smoke from 2003 Al-Mishraq Sulfur Plant fire. *J Occup Environ Med.* 2012;54:717–723.

15. Szema AM, Salihi W, Savary K, Chen JJ. Respiratory symptoms necessitating spirometry among soldiers with Iraq/Afghanistan war lung injury. *J Occup Environ Med.* 2011;53:961–965.

16. Public Law No. 112-260, Section 201: Establishment of Open Burn Pit Registry (enacted in January 2013).

17. King MS, Eisenberg R, Newman JH, et al. Constrictive bronchiolitis in soldiers returning from Iraq and Afghanistan. *N Engl J Med.* 2011;365:222–230.

18. Morris MJ, Zacher LL. Constrictive bronchiolitis in soldiers. *N Engl J Med.* 2011;365:1743–1745.

19. Morris MJ, Banks DE. Personnel with postdeployment dyspnea: chronic lung disease and the role of surgical lung biopsy. In: Harkins DK, ed. *Airborne Hazards Related to Deployment.* Washington, DC: Department of the Army, Office of The Surgeon General, Borden Institute; 2014. Chap 16.

20. Rose C, Abraham J, Harkins D, et al. Overview and recommendations for medical screening and diagnostic evaluation for postdeployment lung disease in returning US warfighters. *J Occup Environ Med.* 2012;54:746–751.

21. Zacher LL, Browning R, Bisnett T, Bennion JR, Postlewaite RC, Baird CP. Clarifications from representatives of the Department of Defense regarding the article "Recommendations for medical screening and diagnostic evaluation for postdeployment lung disease in returning US warfighters." *J Occup Environ Med.* 2012;54:760–761.

22. Morris MJ, Negrescu C, Bell DG, Tinkelpaugh CN. Summary: basic diagnosis and workup of symptomatic individuals. In: Harkins DK, ed. *Airborne Hazards Related to Deployment.* Washington, DC: Department of the Army, Office of The Surgeon General, Borden Institute; 2014. Chap 11.

23. Eschenbacher W. Pulmonary function testing—spirometry testing for population surveillance. In: Harkins DK, ed. *Airborne Hazards Related to Deployment.* Washington, DC: Department of the Army, Office of The Surgeon General, Borden Institute; 2014. Chap 8.

24. Kreiss K. Experience with emerging lung diseases from the National Institute for Occupational Safety and Health. In: Harkins DK, ed. *Airborne Hazards Related to Deployment.* Washington, DC: Department of the Army, Office of The Surgeon General, Borden Institute; 2014. Chap 18.

25. US Department of Veterans Affairs, Department of Defense. *Combined Analysis of the VA and DoD Gulf War Clinical Evaluation Programs: A Study of the Clinical Findings from Systematic Medical Examinations of 100,339 U.S. Gulf War Veterans.* Washington, DC: DVA, DoD; 2002.

26. Dick WJ. Lessons learned from self-selected registries (Agent Orange Registry). In: Harkins DK, ed. *Airborne Hazards Related to Deployment.* Washington, DC: Department of the Army, Office of The Surgeon General, Borden Institute; 2014. Chap 26.

AIRBORNE HAZARDS RELATED TO DEPLOYMENT

Section IV: Health Communication and Outreach

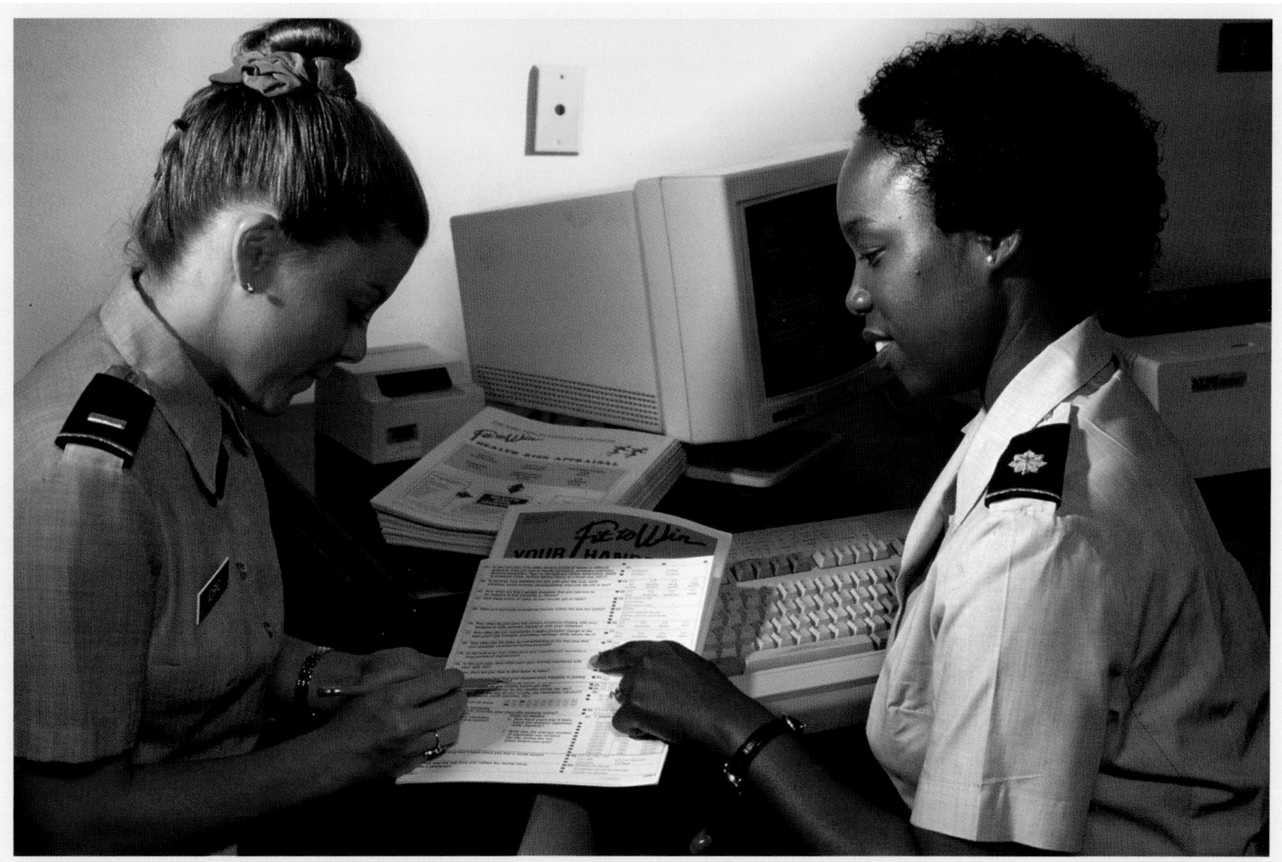

A physician communicating health information to a patient.

Photograph: Courtesy of the US Army Public Health Command (Aberdeen Proving Ground, Maryland).

Chapter 23

RISK COMMUNICATION: AN ESSENTIAL ELEMENT OF EFFECTIVE CARE

CONNIE RAAB, BA*; DEANNA K. HARKINS, MD, MPH†; MICHELLE KENNEDY PRISCO, MSN‡; AND BETHNEY A. DAVIDSON, BS§

*Director, Public Health Communications, Office of Public Health, Veterans Health Administration, US Department of Veterans Affairs, 810 Vermont Avenue, NW, Washington, DC 20420

†Occupational Medicine Physician, Environmental Medicine Program, US Army Public Health Command, 5158 Blackhawk Road, Aberdeen Proving Ground, Maryland 21010-5403

‡Nurse Practitioner, Washington DC Veterans Administration Medical Center, US Department of Veterans Affairs, 810 Vermont Avenue, NW, Washington, DC 20420

§Health Risk Communication Specialist, Army Institute of Public Health, US Army Public Health Command, 5158 Blackhawk Road, Aberdeen Proving Ground, Maryland 21010-5403

INTRODUCTION

Risk communication is a critical foundation of the communication process used by healthcare providers who encounter service members and veterans with deployment health concerns. Effective risk communication is essential in establishing a trusting relationship between the provider and patient. It is a valuable tool for facilitating effective dialogue as they work together to assess the potential health risks that may be present as a result of deployment.

This chapter explains the science of risk communication—what it is, its benefits, and how to apply it in a clinical setting.

WHAT IS RISK COMMUNICATION?

Several well-regarded sources have defined risk communication; the most quoted is probably the 1989 National Research Council (NRC) report *Improving Risk Communication.*[1] This report notes that in the past, risk communication had often been thought of as a one-way process of experts informing nonexperts. Following an in-depth review, however, the NRC concluded that risk communication should be defined as a *two-way process*, that is: "an interactive process of exchange of information and opinions among individuals, groups, and institutions"[1(p21)] concerning a risk or potential risk to human health or the environment. Risk communication "involves multiple messages about the nature of risk and other messages not strictly about risk that express concerns, opinions, or reactions to risk messages or to legal and institutional arrangements for risk management."[1(p21)]

This two-way process definition has been reinforced many times since then. In 1995, the US Public Health Service defined risk communication as a "complex, multidisciplinary, multi-dimensional, and evolving process…used to give citizens necessary and appropriate information and to involve them in making decisions that affect them… ."[2(p1)]

The two-way risk communication process is also central to the work of Dr Vincent Covello, whose endeavor in this field is extensive. In a 2008 brief for the US Agency for International Development, Dr Covello defined risk communication as "…the two-way exchange of information about threats, including health threats… . The goals of risk communication are to enhance knowledge and understanding, build trust and credibility, encourage dialogue, and influence attitudes, decisions, and behaviors. These goals apply to all four major types of risk communication: 1) information and education; 2) behavior change and protective action; 3) disaster warning and emergency notification; and 4) joint problem-solving and conflict resolution."[3]

In a 2012 article that discussed using risk communication to address deployment-related exposure concerns, Dr Susan Santos reinforced the NRC's definition of risk communication and stated that "on a practical level, risk communication is needed when there is 1) complex health- or risk-related information being communicated; 2) a high level of concern; 3) expert disagreement or high uncertainty; and 4) low trust in those seen as responsible for the risk or for providing protection against a risk."[4(p753)]

The scientific discipline of risk communication is supported by several theories. Understanding risk perception is essential to understanding and using risk communication principles. The work of Slovic et al[5] and other social psychologists has yielded a core set of risk perception factors that help shape understanding of risk and that reflect a very different view of risk than that of medical and scientific experts. As Dr Santos notes, the public's responses to risk should not be viewed as misperceptions, just different perceptions. She also stresses that instead of trying to correct what experts in the scientific or medical realm believe are "incorrect perceptions," the goal of risk communication should be to understand concerned stakeholders' attitudes, knowledge levels, perceptions, and beliefs that support the underlying perceptions. By understanding and acknowledging the perceptions held by service members and veterans, healthcare providers can better discuss and address them in the clinical setting. The primary risk perception factors are listed below. For each factor, the version given first is more likely to provoke anxiety and feelings of great risk in the public than the version given second. For example, media attention is more likely to be perceived as a greater risk than is lack of media attention.

Primary Risk Perception Factors:

- involuntary versus voluntary risks; that is, risks wherein one had no choice (such as exposure to airborne hazards while deployed) appear more dangerous than those chosen voluntarily,
- control by the system versus control by the individual,
- exotic versus familiar,
- dreaded versus not dreaded,
- uncertainty versus certainty,
- media attention versus lack of media attention,
- human origin versus naturally occurring,
- benefits unclear versus benefits understood, and
- low trust and credibility versus high trust and credibility.

As Dr Santos discusses, "empowering veterans with information that addresses their concerns and reflects what we know about risk perception and what we do and do not know about possible health risks will set the stage for meaningful communication and empower veterans to better manage their health."[4(p758)] The remainder of this chapter provides further information about what providers can do to address the concerns of service members and veterans about exposures, including those from airborne hazards and burn pits.

EXHIBIT 23-1

EXPOSURE AND RISK COMMUNICATION RESOURCES

Federal Resources

- Risk Communication in the Healthcare Setting, Deployment Health Clinical Center, Department of Defense
  https://www.pdhealth.mil/508/clinicians/risk_comm.asp
- Health Risk Communication Training, US Army Public Health Command
  http://phc.amedd.army.mil/topics/envirohealth/HRC/Pages/HealthRiskCommunicationTraining.aspx
- VA Military Exposures Website
  http://www.publichealth.va.gov/exposures/index.asp
- Centers for Disease Control and Prevention, Risk Communication Website
  http://www.cdc.gov/healthcommunication/Risks/index.html
- Agency for Toxic Substances and Disease Registry (ATSDR), A Primer on Health Risk Communication
  http://www.atsdr.cdc.gov/risk/riskprimer/index.html
- Argonne National Laboratory, Risk Communications Training
  http://www.dis.anl.gov/groups/riskcomm/services/courses.html
- US Food and Drug Administration Risk Communication Resources
  http://www.fda.gov/AboutFDA/ReportsManualsForms/Reports/ucm268041.htm
- Nuclear Regulatory Commission, Effective Risk Communication
  http://www.nrc.gov/reading-rm/doc-collections/nuregs/brochures/br0308/br0308.pdf 2004
  http://www.nrc.gov/reading-rm/doc-collections/nuregs/brochures/br0308/
- World Health Organization, Outbreak Communication Guidelines
  http://www.who.int/infectious-disease-news/IDdocs/whocds200528/whocds200528en.pdf

Academic Resources

- Cornell University Risk Communication Courses
  http://www.risk.comm.cornell.edu/Courses.html
- Johns Hopkins University, Risk Communication Strategies for Public Health Preparedness
  http://www.jhsph.edu/research/centers-and-institutes/johns-hopkins-center-for-public-health-preparedness/training/online/riskcomm.html
- Harvard University School of Public Health, Effective Risk Communication—Theory, Tools, and Practical Skills for Communicating About Risk
  https://ccpe.sph.harvard.edu/programs.cfm?CSID=RCC0000&pg=cluster&CLID=1
- University of North Carolina, Gillings School of Global Public Health, Risk Communication
  http://cphp.sph.unc.edu/training/HEP_RISKC/certificate.php
- George Mason University, Center for Health and Risk Communication
  http://chrc.gmu.edu/
- University of Maryland, Center for Health and Risk Communication
  http://www.healthriskcenter.umd.edu/

Other Resources

- Dr Vincent Covello, Center for Risk Communications Training
  http://centerforriskcommunication.org/
- The Peter M. Sandman Risk Communication website
  http://psandman.com/

WHY RISK COMMUNICATION IS IMPORTANT

In recent years, the fears and concerns of service members and veterans about exposures to environmental, safety, and health hazards have increased along with a corresponding demand for risk information.[4] It is critically important that information disclosed or discussed with service members and veterans is both appropriate and helpful. Planning for how to handle the concerns of service members, veterans, the public, and the media is key to establishing trust and credibility while preventing unnecessary confusion and misunderstanding.

There are several reasons why effective risk communication techniques are important to healthcare providers encountering service members and veterans who have deployment health concerns:

- Good risk communication skills can help to control the message and address misinformation. Providers should focus on developing clear messages supported by facts that address the concerns of targeted stakeholders, as well as the sponsoring entity's goals.
- Given that some surveys have suggested that approximately 33% of service members and veterans have deployment health concerns,[4] good risk communication skills can help to address those concerns in a more timely manner before they become self-fulfilling prophecies or deeply entrenched beliefs.
- Effective risk communication can help create an environment of caring and trust between healthcare providers and their patients as the deployment health concerns are being addressed.
- Risk communication can play an important role in addressing missteps that may have occurred in the past and/or corrective actions currently being undertaken.[4]

Given the high percentage of service members and veterans concerned about potential airborne hazard exposures, utilizing risk communication tools prior to, during, and after deployments will serve to foster a better understanding of the known and unknown effects of potential exposures. Ideally, the US Department of Defense and the US Department of Veterans Affairs should collaborate to develop meaningful information and communication materials that reflect risk communication principles. In the absence of this critical dialogue, service members and veterans may fill the information gaps with incorrect information or may believe information that is inaccurate, thus providing fertile ground for misconception, rumor, and anger.[4] Science and research do not keep up with all of the potential exposures and combinations of exposures that service members and veterans may encounter during their deployments. Consequently, involving these personnel in the risk communication process from beginning to end supports a *partnership* in the process and acknowledges that a process is in place to address their concerns.[6–8]

PRINCIPLES OF EFFECTIVE RISK COMMUNICATION

Effective risk communication is necessary as new threats of deployment hazards surface in deployment and nondeployment settings. As a result of concerns by service members and veterans about the health risks associated with possible deployment-related exposures, primary care providers must learn and exercise effective risk communication methods to better inform these personnel and address their concerns. Employing effective risk communication strategies is not always easy; however, adhering to the following *seven cardinal rules* of effective risk communication[3] should assist healthcare providers:

1. Accept and involve the service member or veteran as a partner. The goal is to produce an informed individual, not to diffuse the concern or replace actions.
2. Plan carefully and evaluate your efforts. Different goals may require different actions.
3. Listen to the concerns of service members and veterans. People often care more about trust, credibility, competence, fairness, and empathy than about statistics and details.
4. Be honest, frank, and open. Trust and credibility are difficult to obtain; once lost, they are almost impossible to regain.
5. Work with other credible sources. Conflicts and disagreements among organizations make communication much more difficult.
6. Meet the needs of the media. They are usually more interested in politics than risk, simplicity than complexity, and danger than safety. These concerns are different from those of the public, so preparing to communicate with the media is different.
7. Speak clearly and with compassion. Never let your efforts prevent acknowledging a concern of service members or veterans or the tragedy of an illness, injury, or death. Service members and veterans can understand risk information, but they may still not agree with the information being conveyed. Realize that some people may not be satisfied.

Each of these rules is important for a variety of reasons.

Rule 1: Accepting and involving service members and veterans as partners demonstrates respect for them by engaging them early, before important decisions are made. Service members and veterans have the right to participate in decisions that affect their lives, their health, and the things they value.

Rule 2: Planning carefully and evaluating one's efforts support flexibility in using different risk communication strategies among service members and veterans. Beginning with clear objectives and evaluating technical information about risks help to direct specific communications to the individual patient who may have political, cultural, or agenda-driven concerns.

Rule 3: Listening to the specific concerns of service members and veterans allows healthcare providers to open a two-way dialogue that facilitates trust and credibility, as well as fosters compassion and competence. Gathering information about the values and beliefs of service members and veterans through interviews, discussion groups, and surveys allows for identification of what really matters to them and supports addressing their concerns. Such information gathering also aids providers in identifying the scientific and medical information that need to be shared with their patients.

Rule 4: Honesty, frankness, and openness must be present to establish trust and credibility with the patient. The patient's expectation that the healthcare provider will be credible based on his or her credentials alone provides a false sense of comfort. Providers should express willingness to answer questions and correct errors that may have been made. Do not minimize or exaggerate the level of risk; always lean toward sharing more information, not less.

Rule 5: Coordination and collaboration with credible sources help to build trust and communicate risk-related information. Conflict and disagreements, as well as inconsistency, among various experts and sources of information may lead to confusion and frustration, and may heighten uncertainty and raise concern (even outrage) among service members and veterans. Interorganizational coordination and communication foster a *team* approach in responding to service members and veterans. Efforts of healthcare providers to partner with other communication sources, both internally and externally, will go a long way toward establishing effective risk communication strategies.

Rule 6: Meeting the needs of the media is often critical in communicating information on risks. Today's media contributes significantly to setting the tone for how service members, veterans, and the general public view health, safety, and environmental risks. On the one hand, science and the media may be at odds, and the media may be more skeptical and more interested in the sensational than in the technical. Yet, on the other hand, experts too often do not present concise or clear messages, thus adding to the distortion that can occur. Working with the media to convey helpful and accurate information as a partner is imperative and will help to minimize potential misinformation. Because the media covers various viewpoints, it needs input from subject matter experts to provide the public with information that is useful, factual, and reliable.

Rule 7: Speaking clearly, with compassion, and minimizing the use of technical language and jargon can help to bridge the gap of understanding between the healthcare provider and the service member or veteran. Foremost, in any discussion of risk and benefits, empathy and caring should carry more weight than numbers, statistics, and technical facts.

HOW TO APPLY RISK COMMUNICATION TO THE CLINICAL ENCOUNTER

In many instances, primary care providers are the first point of contact for service members and veterans who have questions about deployment exposures. For this reason, it is important that primary care providers be familiar with risk communication principles when addressing deployment exposure concerns. Trying to follow risk communication principles during busy primary care encounters is not always easy. Several concrete and actionable items[4,9–13] are listed below to assist busy clinicians with addressing these concerns more effectively:

- Emphasize compassion, empathy, and concern at the outset of the interview.
- Work to establish trust and credibility with the service member and veteran.
- Gain an understanding of the perception of the service members or veterans about the potential health effects that may be related to an exposure.
- Acknowledge what you do not know.
- Recognize that there may be conflicting information about potential health effects regarding a particular exposure.
- Keep the message simple about what is and is not known about potential health effects related to an exposure.
- Realize that service members and veterans may be more concerned about exposures they cannot control versus exposures they can control.

Emphasize Compassion, Empathy, and Concern at the Outset of the Interview

Set aside any preconceptions regarding whether or not deployment-related exposures are a legitimate cause of the health concerns of the service members or veterans, and emphasize respect and gratitude for the patient's military service. Validating the patient's health concerns will help reassure the patient that the provider understands the patient's perspective. This, in turn, will instill the patient's confidence in the provider and enhance the rapport and trust between the two parties. The primary care provider must also be aware that unspoken factors may be present that may hinder trust-building. For example, service members or veterans may not trust their healthcare providers to diagnose a health problem that may implicate the military. Such a patient may fear being labeled as a troublemaker and possibly losing his or her military benefits as a result. The primary care provider should diffuse any potential for any such clinician–patient contests before they occur. Challenging or debating the validity, legitimacy, or cause of a service member's or veteran's deployment-related health concerns erodes trust, may cause the patient to worsen, and may lead to clinical miscues. It is honest and reasonable to respectfully acknowledge and explain to the patient that some of the symptoms or health effects causing service members or veterans to seek care may not be the result of exposures in the military and/or may ultimately lack clinical explanations. The primary care provider's focus should be on using his or her skills in advocacy, explanation, and compassion to fulfill the provider's duty and obligation to help the service member or veteran.

Work to Establish Trust and Credibility With the Service Member and Veteran

Establish trust and credibility early in the provider–patient relationship by agreeing on an agenda for the initial interview. Encourage the service member or veteran to offer his or her concerns about deployment-related illnesses. Given the potential for mistrust, service members and veterans may not share the connections they have made between their symptoms and their deployment unless the primary care provider asks about them directly and specifically. At the beginning of the interview, the provider should ask the service member or veteran to name his or her top one or two health concerns. If time constraints are present, acknowledge this fact and address it. To save time and facilitate a more productive interview, the patient's top health concerns can either be recorded by the medical assistant conducting the intake interview or collected on an intake form that is reviewed prior to the interview. After the initial greetings and introductions have been made, the healthcare provider could begin the conversation with: *My understanding is that you have some health concerns about nerve agent use at Khamisiyah. During the next 5 to 10 minutes, I would like to discuss with you what we know about this.* Engage the patient in establishing an agreed-upon agenda for the time available, and offer to schedule follow-up phone calls or longer appointments with the patient if he or she has additional questions, or if the complexity of the concerns necessitates further discussion.

Gain an Understanding of the Perception of the Service Members or Veterans About the Potential Health Effects That May Be Related to an Exposure

The provider needs to understand *why* the service member or veteran links the concern to deployment and what sources of information he or she is relying on. A prompt for this conversation could be: *Tell me what you know about what happened at Khamisiyah.* Gaining insight into a service member's or veteran's preexisting views about potential health risks is important, because such information often helps to guide the message. In some cases, the service member or veteran may be more receptive to hearing certain messages once his or her viewpoint has been acknowledged. In other instances, healthcare providers must recognize strongly entrenched beliefs held by service members and veterans. These viewpoints may prove more difficult to change even in the presence of conclusive scientific evidence.

Acknowledge What You Do Not Know

In some instances, primary care providers may not be familiar with the environmental exposure concern that a service member or veteran wishes to discuss, or the provider may need more information to obtain clarity as to exactly what transpired. This is particularly true for exposures that may not occur very frequently or that may have occurred in the remote past. In these cases, it is important to acknowledge that you do not have the information and to reassure the service member or veteran that you will follow up with the patient after you have researched the issue and, if needed, consulted with specialists. For example, suggested language could be: *I am not familiar with this particular exposure, but I will talk to some of my colleagues who may be more knowledgeable about it. I would like to schedule a time to meet with you again in 2 weeks to discuss what I find out.* It is important to schedule the follow-up appointment with the service member or veteran to ensure that a timeline is established for addressing the concern. Additionally, following up within a designated timeframe helps to further establish the provider–patient trust and rapport that are so critical when risk communication principles are being used. Depending on the exposure or particular health issue, the primary care provider may choose to consult with the local environmental health clinician or an occupational and environmental medicine specialist at the War Related Illness and Injury Study Center or the US Army Public Health Command. These personnel may have helpful information about potential deployment-related exposures and health effects.

Recognize That There May Be Conflicting Information About Potential Health Effects Regarding a Particular Exposure

Often, a reasonable uncertainty exists as to whether a given exposure occurred or, if it did, the magnitude of the exposure (dose). In other instances, uncertainty exists as to whether a given exposure or dose can lead to illness, and, if so, what symptoms would potentially indicate such an exposure having taken place. Acknowledge the existence of a *reasonable clinical uncertainty*, that is, an expert consensus may not be present, and the exposure data or information may be limited. For example, suggested language could be: *There is a great deal of information about Agent Orange on the Internet, and some of the reports are conflicting. A number of studies are currently looking at this issue to review the data and try to improve the certainty of the results. At this point in time, based on the research reviewed, we believe that. ...* The healthcare provider is best advised to acknowledge uncertainty rather than using exaggerated or demeaning expressions of certainty, or relying on bias or preconception. It is honest and reasonable to acknowledge that some of the symptoms causing service members or veterans to seek care may ultimately lack clinical explanations.

Keep the Message Simple About What Is and Is Not Known About Potential Health Effects Related to an Exposure

Ask the service member or veteran to rephrase what he or she thinks the *take-home message* is as it relates to the exposure concern. For example, suggested language could be: *We have discussed a lot today. What is your understanding of what depleted uranium is and how it may affect you?* Provider–patient collaboration, both in communication and the patient's care, is key to fostering rapport. After learning how the patient prefers to receive health information, try to accommodate that preference. Provide printed handouts and web resources from reputable sources, such as the Centers for Disease Control or the Agency for Toxic Substances and Disease Registry, to reinforce the discussion that took place during the clinical encounter. Providers should strive to provide resources that are tailored for a general audience and are easy to understand.

Realize That Service Members and Veterans May Be More Concerned About Exposures They Cannot Control Versus Exposures They Can Control

Empower service members and veterans with the realization that while some past exposures cannot be changed, steps can be taken to minimize potential future harmful exposures. For example, suggested language could be: *I understand that you are concerned about airborne pollutants that you may have been exposed to while in Iraq. We have discussed what we currently do know and what we are doing to better understand the potential health effects. While we are trying to better understand some of these exposures, your current health is important, so we need to do whatever we can to help you manage your current symptoms. At our next visit, we should also talk about general things you can do to protect/improve your health.*

At the next follow-up visit, the provider should inform the patient about measures that can reduce future exposures and provide advice about personal exposures that may impact the patient's health. For example, suggested language could be: *Let us now talk about ways that we can try to minimize future harmful exposures to airborne pollutants. ... I am also concerned about your continued smoking and how this may affect your health. Maybe we can discuss some ways to work on this.* Discussion should take place between the provider and patient to determine how best to work together to promote the patient's overall health, as well as provide the patient with the necessary resources (Exhibit 23-1) and support to develop and maintain a healthy lifestyle.

SUMMARY

Good risk communication techniques do not alleviate all exposure concerns. However, poor risk communication almost always exacerbates the concern. For this reason, following the previously described principles and interacting with service members and veterans in an honest, caring, and compassionate manner may help to provide them with the important health information they need to improve their overall quality of life.[4,10–13]

REFERENCES

1. National Research Council Committee on Risk Perception and Communication. *Improving Risk Communication.* Washington, DC: The National Academies Press; 1989.

2. US Department of Health and Human Services, US Public Health Service. *Risk Communications: Working With Individuals and Communities To Weigh the Odds. Prevention Report.* Washington, DC: DHHS-PHS; February/March 1995.

3. Covello VT. *Risk Communication: Principles, Tools, and Techniques. Global Health Technical Briefs*. Washington, DC: US Agency for International Development; 2008.

4. Santos SL, Helmer D, Teichman R. Risk communication in deployment-related exposure concerns. *J Occup Environ Med*. 2012;54:752–758.

5. Slovic P, Fischhoff B, Lichtenstein, S. Rating the risks. *Environment*. 1979;21:14–39.

6. US Department of Health and Human Services, Centers for Disease Control and Prevention. *Crisis and Emergency Risk Communication*. Washington, DC: DHHS-CDC; 2013.

7. US Department of Health and Human Services, Agency for Toxic Substances & Disease Registry. *A Primer on Health Risk Communication. Principles and Practices Overview of Issues and Guiding Principles*. Washington, DC: DHHS-ATSDR; 1994.

8. Sandman PM. Risk communication: facing public outrage. *EPA J*. 1987;13:21–22.

9. Frewer LJ, Scholderer J, Bredahl L. Communicating about the risks and benefits of genetically modified foods: the mediating role of trust. *Risk Anal*. 2003;23:1117–1133.

10. Peters RG, Covello VT, McCallum DB. The determinants of trust and credibility in environmental risk communication: an empirical study. *Risk Anal*. 1997;17:43–54.

11. Weinstein ND, Nicolich M. Correct and incorrect interpretations of correlations between risk perceptions and risk behaviors. *Health Psychol*. 1993;12:235–345.

12. US Department of Health and Human Services, Substance Abuse and Mental Health Services Administration. *Communicating in a Crisis: Risk Communication Guidelines for Public Officials*. Washington, DC: DHHS-SAMHS; 2002.

13. Santos SL. *Risk Communication and Communicating with Patients*. Washington, DC: Department of Veterans Affairs, War Related Illness and Injury Study Center; 2011.

Chapter 24

COMMUNITY-BASED PARTICIPATORY RESEARCH: AN OVERVIEW FOR APPLICATION IN DEPARTMENT OF DEFENSE/VETERANS AFFAIRS RESEARCH

ERIN N. HAYNES, DRPH, MS*

*Assistant Professor, Department of Environmental Health, Division of Epidemiology and Biostatistics, University of Cincinnati College of Medicine, 3223 Eden Avenue, Cincinnati, Ohio 45267-0056

INTRODUCTION

Community-based participatory research (CBPR) is an approach to research that promotes active involvement with community partners or stakeholders. It begins at the generation of a research question and continues through dissemination of results, policy decisions, and/or interventions. CBPR fosters collaboration among research scientists and people affected by the issue under investigation (eg, community members, active military personnel, veterans, and patients with a particular disease). Decision makers (public health policymakers and organizational leaders) who can apply research findings for the benefit of all research partners typically join these partnerships. Proponents of participatory research have reported that these partnerships have yielded great benefits to the research study, including

- increasing the capacity for data collection, analysis, and interpretation;
- reducing the "iatrogenic" effects of research;
- enhancing the relevancy of research questions; and
- maximizing the return of research to improve policy and practice.[1–6]

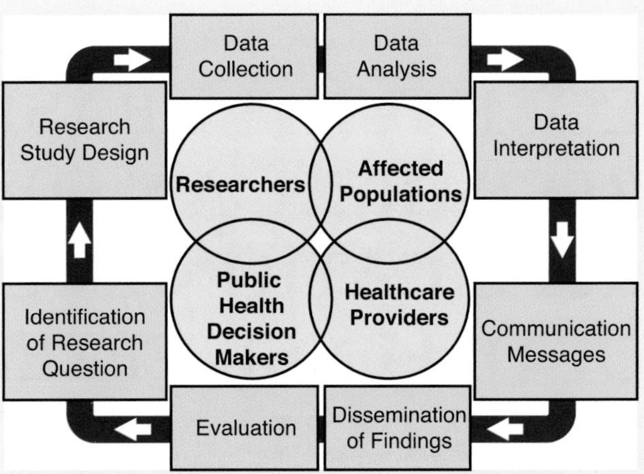

Figure 24-1. Overview of the process of community-based participatory research. Key steps of the cyclical research process are outlined and demonstrate that the research study team includes researchers, affected populations, public health decision makers, and healthcare providers. Their input is needed throughout the research process.

Over the past few decades, participatory research has gained momentum across academic institutions, community-based organizations, and federal agencies. The National Institute of Environmental Health Sciences (NIEHS) has taken a lead within the National Institutes of Health in applying and funding active community/stakeholder participation in research.[7,8] NIEHS recently initiated the Partnerships for Environmental Public Health umbrella program.[9] The goal of this program is to engage communities in all stages of research, outreach, and educational activities to prevent, reduce, or eliminate environmental exposures that may lead to adverse health outcomes, with particular emphasis on populations at highest risk. Within the NIEHS portfolio of research funding announcements, community participation in research is either strongly encouraged or is a required element of the research proposal. For example, in 2012, NIEHS launched a funding opportunity titled *Research to Action: Assessing and Addressing Community Exposures to Environmental Contaminants.* Engagement of those affected by exposures is a requirement of the funding announcement. As illustrated in Figure 24-1, participatory research calls on the skill of individuals with diverse expertise, including members of the affected population, public health decision makers, healthcare providers, and scientific researchers. These individuals are part of the collaborative research team that is involved in the research process from conception of the research question, study design, conduct, analysis, interpretation, and conclusions to communication of results.

CBPR stemmed from the understanding that communities of disadvantage have higher morbidity and mortality as a result of socioeconomic status. Participatory research was initially conceived to improve the health of disadvantaged populations, as defined by socioeconomic status, race, or location. The guiding principles of CBPR can be useful when developing research involving active military and veterans. Therefore, the principles of CBPR are explained herein with relevance to active military and veterans research.

NINE PRINCIPLES OF COMMUNITY-BASED PARTICIPATORY RESEARCH

In 1988, Dr Barbara Israel and colleagues[1] identified nine guiding principles of CBPR to help guide the CBPR process. These principles are outlined in Exhibit 24-1 and are general guidelines that can be adapted to fit a particular research project. Although they are presented in this chapter as distinct items, their collective integration is essential to the conduct of participatory research. Because each research study is unique and requires multidisciplinary expertise, each partnership is also unique and requires a tailored approach. Even though all nine principles of participatory research are described in this chapter, it is anticipated that a subset of these principles will be modified and selected for effective implementation of participatory research within Department of Defense (DoD) and Department of Veterans Affairs (VA) funded research.

Principle 1: Recognize That the Community Is a Unit of Identity

The concept of community as a separate entity is critical to CBPR.[1] A community extends well beyond a neighborhood and is defined based on the perception of the community. For example, a community may be defined as a group of individuals who have a shared set of values and norms, common symbol systems, common environmental exposures, common disease, emotional connection to each other, and commitment to shared goals. With respect to the military, a community may represent a group with a particular exposure, disease, or service during a particular timeframe.

To conduct the research effectively, individuals and organizations outside of the identified community may need to be included in the research partnership. These may include community-based organizations, representatives from health service organizations, healthcare professionals, academia, or others identified by the community who can provide useful resources and skill sets to the research agenda.

Principle 2: Identify and Build on Strengths and Resources Within the Community

Each community has unique strengths and resources that can be useful to the research study. Recognition and implementation of this principle enlighten not only the scientific researcher, but also the community itself to these potential resources and strengths. Community members have expertise and vast social experiences that may not be found in the scientific researcher. CBPR recognizes that the expertise of the community members is equally as beneficial to the research study as the knowledge of the research scientist. Participatory research recognizes the value in each partner's expertise and their view of the problem.

Community members or affected individuals should be regarded as experts. Affected individuals understand the community better than the scientist. They can provide expertise in sources of exposure, timing of exposure, and potential confounders. For example, in a study of air pollution, affected individuals would know when exposures would most likely occur, who might be most exposed, and characteristics about the affected population that may increase exposure. In addition, members of the affected community can also provide expertise in how results are communicated back to the community and through what mechanisms. Inclusion of this expertise enhances the relevance of the research study in its potential to decrease exposure and improve the health of the population. A

EXHIBIT 24-1

NINE GUIDING PRINCIPLES OF COMMUNITY-BASED PARTICIPATORY RESEARCH

Principle 1
Recognize that the community is a unit of identity

Principle 2
Identify and build on strengths and resources within the community

Principle 3
Facilitate a collaborative, equitable partnership throughout all phases of research

Principle 4
Foster co-learning and capacity building among all partners

Principle 5
Integrate and achieve balance between knowledge generation and intervention for the mutual benefit of all partners

Principle 6
Realize that research should be driven by the community addressing locally relevant public health problems

Principle 7
Develop a system to encourage a cyclical, iterative process

Principle 8
Make sure that communication of research findings is disseminated to all partners and that partners are involved in the wider dissemination of results

Principle 9
Understand that community-based participatory research involves a long-term process and a commitment to sustainability

literature review of CBPR intervention studies by the Agency for Healthcare Research and Quality found that community involvement enhanced the element of intervention quality, such as enhanced recruitment efforts, improved research methods and dissemination, and improved descriptive measures.[10]

Principle 3: Facilitate a Collaborative, Equitable Partnership Throughout All Phases of Research

It is well recognized that the successful conduct of research requires a multidisciplinary approach, in which experts are invited to participate in the research to benefit scientific discovery with the ultimate goal of improving public health. Once community partners are regarded as experts, then their role in the conduct of the research study becomes equitable. This principle ensures that expertise from the affected community is included in all phases of the research study. Community partners become equally important in the decision-making processes that frame the research study as the scientific experts.

Scientists can facilitate this equality by including members of the affected community on the research study team. During research study meetings, community partners should be encouraged to contribute to each phase of the research study, including identification of the problem or issue that needs to be addressed through research; how data are collected; interpretation of results; and communication of research findings to study participants and others. The advice of partners should be sought as questionnaires are developed, biological and environmental data collection are being planned, potential confounds are being discussed, etc. Once the study is launched, the community partner still remains integral to the research study team. The partner can provide insight into effective study recruitment mechanisms and assist in troubleshooting data collection issues. Also, the expertise of the partner is critical to the interpretation of data analyses and identification of the public at large.

Principle 4: Foster Co-learning and Capacity Building Among All Partners

Co-learning occurs as scientists and community partners begin to share their experiences in the context of the research study. For example, if a research scientist investigated the health impacts associated with carpentry, the scientist would highly benefit from learning about the lifestyle and work experiences of a carpenter. These may include work hours, ergonomic issues, or other hazards on the job not previously considered by the researcher. In turn, the carpenter would gain knowledge on the conduct of research and, ultimately, how to improve working conditions and practices to improve occupational health and safety. This co-learning occurs when representatives of the study population become integral members of the research team.

To foster co-learning in the research collaboration, the capacity of each—the scientist and the carpenter—needs to be enhanced. To build capacity of the scientist in this example, he/she may need to visit the carpentry site to witness the potential exposures and customary practices of carpenters and learn the names of trade tools. The carpenter will need to understand the purpose of the research, what is involved in conducting a research study, and how funding is obtained to support the research. Community partners should be part of the decision-making process for selecting what capacity they need built. For example, in a CBPR research study in Marietta, OH, where residents were concerned about air quality and health, the community partners asked for workshops on air particles and health to further understand air sampling and the potential health impacts of various-sized particles.[11]

Principle 5: Integrate and Achieve Balance Between Knowledge Generation and Intervention for the Mutual Benefit of All Partners

Within CBPR, it is anticipated that the research conducted is beneficial for all partners. Research scientists add to the scientific literature and expand their specific fields, whereas community partners have an improved understanding of their particular concern. CBPR highlights the importance of applying the knowledge gained from research into an intervention that will help solve the community's initial concerns. This integration or application of the science into appropriate interventions provides a win–win situation in which scientists walk away with a better-conducted study because of the contribution of the community partners, whereas community members receive a solution to their problem.

Community organization has been identified as an essential element for successful implementation of community-based cardiovascular disease prevention programs.[12] When key community leaders and community organizations are mobilized, health promotion becomes a community theme, and time and resources are more readily available for prevention activities.

Principle 6: Realize That Research Should Be Driven by the Community Addressing Locally Relevant Public Health Problems

The conduct of science is the systematic investigation of a question. In CBPR, the scientific research question is identified by the community and that question has arisen from their concern or problems with a particular exposure or health outcome. In participatory research, the community's struggle with understanding the issue or problem is co-shared with scientists and jointly investigated. Addressing a community-driven issue is integral to CBPR. It ensures that the research is community relevant and will potentially result in mitigation of the exposure or other intervention that will negate the problem.

Principle 7: Develop a System to Encourage a Cyclical, Iterative Process

Implementing CBPR is not a one-time meeting of scientists and community partners. CBPR requires multiple meetings throughout the research study to ensure that the needs of all partners are being met. This cyclical, iterative process ensures that all research team members have an equal opportunity to contribute during each phase of the research study from problem definition to dissemination of results and action taken, if appropriate. This also ensures that the action taken as a result of the research is acceptable and appropriate for all partners.

Principle 8: Make Sure That Communication of Research Findings Is Disseminated to All Partners and That Partners Are Involved in the Wider Dissemination of Results

Communication of study results is an essential outcome of the community–scientist collaborative research process. All study partners should have access to study results, and great care should be taken to develop communication mechanisms that are appropriate, accessible, and respectful of all partners. This principle also extends to the involvement of community research partners as co-authors of publications, scientific reports, abstracts, and co-presenters at scientific meetings and conferences.

Community partners provide expertise in guiding the development of effective communication messages and strategies for the target population, including study participants and the public at large. As members of the affected community, they can best identify the messages and determine which strategies to deliver those messages would be the most effective.

Principle 9: Understand That Community-Based Participatory Research Involves a Long-Term Process and a Commitment to Sustainability

Development of community-based partnerships necessitates the building of mutual trust and respect. CBPR is a long-term process and requires a commitment to the partnership from all members. When CBPR is implemented, the community partners have identified the research question, provided their expertise for the enhancement of the project, and assisted in the conduct of research and study results dissemination; they are truly vested in the research. Arguably, they have a greater investment in the research than the scientist because the issue under investigation is one that directly affects the health and safety, livelihood, and well-being of their families. Thus, once the research study is complete, it is critical that the partnership does not end. Scientists need to retain the commitment to the partnership even when funding is not available. Maintenance of the partnership requires sustained communication and capacity building for the partners.

A research study operating under CBPR guidelines will not end the partnership once data are collected. As described in Principle 5, the research scientist would also work with the affected community to use the information gained from the study to improve the working or living conditions of research partners. This could be in the form of participating in advocacy for policy change, publishing research findings in peer-reviewed journals to demonstrate credibility of the work, and sharing these results in the form of publications with public health decision-makers engaged in policy decisions relevant to the issue. This step is critical because it sustains the community's trust in the research scientists and the research process.

SUMMARY

Participatory research is a partnership approach that provides an equitable foothold in the research process for all involved. The participatory research approach recognizes that every member of the research team, including representatives from the community, have unique strengths and expertise. Although nine participatory research principles were described, it is not anticipated that the DoD/VA will endorse all of them. For example, the NIEHS endorses only six of the nine guiding principles of CBPR:

1. promotes active collaboration and participation at every stage of research,
2. fosters co-learning,
3. ensures that projects are community-driven,
4. ensures that research and intervention strategies are culturally appropriate,
5. defines community as a unit of identity, and
6. disseminates results in useful terms.[6]

Because the nature of research conducted and funded by the DoD/VA and NIEHS have strong similarities, it is recommended that at least the six principles endorsed by NIEHS be considered for implementation in active military and veteran research. The selection process should be a participatory process involving active military and veterans, as well as research scientists within the DoD/VA. It is also recommended that at least one member of the selection committee have expertise in CBPR. Strong consideration should be made to determine which of the guiding CBPR principles would best serve their research mission. There is little doubt that application of these principles will significantly

- increase research study relevance;
- enhance data collection, interpretation, and analysis;
- improve the capacity of all research partners;
- improve communication of research findings; and
- improve the health and well-being of active military and veterans as the findings are implemented into effective policy and practice.

REFERENCES

1. Israel BA, Schulz AJ, Parker EA, Becker AB. Review of community-based research: assessing partnership approaches to improve public health. *Annu Rev Public Health.* 1998;19:173–202.

2. Israel BA, Eng E, Schulz AJ, Parker EA, Satcher D. *Methods in Community-Based Participatory Research for Health.* San Francisco, CA: Jossey-Bass; 2005.

3. Israel BA, Schulz AJ, Parker EA, Becker AB. Community-based participatory research: policy recommendations for promoting a partnership approach in health research. *Edu Health (Abingdon).* 2001;14:182–197.

4. Macaulay AC, Commanda LE, Freeman WL, et al. Participatory research maximizes community and lay involvement. North American Primary Care Research Group. *Br Med J.* 1999;319:774–778.

5. Minkler M, Wallerstein N, eds. *Community-Based Participatory Research for Health: From Process to Outcomes.* 2nd ed. San Francisco, CA: Jossey-Bass; 2008.

6. O'Fallon LR, Dearry A. Community-based participatory research as a tool to advance environmental health sciences. *Environ Health Perspect.* 2002;110(suppl 2):155–159.

7. O'Fallon LR, Tyson F, Dearry A, eds. Executive summary. In: *Successful Models of Community Based Participatory Research: Final Report.* Research Triangle Park, NC: National Institute of Environmental Health Sciences; 2000: 1–3.

8. O'Fallon LR, Dearry A. Commitment of the National Institute of Environmental Health Sciences to community-based participatory research for rural health. *Environ Health Perspect.* 2001;109(suppl 3):469–473.

9. Birnbaum LS. NIEHS supports partnerships in environmental public health. *Prog Community Health Partnersh.* 2009;3:195–196.

10. Viswanathan M, Ammerman A, Eng E, et al. Community-based participatory research: assessing the evidence. *Evid Rep Technol Assess (Summ).* 2004;August:1–8.

11. Haynes EN, Beidler C, Wittberg R, et al. Developing a bidirectional academic-community partnership with an Appalachian-American community for environmental health research and risk communication. *Environ Health Perspect.* 2011;119:1364–1372.

12. Mittelmark MB, Hunt MK, Heath GW, Schmid TL. Realistic outcomes: lessons from community-based research and demonstration programs for the prevention of cardiovascular diseases. *J Public Health Policy.* 1993;14:437–462.

Chapter 25

TOXIC EMBEDDED FRAGMENTS REGISTRY: LESSONS LEARNED

JOANNA M. GAITENS, PhD, MSN/MPH, RN*; and MELISSA A. McDIARMID, MD, MPH†

*Research Nurse Associate, Baltimore Veterans Affairs Medical Center, 10 North Greene Street, Baltimore, MD 21201; Assistant Professor, Department of Medicine, Occupational Health Program, University of Maryland School of Medicine, 11 South Paca Street, Suite 200, Baltimore, MD 21201

†Medical Director, Baltimore Veterans Affairs Medical Center, 10 North Greene Street, Baltimore, MD 21201; Professor of Medicine and Epidemiology & Public Health, and Director, Division of Occupational and Environmental Medicine, University of Maryland School of Medicine, 11 South Paca Street, Suite 200, Baltimore, MD 21201

INTRODUCTION

In 2008, the US Department of Veterans Affairs (VA) established the Toxic Embedded Fragment Surveillance Center (TEFSC; Baltimore, MD) in response to the growing number of service members who served in Iraq and Afghanistan and sustained an injury after contact with an improvised explosive device. At that time, it was estimated that 5,000 service members potentially had a retained embedded fragment as the result of such an injury.[1] As the conflicts continued, this number continued to grow, with one estimate reaching more than 40,000 service members (C. Perdue, personal e-mail communication, December 2009). In this context, the overall mission of the TEFSC is to

- identify veterans from these conflicts who may have retained fragments as a result of an injury they sustained while serving and
- conduct long-term medical surveillance of this population because of concern about potential local and systemic health effects related to the fragments.

Over the past several decades, there has been controversy about whether retained embedded fragments adversely impact health and warrant removal. In the past, retained embedded fragments were thought not to pose a significant health risk and, therefore, were often not surgically removed unless they caused the patient discomfort or were located in a joint space. For example, Machle[2] reviewed 40 bullet injury cases documented in the literature during the late 1800s and early 1900s. He reported that systemic lead absorption could occur from retained bullets, but that "lead poisoning" was a rare occurrence unless the fragment was located in a joint space.[2] It is important to recognize that, during this period, the ability to quantitatively measure lead exposure was limited. However, lead poisoning was defined then as having clinically overt symptoms related to exposure, including the presence of lead lines and visible central nervous system effects such as ataxia, memory loss, and convulsions. With significant improvements in exposure assessment methodology and a shift toward detecting preclinical disease, the definition of lead poisoning has changed dramatically. As a result, significantly lower lead concentrations have been associated with preclinical adverse health effects, thus raising the question about potential long-term health consequences related to systemic absorption of metal ions from lead fragments and, by inference, fragments of a different composition.

A more recent experience with embedded fragments of long residence time in the body was presented by the friendly fire incidents during the first Gulf War in 1991. During this war, depleted uranium (DU; a byproduct of the uranium enrichment process) was first used in the armor of tanks and in munitions used to destroy enemy tanks. Unlike lead, DU has radiological properties, as well as chemical properties, rendering it a dual health hazard.[3–5] During the 1991 Gulf War, a cohort of service members involved in friendly fire incidents was exposed to DU through inhalation, ingestion, and wound contamination when DU rounds were mistakenly fired upon their tanks.[6–11] Although there was the potential for adverse health effects related to short-term DU inhalation exposure and long-term DU exposure related to embedded fragments, service members involved in the friendly fire incidents were not immediately identified and followed as a cohort until the VA established a medical surveillance program in 1993.[6,7] Within this cohort of 80 individuals, urine measurements have consistently shown that service members and veterans with a retained DU fragment excrete higher concentrations of total uranium in their urine than those without fragments; these veterans have an isotopic DU signature (as opposed to a natural uranium signature), thus raising concern about target organ effects from systemic absorption of DU.[6–11] In addition, there is concern about local effects in areas surrounding fragments because research conducted in laboratory animals implanted with DU pellets has shown the formation of soft-tissue sarcomas in proximity to the implanted pellets.[11] Fortunately, more than 40 years of epidemiological evidence showing no increase in cancer rates in uranium fabrication workers[12] and more than 20 years of medical surveillance in the DU-exposed population have shown no clinically significant uranium-related adverse health effects.[13] Despite these findings, the initial delay in identifying those at risk for DU exposure led to criticism of the VA and raised concerns about whether critical windows of opportunity were missed to fully assess a veteran's exposure to DU early on.

Beyond the DU fragment example, other types of munitions have also raised concerns as potential long-residence, time-embedded fragments, including a recently introduced tungsten, nickel, and cobalt alloy. Although there have been no known friendly fire incidents resulting in embedded fragments of this type, Kalinich et al[14] found that laboratory animals implanted with pellets of this alloy excreted elevated concentrations of tungsten, nickel, and cobalt in their urine and developed rhabdomyosarcomas that quickly metastasized to the lung. This finding, combined with the experiences previously described, emphasized the need to better understand the types of exposures and potential human health effects that occur from materials embedded in the body. Thus, the VA established the TEFSC (at the Baltimore VA Medical Center) to address the following:

- limited information available regarding fragment composition related to improvised explosive device injuries,
- local and systemic adverse health effects resulting from embedded fragments, and
- delays in identifying and responding to potential hazards that could result in the loss of critically important, time-sensitive exposure information early after initial exposure.

In order to appropriately identify and conduct surveillance of veterans with embedded fragments, it is important to:

- anticipate the hazard and provide a timely response,
- recognize that exposure assessment is critical,
- obtain baseline biomonitoring data, and
- link surveillance data to clinical decision-making and medical management.

LESSON 1: ANTICIPATE THE HAZARD AND PROVIDE A TIMELY RESPONSE

Establishment of the Embedded Fragments Registry

To achieve its mission to identify affected veterans and to conduct medical surveillance of the population of veterans who have embedded fragments, the TEFSC established the Embedded Fragments Registry. In general, public health registries capture data in a systematic fashion to allow for population-level surveillance and identification of patterns and trends related to health status over time.[15] Historically, registries have been disease-focused, meaning data were collected on individuals who had a specific disease or health outcome of interest (ie, cancer). More recently, exposure registries that focus on the collection of data from populations with known exposures have also arisen.[16] Exposure registries are often established when specific health outcomes associated with an exposure are not well-characterized. Because long-term potential health outcomes associated with fragments are not well understood and the case definition for inclusion into the registry requires an indication that a veteran may have a fragment, the Embedded Fragments Registry is classified as an exposure registry.

Case Finding

As described by Gaitens et al,[17] the Veterans Health Administration developed a two-step screening process, which was fully implemented nationwide in 2009, to actively identify veterans who have embedded fragments and who receive care at a VA medical facility. Local VA healthcare providers are responsible for screening all veterans who served in Operation Iraqi Freedom, Operation Enduring Freedom, and Operation New Dawn using a series of questions that are incorporated into the Computerized Patient Record System. These questions appear as "clinical event reminders" within the veterans' electronic health records and are automatically triggered based on the veterans' dates of service, thus alerting providers of the need to screen individual patients and allowing for more rapid identification of those at risk.

Screening Results

As shown in Figure 25-1, between November 2008 and June 2012 approximately one-half million veterans who served in Iraq and/or Afghanistan completed the *first phase* of the clinical reminder screening process, with 3.5% of these veterans indicating that they may have an embedded fragment as the result of an injury they received while serving in the area of conflict. The *second phase* of the screening process, which is also described in detail by Gaitens et al,[17] was initiated in October 2009 and contains questions regarding the cause of the injury (ie, bullet and/or blast or explosion), history of fragment removal and analysis, and identification of fragments that remain in the body. Responses to these questions trigger automatic inclusion in the Embedded Fragments Registry and are used to classify veterans into four exposure risk categories:

1. has/had a fragment,
2. has a high probability of having a fragment,
3. possibly has a fragment, or
4. likely does not have a fragment.

The automatic transfer of data into the Embedded Fragments Registry when the second phase of the screening process is complete alleviates reliance on providers to alert Center staff of individuals who are eligible for inclusion into the registry. As shown in Figure 25-1, almost 7,900 veterans potentially have a fragment and warrant further evaluation and follow-up. In addition to capturing responses to the screening questions for each veteran, the Embedded Fragments Registry captures other critical pieces of health and exposure-related information, such as fragment composition data and urine biomonitoring results from electronic medical record systems, as well as other available data sources.

Surveillance Protocol

Currently, the medical surveillance protocol—that includes fragment analyses, urine biomonitoring, and imaging of the fragment—is recommended for all veterans who may

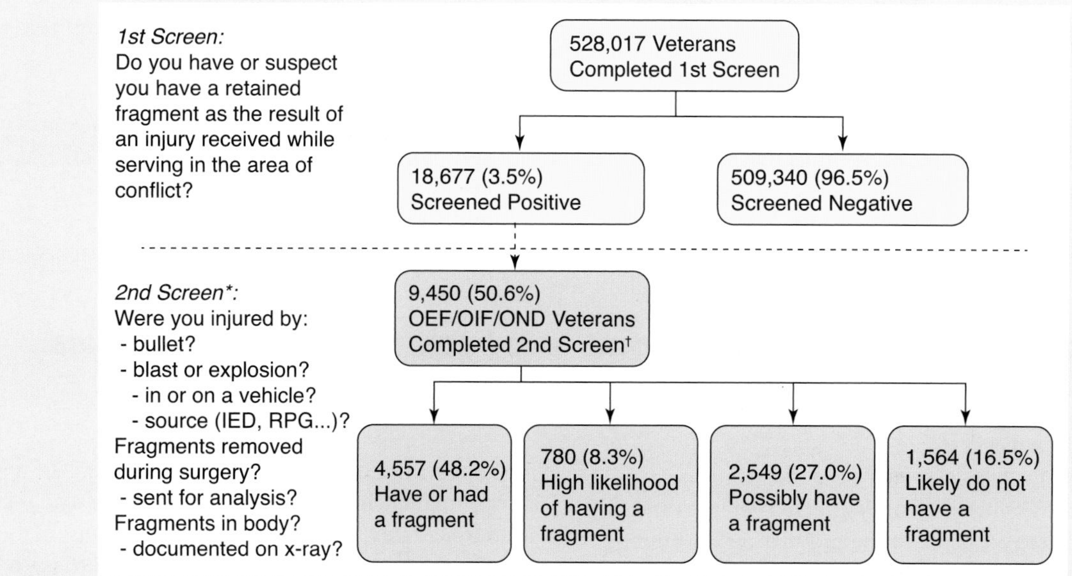

Figure 25-1. Screening results per June 30, 2012.
*Completion of the 2nd screen triggers inclusion in the Embedded Fragments Registry.
†486 of 9,450 (5%) veterans completed the 2nd screen, but had no indication of a positive 1st screen included in their electronic medical record.
IED: improvised explosive device; OEF: Operation Enduring Freedom; OIF: Operation Iraqi Freedom; OND: Operation New Dawn; RPG: rocket-propelled grenade

have a retained fragment. Analyses of the results from these activities, combined with other surveillance data captured in the Embedded Fragments Registry, will allow the VA to

- describe the population at risk for embedded fragments,
- characterize exposure related to retained fragments,
- consider potential health effects associated with specific fragment exposure, and
- utilize medical management guidelines to provide care for these veterans.

Fragment Analysis

In uncontrolled environments, such as war zones, it is often difficult to clearly identify and assess exposures at the individual level. In the case of embedded fragments, fragments that are removed during surgery or superficial fragments that work their way out of the body can be analyzed for composition to help characterize a veteran's exposure. Working with a specialized laboratory at the Joint Pathology Center (formerly located within the Armed Forces Institute of Pathology), the VA has established a process that permits VA providers to send such fragments for analyses to determine the composition of its inner and outer cores.[11] Working under the assumption that fragments remaining in the body are similar in composition to those that were removed, identification of the removed fragment materials provides crucial information needed to identify potential health outcomes of interest for an individual veteran and possibly to allow tailored surveillance for toxicants not typically included in a surveillance battery.

Understanding the importance of fragment composition data, in 2007, the Department of Defense (DoD) established a requirement for all military medical treatment facilities to send fragments removed during surgery to specified laboratories for content analyses in an effort to better characterize exposures and identify potentially hazardous embedded fragments.[18] The TEFSC reviewed aggregated fragment composition data from this effort to help develop their surveillance protocol and identify other methods for assessing fragment-related exposure when fragment composition data are not known for an individual service member. Knowing that the majority of fragments contain metals (eg, iron, lead, copper, aluminum, lead, and zinc) allowed the VA to develop a urine biomonitoring panel for toxicants of concern and to identify potential target organs at risk for adverse effects.[17]

The DoD and VA also established processes to allow for the transfer of fragment composition data at the individual level from the DoD to the VA's Embedded Fragments Registry. Currently, the registry is able to identify if a veteran has had a fragment removed and analyzed by the DoD and the results of the fragment analyses. This allows the medical surveillance protocol to be "tailored" to the individual and provides additional information that can be used for interpreting urine biomonitoring results.

LESSON 2: RECOGNIZE THAT EXPOSURE ASSESSMENT IS CRITICAL

Urine Biomonitoring

Urine biomonitoring offers several advantages for assessing fragment-related exposure. First, urine samples are noninvasive, posing no risk to the veteran submitting the sample. Second, monitoring the urine for concentrations of metals frequently found in fragments provides insight into exposure when specific fragment composition for an individual veteran is not known. Third, it helps determine the overall body burden of metals potentially related to fragments.

The TEFSC currently recommends that all veterans who may have an embedded fragment submit a 24-hour urine sample for analysis of concentrations of 14 metals; these metals have been found in fragments that have been removed during surgery from service members who served in the recent conflicts and/or are metals known for their toxicity.[17] All urine samples are submitted to the Baltimore VA Medical Center for creatinine analyses and to the Joint Pathology Center for measurement of the metal concentrations listed in Exhibit 25-1. The Embedded Fragments Registry electronically receives urine biomonitoring results—including creatinine concentrations, metal concentrations, and creatinine-adjusted concentrations—directly from the Baltimore VA Medical Center's laboratory system.[17]

Once results are obtained, creatinine-adjusted concentrations of the metals measured are compared with established reference values to gain insight into the composition of fragments that remain in the body.[11,17] For example, if a veteran's urine sample has a concentration of aluminum above what would be expected to occur in the general population and other sources of aluminum exposure have been ruled out, it is thought that the elevated aluminum concentration may be related to the composition of the fragment.

Over time, as fragments begin to oxidize in the body and changes to the fragments shape are detected on imaging, it is anticipated that higher concentrations of metals released from the fragments will be detected in the urine. Therefore, obtaining a "baseline' urine sample, as well as an X-ray film image of the area surrounding the fragment, as soon as possible after time of injury (or when the veteran transitions from active duty and presents to his/her local VA facility initially for care) are important factors in assessing long-term exposure risks. Although it can be difficult to obtain such data, because a veteran may not be currently experiencing health concerns and therefore not see the value in seeking care, waiting until a health concern presents may lead to more unanswered questions and difficulties in interpreting future urine biomonitoring results.

EXHIBIT 25-1

METALS INCLUDED IN THE URINE BIOMONITORING PANEL

Arsenic
Cadmium
Chromium
Cobalt
Copper
Iron
Lead
Manganese
Molybdenum
Nickel
Tungsten
Uranium
Zinc

LESSON 3: OBTAIN BASELINE BIOMONITORING DATA

Follow-up Actions Triggered by Urine Results

For all veterans who submit a urine sample or fragment for analysis, the TEFSC provides a letter of interpretation for the veteran and the veteran's VA care provider. Letters detailing urine biomonitoring result provide the creatinine-adjusted urine concentrations of each metal, as well as additional details about other potential sources of exposure, whether or not the levels found raise any health concerns, and describe how the urine results compare with fragment composition data, if available. Additionally, the provider letters contain specific recommendations for patient follow-up that include:

- imaging the fragment location with an X-ray film so that a baseline is obtained for future comparisons,
- assessing other potential sources of exposure (ie, occupation, hobby, dietary supplements),
- obtaining additional testing if necessary (ie, performing a blood lead test if urinary lead concentrations are elevated above the reference value), and
- describing a recommended timeframe for repeating urine biomonitoring.

The urgency of these actions depends on the magnitude of the excursion for a specific metal in relation to the reference value and how the result compares with levels linked to health effects in the literature.

The importance of a registry and continued follow-up may not be recognized by some individuals, clinicians included, because those individuals for whom data are collected often do not see the immediate benefits of such an endeavor. However, linking surveillance data to clinical decision-making and medical management provides the veteran and his/her healthcare provider with the information needed to anticipate potential health, possibly by taking preventive action or by detecting early health consequences of fragment-related injury.

LESSON 4: LINK SURVEILLANCE DATA TO CLINICAL DECISION-MAKING AND MEDICAL MANAGEMENT

Target Organ Surveillance

In addition to collecting the exposure data described previously, the Embedded Fragments Registry captures *International Classification of Diseases*, Ninth Revision, codes and clinical laboratory tests of interest directly from the patient's electronic medical record.[17] These measures were chosen by mapping the list of metals frequently found in fragments and including them in the biomonitoring panel to potential health effects and key target organs and systems (eg, the kidney, the immune system, and the reproductive system).[16] In the future, these health outcomes will be examined to detect patterns and trends in disease among those who have embedded fragments of known composition.

SUMMARY

Health concerns related to military deployment can be challenging to address, as potential hazards may not be immediately identified and individual exposures are often not well-characterized. Whenever possible, deployment-related hazards should be anticipated so that affected service members are easily identified and a response is implemented in a timely fashion. Assessing a service member's exposure to a hazard and obtaining baseline biomonitoring data can provide crucial information for determining the appropriate short- and long-term actions needed to mitigate potential health effects related to deployment. Based on these lessons learned from previous incidents, the VA established the Toxic Embedded Fragment Surveillance Center and the Embedded Fragments Registry to identify and conduct long-term medical surveillance of veterans who have embedded fragments. This exposure registry, which links surveillance data to clinical decision-making, will provide the VA with information needed to care for veterans with retained embedded fragments.

Acknowledgments

This work is supported by the US Department of Veterans Affairs and approved by the Baltimore Veterans Affairs Medical Center's Office of Research and Development and the University of Maryland School of Medicine's Institutional Review Board.

REFERENCES

1. United States Department of Veterans Affairs. *Task Force Report to the President: Returning Global War on Terror Heroes, April 2007.* Washington, DC: United States Department of Veterans Affairs; 2007.

2. Machle W. Lead absorption from bullets lodged in tissues: report of two cases. *JAMA.* 1940;115:1536–1541.

3. The Royal Society. *The Health Hazards of Depleted Uranium Munition: Part 1.* London, UK: The Royal Society; 2001. Policy document 6/01.

4. The Royal Society. *The Health Hazards of Depleted Uranium Munitions: Summary.* London, UK: The Royal Society; 2002. Policy document 6/02.

5. National Research Council of the National Academies. *Review of Toxicologic and Radiologic Risks to Military Personnel from Exposure to Depleted Uranium During and After Combat.* Washington, DC: The National Academies Press; 2008.

6. Hooper FJ, Squibb KS, Siegel EL, McPhaul K, Keogh JP. Elevated urine uranium excretion by service members with retained uranium shrapnel. *Health Physics.* 1999;77:512–519.

7. Squibb KS, McDiarmid MA. Depleted uranium exposure and health effects in Gulf War veterans. *Phil Trans R Soc B.* 2006;361:639–648.

8. McDiarmid MA, Squibb K, Engelhardt S, et al. Surveillance of depleted uranium exposed Gulf War veterans: health effects observed in an enlarged "friendly fire" cohort. *J Occup Environ Med.* 2001;43:991–1000.

9. McDiarmid MA, Engelhardt SM, Dorsey CD, et al. Longitudinal health surveillance in a cohort of Gulf War veterans 18 years after first exposure to depleted uranium. *J Toxicol Environ Health Part A.* 2011;74:678–691.

10. Squibb K, Gaitens J, Engelhardt S, et al. Surveillance for long-term health effects associated with depleted uranium exposure and retained embedded fragments in US veterans. *J Occup Environ Med.* 2012;54:724–732.

11. Hahn FF, Guilmette RA, Hoover MD. Implanted depleted uranium fragments cause soft tissue sarcomas in the muscles of rats. *Environ Health Perspect.* 2002;110:51–59.

12. Boice JD Jr, Cohen SS, Mumma MT, Chadda B, Blot WJ. A cohort study of uranium millers and miners of Grants, New Mexico, 1979–2005. *J Radiol Prot.* 2008;28:303–325.

13. McDiarmid MA, Gaitens JM, Hines S, et al. The Gulf War depleted uranium cohort at 20 years: bioassay results and novel approaches to fragment surveillance. *Health Phys.* 2013;104;347–361.

14. Kalinich JF, Edmond CA, Dalton TK, et al. Embedded weapons-grade tungsten alloy shrapnel rapidly induces metastatic high-grade rhabdomyosarcomas in F344 rats. *Environ Health Perspect.* 2005;113:729–734.

15. US Department of Health and Human Services, National Committee on Vital and Health Statistics. *Frequently Asked Questions About Medical and Public Health Registries.* http://www.ncvhs.hhs.gov/9701138b.htm. Accessed December 13, 2012.

16. Schulte PA, Kaye WE. Exposure registries. *Arch Environ Health.* 1988;43:155–161.

17. Gaitens JM, Dorsey CD, McDiarmid MA. Using a public health registry to conduct medical surveillance: the case of toxic embedded fragments in U.S. military veterans. *Eur J Oncol.* 2010;15:77–89.

18. United States Department of Defense, Assistant Secretary of Defense. *Policy on Analysis of Metal Fragments Removed from Department of Defense Personnel*, December 18, 2007. http://www.health.mil/libraries/HA_Policies_and_Guidelines/07-029.pdf. Accessed December 3, 2012. HA Policy 07-029.

Chapter 26

LESSONS LEARNED FROM SELF-SELECTED REGISTRIES (AGENT ORANGE)

WENDI J. DICK, MD, MSPH, MCRP*

Senior Advisor to the Afghanistan Assistant Minister of Defense for Health Affairs, Office of the Command Surgeon, NATO Training Mission-Afghanistan, International Security Assistance Force, Kabul, Afghanistan; Former Director, Environmental Health Program, Pre-9/11 Era, Post-Deployment Health, Office of Public Health, Veterans Health Administration, US Department of Veterans Affairs, 810 Vermont Avenue, NW, Washington, DC 20420

INTRODUCTION

During the Vietnam War, the US military sprayed noncommercial herbicides, such as the phenoxy herbicide blend Agent Orange, to gain a tactical advantage by defoliating jungle that provided enemy cover. Veterans and others returning from Vietnam have attributed a wide range of illnesses to exposure to Agent Orange and the dioxin it contained. In April 1970, Congress held the first of many hearings on herbicide health effects. In 1978, the US Department of Veterans Affairs (VA) created the Agent Orange Registry for Vietnam veterans who were concerned about possible adverse health effects from exposure.

HISTORY OF THE AGENT ORANGE REGISTRY

Agent Orange is the main "tactical" (noncommercial) herbicide the US Air Force sprayed as part of Operation Ranch Hand (1962–1971) during the Vietnam War to destroy food crops and enemy cover.[1,2] Although a number of different herbicides blends were used, Agent Orange comprised the majority. Agent Orange got its name from the color of the stripe on its storage drum. Its active ingredients were a 50:50 mixture of two phenoxy herbicides: 2,4-dichlorophenoxyacetic acid and 2,4,5-trichlorophenoxyacetic acid. Both were common weed killers during the 1950s–1970s, and 2,4-dichlorophenoxyacetic acid is still in use today. The US Department of Defense (DoD) suspended Operation Ranch Hand in early 1971 after Agent Orange was found to be contaminated with 2,3,7,8-tetrachlorodibenzo-*p*-dioxin (TCDD), an unintentional dioxin byproduct of the manufacturing process. Evidence emerged that dioxin caused birth defects in laboratory mice.[3] Returning Vietnam veterans and others have attributed a wide range of illnesses, including birth defects among their children, to exposure to Agent Orange and the dioxin it contained. In April 1970, Congress held the first of many hearings on herbicide health effects. In 1978, the VA created the Agent Orange Registry for Vietnam veterans who were concerned about possible adverse health effects from exposure to Agent Orange during the war. According to Han Kang, PhD (former Director of the Environmental Epidemiology Service, Washington, DC), the VA also initiated this registry as a means to increase access for Vietnam veterans to the VA healthcare system.

In 1994, the Institute of Medicine (IOM) issued its first report titled *Veterans and Agent Orange: Health Effects of Herbicides Used in Vietnam.* This report reviewed the scientific and medical literature regarding the health effects of exposure to Agent Orange and other herbicides used in Vietnam. Reports have been completed every 2 years hence, and the most current update was released on December 3, 2013 (titled *Veterans and Agent Orange: Update 2012).*[4] The VA also asked IOM to determine the level of association between specific health outcomes and exposure to herbicides, including the TCDD contaminant in Agent Orange. Many of the studies reviewed by IOM looked at Agent Orange or its components because it constituted the majority of what was sprayed in Vietnam; the science linking TCDD to adverse health outcomes is well known. The IOM also reviewed the chemicals in herbicides other than Agent Orange, including picloram (Agent White) and cacodylic acid (Agent Blue). Cacodylic acid contains an organic form of arsenic that is a known carcinogen (based on animal studies). The variation in tumor formation caused by arsenic among different animal species is thought to be strongly influenced by genetic differences. The 1994 report identified five diseases with sufficient evidence of an association between the disease and exposure to herbicides or TCDD:

1. chloracne,
2. Hodgkin's disease,
3. non-Hodgkin's lymphoma,
4. porphyria cutanea tarda, and
5. soft-tissue sarcoma.

The report also identified three diseases with limited or suggestive evidence:

1. multiple myeloma,
2. prostate cancer, and
3. respiratory cancers.

When the 2008 update was published, an additional seven diseases or conditions were added to the category of limited/suggestive evidence:

1. amyloid light-chain amyloidosis,
2. chronic B-cell leukemia,
3. hypertension,
4. ischemic heart disease,
5. Parkinson's disease,
6. peripheral neuropathy, and
7. type 2 diabetes mellitus.

Reliable measures of Agent Orange exposure are not available. The VA defined any veteran as "exposed" for the purpose of VA healthcare benefits and disability compensation if they served any length of time in Vietnam.

The Secretary of the VA considers the IOM's findings when determining which health conditions will be presumed as related to Agent Orange exposure ("presumptive" diseases) for the purpose of disability compensation. As of December 22, 2012, the VA considers the following 14 diseases as presumptive for being linked to Agent Orange exposure[1]:

1. amyloid light-chain amyloidosis,
2. chloracne,
3. chronic B-cell leukemias,
4. early-onset peripheral neuropathy,
5. Hodgkin's disease,
6. ischemic heart disease,
7. multiple myeloma,
8. non-Hodgkin's lymphoma,
9. Parkinson's disease,
10. porphyria cutanea tarda,
11. prostate cancer,
12. respiratory cancers,
13. soft-tissue sarcomas, and
14. type 2 diabetes mellitus.

AGENT ORANGE REGISTRY PROGRAM AND ELIGIBILITY

The program offers a medical evaluation available at most VA healthcare facilities. The registry examination provides an opportunity for veterans to obtain a physical examination, discuss their exposure concerns with a knowledgeable healthcare provider, ask questions, and learn about benefits for which they may be eligible.

The Agent Orange Registry is a computerized record of these examinations. Clinicians performing the registry examination follow a comprehensive protocol described in the *Veterans Health Administration Handbook 1302.01*.[5]

Regarding eligibility, any veteran—male or female—who had active military service in the Republic of Vietnam between 1962 and 1975, and who expresses a concern relating to exposure to herbicides may participate in the registry and receive a free examination. Eligible veterans who want to participate in this program are instructed to contact their nearest VA medical facility for an appointment. There is no minimum period of service in Vietnam. Initially, veterans who did not serve in Vietnam were not eligible for the Agent Orange Registry Health Examination even if they could have been exposed to herbicides elsewhere during military service. Beginning in early 2011, veterans who served along the Korean Demilitarized Zone between 1968 and 1971 are also eligible. Additional groups of veterans who are eligible include those who served in certain units in Thailand, and those who were involved in the testing, transporting, or spraying of herbicides for military purposes. Although children of Vietnam or Korean Demilitarized Zone veterans with spina bifida are eligible for certain VA benefits because of an association with herbicide exposure, spouses of veterans are not eligible for this examination. Veterans do not need to enroll in VA healthcare to receive a registry examination because the examination is free.

AGENT ORANGE REGISTRY HEALTH EXAMINATION

Data collection begins prior to the examination with veteran demographics and other information recorded on an Agent Orange Registry Health Examination worksheet. The veteran is encouraged to share concerns about his/her exposures during the examination. Educational materials, such as the most current *Agent Orange Review Newsletter*, are provided. In general, the examining clinician evaluates each veteran's military history and other relevant exposure history, signs, and symptoms. Then, an appropriate examination is performed. In the past, baseline laboratory tests were recommended, but this is no longer the case. There are no specific diagnostic tests or treatments generally recommended specifically for Vietnam veterans or others who served in areas where military herbicides were used. Guidance for clinicians regarding the physical examination is to focus on systems that have been found to have an association with herbicide or TCDD exposure (which may include the skin, lymph nodes, respiratory system, cardiovascular system, hematological system, bone, endocrine, peripheral nerves, and prostate). The examination is documented in the VA's electronic health record (Computerized Patient Record System; CPRS). Worksheet data are entered in a separate online database that is not connected to the medical record. Longstanding VA policy requires that this information be provided to the veteran in a face-to-face discussion with the clinician and that a follow-up letter summarizing the results of the registry examination be mailed to the veteran within 2 weeks. If health problems are detected during the examination, veterans are encouraged to enroll for VA healthcare if they have not already done so or to follow-up with their private provider. Veterans may receive a follow-up evaluation if necessary.

VETERANS AFFAIRS ENVIRONMENTAL HEALTH CLINICIANS AND COORDINATORS

Each VA medical center has an assigned Environmental Health Clinician who is responsible for the conduct of Agent Orange Registry Health Examinations (as well as for other special registry and deployment-related environmental and occupational health issues). Each VA medical center also has an Environmental Health Coordinator who is responsible for coordinating Agent Orange Registry Health Examinations (ie, scheduling appointments, providing educational materials, collecting nonclinical data, ensuring that follow-up letters are completed, and managing data entry).

AGENT ORANGE REGISTRY DATA

The Agent Orange Registry program is not a research program. Because of the self-selected nature of the veterans who present for the voluntary examination program, as well as the lack of any controls, the registry is no substitute for a properly designed epidemiological study. However, data from the Agent Orange Registry database can be helpful to track patterns of veterans completing these examinations. The registry can also be utilized to answer queries about the number of veterans who reported exposure outside of Vietnam or other data of interest. Even if all of the veterans completing registry examinations were not exposed to military herbicides, the database can serve as a list of veterans who have concerns about exposure.

VETERANS' UTILIZATION OF THE AGENT ORANGE REGISTRY HEALTH EXAMINATION

Table 26-1 shows the number of veterans who received Agent Orange Registry Health Examinations since the program started in 1978. As of September 30, 2012, a total of 573,088 veterans have completed an evaluation.[6] Assuming there were approximately 2.7 million Vietnam veterans, this means that about 21% have had an Agent Orange registry evaluation.[7]

It is important to note that even though the program is more than 3 decades old, many veterans are still contacting the VA each week for their initial Agent Orange Registry Health Examination. A query of registry data through early 2012 showed that approximately 98% of the registry participants identified their exposure location as Vietnam. Exposure data are based on self-reports from veterans and have not been verified by the DoD Manpower Data Center (Washington, DC) or the National Personnel Records Center (St Louis, MO). A number of the registry participants identified sites that had not been identified by the DoD as a location where Agent Orange was sprayed, tested, or stored (eg, Okinawa, Guam, and Alabama).

TABLE 26-1

AGENT ORANGE REGISTRY EVALUATIONS (SEPTEMBER 30, 2013)

Evaluations	No.
Initial	573,088
Follow-up	65,758
Total (Initial + Follow-up)	**638,846**

OUTREACH TO VETERANS

Participation in the Agent Orange Registry offers an opportunity for the veteran to discuss his/her exposure concerns and provide information about research studies, VA healthcare, and other benefits. Veterans who complete an Agent Orange Registry Health Examination are automatically added to the mailing list for the *Agent Orange Review*, a hard-copy newsletter with updates on IOM studies and other research and veteran benefits. Recipients are encouraged to share information in the newsletter with other veterans.

The VA also provides newsletters to all of its healthcare facilities and veterans centers for distribution to veterans and the VA staff. The VA Office of Public Health posts current and archived *Agent Orange Review* newsletters on its website.[8]

LESSONS LEARNED

Numerous limitations have been identified for the Agent Orange Registry. A key one is that as a self-registry, veterans report exposure to Agent Orange without verification that they meet eligibility criteria for having served in an area that DoD identified as a location where Agent Orange was sprayed, stored, or tested. For veterans who do not receive care through the VA healthcare system, it may not be possible for the clinician performing the examination to validate the symptoms or diagnoses that veterans report.

Not all veterans potentially exposed to Agent Orange are aware of the registry. The VA has estimates for the number of veterans who served in Vietnam, but does not possess a master list of all veterans who were potentially exposed. Therefore, the VA relies on veterans to self-identify.

An ongoing area of substantial confusion for veterans is that the registry examination is not a Compensation and Pension Examination for disability compensation. Some veterans mistakenly believe that completing a registry examination will initiate a disability claim, provide medical treatment, or open the door to other benefits.

For the VA staff, Agent Orange Registry Health Examinations can be quite burdensome. Multiple steps are involved in the registry examination process and require two staff members to complete the following:

- scheduling the examination and collecting information via the worksheet prior to it (usually done by the Environmental Health Coordinator);
- documenting medical information on the worksheet during the examination, as well as entering the physical examination into CPRS (usually done by the Environmental Health Clinician); and
- entering worksheet data into the registry database, which is separate from CPRS and requires a username and password, and issuing the follow-up letter (both tasks are usually done by the Environmental Health Coordinator).

Training of Environmental Health Coordinators and Environmental Health Clinicians on the registry process may vary from facility to facility. Often, these staff have multiple, varied responsibilities, and the clinicians and coordinators are not always co-located in the same facility. Environmental Health Coordinators may lack understanding about eligibility criteria and scheduling guidelines. Some facilities have long waits (greater than the recommended 30 days) for registry appointments. For clinicians, a number of facilities have created a built-in Agent Orange Registry template to help guide them through the examination, whereas others may record the examination on a generic physical examination paper form to scan into CPRS later.

Delays of data entry and omission may occur for several reasons. First, registry staff often shoulder a variety of responsibilities and thus may have competing time priorities. Second, the dual-data entry that is necessary because of the database being separate from the electronic health record means that some veterans' data may get entered incompletely, late, or not at all. The VA staff may also not understand the importance of entering the data (eg, that the database is used to monitor trends). Examples include providing newsletters with Agent Orange updates to veterans and being a source of information for responding to congressional or veterans service organization inquiries regarding veterans characteristics in the database. The only way to identify a discrepancy between registry examinations conducted and entries in the registry database would be through a manual process.

The quality, consistency, and usability of registry data are limited by many factors. Quality is limited by the unverified self-reported data. A substantial barrier to consistency exists because many of the data fields take free-form text versus categorical data, which also limits their use for epidemiological studies.

Timeliness is another issue. The lag time between herbicide exposure and completion of the registry examination is 7 years at the least and more than 30 years for veterans currently pursuing a registry examination. Decrements in recall, lack of exposure data, and the unavailability of electronic service records during most of the Vietnam War era limit the validity of information entered into the registry database.

The utility of any database depends on the quality and completeness of the data being entered. As previously described, the Agent Orange Registry has substantial challenges in both regards, restricting meaningful analyses. The ability to evaluate and draw conclusions from the registry is also made more difficult because of the immense size of the database (with over half a million veterans and counting), and many data fields accepting open-ended responses. User-friendly procedures and data entry are important. Less is often more, meaning that the more data requested, the greater the workload and a higher likelihood for incomplete or missing data.

Integration of the Agent Orange Registry Health Examination into the VA's electronic health record would have several advantages to the current system; it could assist eligibility determination, verify self-reported data for veterans who receive their healthcare through the VA, and eliminate the need for dual-data entry. This in turn would improve data timeliness, quality, and consistency. Incorporation into the electronic health record also opens the door for clinicians or other VA staff to run their own data queries on veterans who have completed registry examinations, which enhances the meaningfulness of capturing the data. Having procedures for registry examinations that are different from other examinations steepens the learning curve, impairs clinical workflow, diminishes the ability to identify VA-wide best practices, and makes it more difficult for facilities to adopt them.

The VA will explore integration of registry examinations and data into the electronic health record as resources become available. Another area that could be investigated would be an evaluation of the health benefits and any harm for veterans who receive Agent Orange Registry Health Examinations. The VA has not conducted such an assessment to date, but it would be important to consider before embarking on changes to the current registry process.

SUMMARY

The VA initiated the Agent Orange Registry Health Examination program to respond to veterans' health concerns about possible exposure to Agent Orange and to improve the access of Vietnam veterans to the VA services. More than 30 years later, the registry program is still active, and the number of veterans completing registry examinations continues to grow. The main limitations of the Agent Orange Registry from a research perspective are that veterans self-select to participate, and exposure and health data are not confirmed. The Agent Orange Registry benefits veterans by providing a free evaluation that includes a physical examination, discussion of their exposure concerns with a clinician, and a means for outreach to these veterans by providing updates about relevant health studies and veteran benefits. Integration into the electronic health record could streamline the registry examination process for veterans, improve morale and productivity for clinic staff, increase the quality of examinations, and yield usable data for researchers.

REFERENCES

1. US Department of Veterans Affairs. *Military Exposures—Agent Orange*. Veterans Affairs Office of Public Health website. http://www.publichealth.va.gov/exposures/agentorange/index.asp. Accessed December 14, 2012.

2. Buckingham WA. *Operation Ranch Hand: Herbicides in Southeast Asia*. Air & Space Power Journal website. http://www.airpower.maxwell.af.mil/airchronicles/aureview/1983/jul-aug/buckingham.html. Accessed December 14, 2012.

3. Young AL. The military use of tactical herbicides in Vietnam. In: Young AL. *The History, Use, Disposition and Environmental Fate of Agent Orange*. New York, NY: Springer; 2009: 57–115.

4. Institute of Medicine. *Veterans and Agent Orange: Update 2010*. Washington, DC: The National Academies Press; 2012.

5. US Department of Veterans Affairs. *Veterans Health Administration Handbook 1302.01*. Agent Orange Registry (AOR) Program Procedures to Include All Veterans Exposed to Agent Orange: September 5, 2006. http://www.va.gov/vhapublications/ViewPublication.asp. Accessed December 14, 2012.

6. US Department of Veterans Affairs. Austin Information Technology Center website. http://www.aac.va.gov/aboutaac.php. Accessed November 26, 2012.

7. US Department of Veterans Affairs. *Vietnam Veterans*. Veterans Benefits Administration website. http://benefits.va.gov/PERSONA/veteran-vietnam.asp. Accessed December 19, 2012.

8. US Department of Veterans Affairs. *Publications & Reports on Agent Orange*. Veterans Affairs Public Health website. http://www.publichealth.va.gov/exposures/agentorange/publications/index.asp. Accessed March 11, 2014.

AIRBORNE HAZARDS RELATED TO DEPLOYMENT

Section V: Research Initiatives

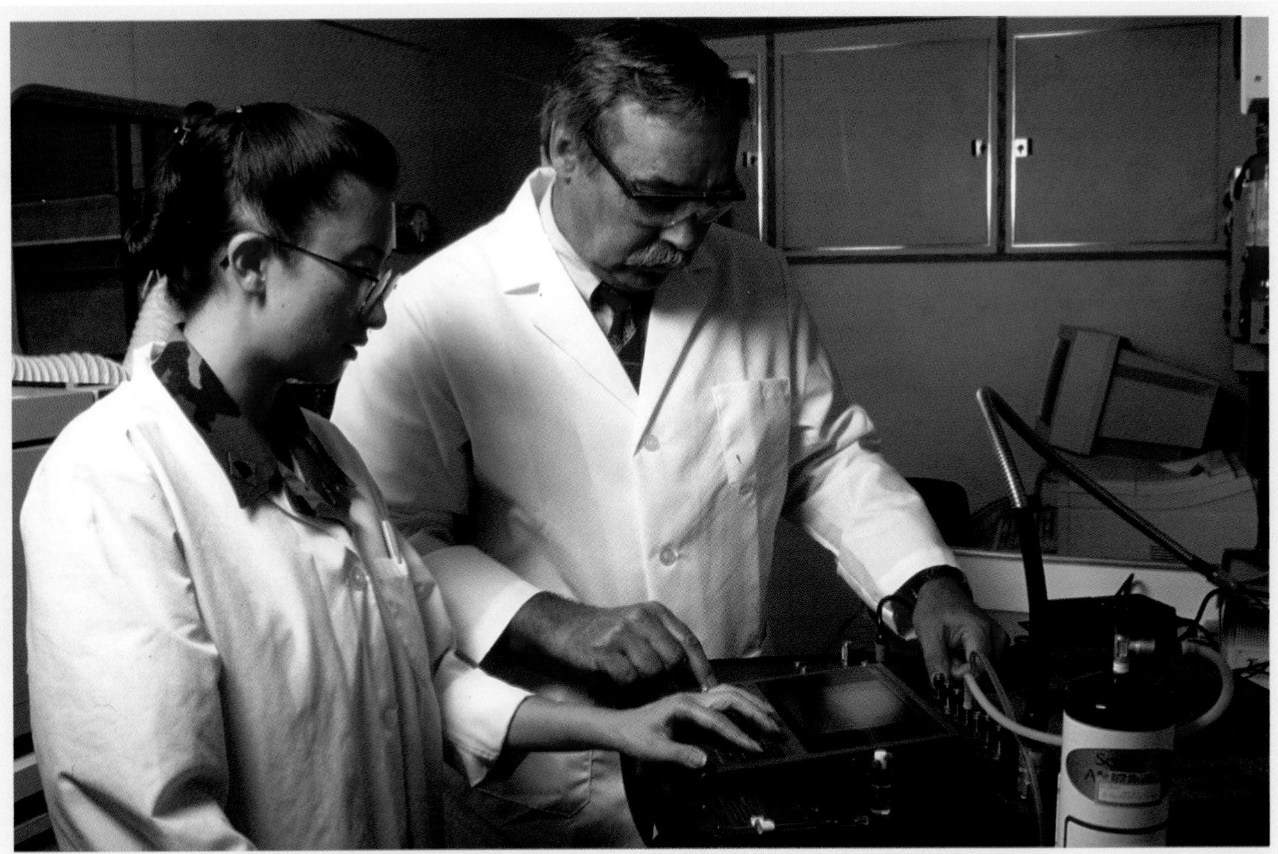

Two researchers conducting laboratory testing.

Photograph: Courtesy of the US Army Public Health Command (Aberdeen Proving Ground, Maryland).

Chapter 27

RESEARCH STUDIES: OVERVIEW AND FUTURE DIRECTIONS

DAVID A. JACKSON, PHD*

**Director, Pulmonary Health Program, US Army Center for Environmental Health Research, 568 Doughten Drive, Fort Detrick, Maryland 21702-5010*

INTRODUCTION

It has been known that service members deployed to southwest Asia (SWA) are exposed to extremely high levels of airborne particulate matter (PM) since early in Operation Iraqi Freedom/Operation Enduring Freedom.[1] The US Army Center for Health Promotion and Preventive Medicine (now the US Army Public Health Command [USAPHC; Aberdeen Proving Ground, MD]) conducted the Enhanced Particulate Matter Survey Program (EPMSP) that analyzed the ambient concentrations and composition of PM at 15 sites throughout SWA. USAPHC also showed that ambient levels of PM in SWA far exceed US Environmental Protection Agency environmental guidelines, National Institute for Occupational Safety and Health (NIOSH; Washington, DC) and Occupational Safety and Health Administration occupational levels, and military exposure guidelines.[2] Adverse health effects, including cardiovascular and pulmonary diseases, are well-established consequences of exposure to high levels of PM, with aerodynamic diameters of <10 μm (PM_{10}) and especially less than 2.5 μm ($PM_{2.5}$).[3] The severity of the effects depends on the amount and duration of the exposure, the physical and chemical characteristics of the PM, and the health of the exposed individuals. In addition to exposure to high levels of ambient PM in theater, many service members have been exposed to combustion products from burn pits in which shipping materials, and occupational, food, and residential wastes were incinerated. Exposure to the smoke has been associated with dermal and respiratory irritations.[4] Although there is reasonable cause for concern that these exposures might result in long-term adverse health effects, at present there is neither clear evidence that disease is associated with these exposures nor adequate data to develop reliable risk assessments.

In 2004, Shorr and coworkers[5] reported on an 18-case cluster of acute eosinophilic pneumonia with two mortalities among soldiers deployed to Iraq. They were unable to determine a likely cause for the cluster of this rare disease, although ~80% of patients had recently begun to smoke, and acute eosinophilic pneumonia has been reported to be associated with smoking in a small number of cases.[6] One distinguishing feature of this cohort was that all but one of the patients reported exposures to high levels of ambient dust.

In 2011, King and colleagues[7] described a case series of 80 soldiers from Fort Campbell, KY, who were referred to Vanderbilt University Medical Center (Nashville, TN) between February 2004 and December 2009 for evaluation of exertional dyspnea. Forty-nine of these patients received thoracoscopic lung biopsies. All biopsied patients exhibited lung abnormalities, and 38 of the 49 patients were diagnosed as having a rare condition: constrictive bronchiolitis (CB). The CB patients were described as having experienced exposure to dust storms (33/38); exposure to the sulfur fire at the Al Mishraq sulfur mine in 2003 (28/38); as well as exposure to burn pit, human waste, and combat smoke.

Epidemiological studies have suggested that there are modest increases in respiratory symptoms among service members and veterans who have deployed to SWA.[8–10] The Armed Forces Health Surveillance Center (Silver Spring, MD) performed a large epidemiological study of service members stationed in operating bases with and without burn pits, and also performed a study of personnel stationed near civilian incinerators. At most, the study found limited evidence of association between living in proximity to an incineration site and increased risk of adverse health outcomes[4] (see Chapter 6: Epidemiology of Airborne Hazards in the Deployed Environment and Chapter 7: Discussion Summary: Defining Health Outcomes in Epidemiological Investigations of Populations Deployed in Support of Operation Iraqi Freedom and Operation Enduring Freedom).

In contrast, reports in the popular press ascribe diseases in service members and veterans, ranging from cancers to substantial impairments in respiratory function to exposure to PM and burn pit smoke.[11–13] Advocacy groups such as Burnpits 360° (Robstown, TX)[14] and the Sergeant Thomas Joseph Sullivan Center (Washington, DC)[15] also assert that exposures to dust and smoke during deployment to SWA have resulted in ill health of service members and veterans.

In response to concerns about potential health issues arising from inhalational exposures in SWA, a number of working groups (WGs) have been convened in efforts to develop frameworks for understanding risks and developing solutions. The Joint Particulate Matter Working Group, charted by the US Department of Defense, met at the NIOSH in 2005 to investigate potential health issues related to this ongoing PM exposure. The group identified a number of knowledge gaps that included the physical and chemical characteristics of ambient PM in SWA and assessment of its toxicity.[1] In 2010, Dr Cecile Rose (Director, Occupational and Environmental Medicine Clinic) at National Jewish Health in Denver, CO, organized a meeting attended by representatives of the Army, Navy, and Veterans Affairs, as well as private and academic healthcare providers. In addition to considering the state of science related to deployment-related pulmonary health threats, participants also considered approaches for performing surveillance and evaluating respiratory health in the context of deployment. Like the Joint Particulate Matter Working Group, this body concluded that there was not adequate toxicological, epidemiological, or clinical data to adequately evaluate either the scope or severity of adverse effects of inhalational exposures in troops deployed to SWA. Outcomes and recommendations of this meeting are reported and expanded on in a special issue of the *Journal of Occupational and Environmental Health.*[16]

In addition to the WGs previously described, two independent reviews of the state of knowledge about airborne hazards in SWA were commissioned from the National Academy of Science (Washington, DC). The USAPHC commissioned an independent review of the EPMSP by the Committee on Toxicology of the National Academy of Sciences that was published in 2010.[17] Despite the breadth of the EPMSP, the Committee concluded that there was not enough data relating the knowledge of the chemistry and abundance of ambient PM to health effects to provide a foundation for health risk assessment. Similarly, a 2011 report—commissioned from the Institute of Medicine (Washington, DC) by the US Department of Veterans Affairs on the possible effects of exposure to burn pit smoke in Iraq and Afghanistan—failed to find sufficient evidence to evaluate possible risks from exposures to burn pit combustion products.[18]

Following the National Jewish Health Working Group, it was clear that a coordinated effort to resolve issues related to deployment-related respiratory disease would be required because available data were limited, conflicting, and drawn from diverse sources. In response to this problem, a new Pulmonary Health Task Area was proposed by the Military Operational Medicine Research Program (MOMRP; Fort Detrick, MD) of the US Army Medical Research and Materiel Command (MRMC; Fort Detrick, MD) with the support of the MRMC commander. In June 2010 and December 2011, MOMRP brought together diverse groups of experts to examine the current medical and scientific evidence and to formulate an integrated, multidisciplinary research plan to address the issue of deployment-related respiratory disease. These WGs, chaired by the author, included representatives of all four services; the Department of Veterans Affairs; and academic experts in pulmonary medicine, toxicology, pulmonary pathology, occupational and preventive medicine, computer science, and epidemiology. The WGs considered the available scientific, epidemiological, and medical evidence, and provided a gap analysis and recommendations for the prioritization of research.

Although the relevant epidemiological and clinical data are presented elsewhere in this book (see Chapter 6: Epidemiology of Airborne Hazards in the Deployed Environment, Chapter 7: Discussion Summary: Defining Health Outcomes in Epidemiological Investigations of Populations Deployed in Support of Operation Iraqi Freedom and Operation Enduring Freedom, and Chapter 31: Update on Key Studies), the current research discussed herein focuses primarily on data from experimental toxicology studies that are largely complete. This chapter also briefly covers some ongoing research that has not been described elsewhere. The Future Research section of this chapter presents the proposed clinical research summaries of the MOMRP WGs.

CURRENT RESEARCH

A number of research projects have been undertaken by US Department of Defense-funded researchers in response to historical concerns about exposures to PM in SWA and in response to concerns expressed by the WGs. These projects will fall within the scope of future research areas proposed by the MOMRP WGs, but it is worth noting that some of them had already commenced before those WGs met.

Several studies have addressed the toxicity of dusts from SWA. Wilfong and coworkers[19] at the Naval Health Effects Laboratory at Wright-Patterson Air Force Base (now the Naval Medical Research Unit-Dayton; NAMRU-D) exposed rats to PM collected at Camp Buehring, Kuwait. PM was collected inside closed tents from precleaned surfaces and sieved to ≤10 μm in diameter. In addition, PM was suspended in phosphate-buffered saline, and 1, 5, or 10 mg of PM in buffer was injected intratracheally into the lungs of rats. Control exposures were performed with equal masses of titanium dioxide (negative control) and silica (positive control) particles of similar size. Animals were harvested at 1, 3, and 7 days and 6 months postexposure. Based on biochemical, histological, and cell profile data, both the Camp Buehring PM and titanium dioxide particles provoked a mild transient inflammatory response in the lungs that was largely resolved in 7 days and completely resolved in 6 months. Positive control silica particles provoked a lasting inflammatory response that persisted through the 6-month experiment. The authors also examined the histology of the spleen, testis, and kidney, but found no abnormalities attributable to exposure to the PM.

A second study led by NAMRU-D (Dorman et al[20]) investigated the effects of the pulmonary health threats of tobacco smoking and inhalational exposure to PM from Iraq singly and in combination in rat studies. As noted previously, exposure to fine PM is common for service members deployed to SWA, and there is an increased incidence of new-onset and recidivist smoking in active duty military personnel.[21] Rats were exposed to mainstream cigarette smoke or air using a nose-only exposure system for 3 hours/day, 5 days/week for 4 weeks. At this time, rats also began to be exposed to aerosolized silica particles (positive control) or surface soil collected at Camp Victory near Baghdad, Iraq, for 19 hours/day for 2 weeks in whole-body inhalation chambers. Although the soil used in this study was not extensively characterized, it is reasonable to assume that it is substantially similar to the Camp Victory soil analyzed in the EPMSP that contained chiefly clay minerals and low amounts of silica.[2] Soil and silica particles were size fractionated and blown into the inhalation chambers at approximately 1 mg/m^3, with mean aerodynamic diameters of 1.7 and 1.4 μm, respectively.

This study examined a large number of variables, including

- standard clinical parameters,
- plethysmography,
- histopathology,
- bronchiolar lavage biochemistry,
- cell profiles and proteomics, and
- global gene expression in the lung.

Despite the comprehensiveness of this study, few responses attributable to soil particle exposure were identified. Inflammation was minimal in either soil- or silica-exposed animals based on histopathological assessment, although the prevalence of indicators of inflammation was greater in animals exposed to silica. Similarly, gene expression and proteomics data are suggestive of mild inflammation in exposed animals, with silica eliciting somewhat greater responses. No statistically significant differences from control in lung function measures were found for soil- or silica-exposed animals.

The findings with particle exposures alone contrast strongly with the results of mainstream cigarette smoke exposures either in combination with soil or silica particles or alone. Histological lesions, alterations in cell profiles in lavage fluid, reduced body weight, and abnormal plethysmographic results were apparent. Although there was some evidence of interaction between particle and smoke exposures, particularly in the gene and protein expression data, the largest effects throughout the experiment resulted from cigarette smoke exposure. The authors concluded that pulmonary toxicity of the Camp Victory surface soil is qualitatively similar to, but less than, the toxicity of silica.

Two roughly parallel studies, conducted by the author's research program at the US Army Center for Environmental Health Research and NIOSH, attempted to address the toxicity of PM from SWA (A. Jackson, personal communication, 2013) by examining the effects of a single intratracheal instillation in rats of ambient PM collected at Camp Victory. PM was collected using high-volume air samplers designed to capture airborne particles 10 µm in diameter and smaller at Camp Victory during the spring of 2008 and the spring of 2009 by US Army Center for Health Promotion and Preventive Medicine (now USAPHC) personnel. In the first study, rats were exposed to 2.5, 5.0, or 10 mg/kg PM collected in 2008 or a fine, standard, freshly fractured silica (obtained from Dr Vince Castranova at NIOSH) in buffered saline and examined 3, 7, 30, 60, 120, or 150 days later. The control was buffer only. The 2008 dust-exposed animals showed early evidence of inflammation and tissue damage in the lung as judged by cell counts and the presence of lactate dehydrogenase and albumin in the bronchiolar lavage fluid collected from the animals. However, inflammation largely abated in 7 days and was not evident at the longest time tested (120 days). In contrast, silica-exposed animals showed persistent inflammation by these measures up to 120 days. Histological examination of lung tissue from the animals extending to 150 days was consistent with the biochemical and cell profile analyses, and the animals exposed to silica-positive control showed fibrotic and potentially neoplastic changes.

The second exposure study had several aims:

- to determine whether their observations with the 2008 PM were reproducible and whether the ambient environmental dust was similar toxicologically over time;
- to compare the toxicity of the 2008 and 2009 dust samples with a standard reference material that had some similarity to a well-studied US exposure and was less toxic than the silica control typically used in this type of study; and
- to make a head-to-head comparison of the Camp Victory PM with the Camp Buehring dust tested by Wilfong and coworkers (generously provided by V Mokashi, NAMRU-D).

A well-characterized US urban PM (or USPM) collected in the St. Louis, MO, area during the 1970s was selected as a reference material.[22] Rats were exposed by intratracheal instillation to 2.5, 5.0, and 10.0 mg/kg environmental PM in buffered saline. Again, silica served as a positive control, and the buffer served only as a negative control. Histology of lung tissue from the rats was evaluated at 60, 120, and 150 days (silica, 2009 dust, USPM). Because the 2008 Camp Victory and Camp Buehring sample materials were limited, animals exposed to these PMs were examined only at 120 and 150 days.

Results of this follow-on experiment were consistent with the earlier ones. Mild small airway changes (distortion and fibrosis of terminal bronchioles) and centriacinar emphysematous lesions were associated with exposure to all the dusts in this experiment. Emphysematous changes were most severe in animals exposed to the USPM, which has a high combustion product content[22] rather than mineral materials like the Camp Victory[20] and Camp Buehring PMs.[19] Because of the report of CB in troops returning from SWA by King and coworkers,[7] airways 180 to 360 µm in diameter were given careful attention in a reexamination of histological materials. However, no evidence of CB is in the sense of circumferential fibrosis with luminal constriction was observed.

Environmental PM tested from Iraq and Kuwait does not appear to be highly acutely toxic, although repeated exposure might lead to obstructive disease or allergic lung disease (eg, hypersensitivity pneumonitis or asthma in some individuals). However, differences between human and rat anatomies and between experimental rat exposure and environmental exposure conditions experienced by soldiers do not permit definitive conclusions to be drawn.

A number of studies at Brooke Army Medical Center (Fort Sam Houston, TX), funded in whole or in part through MOMRP, have been undertaken in an attempt to determine the prevalence of pulmonary disease in active duty military, develop case definitions, evaluate pre-/postdeployment spirometry for health surveillance, and improve clinical characterization of patients complaining primarily of exertional dyspnea. These studies will not be addressed further here because they are discussed in Chapter 6: Epidemiology of Airborne Hazards in the Deployed Environment, Chapter 8: Pulmonary Function Testing—Spirometry Testing for Population Surveillance, and Chapter 31: Update on Key Studies.

The cluster of CB cases diagnosed at Vanderbilt Medical Center and controversy surrounding them[23,24] highlighted the need for an objective system for diagnosing small airways disease. The MOMRP of the MRMC awarded a 3-year grant to investigators at National Jewish Health and Vanderbilt University to develop a standardized method for quantifying small airways abnormalities. This study is ongoing and has assembled a team of pathologists, established scoring criteria, and prepared test sets of slides for evaluation that include the CB specimens from Vanderbilt Medical School, CB lung samples from the Lung Tissue Research Consortium (National Heart, Lung, and Blood Institute [Bethesda, MD]), and normal lung tissue from the International Institute for the Advancement of Medicine (Edison, NJ).

The possible role of exposure to combustion products from open burn pits in the pathogenesis of a variety of disease states is a matter of some concern to service members and families,[13,14] as well as the military and US Department of Veterans Affairs medical communities. This has been evidenced by the Armed Forces Health Surveillance Center epidemiological study[4] of possible effects of burn pit exposure and by the Institute of Medicine report[18] on the issue commissioned by the Department of Veterans Affairs. In July 2012, according to Commander Daniel Hardt, NAMRU-D had undertaken direct studies to assess the toxicity of burn pit smoke using cell culture exposures to combustion products from reconstituted burn pit material mixtures. Composition of the combustion plume had been analyzed, and evaluation of the toxic responses of the exposed cells was under way. NAMRU-D has recently obtained funding to extend its research to more relevant animal experiments.

In an effort to develop an understanding of the types of lung disease that may be associated with deployment, the Joint Pathology Center (Silver Spring, MD) has initiated efforts to investigate pathologies evident in surgical lung specimens from deployed service members. In March 2013, Dr Michael Lewin-Smith acknowledged that the study would also investigate whether there is evidence of an association between pulmonary lesions and the composition of PM in lung specimens.

In a 2012 presentation to the Pulmonary Health in Deployed Environments In-Process Review, Drs Bora Sul and Jaques Reifman described how the MRMC's Bioinformatics High Performance Computing Software Applications Institute (Fort Detrick, MD), with the assistance of Brooke Army Medical Center, has undertaken a combined computational and physical modeling effort to ascertain whether obstructions and functional alterations in the small branches of the bronchial tree perturb air flow in ways that may be detectable using magnetic resonance imaging. Such an approach could significantly improve diagnostics and potentially reduce the number of thoracoscopic biopsies that are necessary for diagnosis of lung disease.

FUTURE RESEARCH

On June 22–23, 2010 and December 1–2, 2011, the Military Operational Medicine Research Area Directorate convened a WG of military service, Veterans Affairs, and extramural experts to provide direction for a proposed Defense Health Program-funded task area that would manage a structured research effort investigating pulmonary health threats of deployed service members. It should be noted that a few of the studies discussed herein have actually begun since the WGs met. It is currently expected that the task area will be funded and begin studies in federal Fiscal Year 2014.

The WGs were charged with the following:

- identifying data gaps or threats related to respiratory health risks for service members in SWA,
- determining research approaches to address data gaps,
- indicating competencies or capabilities required to address threats, and
- prioritizing efforts to address the data gaps and required competencies.

Both WGs recognized four broad areas of research:

1. clinical studies,
2. animal studies,
3. biomarkers, and
4. epidemiology/exposure assessment.

The WGs also recognized four principal knowledge gaps:

1. disease prevalence and severity,
2. disease screening and diagnosis,
3. toxicity/pathogenicity of PM, and
4. intervention and treatment.

The two WGs reached very similar conclusions, and a consensus is presented here. Proposed and prioritized projects (in order of decreasing priority within sections) are also described. It is expected that the findings of these projects will form the basis for initial decision-making when the task area is implemented.

Clinical Studies

Clinical studies were recognized as foundational for establishing case definitions of deployment-related pulmonary disease and for determining its prevalence and severity. Several types of studies were proposed to address the issue of disease prevalence and severity. A retrospective chart review study and a postdeployment respiratory health study of service members with dyspnea were put forward because they could be rapidly initiated and executed. The postdeployment study could also serve as a pilot/feasibility study for a larger pre- and postdeployment assessment of pulmonary health in deployed service members. Both patient studies would include collecting biosamples for a proposed repository and collecting biosamples for biochemical biomarker discovery, along with patient histories, pulmonary function, and imaging data. A number of these studies have begun, and preliminary findings are described elsewhere in this book.

In addition, provided that data of sufficiently high quality could be collected, a study of indigenous Iraqis who were continuously exposed to the SWA environment might reveal long-term effects that are difficult to discern in deployed service members in the short term. Analysis of lung samples taken at autopsy from deployed service members might reveal undiagnosed and/or subclinical disease that foreshadow later health outcomes.

A final issue was the well-publicized diagnosis of CB in some soldiers by open lung biopsy at Vanderbilt University Medical Center. A careful, independent study of these patients and controls was proposed to assess the association of the morphological features seen in these patients with disease. This study has already begun.

The following nine summary points of the proposed clinical research is provided here in order of decreasing priority (based on a tradeoff of cost, feasibility, and importance for filling the identified data gaps):

1. perform a retrospective chart study of active duty military personnel diagnosed with chronic lung disease;
2. create a registry of all military personnel diagnosed with chronic pulmonary disease (see section on Biomarkers);
3. evaluate postdeployment military personnel with complaints of new-onset dyspnea to determine the etiology of pulmonary disease and the utility of clinical evaluation (see section on Biomarkers);
4. carry out a pre- and postdeployment evaluation of military personnel to determine the incidence of postdeployment disease (see section on Biomarkers);
5. complete a pre- and postdeployment screening to determine whether spirometry can serve as a sensitive measure of underlying lung disease;
6. standardize diagnostic methods for patients with small airways disease, including the CB cases seen at Vanderbilt University Medical Center;
7. perform a review of lung specimens from autopsies to determine whether there is undiagnosed lung disease in deployed, compared with nondeployed, military personnel (if available);
8. evaluate the respiratory health of the native Iraqi/Afghanistan population to determine the incidence and severity of background pulmonary disease; and
9. test whether spirometry and chest X-ray film screening on entry to service can predict lung disease in a longitudinal pre-/postdeployment study.

Animal Studies

Because clinical studies are limited by standard-of-care considerations and are largely descriptive, the WGs discussed a number of animal studies for the direct determination of the toxicity and pathogenicity of PM and sulfur fire combustion products, development of biomarkers of disease, and studies of the mechanisms of pulmonary disease to address the toxicity/pathogenicity and disease screening/diagnosis gaps. In particular, WGs recommended rodent toxicity studies and studies of the pulmonary health of working dogs. The WGs proposed studying the toxicity of PM from several localities and the effects of repeated PM exposures. Several of these studies have begun and have been described previously.

The WG also proposed examining the pulmonary health of deployed working dogs exposed to the same environmental conditions as deployed service members over substantial periods of time. The dogs receive comprehensive veterinary workups, and a large number of tissue samples collected at necropsy are available. During checkups or at necropsy, collection of biosamples for biomarker studies may be possible.

Both the dog and rat populations are more homogeneous than humans and are likely to support small studies with useful statistical power.

The following five summary points of the proposed clinical research is described here in order of decreasing priority:

1. determine the toxicity/pathogenicity of ambient SWA PM collected from multiple sites in rat single intratracheal instillation studies;

2. complete a longitudinal study of the pulmonary health of working dogs,
3. perform a lung necropsy study of deployed/non-deployed working dogs for toxicity and pathology,
4. carry out experiments with repeated exposures of rats to PM from SWA to test the toxic effects of chronic exposure in contrast to single exposure studies, and
5. determine the mechanism and pathogenesis of lung injury using a known lung toxicant (eg, crystalline silica).

Biomarkers, Biosample Repository, and Chronic Pulmonary Injury Registry

Practically speaking, the biomarkers focus area cannot readily be separated from the clinical and animal studies that will provide the samples and raw data for its studies. However, the research methods and aims are sufficiently different to warrant a separate discussion. Data and samples will be acquired from the clinical and animal studies described herein.

Developing biomarkers to improve the diagnosis of pulmonary disease and to monitor disease progression was recognized as a high priority need for both the disease prevalence and severity gap and the disease screening and diagnosis gap. Two types of biomarkers were identified: (1) molecular and (2) physiological. Molecular biomarkers are biochemical entities; ribonucleic acid molecules; proteins; or small molecules that can be measured in blood, bronchoalveolar lavage fluid (BALF), or other biological matrices to improve diagnosis and monitor disease progression. Physiological biomarkers represent information derived from functional measurements of the mechanics or effectiveness of respiration. Such biomarkers would be based on pulmonary function tests, impulse oscillometry, bronchoprovocation, or other functional or mechanical data sources.

A prospective registry of data from current military personnel with diagnosed postdeployment lung disease and a repository for biosamples were also recognized as high priority needs. The registry would permit tracking the progression of disease and could be potentially mined for common factors associated with the development of respiratory disease. A biosample repository containing samples from individuals in the registry and from clinical studies (eg, postdeployment evaluations of dyspneic service members or pre-/post-deployment evaluations of military personnel) could provide materials for biomarker validation and, potentially, even discovery since the emergence and diagnosis of progressive pulmonary disease could be delayed for months or years. Relevant biosamples could include blood, urine, and BALF. The registry of patients with chronic respiratory disease should include deployment and occupational history, as well as demographic and clinical data (including high-resolution computed tomography scans, baseline pulmonary function tests, and physical fitness test data).

The following four summary points of the proposed clinical research is described here in order of decreasing priority:

1. establish a prospective US Department of Defense registry, including current military personnel with diagnosed postdeployment lung disease and a biomarker repository (see section on Clinical Studies);
2. identify/validate molecular and physiological biomarkers of disease and disease progression in military personnel participating in the postdeployment STAMPEDE 1 (Study of Active-Duty Military for Pulmonary Disease Related to Environmental Dust Exposure-1) study of service members with dyspnea using biosamples and physiological data (see section on Clinical Studies);
3. identify/validate molecular and physiological biomarkers in a pre-/postdeployment clinical study of service members with a comprehensive pulmonary evaluation using physiological measurements and biosamples (see summary point 2; also see section on Clinical Studies); and
4. identify candidate molecular and physiological biomarkers of lung injury and disease progression in BALF, blood, urine, and physiological measurements in controlled lung injury studies in rats (see section on Animal Studies).

Epidemiology/Exposure Assessment

Because the Clinical Studies focus area does not have the ability to examine large numbers of service members, epidemiological and exposure assessment methods are required to capture subtle and rare effects of deployment on respiratory health. In addition, by taking advantage of existing databases (eg, the Millennium Cohort Study, Military Health System, TRICARE, and The Total Army Injury and Health Outcomes Database) with time depth, a historical perspective on pulmonary disease diagnoses among service members can be generated. Building on the historical perspective, prospective continuing epidemiological studies may provide insights into the chronicity of deployment-related respiratory disease. Thus, the Epidemiology/Exposure Assessment focus area provides expeditious and cost-effective tools for identifying possible associations among deployment, disease, and PM exposures.

The WGs proposed several Epidemiology/Exposure Assessment studies to address the identified data gaps. A retrospective overview of pulmonary health in deployed service members could be developed to serve as a baseline for contemporary and prospective evaluations of respiratory disease related to deployment. Possible adverse effects of PM exposure on deployed service members could be examined by linking demographic and personnel details with medical information in the Military Health System (MHS; inpatient and outpatient data, TRICARE encounter data) to PM and other exposure data (country of deployment, proximity to large burn pits). Because the Millennium Cohort Study is planned to extend until 2022, studies to evaluate the chronicity of deployment-related disease that extend well beyond the limits of the active military career could be performed. Although none of the currently available resources addresses all possible service members—eg, Reserve and National Guard members are underrepresented—and none of the databases contain all service member information, the WG considered that there was a sufficient wealth of facts and figures relevant to the data gaps that the epidemiology and exposure assessment will play critical roles in eliminating the identified knowledge gaps.

The following five summary points of the proposed clinical research is described here in order of decreasing priority:

1. examine historical trends in ICD-9 (*International Classification of Diseases, Ninth Revision*) pulmonary diagnoses among active duty US Army soldiers since 1985;
2. perform a historical prospective study of service member post-deployment, and examine the relationship between PM exposures, deployment, and pulmonary disease using USAPHC surveillance data, MHS healthcare (ICD-9 pulmonary diagnostic codes), personnel, and deployment records;
3. complete a study of the relationship between PM exposures, deployment, and pulmonary health using USAPHC surveillance data, MHS, deployment, and personnel records for active duty participants in the Millennium Cohort Study;
4. perform a 10-year longitudinal study to establish the chronicity of pulmonary disease in deployed service members using USAPHC PM surveillance data, MHS, personnel, and deployment records for participants in the Millennium Cohort Study; and
5. develop and validate an improved exposure assessment survey instrument to more effectively identify exposures and high-risk service members.

SUMMARY

These WGs and independent committees reached substantially consonant conclusions about the state of knowledge of health risks associated with exposure to ambient PM in SWA. The MOMRP Pulmonary Health Task Area Working Group identified four major data gaps:

1. prevalence and severity of deployment-related disease,
2. methods for diagnosis and screening,
3. intervention and treatment, and
4. toxicity and pathogenicity of SWA PM.

The WG also proposed priorities for research in four specific focus areas:

1. clinical research,
2. animal models of toxicity,
3. biomarkers, and
4. exposure assessment.

As new information emerges from ongoing research in both the military and civilian settings, it is certain that the details of the broad research plan described herein will be adapted to account for that new knowledge. Nevertheless, the program as currently envisioned, seems to be well designed to provide answers to critical questions related to airborne hazards experienced by service members deployed to SWA.

Acknowledgment

This research was sponsored by the Military Operational Medicine Research Program of the US Army Medical Research and Materiel Command, Department of the Army, Fort Detrick, MD.

REFERENCES

1. Weese CB, Abraham JH. Potential health implications associated with particulate matter exposure in southwest Asia. *Inhal Toxicol.* 2009;21:291–296.

2. Engelbrecht JP, McDonald EV, Gillies JA, Jayanty RK, Casuccio G, Gertler AW. Characterizing mineral dusts and other aerosols from the Middle East. Part 1. Ambient sampling. *Inhal Toxicol.* 2009;21:297–326.

3. Davidson CI, Phalen RF, Solomon PA. Airborne particulate matter and human health: a review. *Aerosol Sci Technol.* 2005;39:737–749.

4. Armed Forces Health Surveillance Center. *Epidemiological Studies of Health Outcomes Among Troops Deployed to Burn Pit Sites.* San Diego, CA: The Naval Health Research Center (and the U.S. Army Public Health Command–Provisional, Edgewood, MD); May 2010.

5. Shorr AF, Scoville SL, Cersovsky SB, et al. Acute eosinophilic pneumonia among US military personnel deployed in or near Iraq. *JAMA.* 2004;292:2997–3005.

6. Galvin JR, Franks TJ. Smoking–related lung disease. *J Thorac Imaging.* 2009;24:274–284.

7. King MS, Eisenberg R, Newman JH, et al. Constrictive bronchiolitis in soldiers returning from Iraq and Afghanistan. *N Engl J Med.* 2011;365:222–230.

8. Smith B, Wong CA, Smith TC, Boyko EJ, Gacksetter GS, Ryan MAK. Newly reported respiratory symptoms and conditions among military personnel deployed to Iraq and Afghanistan: a prospective population-based study. *Am J Epidemiol.* 2009;170:1433–1442.

9. Szema AM, Peters MC, Weissinger KM, Gagliano CA, Chen JJ. New-onset asthma among soldiers serving in Iraq and Afghanistan. *Allergy Asthma Proc.* 2010;31:67–71.

10. Abraham JH, DeBakey SF, Reid L, Zhou J, Baird C. Does deployment to Iraq and Afghanistan affect respiratory health of US military personnel? *J Occup Environ Med.* 2012;54:740–745.

11. Kennedy K. Balad burn pit harmed troops living 1 mile away. *Army Times.* January 23, 2010. http://www.armytimes.com/news/2010/01/military_burn_pit_011810w/. Accessed September 19, 2010.

12. Kennedy K. Lung disease of soldier linked to burn pits. *Army Times.* July 2, 2009. http://www.armytimes.com/news/2009/06/military_burnpits_lungs_063009w/. Accessed September 19, 2010.

13. Peeples L. Gulf war syndrome, other illnesses among veterans may be due to toxic environments. *The Huffington Post.* February 7, 2013. http://www.huffingtonpost.com/2013/02/07/gulf-war-syndrome-veterans_n_2634838.html. Accessed February 22, 2013.

14. Burnpits 360° website. *Invisible Wounds of Toxic Exposure.* http://burnpits360.org. Accessed February 22, 2013.

15. Sergeant Sullivan Center. *He Found a Diagnosis, Solving a Medical Mystery for Veterans: Dr. Robert Miller: Excellence in Post-deployment Health.* http://www.sgtsullivancenter.org/press-release-dr.robert-miller.html. Accessed February 22, 2013.

16. Teichmann R. Health effects of deployment to Afghanistan and Iraq. *J Occup Environ Med.* 2012;54:655–764.

17. National Research Council. *Review of the Department of Defense Enhanced Particulate Matter Surveillance Program Report.* Washington, DC: National Academy Press; 2010: 10–11, 51–56.

18. Baird CP. Review of the Institute of Medicine report: long-term health consequences of exposure to burn pits in Iraq and Afghanistan. *US Army Med Dept J.* 2012;July–Sept:43–47.

19. Wilfong ER, Lyles M, Tietcheck R, et al. The acute and long-term effects of Middle East sand particles on the rat airway following a single intratracheal instillation. *J Toxicol Environ Health A*. 2011;74:1351–1365.

20. Dorman DC, Mokashi V, Wagner DJ, et al. Biological responses in rats exposed to cigarette smoke and Middle East sand (dust). *Inhal Toxicol*. 2012;24:109–124.

21. Poston WS, Taylor JE, Hoffman KA, et al. Smoking and deployment: perspectives of junior enlisted US Air Force and US Army personnel and their supervisors. *Mil Med*. 2008;173:441–447.

22. National Institute of Standards and Technology. *Standard Reference Material 1648a [Certificate of Analysis]*. Gaithersburg, MD: 2012.

23. Morris MJ, Zacher LL. Constrictive bronchiolitis in soldiers [letter]. *N Engl J Med*. 2011;365:1743–1745.

24. Kushner WG. Constrictive bronchiolitis in soldiers [letter]. *N Engl J Med*. 2011;365:1744.

Chapter 28

CONSIDERATIONS REGARDING BIOMONITORING

CAMILLA A. MAUZY, PhD*; LISA M. KIRK BROWN, DrPH†; COLEEN P. BAIRD, MD, MPH‡; AND CAROLE TINKLEPAUGH, MD, MPH§

*Biomarker/Biomonitor Development Project Director, Aerospace Toxicology Program, Molecular Bioeffects Branch (RHDJ), 711th Human Performance Wing, Air Force Research Laboratory, Wright-Patterson Air Force Base, Ohio 45433

†Adjunct Professor, Uniformed Services University of the Health Sciences, 4301 Jones Bridge Road, Bethesda, Maryland 20814

‡Program Manager, Environmental Medicine Program, Occupational and Environmental Medicine Portfolio, Army Institute of Public Health, US Army Public Health Command, 5158 Blackhawk Road, Aberdeen Proving Ground, Maryland 21010-5403

§Occupational Medicine Physician, Environmental Medicine Program, US Army Public Health Command, 5158 Blackhawk Road, Aberdeen Proving Ground, Maryland 21010-5403

INTRODUCTION

Determining Military Exposures

Reliable estimates of acute or chronic exposures of large military populations in constant flux in theater have been difficult, with multiple assessments reporting minimal or no health associations.[1–4] Therefore, the study of exposure/health outcome associations in service members following deployment has been limited by a lack of individual exposure information, as discussed elsewhere in this book. In addition, individual variability, including susceptibility characteristics (eg, genetics and epigenetics, preexisting health conditions, and psychosocial stress) plays a role in the overall risk and development of disease. Strategies to improve exposure monitoring and risk assessment have been suggested in other chapters, including localized or personal detection devices for monitoring of airborne and chemical hazards, optimization of current techniques (eg, spirometry), and new epidemiology approaches. In addition to these strategies, biomonitoring has been proposed as another approach.[5,6] Past utility of biomonitor techniques focused on the determination of the body burden of environmental chemicals (xenobiotics) of interest. For exposures with sufficient dose–response information, the internal dose as determined by this method may correlate with potential health effects. However, a newer and more encompassing definition of biological monitoring includes the quantitative detection of the molecular changes that occur in the body on exposure.[7]

The Exposome

With the described difficulties establishing accurate individual exposure levels using traditional methods, more recent efforts have been focused on determining the body's own molecular signatures to indicate types and levels of exposures.[8–10] The term *exposome*, coined by Dr Christopher Wild in 2005,[11] has come to signify alternations in the body that occur on acute and chronic environmental exposures over a lifetime, as well as individual social determinants that also play a role in outcome.[12] In effect, Wild has suggested that a person's exposome data could be used to track a lifetime of environmental exposures, and used to identify *individualized* risk and disease outcome. Such data could be seen as the exposure ancillary to the personalized medicine thrusts in both military[13] and civilian[14] populations.

WHAT ARE BIOMARKERS?

Definition of the term *biomarker* varies depending on scientific focus and use, but the formal definition recognized by the National Institutes of Health is "a characteristic that is objectively measured and evaluated as an indicator of normal biological processes, pathogenic processes, or pharmacological responses to a therapeutic intervention."[15] With this broad definition, a biomarker would include any molecular entity produced by the body, a xenobiotic or its metabolites inside the body, or even measurement of physical or cognitive attributes. In each case, however, the biomarker will reflect, in a quantitative manner, the interaction between a biological system and an exposure.[16] Thus, within the National Institutes of Health definition, the utility of biomarkers spans a continuum from exposure to physiological effect, as well as susceptibility to exposures or outcomes (Figure 28-1). Desirable biomarkers are accurate, minimally or noninvasive, economical, easily repeated, and accessible.[17] Biomarkers should also be stable with a relatively long half-life in the

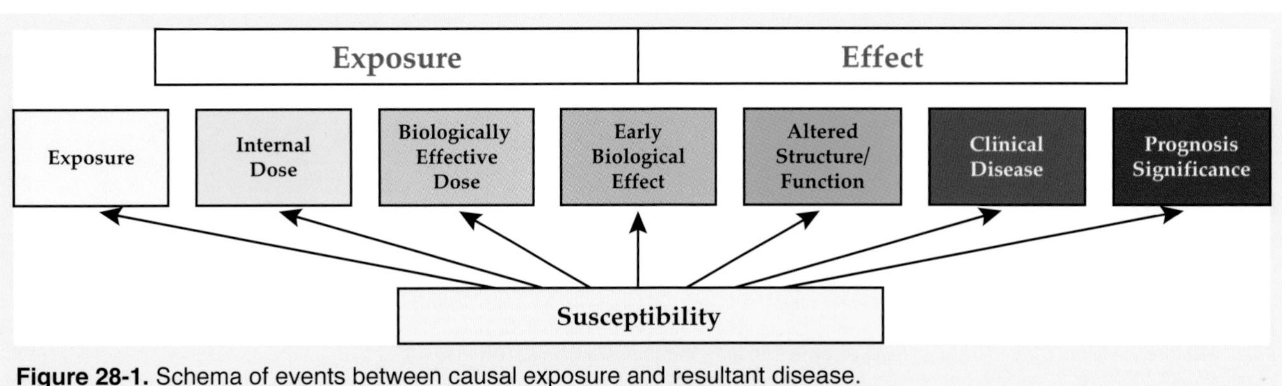

Figure 28-1. Schema of events between causal exposure and resultant disease.

test sample. Optimally, a biomarker should be specific to the exposure or stressor of interest and not confounded by other exposures, although such nonspecificity for molecular markers may be overcome by the use of a test panel rather than usage of a single marker. Biomarkers should be translatable, that is, bridge preclinical research (most likely done in animal models) to clinical results. Desirable biomarkers that indicate susceptibility to a particular condition or exposure should have sufficient prevalence in the population of interest to justify screening or targeted screening, as well as enough data to prompt an action. Finally, in order to utilize biomarkers, there must be a robust technological infrastructure and expertise available. Unlike physiological biomarker testing, detection of specific molecular changes for monitoring may allow early detection of subtle, subclinical changes that occur upon even acute exposures, as well as the possibility of the identification of exposure level/type long after such an event.

TYPES OF BIOMARKERS

Biomarkers of Exposure

Biomarkers of exposure are measured as the unchanged, parent chemical substance; its metabolite; or the product of its interaction with a target within the body.[18] The quantitation of a specific chemical, or a metabolic derivative of that chemical, within a biological sample can provide accurate assessments of systemic exposures for internal or external doses. The merits of baseline and periodic assessment of levels of chemical substances in blood and/or urine have been considered for service members as a group. In 2001, the Military Deployment Human Exposure Assessment compared exposure levels to a variety of chemicals with air and personal monitoring during a deployment.[19,20] Although there were no detections at actionable levels, such measurements could serve as a baseline to detect changes over time, after consideration of other confounding exposures. For the past three decades, the Centers for Disease Control and Prevention (Atlanta, GA) have been measuring biomarkers of exposure for more than 200 chemicals in nonoccupationally exposed populations in the United States as part of the National Health and Nutrition Evaluation Survey.[21] Currently, measured chemicals are associated with pollution in the air, pesticide use, and chemicals that are based on human activities, such as phthalates (found in plastics such as bottles and cups), bisphenyl A, and flame retardants. Although these measured levels usually have no prognostic value, they are assessed to evaluate trends over time and to look at regional or age differences.

Biomarkers of exposure in deployed military populations have been recommended and considered as an approach to understanding complex exposure situations, such as smoke from burning trash, although there are a number of limitations.[22,23] These include a brief window of opportunity for sample collection from rapid metabolism or excretion, a lack of specificity as to the source (ambient air vs smoking, for example, for some metals and volatile organic compounds), and the general lack of prognostic value.[17] The US Department of Defense (DoD) policy addressing the use of exposure biomarkers related to deployment includes the testing of blood for lead levels (when appropriate), as well as a 24-hour urine-depleted uranium bioassay for those considered at high risk based on responses to a screening questionnaire.[24]

Exposure biomonitoring is most frequently done in occupational settings for established medical surveillance programs. In workers with specific exposures due to their work operations, exposure biomarkers, largely in blood or urine, can be useful to evaluate whether exposures to these specific hazards exceed acceptable limits following a shift or at the end of the work week.[25] Currently, DoD occupational medicine guidance recommends hazard-directed medical surveillance, with few occupation-specific requirements.[26] DoD pesticide applicators and technical escort personnel (those who deal with explosive ordinance) are two occupations with specific biomonitoring requirements to address potential deployment-related exposures. Measurement of specific exposures in deployment may follow specific events or incidents. Two examples include (1) the assessment of whole blood chromium levels following a potential exposure to sodium dichromate powder dispersed at a vandalized water treatment plant in Iraq; and (2) lead and zinc protoporphyrin levels following exposure to elevated lead levels in air, potentially from the burning of batteries by local Iraqis outside a base camp.[27,28]

Depending on how biomarkers are categorized, *surrogate biomarkers* or *surrogate endpoint biomarkers* can be considered a type of exposure biomarker.[29] Surrogate biomarkers are used to substitute for a clinical endpoint and can be either intrinsic (blood pressure, protein isoforms) or extrinsic (cigarette consumption).[30] In the DoD, methemoglobin has been used as a surrogate biomarker to indicate cyanide intoxication levels, providing a level of protection by linking physiological/toxicological effects of cyanide to methemoglobin levels.[31]

Biomarkers of Effect

Biomarkers of effect include any measurable biochemical, functional, or structural change associated with exposure to and interaction with an agent. The effect may not be specific to a given exposure or agent. Pulmonary function testing is a familiar example; exposure to inhalation hazards may impact pulmonary function, as can personal habits such as smoking.[6] Application of pulmonary testing as a biomarker of effect in specific cohorts and the relative merits and issues associated with pulmonary function testing are discussed in other chapters in this book.[32]

Biomarkers of Susceptibility

Biomarkers of susceptibility reflect inherent or acquired modifications in the response to exposures or other stressors.[33] Susceptibilities can be disease states, genotypic and phenotypic variants, or the corresponding physiological states. Asthma and other respiratory conditions, cardiorespiratory disease, and other physiological changes associated with disease states are known to be associated with susceptibility to adverse outcomes of exposures. Although several types of molecules (protein, ribonucleic acid [RNA], etc) can serve as susceptibility markers, genome polymorphisms are particularly well suited as indicators of susceptibility. Toxicogenetic studies can lead to the development of new genetic screening tests for susceptibility to specific exposures. An example of such research is the identification of a variant allele in the tumor necrosis factor-α gene. While still in the research phase, studies examining the genotypes of coal workers who have developed silicosis have identified a polymorphism in the tumor necrosis factor-a that seems to be linked to susceptibility in the development of silicosis.[34]

Comparison of Biomarker Types

For exposures with sufficient dose–response information, the internal dose may correlate with potential health effects. *Exposure* biomarkers can integrate and quantify the dose internalized by inhalation, ingestion, and skin absorption routes of exposure. Internal measures of exposure to stressors are closer than external measures are to the targeted site of action for biological effects, potentially reducing confounding factors and consequently strengthening the ability to determine whether exposure correlates with the biological effects.[22] Markers of *effect* may identify subclinical changes from various exposures with the same target organ effect. Biomarkers of *susceptibility* may identify individuals at higher risk for adverse effects, although the prevalence of such susceptibility may be insufficient for screening to be an appropriate use of limited resources. Less frequently used classifications include the role of the biomarker in the pathophysiology of tissue injury (eg, inflammation) or activation of coagulation or fibrosis.

BIOMARKER DISCOVERY AND APPLICATIONS

Omics Technologies

The uses of high-throughput methodologies to examine the global (entire) expression of a given molecule are usually described as "Omics" technologies. These research areas include the following:

- proteomics (proteins),
- metabolomics (metabolites),
- genomics/transcriptomics (deoxyribonucleic acid [DNA] or RNA),
- adductomics (DNA adducts),
- lipidomics (lipids),
- epigenomics (epigenetic changes), and many others.

The ability to examine large sample numbers using analytic methods linked with bioinformatics has led to substantial gains in biomarker discovery in the last 10 years. Omics studies permit an unbiased examination of the expression of a given molecular population under different conditions (exposures, exposure routes, dosages). This *bottom up* approach allows identification of heretofore unlinked and unknown pathways. Although not within the scope of this chapter, excellent reviews on each of these technologies can be found elsewhere. Most of the primary Omics (proteomics/genomics/metabolomics) are currently used in biomarker discovery related to pulmonary diseases.[35]

Test Matrices

Traditional biological sources used for discovery and biomonitoring include whole blood, serum, plasma, urine, saliva (historical, now reemerging), among others (Figure 28-2). Additionally, physiological measurements—including pulmonary function testing, blood pressure, and pulse—can be used.[36,37] All other things being equal, the least invasive of these is preferable if the same quality of information can be obtained from the sample. Of these, blood and urine are commonly examined. Measurements of molecular components or chemicals in blood may indicate exposures, mobilization from stores, or cellular damage. Urinary biomarkers may be indicative of the same, although the response may slightly lag in time compared with those found in blood. Neither may provide information about the whole-body burden or internal dose sequestered in bone, fat, or other tissue.

Saliva is another medium of potential interest for exposure biomonitoring. It is readily accessible by noninvasive methods. Saliva biomarkers produced by healthy or diseased individuals are "sentinel molecules that could be used to scrutinize health and disease surveillance."[36] Levels of therapeutic, hormonal, immunological, or toxicological molecules are reflected in the molecular composition of saliva.

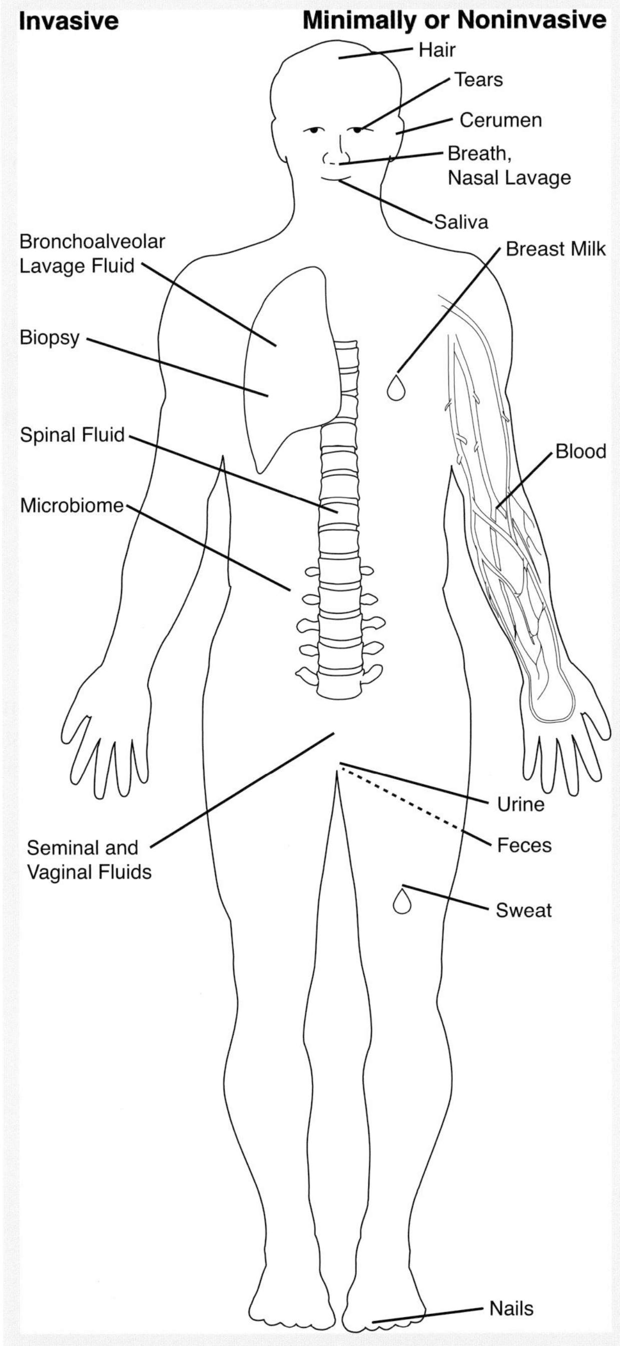

Figure 28-2. Test matrices for biomarker discovery and monitoring.

An example of the use of saliva as a biomarker of exposure uses levels of thiocyanate ions to differentiate smokers from nonsmokers.[38] Compared with urine and blood, saliva was found to be the most sensitive. Currently, saliva analysis for chemical exposures of interest is not common.

Hair or nails are most useful if there is a desire to assess internal dose over time, and the compound is known to be found within the sample. In recent years, the number of sources has expanded to include saliva, induced sputum (cellular or acellular), bronchoalveolar lavage fluid, and others.

Biomarker Detection

Assays for the selected biomarker must be sensitive (few false negatives) because detection levels are most likely low (picogram for proteins) for the marker of choice in the given sample. Such low levels of biomarker detection, for molecular signals, are highly probable given that most acute or chronic exposures will display only subclinical effects. The measurement should have a reference standard in unexposed or healthy populations, provide prognostic information, and be predictive (proportional to the degree of severity of the pathology).[17,36] Once a biomarker has been identified and appropriate assays and baselines developed, a stringent set of prevalidation and validation studies are necessary prior to clinical or biomonitoring uses.[39]

Current Pulmonary Biomarker Discovery Research

The application of Omics technologies for a new molecular signature indicative of lung injury or disease is still relatively recent when compared with analogous studies in kidney and liver diseases.[40] However, several recent studies demonstrate the potential utility of several types of molecules in a wide range of text matrices.[41]

There is a growing inventory of potential biomarkers that can be detected and quantified in exhaled air or exhaled condensate.[42] Breath analysis of exhaled volatile organic compounds may be a quantitative, noninvasive, simple, and safe method of measuring airway inflammation that provides a complementary tool to other methods of assessing airway disease, including asthma.[43] Volatile compounds can be measured directly in expired air, and are currently under examination for the detection of lung inflammation and asthma. Other nonvolatile compounds have been measured almost exclusively in bronchoalveolar lavage fluid. A less invasive approach uses exhaled breath condensate, which is formed by cooling expired air to assess nonvolatile compounds. These include biomarkers of oxidative stress and inflammation, often proteins.

The exhaled breath condensate has also been used as biomarker of exposure to some heavy metals and mineral compounds.[44]

Examination of serum and urine for pulmonary disease biomarkers has identified a number of potential markers in the past few years.[40] Clara cell proteins and surfactant protein A in serum have been examined in several studies for associations with lung injury. Studies of samples taken from multiple cohorts with smoke inhalation exposures indicate that Clara cell proteins and surfactant protein A seem to increase in serum approximately 24 hours postexposure.[45–47] Metabolomic analyses of urine and plasma in chronic obstructive pulmonary disease have identified trigonelline and formate as potential urinary metabolite biomarkers for this condition.[48] The success seen in this study suggests that metabolomic approaches may be successful for other pulmonary diseases.[49]

A large number of transcriptomic analyses of gene expression in the bronchial airway epithelium and lung parenchyma cells has permitted identification of condition-specific genes and molecular pathways modulated by cigarette smoking or as a result of lung function impairment in chronic obstructive pulmonary disease.[50,51] RNA expression studies such as these are used to develop panels of gene expression signatures specific to a given pulmonary injury or disease. In asthma transcriptomics studies, T-cell type 2–mediated inflammation symptoms can be followed by a set of interleukin-13 and interleukin-14–induced genes.[52] In addition, while sample collection via bronchial brushing is invasive, data collected from such studies would be invaluable in gaining a comprehensive understanding of the molecular disease mechanisms initiated by inhalation of airborne hazards.

NEW DIRECTIONS IN PULMONARY INJURY BIOMARKER RESEARCH

Epigenetic Biomarkers

In the past 10 years, the field of epigenetics has expanded with the development of high-throughput multiplex discovery methodologies.[53] For environmental exposures, applicability of epigenetics to environmental exposures is particularly relevant.[54] Indeed, the idea of a "longitudinal epigenome-wide association study" approach has been suggested to allow the examination of influences of various exposures and environmental factors (eg, exercise, diet) on the epigenetic signature.[55] This signature (or the epitype) can and does change during its lifetime, altering gene expression to incur specific pathway alterations.[56,57]

Nasal Lavage Analysis

Although not unknown in allergen testing,[58] the use of nasal lavage as a test matrix for lung injury biomarkers may be a relatively new idea. Biomarker studies in asthma have indicated that monitoring eosinophil-derived neurotoxin in nasal lavage is a useful and noninvasive method to monitor eosinophilic inflammation.[59]

CURRENT USES OF BIOMARKERS IN MONITORING PULMONARY INJURY

Currently, there are few pulmonary biomarkers routinely used in clinical applications. Discussions of the use of spirometry and its limitations in the measurement of lung function are examined in Chapter 8 (Pulmonary Function Testing—Spirometry Testing for Population Surveillance), Chapter 9 (Discussion Summary: Recommendation for Surveillance Spirometry in Military Personnel), and Chapter 10 (Spirometry Monitoring and Prevention Using Spirola Software). One reason for the limited number of clinical biomarkers is the lack of reference values and standardization of known markers. As such, further research, development, and refinement are imperative for pulmonary disease biomarkers to become an integral part of clinical practice. In addition, new pulmonary biomarkers, as previously described, are still in the prevalidation stages or early validation stages, and have yet to be fully evaluated and approved for clinical uses. One exception to the lack of clinical applications is the measurement of fractional exhaled nitric oxide in the evaluation of patients with obstructive airways disease.[42] Fractional exhaled nitric oxide has been shown to reflect an increase in eosinophilic inflammation in the lung, although its use may be limited to specific lung diseases (eg, asthma).[60]

GENETICS IN PULMONARY INJURY RESEARCH

The availability of the Human Genome Sequence, high-throughput capabilities of multiplex, chip-based, genome-wide association screens, and bioinformatics has accelerated discovery of new gene–gene mutations associated with susceptibility to environmental hazards. It is projected that with the increased affordability of whole genome sequencing,[61,62] large cohort studies will link DNA sequence (genotype) to health outcomes and exposures (phenotypes). Genetic research will yield information on new potential biomarkers and, more importantly, specific pathways altered upon specific exposures and dosages. Studies of gene–environment interactions in lung disease have already identified a number of genes that predispose individuals to a higher risk of injury.[63]

Several genes have been shown to act as modifiers of response to exposures making an individual more susceptible. For example, polymorphisms in oxidative stress genes (*GSTM1*, *GSTP1*, *NQ01*) have been shown to modify response to particulate matter and ozone.[64] Diet and genes influencing metabolism have been shown to influence closing volume response to pollution, thus indicating protective effects for n-3 fatty acids, antioxidants, and methyl nutrients.[65–67] Another polymorphism of cellular DNA has been associated with susceptibility to silicosis.[68] Response to inhaled silicon dioxide nanoparticles in animal studies demonstrated that toxicity varied with age, and different biomarkers of susceptibility may exist at different stages.[11]

Current research strategies are exploring gene–environment interactions. One research strategy studied subjects exposed to airborne endotoxins and potential genotype signatures. It was seen that three single nucleotide polymorphisms in the *CD14* gene and one in the *MD2* gene could modify asthma symptoms generated in response to endotoxin exposure, indicating that carriers of these major allele variants were at greater risk than homozygotes.[69]

Although genetic research is helpful in understanding lung injury, its use for susceptibility screening in the military may be of limited value and only under specific conditions. Such tests may only be cost-effective when the prevalence of the genetic mutation is moderately high and the susceptibility difficult or impossible to ascertain otherwise. In addition, validated linkage of genotype to health decrement caused by exposures is essential, with a clear plan of action to advert adverse outcomes with intervention.

An example of a current military screening program for genetic susceptibility is the genetically based test for glucose-6-phosphate dehydrogenase (G6PD) deficiency.[70] The Army screens for G6PD deficiency prior to deployment to malarious regions, as deficiency is associated with adverse reactions to some medications, one of which is the antimalarial primaquine. Worldwide, G6PD deficiency occurs in approximately 1 in 16 individuals (6.25%). In US military personnel, prevalence was found to be 2.5% in males and 1.6% in females, and overall most common in African Americans, Asian, and Hispanic individuals. Screening for this susceptibility is considered clinically warranted due to the prevalence rate and the fact that the finding is actionable because specific drugs cannot be administered to these individuals.

SUMMARY

It has been broadly recognized that to understand the potential implications of deployment exposures on service member health, improvements in exposure science are needed.[71,72] Accurate exposure information is critical in epidemiology studies to compare outcomes in populations that have different exposure levels,[27] and it has been seen that questionnaires have known limitations and do not accurately access past exposure levels. Better exposure data can provide more precise risk estimates that may lead to public health actions. Biological monitoring is one tool for improved exposure assessment and has the potential for accurate, on-site, real-time monitoring (Figure 28-3). It can also identify effects of exposure and populations at potentially higher risk from exposures. The concept of the exposome has been proposed as a research challenge equivalent to the Human Genome Project.[11] Using a combination of high-throughput Omics technologies, efforts are now being directed at the evaluation of the exposome, which would evaluate the entire internal biochemical environment, including natural and disease processes and absorbed doses from xenobiotics and their effects on metabolism, gene and protein expression, and damage to biological molecules.

One approach might use high-resolution mass spectroscopy or ^{1}H-NMR (proton nuclear magnetic resonance) to identify chemicals and their metabolic signatures in multiple test matrices. This may detect low levels of exposure to anticipated and unanticipated exposures, identify changes in normal cellular metabolism, or identify trends over time and space. Proteomics could also be used to perform global scans for alterations in protein levels of pre- and

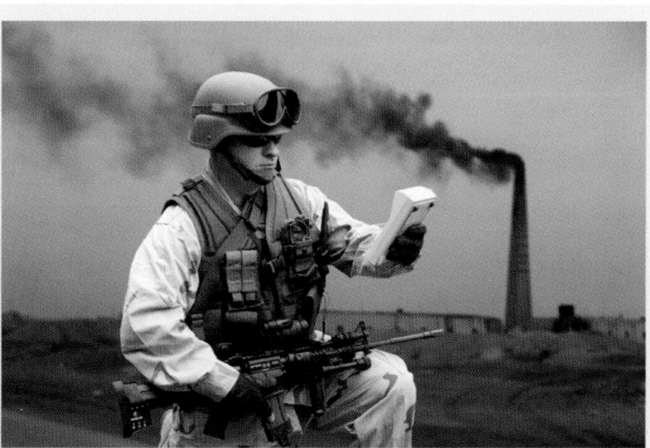

Figure 28-3. Conceptual field monitoring for exposures. Photograph: Reproduced from *Air Force Research Laboratory Technical Report,* AFRL-RH-WP-TR-2009-0106.

postdeployment samples. Such analyses could examine expression changes in immunoglobulins and other proteins known to modulate on exposure to allergens, for example, or even determine unique protein "signature" patterns indicative of specific chemical exposures or specific organ effects. Beyond the use of serum, whole blood and other specimens may allow the detection of changes in cells, genetic material, and transcription products. Additionally, changes following exposure to vaccinations or stress may be identified beyond changes associated with exposure to toxic compounds.

The DoD is assessing the progress of this field and hopes to initiate at least one pilot project to assess the feasibility of Omics techniques on serum from the DOD Serum Repository (DoDSR) to increase understanding of the environment–effect relationship, particularly as it relates to deployment. In 1989, the DoDSR was established for storing the serum that remained from mandatory human immunodeficiency virus testing.[73] Serum may be utilized to evaluate exposures by examination of a number of potential molecular marker patterns. The DoDSR has expanded to include the storage of operational deployment specimens, and now contains more than 50 million specimens representing pre- and postdeployment specimens, as well as serum remaining from human immunodeficiency virus testing. It has serial specimens on active and reserve components of Army, Navy, Air Force, and Marines, as well as the ability to link to demographic and health outcome data.

Significant challenges remain in the field of exposomics.[11,64,74] The exposome can vary over time for poorly understood reasons, such as aging and general environmental conditions. Therefore, large cohort processing of a large number of specimens is needed to eliminate experimental noise and pick up the low level signals of interest. If DoD supports efforts to move the suggested initiatives forward, it will likely be some time before the efforts yield practical information and clinical utility. Many of the biomarkers of the past were limited by difficulties in their interpretability to identify changes early enough to initiate preventive measures, as well as provide limited prognostic information. Even new biomarkers have limitations in their use.[75] However, the full scope of benefits from new biomarker discovery efforts will not be revealed for several years. The question of exposure and effect is a very old one that continues to be asked, but new technologies in biomonitoring may contribute to the answer.

REFERENCES

1. Powell TM, Smith TC, Jacobson IG, et al. Prospective assessment of chronic multisymptom illness reporting possibly associated with open-air burn pit smoke exposure in Iraq. *J Occup Environ Med.* 2012;54:682–688.

2. Jones KA, Smith B, Granado NS, et al. Newly reported lupus and rheumatoid arthritis in relation to deployment within proximity to a documented open-air burn pit in Iraq. *J Occup Environ Med.* 2012;54:698–707.

3. Smith B, Wong CA, Boyko EJ, et al. The effects of exposure to documented open-air burn pits on respiratory health among deployers of the Millennium Cohort Study. *J Occup Environ Med.* 2012;54:708–716.

4. Rose CS. Military service and lung disease. *Clin Chest Med.* 2012;33:705–714.

5. Institute of Medicine of the National Academies. *Protecting Those Who Serve: Strategies to Protect the Health of Deployed US Forces.* Washington, DC: National Academies Press; 2000.

6. Mayr M. Metabolomics: ready for the prime time? *Circ Cardiovasc Genet.* 2008;1:58–65.

7. Juberg DR, Bus J, Katz DS. *The Opportunities and Limitations of Biomonitoring.* Midland, MI: Mackinac Center for Public Policy; 2008. Policy brief.

8. Kerns RT, Bushel PR. The impact of classification of interest on predictive toxicogenomics. *Front Genet.* 2012;3:14.

9. McHale CM, Zhang L, Hubbard AE, Smith MT. Toxicogenomic profiling of chemically exposed humans in risk assessment. *Mutat Res.* 2010;705:172–183.

10. George J, Singh R, Mahmood Z, Shukla Y. Toxicoproteomics: new paradigms in toxicology research. *Toxicol Mech Methods.* 2010;20:415–423.

11. Wild CP. Complementing the genome with an "exposome": the outstanding challenge of environmental exposure measurement in molecular epidemiology. *Cancer Epidemiol Biomarkers Prev.* 2005;14:1847–1850.

12. Wild CP. The exposome: from concept to utility. *Int J Epidemiol*. 2012;41:24–32.

13. Bradburne CE, Carruth LM, Lin JS, Sivakumar A, Benson JH, Vogel RA. Implementing genome-informed personalized medicine in the U.S. Air Force Medical Service via the Patient-Centered Precision Care Research (PC2-Z) Program. *Johns Hopkins APL Tech Dig*. 2013;31:333–344.

14. Miranda DM, Mamede M, Souza BR, et al. Molecular medicine: a path towards a personalized medicine. *Rev Bras Psiquiatr*. 2012;34:82–91.

15. Biomarkers Definitions Working Group. Biomarkers and surrogate endpoints: preferred definitions and conceptual framework. *Clin Pharmacol Ther*. 2011;69:91.

16. World Health Organization International Programme on Chemical Safety. *Biomarkers in Risk Assessment: Validity and Validation*. Geneva, Switzerland: World Health Organization; 2001.

17. Weese CB. Deployment exposure assessment and the role of biomonitoring. *US Army Med Dept J*. 2004;January–March;60–67.

18. Silins I, Högberg J. Combined toxic exposures and human health: biomarkers of exposure and effect. *Int J Environ Res Public Health*. 2011;8:629–647.

19. May LM, Weese C, Ashley DL, Trump DH, Bowling CM, Lee AP. The recommended role of exposure biomarkers for the surveillance of environmental and occupational chemical exposures in military deployments: policy considerations. *Mil Med*. 2004;169:761–767.

20. May LM, Heller J, Kalinsky V, et al. Military deployment human exposure assessment: urine total and isotopic uranium sampling results. *J Toxicol Environ Health A*. 2004;67:697–714.

21. Centers for Disease Control and Prevention, National Center for Environmental Health, and National Biomonitoring Program. *Fourth National Report on Human Exposure to Environmental Chemicals: Updated Tables*. http://www.cdc.gov/exposurereport/. Accessed March 2013.

22. National Research Council and Committee on Human and Environmental Exposure Science in the 21st Century. *Exposure Science in the 21st Century: A Vision and a Strategy*. Washington, DC: National Academies Press; 2012.

23. Lioy PJ, Smith KR. A discussion of exposure science in the 21st century: a vision and a strategy. *Environ Health Perspect*. 2013;121:405–409.

24. US Department of Defense, Undersecretary for Defense (Personnel and Readiness). *DoD Deployment Biomonitoring Policy*. Washington, DC: DoD; February 6, 2004. HA policy 04-004.

25. American Conference of Governmental Industrial Hygienists. *Documentation of Threshold Limit Values and Biological Exposure Indices*. 7th ed. Cincinnati, OH: ACGIH; 2001.

26. US Department of Defense. *US Department of Defense Instruction Manual 6055.05 M. Occupational Medical Examinations and Surveillance Manual*. Washington, DC: Under Secretary of Defense for Acquisition, Technology and Logistics; May 2, 2007.

27. Baird C. The basis for and uses of environmental sampling to assess health risk in deployed settings. *Mil Med*. 2011;176(suppl 7):84–90.

28. Brix K, O'Donnell FL. Panel 1. Medical surveillance prior to, during, and following potential environmental exposures. *Mil Med*. 2011;176(suppl 7):91–96.

29. Boone CW, Kelloff GJ. Intraepithelial neoplasia, surrogate endpoint biomarkers, and cancer chemoprevention. *J Cell Biochem Suppl*. 1993;17F:37–48.

30. Aronson JK. Biomarkers and surrogate endpoints. *Br J Clin Pharmacol*. 2005;59:491–494.

31. Marino MT. Use of surrogate markers for drugs of military importance. *Mil Med*. 1998;163:743–746.

32. Rose C, Abraham J, Harkins D, et al. Overview and recommendations for medical screening and diagnostic evaluation for postdeployment lung disease in returning US warfighters. *J Occup Environ Med*. 2012;54:746–751.

33. National Research Council, Subcommittee on Reproductive and Neurodevelopmental Toxicology, and Committee on Biologic Markers. *Biological Markers in Pulmonary Toxicology*. Washington, DC: National Academies Press; 1989.

34. Gulumian M, Borm PJ, Vallyathan V, et al. Mechanistically identified suitable biomarkers of exposure, effect, and susceptibility for silicosis and coal-worker's pneumoconiosis: a comprehensive review. *J Toxicol Environ Health B Crit Rev*. 2006;9:357–395.

35. Wheelock CE, Goss VM, Balgoma D, et al. Application of omics technologies to biomarker discovery in inflammatory lung diseases. *Eur Respir J*. 2013;42:802–825.

36. Wong DT, Xiao H, Zhang L. Salivary biomarkers for clinical applications. *Molec Diag Ther*. 2009;4:245–269.

37. Harkins DK, Susten AS. Hair analysis: exploring the state of the science. *Environ Health Perspect*. 2003;111:576–578.

38. Maliszewski TF, Bass DE. True and apparent thiocyanate levels in body fluids of smokers and nonsmokers. *J Appl Physiol*. 1955;8:289–291.

39. Goodsaid FM, Frueh FW, Mattes W. Strategic paths for biomarker qualification. *Toxicology*. 2008;245:219–223.

40. Nicholas BL. Search for biomarkers in chronic obstructive pulmonary disease: current status. *Curr Opin Pulmon Med*. 2013;19:103–108.

41. Jain KK. *Technologies for Discovery of Biomarkers*. In: Jain KK, ed. *The Handbook of Biomarkers*. New York, NY: Humana Press; 2010: 23–71. Chap 2.

42. American Thoracic Society and European Respiratory Society. ATS/ERS recommendations for standardized procedures for the online and offline measurement of exhaled lower respiratory nitric oxide and nasal nitric oxide, 2005. *Am J Respir Crit Care Med*. 2005;171:912–930.

43. Dweik RA, Boggs PB, Erzurum SC, et al. An official ATS clinical practice guideline: interpretation of exhaled nitric oxide levels (FENO) for clinical applications. *Am J Respir Crit Care Med*. 2011;184:602–615.

44. American Thoracic Society and European Respiratory Society. Measurement of exhaled lower respiratory nitric oxide and nasal nitric oxide (FENO). *Am J Respir Crit Care Med*. 2005;171:912–930.

45. Stockfelt L, Sallsten G, Olin AC, et al. Effects on airways of short-term exposure to two kinds of wood smoke in a chamber study of healthy humans. *Inhal Toxicol*. 2012;24:47–59.

46. Greven F, Krop E, Burger N, Kerstjens H, Heederik D. Serum pneumoproteins in firefighters. *Biomarkers*. 2011;16:364–371.

47. St Helen G, Holland NT, Balmes JR, et al. Utility of urinary Clara cell protein (CC16) to demonstrate increased lung epithelial permeability in non-smokers exposed to outdoor secondhand smoke. *J Expo Sci Environ Epidemiol*. 2013;23:183–189.

48. McClay JL, Adkins DE, Isern NG, et al. $^{(1)}$H nuclear magnetic resonance metabolomics analysis identifies novel urinary biomarkers for lung function. *J. Proteome Res*. 2010;9:3083–3090.

49. Hu JZ, Rommereim DN, Minard KR, et al. Metabolomics in lung inflammation: a high-resolution $^{(1)}$H NMR study of mice exposed to silica dust. *Toxicol Mech Methods*. 2008;18:385–398.

50. Steiling K, Kadar AY, Bergerat A, et al. Comparison of proteomic and transcriptomic profiles in the bronchial airway epithelium of current and never smokers. *PLoS One*. 2009;4:e5043.

51. Gower AC, Steiling K, Brothers JF 2nd, Lenburg ME, Spira A. Transcriptomic studies of the airway field of injury associated with smoking-related lung disease. *Proc Am Thorac Soc*. 2011;8:173–179.

52. Woodruff PG, Modrek B, Choy DF, et al. T-helper type 2-driven inflammation defines major subphenotypes of asthma. *Am J Respir Crit Care Med*. 2009;180:388–395.

53. Etheridge A, Lee I, Hood L, Galas D, Wang K. Extracellular microRNA: a new source of biomarkers. *Mutat Res*. 2011;717:85–90.

54. Jirtle RL, Skinner MK. Environmental epigenomics and disease susceptibility. *Nat Rev Genet*. 8:253–262.

55. Lahiri DK, Maloney B. Gene × environment interaction by a longitudinal epigenome-wide association study (LEWAS) overcomes limitations of genome-wide association study (GWAS). *Epigenomics*. 2012;4:685–699.

56. Perdomo C, Spira A, Schembri F. MiRNAs as regulators of the response to inhaled environmental toxins and airway carcinogenesis. *Mutat Res*. 2011;717:32–37.

57. Vaporidi K, Vergadi E, Kaniaris E, et al. Pulmonary microRNA profiling in a mouse model of ventilator-induced lung injury. *Am J Physiol Lung Cell Mol Physiol*. 2012;303:L199–L207.

58. Koren HS, Hatch GE, Graham DE. Nasal lavage as a tool in assessing acute inflammation in response to inhaled pollutants. *Toxicology*. 1990;60:15–25.

59. Kim CK. Eosinophil-derived neurotoxin: a novel biomarker for diagnosis and monitoring of asthma. *Korean J Pediatr*. 2013;56:8–12.

60. Barnes PJ, Dweik RA, Gelb AF, et al. Exhaled nitric oxide in pulmonary diseases: a comprehensive review. *Chest*. 2010;138:682–692.

61. McMorrow D. *The $100 Genome: Implications for the DoD*. McLean, VA: Mitre Corporation; December 2010. JASON Technical Report JSR-10–100.

62. Cyranoski D. Chinese bioscience: the sequencing factory. *Nature*. 2010;464:22–24.

63. Kleeberger SR, Cho HY. Gene-environment interactions in environmental lung diseases. *Novartis Found Symp*. 2008;293:168–178.

64. Utell M. *Biomarkers and Genetics in Pulmonary Disease Research*. Presentation at the Joint VA/DoD Airborne Hazards Symposium, Arlington, VA, August 2012.

65. Romieu I, Trenga C. Diet and obstructive lung diseases. *Epidemiol Rev*. 2001;23:268–287.

66. Shi Q, Zhang Z, Li G, et al. Sex differences in risk of lung cancer associated with methylene-tetrahydrofolate reductase polymorphisms. *Cancer Epidemiol Biomarkers Prev*. 2005;14:1477–1484.

67. Bentley AR, Emrani P, Cassano PA. Genetic variation and gene expression in antioxidant related enzymes and risk of COPD: a systematic review. *Thorax*. 2008;63:956–961.

68. Yucesoy B, Vallyathan V, Landsittel DP, Simeonova P, Luster MI. Cytokine polymorphisms in silicosis and other pneumoconioses. *Mol Cell Biochem*. 2002;234-235:219–224.

69. Smit LA, Heederik D, Doekes G, et al. Endotoxin exposure, CD14 and wheeze among farmers: a gene–environment interaction. *Occup Environ Med*. 2011;68:826–831.

70. Chinevere TD, Murray CK, Grant E Jr, et al. Prevalence of glucose-6-phosphate dehydrogenase deficiency in U.S. Army personnel. *Mil Med*. 2006;171:905–907.

71. Institute of Medicine of the National Academies. *Long-Term Health Consequences of Exposure to Burn Pits in Iraq and Afghanistan.* Washington, DC: National Academies Press; 2011: 1–9, 31–44, 117–129.

72. Institute of Medicine of the National Academies. *Protecting Those Who Serve: Strategies to Protect the Health of Deployed US Forces.* Washington, DC: National Academies Press, 2000.

73. Rubertone MV, Brundage JF. The Defense Medical Surveillance System and the Department of Defense Serum Repository: glimpses of the future of public health surveillance. *Am J Public Health.* 2002;92:1900–1904.

74. Davis M, Boekelheide K, Boverhof DR, et al. The new revolution in toxicology: the good, the bad, and the ugly. *Ann N Y Acad Sci.* 2013;1278:11–24.

75. Mayeux R. Biomarkers: potential uses and limitations. *NeuroRX.* 2004;1:182–188.

Chapter 29

DISCUSSION SUMMARY: EXPOSURE CHARACTERIZATION—QUESTIONNAIRES AND OTHER TOOLS

JOEL C. GAYDOS, MD, MPH*; AND KATHLEEN KREISS, MD†

*Colonel (Retired), Medical Corps, US Army; Science Advisor, Armed Forces Health Surveillance Center, 11800 Tech Road, Suite 220, Silver Spring, Maryland 20904
†Field Studies Branch Chief, Division of Respiratory Disease Studies, National Institute for Occupational Safety and Health, Centers for Disease Control and Prevention, Mailstop H-2800, 1095 Willowdale Road, Morgantown, West Virginia 26505

INTRODUCTION

Members of the US uniformed services are occupationally exposed to a very large number of potentially hazardous agents.[1] These agents may be associated with the use and maintenance of their own equipment, the result of other human activity, or naturally occurring.[1,2] These military exposures have occurred for thousands of years.[1] However, in the last 40 years in the US military, exposures to defoliants (Agent Orange) and oil well fires have caused considerable concern.[3–5] In the recent wars in Afghanistan and Iraq, US military personnel have been diagnosed with unusual conditions, such as eosinophilic pneumonia and constrictive bronchiolitis.[6,7] The possibility looms that unidentified exposures may have contributed to these conditions and that these exposures persist. Concern about occupational exposures and potential chronic adverse effects in the recent wars has also been fueled by reports of large numbers of troops living and working for long periods near open burn pits covering many acres, exposures to severe sandstorms, and US military members fighting a sulfur plant fire that burned continuously for almost a month.[8–12] Recently, two medical journals devoted entire volumes to potentially hazardous exposures of military personnel.[13,14]

Recognizing and mitigating potentially hazardous exposures, identifying those possibly exposed in Afghanistan and Iraq, characterizing their exposures (consisting of primarily airborne hazards), and developing and implementing long-term programs to deal with the consequences of the exposures continue to be challenging.[15] To assess the current situation and develop plans for the future, the US Department of Veterans Affairs (VA) and the US Department of Defense (DoD) partnered to conduct a symposium during August 21–23, 2012 in Crystal City, VA. Major objectives of the Joint VA/DoD Airborne Hazards Symposium were to develop an overview of potential health effects (short-term and long-term) related to airborne hazards for Operation Enduring Freedom (Afghanistan, October 2001–present), Operation Iraqi Freedom (March 2003–August 2010), and Operation New Dawn (Iraq, September 2010–present) and to summarize current epidemiological evidence on the deployment health effects of interest. Another objective was to foster discussion of potential actions for the DoD and VA to improve surveillance, standardize evaluations, and increase communication and collaboration.[1] The symposium consisted of didactic presentations, discussions, and focused work groups. This chapter summarizes the discussion and findings of Work Group B. Members of this group were tasked with identifying and assessing the available tools for exposure characterization (placing emphasis on the use of questionnaires), and with providing recommendations to improve exposure characterization in the future.

IMPORTANCE OF EXPOSURE CHARACTERIZATION

In referring to exposures of military members, some have used the term *exposure characterization*. Ideally, characterization of an actual or potential exposure would include the following:

- potentially harmful agent or agents,
- reliable and meaningful measurements of the agents' concentrations in time and space,
- identifying information on the people who may have been exposed and their duration and manner of exposure (exposure pathways),
- absorbed doses,
- target organs and disease states that may result, and
- available tests to document the absorbed dose and to detect pathological changes resulting from the exposure.

Others have used the term *exposure assessment*. Exposure assessment has been defined as the quantitative or qualitative evaluation of human contact with a potential toxicant that includes the intensity, frequency, and duration of contact, and may include evaluations of the following:

- rates at which the chemical crosses an internal or external boundary of the human body (chemical intake or uptake rates),
- route by which it crosses the boundary (dermal, oral, or respiratory exposure route),
- amount of the chemical that actually crosses the boundary (a dose), and
- amount absorbed (internal dose).[16]

Whether speaking of exposure characterization or exposure assessment, the ability to identify and measure exposures of military forces, to identify those potentially exposed, and to generate reliable estimates of risk for acute or chronic health effects are of great importance for several reasons:

- to minimize or reduce acute health effects that may result in decrements in job performance, thereby placing the success of the military mission at risk;
- to reduce the loss of trained military personnel who may decide to leave military service because of persistent symptoms associated with their deployment;

- to acknowledge the military's and the nation's duty to prevent injury and illness in uniformed members to the greatest extent possible and to care for those who become ill or injured as a result of their service; and
- to develop research questions and support research related to acute and chronic health effects associated with military exposures to prevent morbidity and mortality in the future.[17]

TOOLS FOR EXPOSURE CHARACTERIZATION

Environmental monitors are used to identify and quantitate agents of concern over time. These devices may be placed on an individual (eg, in the breathing zone area [personal sampling devices]) or situated at critical points in the environment in an attempt to identify the agents present and to provide some indication of concentrations over time in a defined area. Because continuous monitoring for specific individuals over time is unlikely to occur, available sampling data may be entered into models with other related data (eg, wind and additional meteorological data) and estimated exposure values generated for individual service members or entire military units.

Although environmental sampling data are usually incomplete, biomonitoring may be utilized when suitable tests are available. Biomonitoring involves the collection of body fluids or tissues at appropriate times relative to the possible exposure and testing of these for the agent of concern or metabolites that correlate with exposure. Another tool that is commonly used to compensate for inadequate exposure data is the questionnaire. Questionnaires may be general in nature and broadly applied or specifically designed for selected occupational or exposure groups. These usually attempt to obtain self-reported information on exposures and state of health. If the agent or agents of a potential exposure are known—and the target organs and pathological effects are defined—and a reliable test is available to identify those exposed or those who are experiencing a pathological effect, initial medical screening and later periodic medical follow-up may be initiated for the occupational groups of concern.

In a general manner, adverse health effects, including those from hazardous exposures, are monitored through public health surveillance programs that some refer to as medical surveillance programs.[18] All of the uniformed services engage in various types of public health surveillance. "Public health surveillance is the ongoing, systematic collection, analysis, and interpretation of health data, essential to the planning, implementation, and evaluation of public health practice, closely integrated with the dissemination of these data to those who need to know and linked to prevention and control."[19(p1)] For example, respiratory diseases may be monitored closely in groups with known or suspected exposure to respiratory toxicants. In selected situations, the occurrence of respiratory morbidity and mortality in the groups of interest is compared with the occurrence in other similar groups without known or suspected exposure. The value of public health surveillance can be greatly increased if the population of interest is well defined and the exposure of concern is well characterized. The public health practitioner who can reasonably define the population at risk, the adverse outcome of interest, and the probable latency period has a good chance of identifying a problem if a problem does indeed exist.

Environmental Monitoring

The issues related to environmental monitoring during military deployments have been extensively reviewed elsewhere and are only briefly mentioned here.[15,20–22] Environmental monitoring is usually the responsibility of military preventive medicine (PVNTMED) personnel. In recent conflicts, these PVNTMED specialists have been assigned broad areas of responsibility, which has caused them to focus on collecting area samples rather than individual or personal samples.[23] An area sample represents only the situation at the sampling site during the defined period of operation of the sampler. Because meteorological and working conditions may vary considerably over time, extrapolation of these results is often not recommended. Additionally, routine sampling is usually conducted only for particulate matter, metals associated with particulate matter, and sometimes volatile organic compounds.[23] Sampling to detect and identify other compounds of possible concern (eg, semivolatile organics, dioxins, and novel or unknown toxicants) is uncommon.[23]

Getting state-of-the-art sampling equipment and trained operators for this equipment into the areas where monitoring is needed has been challenging. Administrative requirements of the military purchasing and training systems have been an impediment. Transportation to distant areas has also been challenging because warriors, guns, and bullets receive priority on aircraft and other vehicles. Over the last two decades, sampling devices have been greatly improved to include significant reductions in size and weight. However, military commanders have many critical priorities, and the importance of monitoring potential exposures must be explained and emphasized by qualified PVNTMED and other medical personnel. These challenges continue to be frequently encountered.[15] Persistent efforts are needed to:

- improve the US military's ability to monitor the deployment environment,

- identify and characterize actual or potential exposures quickly,
- mitigate their impact on health and performance, and
- facilitate any follow-up actions needed.

Modeling

Modeling by military medical personnel to prevent disease and nonbattle injuries is frequently done prior to a military mission as part of an effort to identify and analyze medical threats and predict disease and exposure risks in different geographic regions at various times of the year.[24] This type of modeling is routinely supported by the National Center for Medical Intelligence (Fort Detrick, MD), the Armed Forces Health Surveillance Center (Silver Spring, MD), and public health organizations in the uniformed services. Results from this work are used to assist military commanders and medical personnel in identifying and responding to the disease and exposure risks, to include implementing specific preventive measures (eg, immunizations and prophylactic drugs) when these are available.

Defining troop exposures through modeling after a potential exposure has occurred is a much more difficult task. A noteworthy example is the modeling of exposures to products of combustion from the demolition of oil wells in Kuwait by Iraqi troops in Operation Desert Storm in early 1991.[5] A major obstacle in completing this project was determining troop locations in time and space. Administrative actions have been initiated to improve the capability of medical personnel to identify individual military members in time and space, relative to a potentially hazardous exposure; but the detail needed for meaningful modeling may not be attainable. Reliable exposure modeling requires adequate amounts of pertinent data; highly trained, experienced people; sophisticated computer hardware and software; and time.

Modeling prior to a military mission and after a potential exposure has occurred can be expected to be used in the future. Therefore, the US military should maintain and improve its expertise in this area. However, it is unlikely that modeling to define possible past exposures would be used effectively on a regular basis.

Biomonitoring

In situations where exposed individuals can be identified and a reliable test exists for the agent of concern, biomonitoring may be implemented. An example is the ongoing evaluation of veterans who were wounded by depleted uranium fragments.[25] However, an attempt to prospectively conduct biomonitoring on members of a defined military unit possibly exposed to the burning oil wells of Operation Desert Storm encountered problems with interpretation of laboratory tests and lost data and information.[26] A large explosion and fire destroyed study logs. In the absence of environmental monitoring results and information on other exposures (eg, food consumed, such as grilled meat), interpreting results for tests such as DNA-polycyclic aromatic hydrocarbon adducts was problematic. In general, attempts to do biomonitoring may not be feasible because the agent is unknown, an appropriate laboratory test may not be readily available or extremely expensive, and the effort may have to be implemented as a research project. It is unlikely that biomonitoring will be used frequently in the military in the immediate future. However, research in this area should be encouraged because this tool could be valuable in selected situations and could possibly have widespread use in the more distant future.

Questionnaires

In an extensive review of the challenges to exposure assessment in Gulf War veterans published in 2006, Glass and Sim[17] concluded that, "Due to the poor quality and accessibility of objective military exposure records, self-assessed exposure questionnaires are likely to remain the main instrument for assessing the exposure for a large number of veterans."[17(p627)]

In the US military, the word "deployment" refers to the relocation of forces and material to desired operational areas. The desired operational areas are generally places where hostile action is occurring or could be expected to occur. The US military currently uses three deployment-related, self-administered questionnaires:

1. the Pre-Deployment Health Assessment (DD Form 2795, September 2012),
2. the Post-Deployment Health Assessment (PDHA; DD Form 2796, September 2012), and
3. the Post-Deployment Health Re-Assessment (DD Form 2900, September 2012).

These questionnaires are 7 to 10 pages long and request information about the service member's state of health, alcohol use, and deployment experiences that include exposures and concerns related to deployment. Some potential exposures are specifically addressed, such as exposures to blasts and explosions, depleted uranium, and animals. Deployment questionnaires contain many items relating to mental health.[27]

The Pre-Deployment Health Assessment questionnaire is administered within 60 days prior to the expected deployment. Completion of the PDHA occurs when an individual is administratively being released from the deployment area or within 30 days after returning to a home base. The

Post-Deployment Health Re-Assessment questionnaire was initiated in 2005 because field research indicated that health concerns, particularly those relating to mental health, occurred more frequently several months after a deployment. It is completed 90 to 180 days after returning to home station. [27]

All three deployment questionnaires were developed as tools to identify and address health issues and concerns, and potentially harmful exposures and concerns. Completion of these questionnaires requires follow-up with a face-to-face encounter with a trained healthcare provider to review and address responses to the questionnaire, as well as related issues and concerns. The DoD deployment questionnaires were developed for implementation as clinical tools. Significant shortcomings with the deployment questionnaires have been identified. In the first case, soldiers in Iraq who may have experienced a potentially harmful exposure to hexavalent chromium were told about their exposure and instructed to report the event in their postdeployment forms (PDHAs).[28,29] Of 227 soldiers with completed PDHA forms filed and available for review, only 55 (24.2%) accurately reported chromium exposure.[29] Only 96 (42.3%) soldiers, including the 55 identified previously, mentioned chemical exposure of any kind.[29]

A second case came to light following the first death of a US service member from rabies after an overseas dog exposure since 1974.[24,30,31] The service member who died was reported to have mentioned being bitten by a dog in Afghanistan on his PDHA form, but the medical officer who reviewed his form took no action.[31] An extensive effort was initiated by the US Army Public Health Command (Aberdeen Proving Ground, MD) to identify other uniformed service members who had contact with wild animals and may be at risk of rabies and in need of treatment.[31] Efforts to identify soldiers at risk for rabies included review of health assessment forms completed following deployment and other medical data bases.[31] Review of health assessment forms and other medical records resulted in well over 100 soldiers receiving rabies postexposure prophylaxis.[31] The outreach effort also identified about 300 soldiers who had never reported the dog bite they received.[31] Approximately 50 of these 300 soldiers were given postexposure prophylaxis.[31]

Investigators have pointed out that data and information from the PDHA must be carefully assessed and used with caution, with consideration that true exposure risks will probably be underestimated.[29] The need for continuous evaluations of the Deployment Health Assessment questionnaires has been identified.[29] Even though the deployment-related questionnaires were developed as tools to facilitate recall and discussion during individual patient encounters and have documented shortcomings, investigators continue to use the responses in these forms to develop population-based data.[32–34] Others have argued that policies and priorities should not be determined solely on the basis of PDHA studies.[29]

WORK GROUP B DISCUSSION

Work Group B members supported positions developed by others and published regarding monitoring for hazardous exposures, such as the following:

- military commanders must be informed about the reasons for monitoring and must provide command support and leadership;
- monitoring must be done with clearly defined objectives and a meaningful plan; and
- efforts must continue to improve military procurement and training systems to facilitate having state-of-the-art equipment and trained operators available when needed.[15,24,35]

Work Group B members did not see postexposure modeling or biomonitoring to be tools that would be readily available and widely used in the near future. However, the need to continue to develop expertise and to do research with these tools was acknowledged.

Members of the group noted that full protection of deployed forces from hazardous exposures cannot be accomplished by monitoring devices and questionnaires. Military leaders must be informed about known and likely exposures, and be alert to the possibility of unanticipated exposures; they must assume their responsibility and take action to avoid or minimize exposures.[15,24] Examples of ongoing exposures in which early interventions could have reduced the possibility of exposure and later concerns about the exposure were identified by: (*a*) the use of large, open burn pits in the recent Iraq war for years; and (*b*) civilian contractors and military units working on a site contaminated with carcinogenic hexavalent chromium, an exposure that persisted through several rotations of military units.[28,29] Prompt recognition of a hazard, followed by a quick response of trained and equipped PVNTMED personnel, should increase the possibility that appropriate monitoring, appropriate use of questionnaires tailored to the situation, and perhaps the use of other tools previously discussed—all specifically designed for the situation at hand—would lead to the best possible exposure characterization. Rapid, reliable exposure characterization would contribute greatly to preventing morbidity and mortality, and would facilitate follow-up of those who may need it.

Considerable time was devoted to the discussion of questionnaires. Work Group B members agreed that questionnaires have value in assisting with patient recall and providing information to providers during clinical encounters. Additionally, the group agreed that questionnaire data could identify the need for new research or support research projects currently underway. However, there was little or no support for the idea that one or a few large questionnaires could cover all possible exposure situations.

One suggestion was to develop a *questionnaire bank*. The bank would contain questions that had been developed and evaluated for various categories of exposures. Responders to situations during deployments, such as clinicians and researchers, could use the bank to find questions pertinent to their work and develop specialized questionnaires for their particular needs. There was strong support for the idea that responding to an incident required a questionnaire tailored to the situation.

The use of large questionnaires that cover a broad range of topics in the US military was discussed. Most thought these questionnaires were too often viewed by service members as simply another requirement that had to be completed. Therefore, the reliability of the responses was unpredictable and depended on the service member's state of mind. Overcoming this situation would require questionnaires that were clear and concise. Additionally, service members and healthcare providers had to be convinced about the importance of the questionnaire and had to feel comfortable that they knew the intent of the questionnaire and the possible outcomes. With regard to possible outcomes, the importance of trained providers evaluating all answers and appropriate follow-up being implemented in a timely fashion was stressed.

SUMMARY

All questionnaires developed should be clear and concise and have:

- the reasons for the questionnaire and the expected outcomes clearly stated;
- the manner in which the questionnaire would be presented to uniformed members described;
- the method, place, and time for administering the questionnaire identified;
- the manner of follow-up of responses by trained personnel stated; and
- the intended use of the data obtained described.

Glass and Sim[17] believed that the practical choice for exposure assessment in military populations is the use of piloted and validated questionnaires that are completed during or soon after exposure. However, they point out the need for built-in checks of reliability, retesting to assess repeatability, and other safeguards.[17] The cautions and checks that they have identified for questionnaires must be considered for implementation by those who develop and administer questionnaires to US military members.[17] Work group B participants recommended the following:

- continue efforts to inform military leaders about hazardous exposures and their leadership responsibility to identify and respond to these;[15,24]
- continue efforts to procure and field state-of-the-art monitoring equipment in a timely fashion and personnel trained to operate the equipment;[15]
- maintain and improve expertise in the modeling of exposures and biomonitoring and support research in the areas that may be of value to the military;
- consider developing a questionnaire bank that would contain questionnaires and questions on various types of exposures and exposure outcomes (DoD and VA clinicians, public health specialists, and environmental scientists should have access to the repository)—the questionnaire bank would facilitate rapid development of questionnaires tailored to specific exposure scenarios; and
- develop checks of reliability and other safeguards for the deployment-related questionnaires currently being used.[17]

Acknowledgment

We thank all the participants of Work Group B: P. Ciminera, N. Desai, S. Gordon, T. Guidotti, D. Hardt, D. Harkins, M. Hodgson, T. Irons, B. Jaeger, S. Jones, J. Kirkpatrick, J. Kolivosky, M. Markiewicz, C. Mauzy, C. McCannon, C. Postlewaite, M. Prisco, R. Przygodzki, G. Reynolds, and J. Sharkey. (This chapter is a report of Work Group B.)

REFERENCES

1. Teichman R. Health hazards of exposures during deployment to war. *J Occup Environ Med.* 2012;54:655–658.

2. Richards EE. Responses to occupational and environmental exposures in the U.S. military—World War II to the present. *Mil Med.* 2011;176(suppl 7):22–28.

3. Young AL, Cecil PF. Agent Orange exposure and attributed health effects in Vietnam veterans. *Mil Med.* 2011;176(suppl 7):29–34.

4. Brown MA. Science versus policy in establishing equitable Agent Orange disability compensation policy. *Mil Med.* 2011;176(suppl 7):35–40.

5. Heller JM. Oil well fires of Operation Desert Storm—defining troop exposures and determining health risks. *Mil Med.* 2011;176(suppl 7):46–51.

6. Shorr AF, Scoville SL, Cersovsky SB, et al. Acute eosinophilic pneumonia among US military personnel deployed in or near Iraq. *JAMA.* 2004;292:2997–3005.

7. King MS, Eisenberg R, Newman JH, et al. Constrictive bronchiolitis in soldiers returning from Iraq and Afghanistan. *N Engl J Med.* 2011;365:222–230.

8. Conlin AM, DeScisciolo C, Sevick CJ, Bukowinski AT, Phillips CJ, Smith TC. Birth outcomes among military personnel after exposure to documented open-air burn pits before and during pregnancy. *J Occup Environ Med.* 2012;54:689–697.

9. Jones KA, Smith B, Granado NS, et al. Newly reported lupus and rheumatoid arthritis in relation to deployment within proximity to a documented open-air burn pit in Iraq. *J Occup Environ Med.* 2012;54:698–707.

10. Smith B, Wong CA, Boyko EJ, et al. The effects of exposure to documented open-air burn pits on respiratory health among deployers of the Millennium Cohort Study. *J Occup Environ Med.* 2012;54:708–716.

11. Abraham JH, DeBakey SF, Reid L, Zhou J, Baird C. Does deployment to Iraq and Afghanistan affect respiratory health of US military personnel? *J Occup Environ Med.* 2012;54:740–745.

12. Baird CP, DeBakey S, Reid L, Hauschild VD, Petruccelli B, Abraham JH. Respiratory health status of US Army personnel potentially exposed to smoke from 2003 Al-Mishraq Sulfur Plant fire. *J Occup Environ Med.* 2012;54:717–723.

13. Department of Defense. Proceedings of the 2010 symposium "Assessing Potentially Hazardous Environmental Exposures Among Military Populations," May 19–21, 2010, Bethesda, Maryland. *Mil Med.* 2011;176(suppl 7):1–112.

14. *Journal of Occupational and Environmental Medicine*. Special issue: health effects of deployment to Afghanistan and Iraq. *J Occup Environ Med.* 2012;54:655–759 (entire issue).

15. Gaydos JC. Military occupational and environmental health: challenges for the 21st century. *Mil Med.* 2011;176(suppl 7):5–8.

16. US Environmental Protection Agency. *Guidelines for Exposure Assessment*. Washington, DC: USEPA; 1992. EPA/600/Z-92/001.

17. Glass DC, Sim MR. The challenges of exposure assessment in health studies of Gulf War veterans. *Philos Trans R Soc Lond B Biol Sci.* 2006;361:627–637.

18. Buehler JW. Centers for Disease Control and Prevention. CDC's vision for public health surveillance in the 21st century. *MMWR Surveill Summ.* 2012;61(suppl):1–2.

19. Thacker SB, Berkelman RL. History of public health surveillance. In: Halperin W, Baker EL, eds. *Public Health Surveillance.* New York, NY: Van Nostrand Reinhold; 1992.

20. Lioy PJ, Rappaport SM. Exposure science and the exposome: an opportunity for coherence in the environmental health sciences. *Environ Health Perspect.* 2011;119:A466–A467.

21. Martin NJ, Richards EE, Kirkpatrick JS. Exposure science in U.S. military operations: a review. *Mil Med.* 2011;176 (suppl 7):77–83.

22. Batts R, Parzik D. Panel 3: conducting environmental surveillance sampling to identify exposures. *Mil Med.* 2011;176 (suppl 7):101–104.

23. Mallon TM. Progress in implementing recommendations in the National Academy of Sciences reports: "protecting those who serve: strategies to protect the health of deployed U.S. forces." *Mil Med.* 2011;176(suppl 7):9–16.

24. Chretien JP. Protecting service members in war—non-battle morbidity and command responsibility. *N Engl J Med.* 2012;366:677–679.

25. Squibb KS, Gaitens JM, Engelhardt S, et al. Surveillance for long-term health effects associated with depleted uranium exposure and retained embedded fragments in US veterans. *J Occup Environ Med.* 2012;54:724–732.

26. Deeter DP. The Kuwait Oil Fire Risk Assessment Biological Surveillance Initiative. *Mil Med.* 2011;176(suppl 7):52–55.

27. US Department of Defense. *US DoD Instruction Number 6490.03, Deployment Health.* http://www.dtic.mil/whs/directives/corres/pdf/649003p.pdf. Accessed December 13, 2012.

28. Weese CB. Evaluation of exposure incident at the Qarmat Ali Water Treatment Plant. *US Army Med Dept J.* 2009;April–June:10–13.

29. Mancuso JD, Ostafin M, Lovell M. Postdeployment evaluation of health risk communication after exposure to a toxic industrial chemical. *Mil Med.* 2008;173:369–374.

30. Centers for Disease Control and Prevention. Imported human rabies in a U.S. Army soldier—New York, 2011. *MMWR Morb Mortal Wkly Rep.* 2012;61:302–305.

31. Montgomery M. Confusion, anger surround report of soldier's rabies death. *Stars and Stripes.* http://www.stripes.com/news/confusion-anger-surround-report-of-soldier-s-rabies-death-1.166967. Accessed January 1, 2012.

32. Helmer DA, Rossignol M, Blatt M, Agarwal R, Teichman R, Lange G. Health and exposure concerns of veterans deployed to Iraq and Afghanistan. *J Occup Environ Med.* 2007;49:475–480.

33. Milliken CS, Auchterlonie JL, Hoge CW. Longitudinal assessment of mental health problems among active and reserve component soldiers returning from the Iraq war. *JAMA.* 2007;298:2141–2148.

34. Heltemes KJ, Holbrook TL, Macgregor AJ, Galarneau MR. Blast-related mild traumatic brain injury is associated with a decline in self-rated health amongst US military personnel. *Injury.* 2012;43:1990–1995.

35. Baird C. The basis for and uses of environmental sampling to assess health risk in deployed settings. *Mil Med.* 2011;176(suppl 7):84–90.

Chapter 30

REVIEW OF EPIDEMIOLOGICAL ANALYSES OF RESPIRATORY HEALTH OUTCOMES AFTER MILITARY DEPLOYMENT TO BURN PIT LOCATIONS WITH RESPECT TO FEASIBILITY AND DESIGN ISSUES HIGHLIGHTED BY THE INSTITUTE OF MEDICINE

JESSICA SHARKEY, MPH*; COLEEN BAIRD, MD†; ANGELIA EICK-COST, PhD, SCM‡; LESLIE CLARK, PhD, MS§; ZHENG HU, MS¥; SHARON LUDWIG, MD, MPH, MA¶; and JOSEPH ABRAHAM, ScD*

*Epidemiologist, Environmental Medicine Program, Occupational and Environmental Medicine Portfolio, Army Institute of Public Health, US Army Public Health Command, 5158 Blackhawk Road, Aberdeen Proving Ground, Maryland 21010-5403

†Program Manager, Environmental Medicine Program, Occupational and Environmental Medicine Portfolio, Army Institute of Public Health, US Army Public Health Command, 5158 Blackhawk Road, Aberdeen Proving Ground, Maryland 21010-5403

‡Senior Epidemiologist, Henry M. Jackson Foundation for the Advancement of Military Medicine, Division of Epidemiology and Analysis, Armed Forces Health Surveillance Center, 11800 Tech Road, Suite 220, Silver Spring, Maryland 20904

§Senior Epidemiologist, General Dynamics Information Technology, Division of Epidemiology and Analysis, Armed Forces Health Surveillance Center, 11800 Tech Road, Suite 220, Silver Spring, Maryland 20904

¥Biostatistician, Henry M. Jackson Foundation for the Advancement of Military Medicine, Division of Epidemiology and Analysis, Armed Forces Health Surveillance Center, 11800 Tech Road, Suite 220, Silver Spring, Maryland 20904

¶Captain, US Public Health Service/US Coast Guard; Director, Division of Epidemiology and Analysis, Armed Forces Health Surveillance Center, 11800 Tech Road, Suite 220, Silver Spring, Maryland 20904

INTRODUCTION

Since military operations began in southwest Asia in 2001, the majority of US military personnel who have served during the last 12 years deployed at least once in support of Operation Enduring Freedom (OEF), Operation Iraqi Freedom (OIF), and/or Operation New Dawn.[1,2] On average, a deployment lasts 9 months. During that time, service members can be exposed to a wide range of environmental hazards that may impact their pulmonary health. Sources for such hazards include particulate matter (PM) indigenous to the desert environment; local industry-related pollutants; and exhaust from the engines of vehicles, machinery, and generators utilized by both military and civilians. It is also possible that deployed service members are at increased risk for both acute and chronic health effects as a result of exposures during deployment, including smoke emitted during the combustion of waste burned in open air burn pits.[3–5]

Prior to 2009, sophisticated solid-waste disposal means (Figure 30-1)—such as the use of incinerators and municipal combustors, containerized removal, or waste segregation for reuse/recycling—were unavailable at many OIF and OEF deployment locations. As a result, burn pits (Figure 30-2) were widely used as the main method for waste management. Defined as "an area, not containing ... an incinerator or other equipment specifically designed ... for burning of solid waste, designated for the purpose of disposing of solid waste by burning in the outdoor air at a location with more than 100 attached or assigned personnel and that is in place longer than 90 days."[6(p9)] Open air burn pits are uncontrolled by nature and are generally characterized by low-temperature burning and smoldering.[7]

The particulates and chemicals emitted by burn pits contribute to the total concentration of environmental pollutants that may have harmful health effects. Components of smoke emitted by burning waste that have the greatest potential to cause health effects include respirable PM of 10 μm in diameter or less (PM_{10}); fine PM of 2.5 μm in diameter or less ($PM_{2.5}$); lead; mercury; dioxins; furans; polycyclic aromatic hydrocarbons; volatile organic compounds (VOCs); and irritant gases.[7] The contribution of burning waste to the environmental concentrations of those contaminants may vary widely and is based on a number of factors; among these are the volume, moisture content, and composition of the materials being burned and meteorological conditions.[8,9]

Anecdotal reports of complaints by service members of respiratory symptoms have been attributed to exposure to burn pit smoke; and news outlets and members of Congress have expressed concern that exposure to burn pit smoke in certain deployed settings is causing adverse health effects.[3,4] In 2009, the Office of the Assistant Secretary of Defense for Health Affairs–Force Health Protection & Readiness tasked the Armed Forces Health Surveillance Center (AFHSC) to support a collaborative multiagency effort to comprehensively evaluate health effects potentially related to burn pit exposures at deployment locations by conducting epidemiological studies using readily available data.

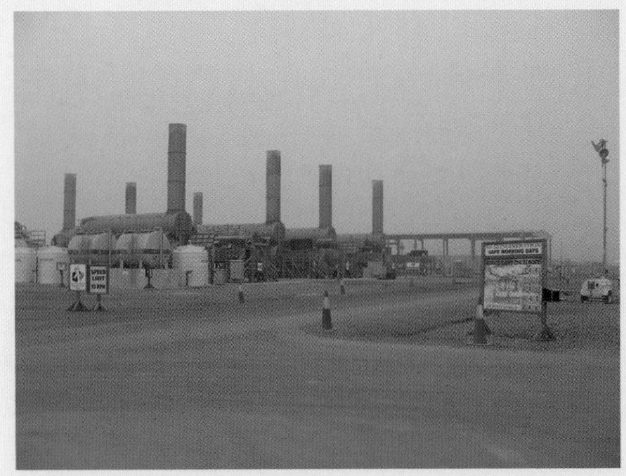

Figure 30-1. Incinerators for solid waste disposal.

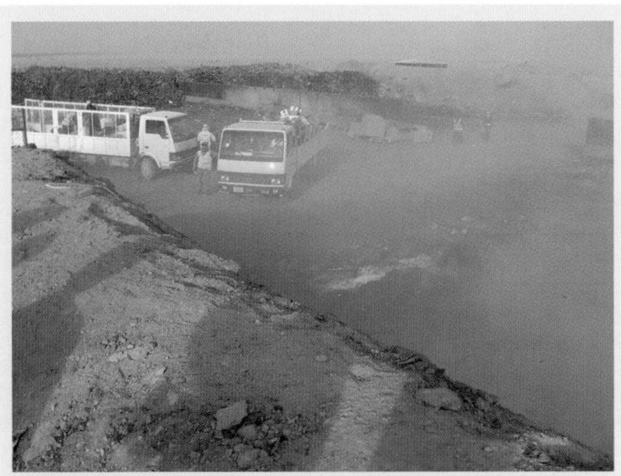

Figure 30-2. Burn pit.

HEALTH EFFECTS AMONG ACTIVE COMPONENT US SERVICE MEMBERS WHO DEPLOYED TO SELECT DEPLOYMENT LOCATIONS: 36 MONTHS' FOLLOW-UP

In response to Force Health Protection & Readiness' inquiry, AFHSC conducted a retrospective cohort study to:

- compare the incidence rates among deployers and nondeployers for respiratory diseases, circulatory disease, cardiovascular disease, ill-defined conditions, and sleep apnea;
- compare the responses on the postdeployment health assessment forms among the individuals deployed to one of several US Central Command (CENTCOM) locations; and
- compare the rates and proportions of medical encounters for respiratory outcomes while assigned to the various US CENTCOM locations.

For the purposes of this discussion, focus will be limited to the primary objective as it relates to respiratory health outcomes. The technical report can be viewed in its entirety, including results from the analyses conducted to address the other objectives and contributions from other collaborating agencies.[10]

Methods

Camp Cohorts

The Defense Manpower Data Center deployment roster was queried for all active duty service members deployed to Joint Base Balad (JBB) or Camp Taji in Iraq, and Camp Buehring or Camp Arifjan in Kuwait for more than 30 days between January 1, 2005 and June 30, 2007. Both Iraqi locations (JBB and Camp Taji) were selected because of the presence of burn pits at those deployment sites, whereas the two camps in Kuwait were selected for the similarity of their environmental characteristics to JBB and Camp Taji without having burn pits on location. During this time period, the population at JBB was as high as 25,000. The burn pit was estimated to be as large as 10 acres,[8,11] although not all areas were burning at any one time. Individuals were required to be at the specific camp at the end of their deployment so that any effects of the location resulting in medical encounters could be accurately captured immediately following the deployment. Personnel who spent time in more than one of the camps or who had multiple, noncontinuous segments in a specific camp during the deployment were excluded. Due to the small number of Marines (<2% of the total camp population) and no Navy personnel identified at these locations, camp cohorts were restricted to service members from the Army and the Air Force.

Comparison Groups

The Defense Medical Surveillance System personnel records were queried for all active duty service members with a history of being stationed in the Republic of Korea for more than 30 days, beginning any time during January 1, 2005 and June 30, 2007. This location was selected for a comparison population because of the meteorological phenomenon known as "yellow dust," which causes annual elevations in geogenic PM in the spring. Additionally, this overseas location was chosen because it requires certain health standards be met at the time of assignment, potentially making for a healthier population when compared with the general military population located in the continental United States (CONUS). The general CONUS military population includes individuals who are convalescing, who are in temporary nondeployable status for a variety of reasons, or who have permanent profiles and/or are in the process of separation from military service. Previously deployed personnel and those already selected for the Iraqi/Kuwait camp cohorts were excluded. A CONUS-based comparison group was also selected, which included all active duty service members who had never been deployed and stationed only in CONUS as of April 15, 2006. Personnel who appeared in any of the Iraqi/Kuwait camp cohorts or the Korea-based comparison group were excluded. Both comparison groups were restricted to service members from the Army and the Air Force because sailors and Marines were not represented in the camp cohorts.

Outcomes of Interest

All medical encounters at a military treatment facility—including both hospitalizations and ambulatory medical encounters—with an *International Classification of Diseases-Clinical Modification, 9th Revision* (ICD-9-CM), code in any diagnostic position indicating a disease of the respiratory system (460–519) during the 36-month follow-up period were captured. Any inpatient or outpatient visit was coded as

- an acute respiratory infection case was noted if ICD-9-CM codes 460–466 were indicated;
- a chronic obstructive pulmonary disease and an allied conditions case were noted if ICD-9-CM codes 490–492 or 494–496 were indicated;
- an asthma case was noted if ICD-9-CM code 493 was indicated; and
- signs, symptoms, and ill-defined conditions involving the respiratory system and other chest symptoms (SSIC [Standard Subject Identification Codes]–respiratory) were noted if ICD-9-CM code 786 was indicated.

Statistical Analysis

Incidence and 95% confidence intervals (CIs) for first diagnoses (number of incident diagnoses per 1,000 person-years) were calculated for each condition for each population. Incidence rate ratios (IRRs) and 95% CIs were calculated to compare the deployed populations to the CONUS-based population. IRRs were adjusted for covariates of importance—specifically age and grade (defined at start of follow-up)—as well as sex, race, and service using Poisson regression models. Negative binomial and zero-inflated negative binomial models were also explored, but provided similar estimates as the Poisson models and are therefore not reported. A service-stratified analysis and stratification by time in location were also conducted, but these results are not shown because they did not yield meaningfully different results from the overall analysis.

Results

Table 30-1 displays a comparison of the demographic and service-related covariates between the five cohorts. There were significant demographic differences in the deployed populations compared with the CONUS-based population. Specifically, the age makeup of the deployed population differed from the CONUS-based cohort, and the gender makeup of the deployed cohorts was different than the Korea and CONUS-based cohorts. JBB has a higher percentage of Air Force personnel, whereas Arifjan and Korea had a higher percentage of Army personnel. The Buehring and Taji cohorts were almost exclusively Army.

Crude unadjusted and adjusted IRRs varied depending on the camp and the outcome of interest (Table 30-2). For all outcomes, subjects from at least one of the camps or Korea had significantly lower incidence rates (*yellow shading*) compared with the CONUS-based cohort. The only outcome and camp with significantly higher unadjusted incidence rate (*green shading*) compared with the CONUS-based cohort was SSIC–respiratory among the Arifjan cohort (IRR = 1.10, 95% CI = 1.02, 1.19); however, this finding was not significant in the adjusted model. Specifically for JBB, adjusted incidence rates compared with the CONUS-based cohort were significantly lower for all outcomes except SSIC–respiratory, which showed no significant difference from the CONUS-based rate.

TABLE 30-1

DEMOGRAPHIC CHARACTERISTICS OF THE STUDY COHORTS: UP TO 36 MONTHS' FOLLOW-UP

	Balad		Taji		Arifjan		Buehring		Korea		CONUS	
	n	%	*n*	%	*n*	%	*n*	%	*n*	%	*n*	%
Total	15,908	100.0	2,522	100.0	4,431	100.0	1,906	100.0	44,962	100.0	237,714	100.0
Age (yrs)												
<20	46	0.3	32	1.3	14	0.3	37	1.9	581	1.3	17,175	7.2
20–29	9,635	60.6	1,695	67.2	2,600	58.7	1,334	70.0	33,086	73.6	141,731	59.6
30–39	4,588	28.8	625	24.8	1,291	29.1	441	23.1	8,574	19.1	50,937	21.4
40+	1,639	10.3	170	6.7	526	11.9	94	4.9	2,721	6.1	27,871	11.7
Sex												
Female	2,478	15.6	317	12.6	554	12.5	205	10.8	9,094	20.2	55,720	23.4
Male	13,430	84.4	2,205	87.4	3,877	87.5	1,701	89.2	35,868	79.8	181,994	76.6
Race												
White	10,967	68.9	1,555	61.7	2,732	61.7	1,218	63.9	25,812	57.4	162,417	68.3
Black	2,388	15.0	581	23.0	971	21.9	345	18.1	10,022	22.3	37,583	15.8
Other	2,553	16.0	386	15.3	728	16.4	343	18.0	9,128	20.3	37,714	15.9
Rank												
E00–E04	6,354	39.9	1,256	49.8	1,707	38.5	988	51.8	26,828	59.7	126,564	53.2
E05–E09	7,092	44.6	1,004	39.8	2,028	45.8	693	36.4	13,546	30.1	62,466	26.3
O01–O10 (including warrant)	2,462	15.5	262	10.4	696	15.7	225	11.8	4,588	10.2	48,684	20.5
Service												
Army	3,989	25.1	2,522	100.0	2,873	64.8	1,904	99.9	32,553	72.4	100,726	42.4
Air Force	11,919	74.9	0	0.0	1,558	35.2	2	0.1	12,409	27.6	136,988	57.6

CONUS: continental United States

TABLE 30-2

INCIDENCE RATE RATIOS OF RESPIRATORY HEALTH OUTCOMES BY COHORT: UP TO 36 MONTHS' FOLLOW-UP

A. Incidence Rate Ratios for Respiratory Diseases (ICD-9-CM: 460–519)

				Unadjusted			Poisson Model		
	Person-years	Incidence	IR*1,000	IRR	95% Lower	95% Upper	IRR	95% Lower	95% Upper
Balad	18,132	6,477	357	0.89	0.87	0.91	0.91	0.88	0.93
Taji	2,866	900	314	0.78	0.73	0.84	0.86	0.81	0.92
Arifjan	4,950	1,847	373	0.93	0.89	0.97	1.00	0.96	1.05
Buehring	1,364	340	249	0.62	0.56	0.69	0.68	0.61	0.75
Korea	49,355	16,661	338	0.84	0.83	0.85	0.83	0.82	0.84
CONUS	272,903	109,563	401		REF			REF	

B. Incidence Rate Ratios of Acute Respiratory Infections (ICD-9-CM: 460–466)

				Unadjusted			Poisson Model		
	Person-years	Incidence	IR*1,000	IRR	95% Lower	95% Upper	IRR	95% Lower	95% Upper
Balad	20,446	4,859	238	0.87	0.84	0.89	0.90	0.88	0.93
Taji	3,128	686	219	0.80	0.74	0.86	0.90	0.83	0.97
Arifjan	5,698	1,333	234	0.85	0.81	0.90	0.95	0.90	1.00
Buehring	1,498	231	154	0.56	0.49	0.64	0.62	0.54	0.70
Korea	54,703	12,615	231	0.84	0.83	0.86	0.82	0.81	0.84
CONUS	311,221	85,382	274		REF			REF	

C. Incidence Rate Ratios of Chronic Obstructive Pulmonary Disease (ICD-9-CM: 490–492, 494–496)

				Unadjusted			Poisson Model		
	Person-years	Incidence	IR*1,000	IRR	95% Lower	95% Upper	IRR	95% Lower	95% Upper
Balad	25,923	564	22	0.84	0.77	0.92	0.91	0.84	0.99
Taji	3,802	93	24	0.95	0.77	1.16	0.83	0.68	1.02
Arifjan	7,174	186	26	1.00	0.87	1.16	0.98	0.85	1.13
Buehring	1,733	31	18	0.69	0.49	0.98	0.62	0.44	0.88
Korea	67,591	1,556	23	0.89	0.84	0.94	0.83	0.78	0.88
CONUS	415,659	10,749	26		REF			REF	

D. Incidence Rate Ratios of Asthma (ICD-9-CM: 493)

				Unadjusted			Poisson Model		
	Person-years	Incidence	IR*1,000	IRR	95% Lower	95% Upper	IRR	95% Lower	95% Upper
Balad	26,164	332	13	0.66	0.59	0.73	0.81	0.73	0.91
Taji	3,815	83	22	1.13	0.91	1.40	0.97	0.78	1.21
Arifjan	7,211	149	21	1.07	0.91	1.26	0.95	0.80	1.11
Buehring	1,720	32	19	0.96	0.68	1.36	0.76	0.53	1.07
Korea	67,638	1,386	20	1.06	1.00	1.12	0.91	0.86	0.96
CONUS	417,579	8,062	19		REF			REF	

(**Table 30-2** *continues*)

Table 30-2 *continued*

E. Incidence Rate Ratios of SSIC–Respiratory Symptoms and Other Chest Symptoms (ICD-9-CM: 786)

				Unadjusted			Poisson Model		
	Person-years	Incidence	IR*1,000	IRR	95% Lower	95% Upper	IRR	95% Lower	95% Upper
Balad	24,036	2,205	92	0.93	0.89	0.97	0.97	0.93	1.01
Taji	3,517	348	99	1.00	0.90	1.11	0.99	0.89	1.10
Arifjan	6,548	712	109	1.10	1.02	1.19	1.07	0.99	1.15
Buehring	1,617	129	80	0.81	0.68	0.96	0.79	0.67	0.94
Korea	32,919	5,931	94	0.95	0.93	0.98	0.91	0.89	0.94
CONUS	382,505	37,772	99		REF			REF	

CI: confidence interval; CONUS: continental United States; ICD-9-CM: *International Classification of Diseases-Clinical Modification, 9th Revision*; IR: incidence rate; IRR: incidence rate ratio; REF: reference value (equal to 1 for the CONUS groups); SSIC: Standard Subject Identification Codes
Notes: For all outcomes, subjects from at least one of the camps or Korea had significantly lower IRs (*yellow shading*) compared with the CONUS-based cohort. The only outcome and camp with significantly higher unadjusted IR (*green shading*) compared with the CONUS-based cohort was SSIC–respiratory among the Arifjan cohort (IRR = 1.10, 95% CI = 1.02, 1.19); however, this finding was not significant in the adjusted model.

Conclusions

The purpose of this analysis was to evaluate post-deployment healthcare encounters among personnel stationed at different in-theater locations in CENTCOM—two locations known to have burn pits and two locations without burn pits—and compare them with a similarly healthy group that may have been exposed to PM levels higher than in the United States (personnel assigned to Korea) and to a CONUS-based group. This study found no evidence that service members at burn pit locations are at an increased risk for the respiratory health outcomes examined up to 36 months' postdeployment. Although this analysis has its limitations, results generally show no impact of burn pit exposure up to 3 years later. Future analyses should focus on improving the quality of individual-level exposure data, including data from additional burn pit sites, and further investigate possible long-term health effects related to burn pit exposure.

LONG-TERM HEALTH CONSEQUENCES OF EXPOSURE TO BURN PITS IN IRAQ AND AFGHANISTAN

Scores of military personnel who served in support of the conflicts in Iraq and Afghanistan have returned home with reported health problems that they attribute to exposure to burn pit emissions during deployment. With concern also coming from families of veterans and Congress, as well as reports from media outlets and the publishing of scientific studies, the US Department of Veterans Affairs (VA) asked the Institute of Medicine (IOM) to form a committee tasked with making a determination of the long-term health effects associated with exposure to burn pits during OEF and OIF. Additionally, the committee was also asked to review feasibility and design issues of future epidemiological studies related to long-term health risks of veterans exposed to the burn pit at JBB. As a part of that effort, the report highlighting the AFHSC's analysis was reviewed, along with other peer-reviewed literature, government documents and data, and relevant reports on the subject. The IOM concluded, "service in Iraq or Afghanistan—that is, a broader consideration of air pollution than exposure only to burn pit emissions—might be associated with long-term health effects, particularly in highly exposed populations (such as those who worked at the burn pit) or susceptible populations (for example, those who have asthma), mainly because of the high ambient concentrations of PM from both natural and anthropogenic, including military, sources."[12(p7)]

In the assessment of the feasibility and design issues of an epidemiological study of veterans exposed to burn pit emissions, the committee concluded that the major challenges of such effort(s) are both exposure assessment and outcome ascertainment. The committee also identified the elements of a well-designed epidemiological study, including

- selection of a relevant study population of adequate size,
- comprehensive assessment of exposure,
- careful evaluation of health outcomes,
- reasonable methods for controlling confounding and minimizing bias,
- appropriate statistical analyses, and
- adequate follow-up time.

Study Design Elements

Study Population Selection

Identified within the IOM report as paramount to the success of an epidemiological study evaluating long-term health risks among veterans exposed to burn pit emissions is the proper selection of both exposed and comparison groups. Ideally, the exposed population is a representative sample of the population of interest, that is, military personnel deployed to locations with burn pits and comparison group(s) should be as similar to the exposed population as possible, with exception of the exposure of interest. Proper study population selection is done to avoid confounding, which occurs when there are differences in baseline characteristics between the groups, as well as bias, including bias related to the selection of exposed and unexposed groups.

In the original analysis conducted by AFHSC, it is not unexpected that one would see lower rates of respiratory health outcomes in the camp cohorts when compared with the CONUS-based population, which includes service members with health profiles considered ineligible for deployment. This issue of noncomparability is referred to as a "healthy warrior" or "healthy deployer" effect, a term used to "designate the selection bias from systematic differences in the health of military personnel who are deployed to a war zone and those who are not deployed due to the selective withholding of chronically ill soldiers from deployment."[13(p316)] To address the issue of noncompatibility, a cohort of military personnel stationed in Korea was selected for its greater degree of similarity in health status to the camp cohorts because service members with certain health problems cannot be supported by the limited healthcare resources found at many sites outside CONUS and therefore remain stationed at CONUS locations. More comparable yet would be a population of OEF/OIF-deployed service members who were located at base camps that utilized other methods of waste management; this would make the most appropriate comparison group for studying long-term health effects associated with exposure to burn pits, as indicated in the IOM report.

Exposure Assessment

According to the IOM report, obtaining accurate exposure profiles is also a key element in any successful environmental exposure-related epidemiological study. As the committee indicates, "exposure assessment characterizes the frequency, magnitude, and duration of exposure to an agent of concern in a population."[12] In an ideal study, exposure assessment would include ascertainment of quantitative exposure data for individual study subjects. Although personal monitors were never utilized and the burn pit at JBB is now closed (therefore, the opportunity to do so is lost), there are ways to estimate levels of exposure for study populations. Other information sources include, but are not limited to, exposure profiles provided on self-reported questionnaires, data from environmental sampling, modeling based on location in relation to the burn pit site, activities performed during deployment, and duration of exposure. Unfortunately, these methods of estimating exposure levels introduce measurement error (misclassification) and potentially bias measures of association between exposure and health outcomes. Differential misclassification would result from measurement errors in exposure that are related to health outcome or vice versa. Nondifferential misclassification describes measurement errors in exposure that are unrelated to health outcome or vice versa. In this case, one would suspect that any misclassification of exposure would occur irrespective of health outcome, resulting in nondifferential misclassification. In instances where self-reported information is used to formulate an exposure assessment, recall bias or the occurrence of exposed cohort study subjects (eg, recalling and reporting subsequent disease(s) more or less so than unexposed subjects) is possible. Recall bias would be an exception to nondifferential misclassification.

Evaluation of Health Outcomes

The IOM report also recognizes accurate ascertainment of health outcomes as just as important as accurate exposure assessment in conducting an epidemiological study examining the association between burn pit emission exposure and long-term health outcomes. As the committee points out, there are several sources of information from which to gather the health status of military personnel, including—but not limited to—electronic medical encounter records containing physician-coded diagnoses; disease registries containing health-related information for veterans and service members; and self-reported questionnaires containing items on postdeployment symptoms and disease. However, there are noted limitations associated with these sources of data. For example, coding errors in the classification of disease or the use of ICD-9-CM codes to describe chief complaints and current symptoms rather than the presence of disease by healthcare providers on electronic medical records would typically result in more cases of disease labeled than actually exist in the population. An illustration of the limitations presented by diagnostic coding is the increased use of bronchitis, not specified as acute or chronic (ICD-9-CM: 490). Although 10-year trends indicate that this code is being used more and more frequently, there is little understanding of what that diagnosis signifies in a clinical sense. Recall bias can occur on questionnaire responses if service members who were exposed to burn pit emissions are more (or less) likely to recall and report subsequent disease than their unexposed counterparts, or if service members with a respiratory diagnosis are more (or less) likely to accurately report past exposures relative to noncases. Use of data from disease registries can also present challenges, such as self-selection and free-text entries, as is the case with the

TABLE 30-3

INCIDENCE RATE RATIOS OF RESPIRATORY HEALTH OUTCOMES BY COHORT: UP TO 48 MONTHS' FOLLOW-UP

A. Incidence Rate Ratios for Respiratory Diseases (ICD-9-CM: 460–519)

				Unadjusted			Poisson Model		
	Person-years	Incidence	IR*1,000	IRR	95% Lower	95% Upper	IRR	95% Lower	95% Upper
Balad	19,425.05	6,798	349.96	0.90	0.88	0.92	0.92	0.90	0.94
Taji	3,029.93	931	307.27	0.79	0.74	0.84	0.86	0.81	0.92
Arifjan	5,287.34	1,916	362.38	0.93	0.89	0.98	1.01	0.96	1.05
Buehring	1,406.61	354	251.67	0.65	0.58	0.72	0.70	0.63	0.78
Korea	53,396.96	17,573	329.1	0.85	0.83	0.86	0.83	0.82	0.85
CONUS	294,779.87	114,579	388.69		REF			REF	

B. Incidence Rate Ratios of Acute Respiratory Infections (ICD-9-CM: 460–466)

				Unadjusted			Poisson Model		
	Person-years	Incidence	IR*1,000	IRR	95% Lower	95% Upper	IRR	95% Lower	95% Upper
Balad	22,180.31	5,173	233.22	0.88	0.85	0.90	0.91	0.89	0.94
Taji	3,336.14	717	214.92	0.81	0.75	0.87	0.90	0.84	0.97
Arifjan	6,182.94	1,399	226.27	0.85	0.81	0.90	0.95	0.90	1.00
Buehring	1,571.03	244	155.31	0.59	0.52	0.66	0.64	0.56	0.72
Korea	59,981.16	13,479	224.72	0.85	0.83	0.86	0.83	0.81	0.84
CONUS	340,952.18	90,461	265.32		REF			REF	

C. Incidence Rate Ratios of Chronic Obstructive Pulmonary Disease (ICD-9-CM: 490–492, 494–496)

				Unadjusted			Poisson Model		
	Person-years	Incidence	IR*1,000	IRR	95% Lower	95% Upper	IRR	95% Lower	95% Upper
Balad	29,254.33	640	21.88	0.85	0.79	0.92	0.91	0.84	0.99
Taji	4,165.45	103	24.73	0.96	0.79	1.17	0.86	0.71	1.05
Arifjan	8,051.75	211	26.21	1.02	0.89	1.17	1.00	0.87	1.15
Buehring	1,873.35	35	18.68	0.73	0.52	1.02	0.66	0.47	0.92
Korea	77,214.95	1,785	23.12	0.90	0.86	0.95	0.84	0.80	0.89
CONUS	477,289.63	12,231	25.63		REF			REF	

D. Incidence Rate Ratios of Asthma (ICD-9-CM: 493)

				Unadjusted			Poisson Model		
	Person-years	Incidence	IR*1,000	IRR	95% Lower	95% Upper	IRR	95% Lower	95% Upper
Balad	29,622.50	361	12.19	0.67	0.60	0.74	0.82	0.74	0.91
Taji	4,194.72	85	20.26	1.11	0.90	1.38	0.95	0.76	1.18
Arifjan	8,137.45	156	19.17	1.05	0.90	1.23	0.92	0.79	1.08
Buehring	1,855.05	33	17.79	0.98	0.69	1.38	0.76	0.54	1.07
Korea	77,477.95	1,504	19.41	1.07	1.01	1.13	0.91	0.86	0.97
CONUS	481,298.15	8,762	18.2		REF			REF	

(Table 30-3 *continues*)

Table 30-3 *continued*

E. Incidence Rate Ratios of SSIC–Respiratory Symptoms and Other Chest Symptoms (ICD-9-CM: 786)

				Unadjusted			Poisson Model		
	Person-years	Incidence	IR*1,000	IRR	95% Lower	95% Upper	IRR	95% Lower	95% Upper
Balad	26,750.12	2,451	91.63	0.93	0.89	0.97	0.96	0.92	1.00
Taji	3,807.19	376	98.76	1.00	0.90	1.11	0.99	0.90	1.10
Arifjan	7,245.26	771	106.41	1.08	1.00	1.16	1.04	0.97	1.12
Buehring	1,723.88	139	80.63	0.82	0.69	0.97	0.80	0.68	0.94
Korea	70,650.63	6,781	95.98	0.97	0.95	1.00	0.93	0.91	0.96
CONUS	431,893.41	42,600	98.64		REF			REF	

CI: confidence interval; CONUS: continental United States; ICD-9-CM: *International Classification of Diseases-Clinical Modification, 9th Revision*; IR: incidence rate; IRR: incidence rate ratio; REF: reference value (equal to 1 for the CONUS groups); SSIC: Standard Subject Identification Codes
Notes: For all outcomes, subjects from at least one of the camps or Korea had significantly lower IRs (*yellow shading*) compared with the CONUS-based cohort. The only outcome and camp with significantly higher unadjusted IR (*green shading*) compared with the CONUS-based cohort was asthma among the Korea cohort (IRR = 1.07, 95% CI = 1.01, 1.13); however, this finding was significantly lower in the adjusted model.

VA registry established to track possible long-term health problems with respect to possible Agent Orange exposure.[14,15] Despite these known potential limitations, AFHSC is not only responsible for maintaining several surveillance databases that store health information for military personnel across the US Department of Defense (DoD), but also they have successfully linked these sources—that contain large amounts of data and have high enough statistical power to detect significant differences across cohorts—to accurately ascertain health outcome. The methodology used and the study findings have been published.[10]

Proposed Approaches to the Study of Health Outcomes From Exposure to Burn Pit Emissions

As part of the task of evaluating the feasibility and design issues of future epidemiological studies on the topic, the IOM committee outlined proposed approaches, organized in several tiers, to address research questions of interest.

Tier 1

The recommendation suggested in Tier 1 focused on the following question: Did proximity to burn pit operations at JBB increase the risk of adverse health outcomes? The proposed approach includes ordinal estimations of individual exposure assessments based on factors such as length of deployment, duties at JBB, distance and location of assigned barracks with respect to the burn pit, and wind dispersion patterns. Although length of deployment can be acquired from existing DoD data sources, there may not be a linear relationship between duration of deployment and burn pit emission exposure, given the truly unique deployment experience each individual service member has, as well as variability in burn pit emissions and meteorological conditions over time. Also readily available in DoD data sources are occupation codes; however, these codes may not reflect true job duties performed during deployment. For example, the burn pit at JBB had guard towers at its periphery to discourage local nationals from going into the pit to secure items still considered to be of value. Due to the nature of their duties, it might be anticipated that these individuals had the highest potential exposure; however, those assigned these duties are not identifiable with a single Military Occupation Series code. Although the importance of this recommendation is acknowledged, for the reasons previously stated, a valid exposure assessment tool would be needed to establish low, medium, or high exposures to burn pit emissions. For more information on exposure characterization and assessment tools, see Chapter 29 (Discussion Summary: Exposure Characterization—Questionnaires and Other Tools).

Tier 2

The recommendation suggested in Tier 2 seeks to address the following question: Did installation of incinerators at JBB reduce the incidence of disease or intermediate outcomes (eg, emphysema or rate of lung function decline)? This recommendation focuses on comparing long-term health outcomes of service members who were deployed to JBB while the burn pits were in full operation with those service members who were deployed to JBB after incinerators were installed. Such a comparison would include several different categories of exposure given the phased-approach taken to transition waste management at JBB from burn pits only to incinerators exclusively. Health risk assessments conducted during time periods of burn pit use (sampling performed in spring and fall 2007) compared with the use of incinerators (sampling performed March–May 2010) identified an increase in the number of samples detecting levels that indicated a potential for respiratory irritation. During open air burn pit operations, two chemicals (acrolein and hexachlorobutadiene) were detected over 1-year Military Exposure Guidelines (MEGs) in 1 of 41 samples in spring 2007, and acrolein detection was estimated to be over 1-year MEGs in 3 of 24 samples in fall 2007. After the burn pit was officially closed in October 2009 and incinerators were installed, a combination of chemicals (primarily acrolein) was detected over 1-year MEGs in 40 of 53 samples. These results may give the impression that there appears to have been a worsening in air quality after the installation of incinerators. However, the increased number and proportion of positive samples are thought to be from a change in laboratory methods used to analyze VOCs in the ambient air samples, from Toxic Organic (TO)-14 to TO-15 between 2007 and 2010 collection efforts. Specifically, the TO-15 method has increased extraction capability for VOCs over the TO-14 method. Consequently, comparing results for the sampling periods using the TO-14 method to the sampling periods using the TO-15 method is somewhat problematic. More work in this area would be needed to determine how these findings correlate with trends in health outcomes. Additional analyses to determine effectiveness of the intervention intended to reduce burn pit emissions exposure (based on rates of respiratory health outcomes) is certainly a worthy endeavor, especially given results from the health risk assessments that were conducted and considering that it was addressed neither by the AFHSC analyses nor any other known research efforts to date.

Tier 3

The research question proposed in Tier 3 is as follows: Did deployment at JBB during full burn pit operation increase risk of adverse health outcomes compared with deployment elsewhere in Iraq or Afghanistan or compared with no deployment? According to the committee, such a question could be addressed assessing exposure to JBB dichotomously. This yes/no exposure categorization broadly indicates exposure to the comprehensive environmental hazards found at JBB rather than serving as a marker for burn pit emission exposure solely. Health outcomes among those who were deployed to JBB while the burn pits were in operation could then be compared with health outcomes of military personnel deployed elsewhere. This proposed approach has been utilized in the past, as described in the assessments conducted by both AFHSC and the Naval Health Research Center (San Diego, CA) as part of the Millennium Cohort Study that were included in the 2010 published technical report *Epidemiological Studies of Health Outcomes Among Troops Deployed to Burn Pit Sites.*[10]

HEALTH EFFECTS AMONG ACTIVE COMPONENT US SERVICE MEMBERS WHO DEPLOYED TO SELECT DEPLOYMENT LOCATIONS: 48 MONTHS' FOLLOW-UP

In the summary of their original analysis, AFHSC acknowledged that future studies should be focused on further investigating possible long-term health effects related to burn pit exposure. The IOM committee also identified adequate follow-up time as a key element of a well-designed epidemiological study. In light of these statements, the first analysis conducted by AFHSC, which included up to 36 months of follow-up postdeployment, has since been updated to include up to 48 months of follow-up postdeployment.

Results

Crude unadjusted and adjusted IRRs varied depending on the camp and the outcome of interest (Table 30-3). For all outcomes, subjects from at least one of the camps or Korea had significantly lower incidence rates (*yellow shading*) compared with the CONUS-based cohort. The only outcome and camp with significantly higher unadjusted incidence rate (*green shading*), compared with the CONUS-based cohort, was asthma among the Korea cohort (IRR = 1.07, 95% CI = 1.01, 1.13); however, this finding was significantly lower in the adjusted model. When compared with the CONUS-based cohort, adjusted incidence rates

TABLE 30-4

MEDIAN AND MEAN FOLLOW-UP TIMES BY COHORT AND ANALYSIS (MONTHS)

	Up to 36 Months' Follow-up		Up to 48 Months' Follow-up	
	Median	Mean	Median	Mean
Balad	1.42	1.67	1.44	1.90
Taji	1.40	1.55	1.41	1.70
Arifjan	1.49	1.67	1.52	1.89
Buehring	0.51	0.93	0.51	1.00
Korea	1.34	1.54	1.41	1.77
CONUS	1.71	1.80	1.74	2.08

CONUS: continental United States

for JBB were significantly lower for all outcomes except SSIC–respiratory, which showed no significant difference from the CONUS-based rate. The median and mean follow-up times for both the original and updated analyses are provided in Table 30-4.

Conclusions

The purpose of this analysis was to increase the follow-up time of the original assessment of health effects among active component service members who deployed to select locations, from 36 months to 48 months. As in the original analysis, this extended analysis found no evidence that service members at burn pit locations are at an increased risk for the respiratory health outcomes examined up to 48 months postdeployment. Furthermore, the extended follow-up analysis showed the same pattern of findings as the original analysis for JBB compared with the CONUS-based cohort, with significantly lower adjusted incidence rates for all respiratory outcomes except SSIC–respiratory that was not significantly different from the CONUS-based rate. Results generally show no impact of burn pit exposure up to 4 years later.

SUMMARY

In addition to outlining proposed questions for future research, the IOM committee highlighted three elements on which to focus when conducting epidemiological studies investigating the association between burn pit emission exposure during deployment and long-term health outcomes:

1. proper study population selection,
2. accurate exposure assessment, and
3. precise ascertainment of health outcomes.

To ensure selection of the most appropriate study population, a cohort of military personnel stationed in Korea was included in these analyses. This was done to address the healthy warrior/healthy deployer effect, providing a group more comparable in health status to the camp cohorts than service members at CONUS locations, as indicated by results presented in Table 30-2 and Table 30-3. Studies conducted to date have typically used deployment to a location with a burn pit as a proxy for exposure to burn pit emissions in the absence of individual-level exposure data. Given the lack of exposure information on a service member-by-service member basis, Korea was also selected to serve as a comparison group due to the potential for exposure to higher PM levels (when compared with a CONUS reference group) as a result of the seasonal yellow dust phenomenon. Despite including a group that may have similar PM exposure to deployed cohorts in the analyses discussed, future efforts should emphasize improved quality of individual-level exposure data.

To improve on health outcome assessment, the original analysis conducted using up to 36 months of follow-up time was extended to include up to 48 months of follow-up. However, median times did not increase notably (Table 30-4), indicating loss to follow-up. Even the follow-up times in the updated analysis would not likely be sufficient time to develop the chronic respiratory health outcomes of interest, which is a limitation that has been noted in previous epidemiological work,[16] highlighting the need for and stressing the importance of a more seamless healthcare system between active duty service and veteran status for truly longitudinal evaluations. Thus, an Integrated Electronic Health Record is currently in development that will combine electronic health record systems of both departments, thus creating a single health record across all DoD and VA medical facilities.[17,18]

These findings should be balanced by the understanding that there are limitations to this study. First, data were not available on individual environmental exposures over time; therefore, all individuals at a location were assumed to have been equally exposed to the conditions of that location. Numerous factors, such as those mentioned by Smith et al,[16] including composition of materials being burned and prevailing wind conditions—as well as deployment duties (apart from or in addition to job classification) and specific duty locations—would have likely had an impact on individual environmental exposures within the camp; however, such data are not available. The bias introduced when such broad exposure definitions are used (exposure misclassification)[16] would weaken the strength of associations found between burn pit emissions exposure and postdeployment respiratory outcomes. Further complicating exposure assessment is the lack of data on where individuals were located prior to being at the camps of interest. If individuals did not spend their entire deployment at one of the specific camps, they may have been exposed to other environmental conditions while at different locations. Second, health outcomes were defined using administrative medical data, which likely resulted in false positives for a variety of reasons, including ICD-9-CM coding errors in the classification of disease and the use of diagnostic codes to describe chief complaints and current symptoms rather than actual disease.

Analyses of postdeployment healthcare encounters are impacted by the fact that all personnel following redeployment are required to have at least one healthcare encounter to complete postdeployment health assessment processing around the time of return, and another visit 3 to 6 months later to complete postdeployment health reassessment processing. This type of mandatory healthcare encounter is not counted as a condition, but may introduce an opportunity to identify a diagnosis. This situation may introduce a surveillance bias that can exaggerate effects observed in deployers when compared with nondeployers. Also, because healthcare during deployment is often limited, "catch up" on requirements such as well-woman examinations, immunizations, and other mandatory visits also occur postdeployment.

Despite efforts to choose cohorts that would be similar to each other, there were significant demographic differences between the study groups necessitating adjustment when comparing results. The question remains if there are unknown/unmeasured determinants of health status that vary between the comparison groups and that may therefore confound the results. Most notable of these would be smoking status, which has significant impacts on respiratory illness and has been shown to increase during deployment. A prospective evaluation performed by the Millennium Cohort Study team found greater percentages of smoking initiation in never-smokers, smoking resumption in past smokers, and increased smoking in current smokers among service members with a history of deployment when compared with nondeployers.[19] Another finding suggests that the prevalence of smoking was found to be 50% higher among deployed versus nondeployed service members.[20] Most recently, Szema et al[21] found that the difference in smoking between deployed and nondeployed military personnel was 16.1% and 3.3%, respectively. Unfortunately, the smoking status of service members is not routinely collected and recorded in any databases readily available to DoD researchers.

Although the results presented are not without limitations and assessment of the feasibility and design issues for epidemiological studies conducted by the IOM highlights areas where improvement is needed for future work, these analyses conducted by AFHSC met all major elements of a well-designed epidemiological study, when possible. Although this study found no evidence that service members at burn pit locations are at an increased risk for respiratory health outcomes on a population level, these findings do not rule out the possibility that certain individuals exposed to smoke from a burn pit may subsequently develop adverse respiratory health conditions. The good health of our active duty service members is needed not only for CENTCOM efforts, but also for every mission and likewise (eg, the well-being of our veterans after serving should be of primary importance). For these reasons, ongoing efforts should continue to focus on further investigating possible long-term health effects related to burn pit exposure, with particular attention aimed at improving the quality of individual-level exposure data in the future.

Acknowledgments

The authors express their sincere appreciation to Robert DeFraites, MD, MPH; Steven Tobler, MD, MPH; Erin Richards, MS; and Robert Lipnick, ScD, of the Armed Forces Health Surveillance Center for previous support of and contribution to this work.

REFERENCES

1. Cavallaro G. If you haven't deployed yet, stand by: search for soldiers without a combat tour could result in break for multiple deployers. *Army Times* [serial online]. February 24, 2008. http://www.armytimes.com/article/20080224/NEWS/802240320/If-you-haven-t-deployed-yet-stand-by. Accessed November 26, 2012.

2. Mitchell B. Army seeks deployment equality. *Military.com News* [serial online]. May 19, 2009. http://www.military.com. Accessed January 28, 2014.

3. Kennedy K. Burn pit at Balad raises health concerns. *Army Times* [serial online]. May 26, 2009. http://www.armytimes.com/news/2008/10/military_burnpit_102708w/. Accessed November 26, 2012.

4. Kennedy K. Lawmakers to hold news briefing on burn pits. *Navy Times* [serial online]. February 4, 2009. http://www.navytimes.com/news/2009/06/military_burn_pit_news_conference_061009w/. Accessed November 26, 2012.

5. US Department of the Army, Public Health Command. *Summary of Evidence Statement: Chronic Respiratory Conditions and Military Deployment*. Aberdeen Proving Ground, MD: US Army Public Health Command; 2011. Factsheet 64-018-1111.

6. US Department of Defense. *Use of Open-Air Burn Pits in Contingency Operations*. February 15, 2011. http://www.dtic.mil/whs/directives. Accessed November 26, 2012. DoD Instruction 4715.19.

7. US Air Force Institute for Operational Health. *Environmental Health Site Assessment, Balad Air Base, Iraq.* Brooks City-Base, TX: AFIOH; 2005.

8. Weese CB. Issues related to burn pits in deployed settings. *US Army Med Dept J.* 2010;Apr–Jun:22–28.

9. Baird CP. Review of the Institute of Medicine report: long-term health consequences of exposure to burn pits in Iraq and Afghanistan. *US Army Med Dept J.* 2012;July–Sept:43–47.

10. U.S. Armed Forces Health Surveillance Center, the Naval Health Research Center, and the U.S. Army Public Health Command. *Epidemiological Studies of Health Outcomes Among Troops Deployed to Burn Pit Sites.* Silver Spring, MD: Defense Technical Information Center; 2010.

11. U.S. Army Public Health Command. *The Periodic Occupational and Environmental Monitoring Summary (POEMS): History, Intent, and Relationship to Individual Exposures and Health Outcomes.* Aberdeen Proving Ground, MD: US Army Public Health Command. Technical Information Paper No. 64-002-1110.

12. Institute of Medicine of the National Academies. *Long Term Health Consequences of Exposure to Burn Pits in Iraq and Afghanistan.* Washington, DC: National Academies Press; 2011: 1–9, 31–44, 117–129.

13. Haley RW. Point: bias from the "health-warrior effect" and unequal follow-up in three government studies of health effects of the Gulf War. *Am J Epidemiol.* 1998;148:315–323.

14. Dick WJ. Oral presentation. *Self-Selected Health Registries at VA & Lessons Learned.* Washington, DC: Joint VA/DoD Airborne Hazards Symposium; August 21, 2012.

15. US Department of Veterans Affairs. *Military Exposures—Agent Orange.* Veterans Affairs Office of Public Health Website. http://www.publichealth.va.gov/exposures/agentorange/index.asp. Accessed December 14, 2012.

16. Smith B, Wong CA, Boyko EJ, et al. The effects of exposure to documented open-air burn pits on respiratory health among deployers of the Millennium Cohort Study. *J Occup Environ Med.* 2012;54:708–716.

17. U.S. Department of Defense and Department of Veterans Affairs (VA). *Fact Sheet: Background on DOD and VA Chicago Announcement on Virtual Lifetime Electronic Record (VLER) and Integrated Electronic Health Record (iEHR).* May 21, 2012. http://www.defense.gov/news/EHRDoDVAFactSheet.pdf. Accessed January 22, 2013.

18. Pellerin C, Marshall TC Jr. *DOD, VA Announce Joint Health Record Milestone.* American Forces Press Service. May 21, 2012. http://www.defense.gov/News/NewsArticle.aspx?ID=116437. Accessed January 22, 2013.

19. Smith B, Ryan MA, Wingard DL, et al. Cigarette smoking and military deployment: a prospective evaluation. *Am J Prev Med.* 2008;35:539–546.

20. Institute of Medicine of the National Academies. *Combating Tobacco Use in Military and Veteran Populations.* Washington, DC: National Academies Press; 2009.

21. Szema AM, Salihi W, Savary K, Chen JJ. Respiratory symptoms necessitating spirometry among soldiers with Iraq/Afghanistan war lung injury. *J Occup Environ Med.* 2011;53:961–965.

Chapter 31

UPDATE ON KEY STUDIES: THE MILLENNIUM COHORT STUDY, THE STAMPEDE STUDY, THE MILLION VETERAN PROGRAM, AND THE NATIONAL HEALTH STUDY FOR A NEW GENERATION OF US VETERANS

NANCY F. CRUM-CIANFLONE, MD, MPH*; MICHAEL J. MORRIS, MD†; DARREL W. DODSON, MD‡; LISA L. ZACHER, MD§; AND RONALD M. PRZYGODZKI, MD¥

*Department Head, Deployment Health Research Department, Naval Health Research Center, 140 Sylvester Road, San Diego, California 92106-3521

†Colonel (Retired), Medical Corps, US Army; Department of Defense Chair, Staff Physician, Pulmonary/Critical Care Medicine and Assistant Program Director, Internal Medicine Residency, San Antonio Military Medical Center, 3551 Roger Brooke Drive, Fort Sam Houston, Texas 78234

‡Colonel, Medical Corps, US Army; Chief, Department of Medicine, Pulmonary/Critical Care Medicine, William Beaumont Army Medical Center, Fort Bliss, 5005 North Piedras Street, El Paso, Texas 79920

§Colonel (Retired), Medical Corps, US Army; Chief, Department of Medicine, Orlando Veterans Administration Medical Center, 5201 Raymond St, Orlando, Florida 32803

¥Acting Director, Biomedical Laboratory Research & Development, Office of Research and Development, US Department of Veterans Affairs, 810 Vermont Avenue, NW, Washington, DC 20420

INTRODUCTION

Several key studies have been initiated by the US Department of Defense (DoD) and the US Department of Veterans Affairs (VA) to provide critical information on the short- and long-term health and well-being of US military service members and veterans. As such, these research studies are vital in understanding emerging health conditions, including respiratory symptoms and conditions, among US military personnel returning from recent conflicts in Iraq, Afghanistan, and neighboring countries. In this chapter, several key epidemiological and clinical studies that can provide critical data in the area of respiratory outcomes among service members and veterans are reviewed. These studies include

- the Millennium Cohort Study (MCS),
- STAMPEDE (Study of Active Duty Military for Pulmonary Disease Related to Environmental Deployment Exposure),
- Million Veteran Program (MVP), and
- National Health Study for a New Generation of US Veterans.

THE MILLENNIUM COHORT STUDY

Overview of the Millennium Cohort Study

The MCS was initiated after the events that followed the 1991 Gulf War—a conflict in which nearly 700,000 US service members[1] were deployed. Thereafter, thousands of service members reported a variety of postdeployment symptoms and illnesses.[2] The DoD subsequently identified the need for a coordinated epidemiological research study to determine if military experiences, including deployments, affect long-term health outcomes. In response to recommendations[3–5] for a large, longitudinal study of US service members, the MCS was launched in July 2001. The primary objective of this ongoing study is to evaluate the impact of military service, including deployments and other occupational exposures, on the long-term health of US service members. Fortuitously, this study was begun prior to the beginning of military operations in Iraq and Afghanistan, thus providing robust baseline predeployment health data and behavioral data for a large cohort of US military service members.[5,6] Given the >2 million service members who have deployed in support of the recent operations in Iraq and Afghanistan this past decade, the MCS offers unprecedented information on the effects of military deployments on both the short- and long-term health outcomes. The study, originally designed for a 21-year period (20 years of military service plus 1 year), is planned to be extended to 67 years to assess the total lifespan of the veteran.

The MCS currently consists of four panels enrolled separately in 2001, 2004, 2007, and 2011, totaling more than 200,000 participants from all five service branches and the Reserve/National Guard. Participants are surveyed at approximate 3-year intervals both during and following service. Participation in the study is by invitation to ensure that a random sample of the military population is enrolled. In 2001, the first panel was a cross-sectional population-based sample of the US military, whereas subsequent panels focused on younger service members with a range of 1 to 5 years of service, varying by panel (Table 31-1). Specific groups were oversampled in the various panels to have adequate sample sizes to access health outcomes in subgroups of interest (eg, Reserves/National Guard, Marines, and women). From 2001 to 2007, approximately 151,000 service members participated in the study, including 67,256 Army, 43,546 Air Force, 27,450 Navy/Coast Guard, and 13,316 Marines. An additional panel (Panel 4) is underway and will enroll an additional ~50,000 participants. Enrollment and follow-up of participants are ongoing and are projected to continue for several decades. As of 2012, 57.5% of participants (Panels 1–3) deployed at least once in support of the wars in Iraq and Afghanistan, 28% deployed multiple times, and 58% of these deployers reported experiencing combat. Currently, 39% of the MCS participants have separated from the military, thus allowing for the evaluation of the health of veterans.

The MCS uses standard methods for conducting its surveys, modeled after the work of Dillman.[7] Mailings (postal and e-mail) are sent out over the course of a survey cycle (typically 18 months) to ensure that deployed service members are able to respond. The survey collects self-reported, individual-level data and consists of 100 items (many with multiple components, a total of >450 questions). The survey collects information on the service member's mental, physical, behavioral, and functional health and uses a variety of standardized instruments. These include the standardized Posttraumatic Stress Disorder (PTSD) Checklist-Civilian Version for assessing PTSD[8–10] and the Patient Health Questionnaire-8 for depression and anxiety symptoms.[11,12] Additionally, the survey captures data on self-reported health symptoms and health professional-diagnosed medical conditions. The survey also collects data on military experiences (including deployments, combat, occupational exposures, and other metrics [eg, sleep, diet, alcohol and tobacco use, and physical activity]). Functional status can be assessed using the Medical Outcomes Study

TABLE 31-1

COMPOSITION OF EACH PANEL IN THE MILLENNIUM COHORT STUDY

Panel	Dates Enrolled	Years of Service at Enrollment	Oversampled Groups	Roster Size (Date)	No. Contacted*	Total Enrolled (% of Those Contacted)
1	July 2001–June 2003	All durations (cross-section of military population)	Females, National Guard/Reserves, and prior deployers†	256,400 (October 2000)	214,388	77,047 (35.9%)
2	June 2004–February 2006	1–2 years	Females and Marine Corps	150,000 (October 2003)	123,001	31,110 (25.3%)
3	June 2007–December 2008	1–3 years	Females and Marine Corps	200,000 (October 2006)	154,270	43,440 (28.2%)
4	April 2011–ongoing	2–5 years	Females and married	250,000 (October 2010)	‡	‡

*Invalid names/postal addresses and duplicates were excluded.
†Deployment to southwest Asia, Bosnia, and/or Kosovo after August 1997.
‡Panel currently being enrolled; ~50,000 service members will be enrolled in Panel 4.

Short Form 36-Item Health Survey, Veterans Version[13,14] with calculation of the mental and physical component scores to determine functional impairment; in addition, general health and employment status are available. Follow-up surveys (administered approximately every 3 years) allow for longitudinal capture of the changing nature of the members' experiences and health symptoms, and their temporal associations.

To complement the measures ascertained on the survey, the MCS data may be linked to a variety of other data sources to provide objective measures of the service members' health and military experiences (Table 31-2). Data linkages include both military and civilian (via TRICARE) inpatient and outpatient care with ICD-9 (*International Classification of Diseases, Ninth Edition*), codes as well as pharmaceutical data from the Pharmacy Data Transaction System. In-theater injury data can be ascertained from the Joint Theater Trauma Registry and the Triservice Combat Trauma Registry-Expeditionary Medical Encounter Database. Environmental exposure data are available through the US Army Public Health Command (Aberdeen Proving Ground, MD). Information can also be obtained from the Career History Archival Medical and Personnel System, a comprehensive database that provides an individually based, longitudinal record of career events from the date of enlistment until the date of separation or retirement. Linkage with the DoD Serum Repository (Silver Spring, MD) provides a potential source of specimens because >99% of MCS members have at least one specimen in the repository.

Numerous published foundational studies have established the MCS as a well-representative sample of the US military and confirmed the excellent reliability of the survey data.[15–21] Additional analyses have also been conducted to investigate the potential for response biases;[22,23] analyses have shown that health, as measured by healthcare use preceding invitation, did not influence responses to participate.[24] Methods to encourage nonbiased responses and retention in the MCS are in place and periodically updated.

Overall, the MCS is an essential component of the DoD's Force Health Protection & Readiness strategy. This large study is setting a new standard for prospective evaluation of the potential short- and long-term health consequences of military occupational exposures, among both active military personnel and the growing number of veterans. Unlike data assembled from Gulf War Veterans, the MCS collects predeployment information and follows service members over time to allow for the longitudinal assessment of military service experiences (eg, deployment), and a variety of mental and physical health outcomes.

Respiratory Outcomes Among Returning Service Members: Data From the Millennium Cohort Study

The MCS has been used to provide critical information on the potential association between deployment experiences and newly reported respiratory outcomes among service members. Data on 46,077 MCS participants from Panel 1 who completed baseline (July 2001–June 2003) and follow-up (June 2004–February 2006) surveys were

TABLE 31-2

LINKAGES OF THE MILLENNIUM COHORT STUDY WITH OTHER DATA SOURCES

Type of Data	Source
Medical record data from military medical facilities world-wide and civilian facilities covered by the DoD insurance system (TRICARE)	Standard Ambulatory Data Record (SADR) and the Standard Inpatient Data Record (SIDR) TRICARE Encounter Data (TED)
Deployment (location and dates) and contact data	Defense Manpower Data Center (DMDC)
Pharmaceutical data	Pharmacy Data Transaction System (PDTS)
Service and medical data from time of enlistment to separation	Career History Archival Medical and Personnel System (CHAMPS)
Injury data from in theater	Joint Theater Trauma Registry (JTTR) and the Triservice Combat Trauma Registry Expeditionary Medical Encounter Database (CTR-EMED); Total Army Injury and Health Outcomes Database (TAIHOD)
Spouse health, behavioral, and relationship data; some child outcomes	The Millennium Cohort Family Study
Environmental exposures	US Army Public Health Command
Links occupational codes between the military services and civilian counterparts	Master Crosswalk File from the DoD *Occupational Conversion Index* manual
Health symptoms and perception, as well as exposure data	Pre- and Post-Deployment Health Assessments (DD 2795 and DD 2796)
Medical status and resource utilization	Health Enrollment Assessment Review (HEAR)
Mortality data	Social Security Administration Death Master File, Department of Veterans Affairs (VA) files, Department of Defense Medical Mortality Registry, and National Death Index
Dates of service, military occupation, and locations	Defense Enrollment Eligibility Reporting System (DEERS)
Medical encounters at the Veterans Administration	Veterans Administration*
Blood samples	DoD Serum Repository

DD: Department of Defense; DoD: US Department of Defense; VA: US Department of Veterans Affairs
*Linkage pending.

used to investigate new-onset respiratory symptoms and conditions.[25] Participants were excluded who either deployed prior to baseline; completed the survey while on deployment; or whose surveys were missing outcome, exposure, or covariate data. Respiratory symptoms evaluated included persistent or recurring cough or shortness of breath, which were self-reported on the MCS survey. Respiratory conditions included asthma, chronic bronchitis, and emphysema that were based on self-reported, health professional-diagnosed conditions. All "newly reported" outcomes were those that were absent at baseline and newly reported at follow-up. Deployments, including the locations and cumulative length, were obtained from the Defense Manpower Data Center (DMDC; Washington, DC). A multivariate logistic regression analysis stratified by service and adjusted by rank, service component, occupation, and smoking status was performed.

In the models examining respiratory symptoms, approximately 24% had deployed. Deployers had a higher frequency of newly reported respiratory symptoms than nondeployers (14% vs 10%), whereas similar frequencies of chronic bronchitis or emphysema (1% vs 1%) and asthma (1% vs 1%) were observed. The incidence rate of chronic bronchitis or emphysema and asthma was 3.3 cases each per 1,000 person-years. An interaction between service branch (but not tobacco use) and respiratory symptoms was noted; hence, models were stratified by branch. Independent of smoking, demographic, and military characteristics, deployment was associated with respiratory symptoms in both Army (adjusted odds ratio [AOR]: 1.73, 95% confidence interval [CI]: 1.57, 1.91) and Marine Corps (AOR: 1.49, 95% CI: 1.06, 2.08) personnel (Table 31-3). Increased deployment length was linearly associated with increased symptom reporting in Army personnel (for deployment lengths from 1 day to >270 days, AORs were 1.59–1.88, $p < 0.0001$), but not among other service branches. Among deployers, elevated odds of respiratory symptoms were associated with land-based deployment—compared with sea-based deployment—with those exclusively deploying to Iraq displaying the largest odds of respiratory symptoms (AOR: 2.16, 95% CI: 1.52, 3.07). There were no statistically significant associations between deployment and the development of any of the newly reported respiratory conditions (asthma, chronic bronchitis, or emphysema) (see Table 30-3). Findings from this study suggested that specific exposures during deployment may be determinants for postdeployment respiratory symptoms (persistent and recurring cough and shortness of breath). Significant associations seen with land-based deployment imply that exposures related to ground combat may be particularly important, but further studies are needed.

A second study was conducted within the MCS to specifically evaluate the effects of potential exposure to an open-air burn pit on respiratory outcomes among deployers to Iraq or Afghanistan.[26] Participants from MCS Panels 1 and 2—who completed surveys from 2004 to 2006 and from 2007 to 2008 and deployed to Iraq or Afghanistan from 2003 to 2008—were included (n = 22,844). Because of the small numbers of deployers in some service branches (Navy, Marines, and Coast Guard), the analyses were restricted to Army and Air Force members. The MCS survey was used to assess respiratory symptoms (ie, persistent or recurring cough or shortness of breath) and conditions (new-onset chronic bronchitis or emphysema, and new-onset asthma). New-onset conditions were defined as reported in the 2007 to 2008 survey with no previous endorsements. Information regarding deployment locations and dates were provided by the DMDC. Potential exposure to an open-air burn pit was defined using the proxy of being deployed within a 3-mile radius of a burn pit at three different camps in Iraq (Joint Base Balad, Camp Taji, and Camp Speicher). Cumulative time near the burn pit (1–56, 57–131, 132–209, ≥210 days) and the specific camp location were also evaluated. The comparison group ("nonexposed") consisted of deployers who were assigned to other areas in Iraq or Afghanistan with no days deployed near a documented burn pit. An alternate comparison group was also established consisting of deployers to Camp Arifjan in Kuwait that does not have documented burn pits. Using separate multivariable logistic regression models, the associations between potential burn-pit exposure (within a 3-mile radius) with newly reported chronic bronchitis or emphysema, newly reported asthma, and self-reported respiratory symptoms were examined. Models were adjusted for the following:

- sex,
- birth year,
- marital status,
- race/ethnicity,
- education,
- smoking,
- aerobic activity,
- service branch,
- service component,
- military rank, and
- occupation.

Of the 22,844 service members evaluated, 3,585 personnel had deployed within a 3-mile radius of a potential burn pit. Similar proportions of exposed and nonexposed groups

TABLE 31-3

ADJUSTED ODDS OF SELF-REPORTED NEW-ONSET* RESPIRATORY SYMPTOMS AND CONDITIONS IN DEPLOYERS COMPARED WITH NONDEPLOYERS: THE MILLENNIUM COHORT STUDY†

	Respiratory Symptoms‡		Chronic Bronchitis or Emphysema		Asthma	
Service Branch	**AOR§**	**95% CI**	**AOR§**	**95% CI**	**AOR§**	**95% CI**
Army	1.73	1.57, 1.91	1.25	0.94, 1.67	1.06	0.77, 1.44
Air Force	1.09	0.95, 1.26	0.93	0.59, 1.47	1.04	0.68, 1.60
Navy / Coast Guard	1.06	0.86, 1.32	0.79	0.42, 1.46	0.90	0.49, 1.65
Marine Corps	1.49	1.06, 2.08	0.94	0.24, 3.75	0.56	0.15, 1.98

AOR: adjusted odds ratio; CI: confidence interval

*New onset was defined as present at follow-up with no previous endorsement of the condition at baseline.

†The number of participants included in each model varied due to exclusion criteria dependent on each specific respiratory outcome.

‡Defined as persistent or recurring cough or shortness of breath reported at follow-up with no previous report at baseline.

§Adjusted for deployment status, sex, birth year, marital status, race / ethnicity, education, smoking status, service branch, service component, military rank, and occupation.

Data source: Smith B, Wong CA, Smith TC, et al. Newly reported respiratory symptoms and conditions among military personnel deployed to Iraq and Afghanistan: a prospective population-based study. *Am J Epidemiol.* 2009;170:1433–1442.

had respiratory outcomes: 1.5% vs 1.6% chronic bronchitis or emphysema; 1.7% vs 1.6% asthma; and 21.3% vs 20.6% respiratory symptoms (16.3% vs 14.6% new-onset respiratory symptoms). In the adjusted model, there was no statistically significant increase in any outcome comparing those potentially exposed to a burn pit with those without a documented exposure, such as:

- chronic bronchitis or emphysema—AOR: 0.91, 95% CI: 0.67–1.24;
- asthma—AOR: 0.94, 95% CI: 0.70–1.27; and
- respiratory symptoms—AOR: 1.03, 95% CI: 0.94–1.13.

Also, there were no statistically significant findings regarding the cumulative days potentially exposed, specific camp sites within a 3-mile radius, or an alternate 5-mile radius on self-reported respiratory symptoms or diagnoses. Only one finding was statistically significant; Air Force personnel deployed within a 2-mile radius of Joint Base Balad had increased odds for respiratory symptoms (AOR: 1.24, 95% CI: 1.01–1.52). However, this finding was marginally significant, with no evidence of trend (ie, no findings with cumulative deployment length), and this group did not have increased odds for any of the other respiratory outcomes. Finally, using the referent group of Camp Arifjan did not significantly change any of the results. In general, these study findings do not support an elevated risk for respiratory outcomes among personnel deployed within proximity of documented burn pits in Iraq.

There are some important limitations of the two studies to consider. All outcomes were self-reported and were not validated by medical record review. Further, the follow-up period was short; hence, long-term outcomes may have been missed. Lastly, the study examining potential burn pit exposures did not use direct quantitative or individual-level exposure data because these data were unavailable; rather, it used a proxy for possible burn pit exposure that has significant potential for misclassification.

Additional studies leveraging the MCS to examine respiratory outcomes are underway. An exploratory study was performed to evaluate the potential association of increasing levels of environmental particulate matter (PM) exposure with the risk of newly reported respiratory symptoms among deployers to southwest Asia. Time-weighted average values of PM_{10} and $PM_{2.5}$ from 15 PM sampling sites in southwest Asia were obtained from the US Army Public Health Command, which resulted from samples that were collected by the DoD Enhanced Particulate Matter Surveillance Program from December 2005 to January 2007. Army participants who completed MCS surveys from 2004 to 2006, from 2007 to 2008, and who deployed to one or more of the sampling sites surveyed by the Enhanced Particulate Matter Surveillance Program were identified. Unfortunately, there were data on only 145 personnel meeting the inclusion criteria and no data on individual-level exposures limiting the ability to study PM levels and respiratory outcomes of interest. If additional environmental exposure data become available, the MCS will explore the potential for additional analyses.

Future studies within the MCS will examine the long-term consequences and the natural history of respiratory symptoms among deployers. Outcomes over time will be determined among those with

- postdeployment respiratory symptoms in terms of resolution or persistence of symptoms,
- development of respiratory diseases (eg, asthma, chronic bronchitis, emphysema, and bronchiolitis),
- medical care visits, and
- quality of life.

Because respiratory diseases may cause substantial healthcare expenditures for the VA and may be of high interest to VA medical planners regarding the potential future health effects of military deployments, respiratory illnesses by deployment and military separation status will be examined. Panel 1 to 3 deployers to Iraq or Afghanistan who completed the baseline and follow-up surveys with up to a decade of data (2001–2013) will be used for these analyses. In addition, because combat deployments are associated with increased mental health outcomes (eg, PTSD and anxiety) and land-based deployers have the highest risk for new-onset respiratory symptoms, future analyses will attempt to explore the relationship of anxiety-related symptoms and combat new-onset respiratory symptoms among land-based deployers to Iraq and Afghanistan.

In summary, the MCS has been used to conduct analyses to examine the potential association between deployment experiences and newly reported respiratory symptoms and conditions. To date, the study results show an increased risk for respiratory symptoms among land-based deployers (Army and Marine Corps), but not among other deployed groups. Of note, no statistically significant associations between deployment and respiratory diseases (chronic bronchitis or emphysema, or asthma) have been found to date. Further, potential exposure (within a 3-mile radius) to an open-air burn pit was not found to be associated with respiratory outcomes, but this study did not include individual-level exposure data. Additional studies are underway to help clarify the role of deployment experiences and respiratory outcomes. In summary, the MCS has prospectively evaluated the impact of military experiences, including deployment, on a variety of health outcomes (including respiratory conditions) among US service members. As the largest study in US military history, the MCS will continue to provide ongoing militarily relevant data on health outcomes of interest to help inform DoD/VA leaders and policies.

THE STAMPEDE STUDY

The objective of the initial STAMPEDE study was to evaluate military personnel who have recently returned from the Operation Iraqi Freedom/Operation Enduring Freedom for evidence of lung disease related to prolonged environmental dust exposure in the current theaters of operation. The study was conducted as a prospective, observational study of active duty military personnel with recent redeployment and consisted of a completed enrollment of 50 patients. Patients were primarily recruited from Fort Hood, TX. Active duty military with redeployment within 6 months and new-onset pulmonary symptoms underwent a standardized evaluation at San Antonio Military Medical Center in San Antonio, TX. All participants completed a respiratory questionnaire with detailed exposure history. Clinical evaluation included the following:

- high-resolution computed tomography (HRCT) of the chest,
- full pulmonary function testing,
- impulse oscillometry,
- methacholine challenge testing, and
- fiberoptic bronchoscopy with bronchoalveolar lavage (BAL) of the right middle lobe.

Transbronchial biopsy was only performed if there was evidence of interstitial changes on chest scanning.

Data analysis is currently ongoing. Current data indicate that 50 patients have been enrolled (80% male, mean age of 31.6 ± 8.2 years) and completed an initial evaluation to include fiberoptic bronchoscopy with BAL. Deployment locations were Iraq (66%), Afghanistan (24%), or both countries (10%) with a mean deployment length of 11.7 ± 3.6 months. This was the first deployment for 50% of the cohort. Chest radiographs were normal in all patients, and HRCT scans of the chest identified minor changes of mild focal airway trapping in three patients, bronchiectasis and emphysematous changes in one patient, and several small subcentimeter nodules in four patients. None of the patients had diffuse infiltrates or parenchymal changes that warranted lung biopsy.

Pulmonary function studies demonstrated normal mean values as shown in Table 31-4. The final diagnosis was

- asthma (16%),
- airway hyperresponsiveness (20%),
- gastroesophageal reflux (4%),
- low diffusing capacity of the lung for carbon monoxide (8%),
- miscellaneous (12%), and
- no diagnosis (42%).

The incidence of lung disease in this patient population was primarily related to asthma-related disorders. There was minimal evidence of chronic inflammatory processes related to deployment based on HRCT or bronchoscopy findings. In this study, military deployment to Operation Iraqi Freedom/Operation Enduring Freedom was not associated with chronic inflammatory changes in the lung based on HRCT imaging and cellular findings in BAL. A significant percentage of patients had no specific pulmonary diagnosis based on normal test results and may have other underlying contributing factors for dyspnea, such as psychological or sleep disorders. Further follow-up is planned to determine continued symptoms in these patients. The suggestion that environmental exposures due to deployment cause interstitial or bronchiolar lung disease cannot be substantiated from this study. A more comprehensive research study is currently being conducted that is enrolling patients with deployment-related respiratory symptoms of any duration. This study will use a more comprehensive panel of testing procedures and provide additional data on longitudinal findings of deployment-related lung disease.

THE MILLION VETERAN PROGRAM: THE VETERANS AFFAIRS OFFICE OF RESEARCH AND DEVELOPMENT MEGACOHORT

Background

The ability to perform excellent large-scale research requires collection of a variety of elements, including well-annotated medical record data, lifestyle/epidemiological data, and genomic data. Although some large biorepositories and centers have begun such ventures—including the Iceland Biobank, United Kingdom Biobank, and Kaiser Biobank—one was not available that would adequately serve the needs of US veterans.[27–29] Fulfilling this need, combined with the efforts of the Veterans Health Administration (VHA) of propelling veteran's genomic healthcare into the 21st century, required the establishment of a Genomics Medicine Program (GMP) within the Office of Research and Development (ORD).

Initially, the ORD established the GMP Advisory Committee (GMPAC) to help guide and advise the Secretary of VA in establishment, directions, assessment, and progress of the GMP and other related genomic initiatives within the VA. The GMPAC is comprised of private and public health;

TABLE 31-4

STAMPEDE PULMONARY FUNCTION STUDIES

PFT Values	Mean ± SD
FEV_1 (% predicted)	87.8 ± 12.9
FVC (% predicted)	91.3 ± 13.5
FEV_1/FVC	79.5 ± 5.9
FEV_1 post-BD (% predicted)	91.1 ± 11.7
Total lung capacity (% predicted)	90.9 ± 13.3
Residual volume (% predicted)	82.9 ± 34.7
DLCO (% predicted)	83.5 ± 19.8

BD: bronchodilator; DLCO: diffusing capacity for carbon monoxide; FEV_1: forced expiratory volume at 1 sec; FVC: forced vital capacity; PFT: pulmonary function testing; SD: standard deviation; STAMPEDE: Study of Active-Duty Military for Pulmonary Disease Related to Environmental Deployment Exposure

scientific; ethical; and legal experts in the field of genetics and veteran representatives, and partners, including but not limited to veterans service organizations, the DoD, and the National Institutes of Health (Bethesda, MD).

Poised against an evolving technological base, an increasing ability to improve healthcare using genomic testing, and an ever-present need to maintain patient privacy concerns, the GMPAC proposed that the VA review the attitudes of veterans toward the use of genomics in research.

Veterans' Attitudes Toward Genomic Research

A pivotal component of the development of the GMP and MVP required the VA to address the attitudes and concerns of veterans toward genomic research. The Johns Hopkins Genetic and Public Policy Center (Baltimore, MD) conducted a survey of veterans that spanned various demographic profiles. The study revealed that 83% of the VHA using veterans supported such a program, and 71% would participate in such program if available.[30] Willingness to participate was correlated with altruistic behavior, such as being a blood or organ donor. Three quarters of the veterans surveyed supported a key linking the individual's findings with their medical record data and themselves. Importantly, 93% revealed concern regarding information privacy and security. Lastly, the survey showed 96% felt that receiving information about their health was important.

The same group was requested to conduct a second survey of veterans to explore the veterans' attitudes pertaining to enrollment models, including opt-in (voluntary participation and enrollment into model) vs opt-out (automatic participation and enrollment model) enrollment. Interestingly, the majority of veterans were comfortable with either enrollment model, with 80% favoring an opt-in and 69% favoring an opt-out approach.[31] Nearly 80% of veterans were also comfortable with the VA using residual clinical samples for research purposes. Overall, both studies reveal strong support for establishment of a GMP program, a biobank for research needs, and support for genomic research.

The Million Veteran Program

Launched in May 2011 by VA Chief of Staff John R. Gingrich, the MVP now includes 50 of the 107 VA medical centers (VAMCs) that have the capacity for research (of 152 VAMCs total). The ultimate goal is to enroll 1 million veterans who use VHA for their healthcare over a 5- to 7-year timeframe. The overarching goal of the MVP is to unite genetic, health and lifestyle, and military exposure data, together within a single database called the Genomic Information System for Integrated Sciences (GenISIS). The VA is ideally poised for such a venture, that is, the VA—one of the largest healthcare systems within the United States—has more than 8.5 million enrollees as of 2012. Any given veteran enrollee has, on average, 15 years of electronic healthcare record data. Further, the VA has embedded within its healthcare system a world-class research program (ORD) with four research services:

- preclinical sciences,
- clinical sciences,
- rehabilitation sciences, and
- health implementation sciences.

ORD has a unifying VA Central Institutional Review Board overseeing large-scale research further streamlining approval from numerous research sites. Embedding the GMP within ORD enables the interdigitation of genomics between the four services, thereby addressing a multitude of questions at various research levels. Importantly, the MVP has strong support by VA leadership. Among the participants within MVP are VA Secretary Eric K. Shinseki, Deputy Secretary W. Scott Gould, and Chief of Staff John R. Gingrich.

Enrollment of veterans into the MVP begins with veterans receiving a letter asking if they would like to join the program. They may either opt into the program, or if they choose not to be asked again, opt out from further being contacted. If they opt in, they fill out a brief health survey and make an appointment at the VAMC to accompany their next medical visit. During this visit, they are educated about the program and given the opportunity to consent to be in the database and to make their medical records available for future unspecified studies. Also during this visit, they have blood drawn. Of note, the participants are identified with a unique number identifier. The GenISIS system provides this unique identifier, which tags all subsequent survey and sample data in a chain of custody. In no way are any Health Insurance Portability and Accountability Act (HIPAA) identifiers available to anyone except for a limited set of individuals who maintain and oversee the database processes.

In addressing the veteran's concerns of data privacy, several safeguards into the MVP and GenISIS have been introduced. For example, all blood samples and products isolated from them (buffy coat, DNA [deoxyribonucleic acid], etc) are stored in a secure manner using bar code technology as the primary identifier. The interlinking of medical record data and genomic data are performed in a similar manner. Access to data for research, when it becomes available, will be provided only to authorized researchers within the VA, other federal health agencies, and academic institutions within the US, in a secure manner. This will entail the use of a computer portal into the GenISIS computing environment. The VA Central Institutional Review Board and the peer-reviewed proposals for these studies will dictate appropriate restrictions and limitations of data access as required. Such a portal will provide a virtual "sandbox" to perform one's research work with specific and limited access to genotypic and phenotypic data, as well as statistical tools to enable the performance of a sound analysis of the research question at hand. Importantly, in no way will the researcher have access to a veteran participant's name, address, social security number, or date of birth at any time. Therefore, data security is upheld.

The goal is for the researcher to work, through the GenISIS secure environment, on relationships of genotypic, phenotypic, and epidemiological data to identify relationships between any combinations of the aforementioned areas. In addition, having access to updated data longitudinally—both genomic as well as health record data—thereby enables the researcher to perform research on the level of epigenetics, microRNA (ribonucleic acid), and the like. Further, the research environment will also allow future repurposing of data points identified in any given study once it is completed and/or published. Additional sampling will be limited to the researcher's ability to implement secondary phenotypic survey requests and the ORD's/GMP's ability to perform genomic-level analytics. Ultimately, associations between genes and health could lead to improved approaches of disease screening, prognosis, diagnosis, and truly personalized care.

Of those responding to the request letter, more than 20% of all mailings (1.3 million recipients) have responded in favor of opting into the MVP, with approximately 10% directly responding not to participate at all. The remaining 70% have neither responded for nor against participation. As of December 7, 2012, the MVP had 114,638 enrollees, with periods of service spanning from World War II to the current conflicts. Remarkably, nearly 14% of the enrollees were veterans who had not received a letter, but who had heard about the program and opted in/enrolled on their own. The program is enrolling in relative alignment to the population seen using the VHA,[32] with more than 7% women participants, and approximately 13% and 6% African Americans and Hispanics participating, respectively. The ability to identify unique subpopulations within the MVP, including the use of additional survey tools and the like to enable additional data gathering (eg, respiratory questionnaire), is a potential strength of the program. Further data on VA sites participating in the MVP, our data security measures, and study status may be seen at the ORD MVP website.[33]

Thus, the VA is uniquely set to succeed with the GMP and MVP because of the altruistic patient and workforce populations. The VA ORD has had a long history of unique, game-changing discoveries that have improved veteran and national healthcare. By using the large longitudinal megacohort MVP, the VA can further improve veterans' healthcare.

SUMMARY

Concerns regarding respiratory symptoms and outcomes have arisen over the past decade—a time in which >2 million service members deployed to Iraq, Afghanistan, and neighboring countries. Several important studies have been initiated by the DoD and VA to provide critical information on the health outcomes, including respiratory conditions, of US military service members and veterans. These include a large epidemiological study consisting of >200,000 service members and veterans with planned longitudinal follow-up over the course of their lifetimes (the MCS); a clinical study among military members returning from deployments with respiratory symptoms (the STAMPEDE); a large ongoing collection of genetic, health, and lifestyle data among approximately 1 million veterans (the MVP); and a 10-year longitudinal study of recent veterans (National Health Study for a New Generation of US Veterans). These research studies represent an invaluable resource for understanding emerging health conditions, including respiratory symptoms and conditions, among US military personnel and veterans.

REFERENCES

1. Institute of Medicine, Committee on Measuring the Health of Gulf War Veterans, Division of Health Promotion and Disease Prevention. *Gulf War Veterans: Measuring Health.* In: Hernandez LM, Durch JS, Blazer DG II, Hoverman IV, eds. Washington, DC: National Academy Press; 1999.

2. Knoke JD, Gray GC. Hospitalizations for unexplained illnesses among U.S. veterans of the Persian Gulf War. *Emerg Infect Dis.* 1998;4:211–219.

3. Secretary of Defense. *Report to the Committee on National Security, House of Representatives and the Armed Services Committee, and the U.S. Senate on the Effectiveness of Medical Research Initiatives Regarding Gulf War Illnesses.* Washington, DC: Department of Defense; 1998.

4. House of Representatives, 105th Congress-2nd Session. *Strom Thurmond National Defense Authorization Act for Fiscal Year 1999 (Conference Report to Accompany H.R. 3616).* Washington, DC: Government Printing Office; 1998. Report 105-736.

5. Gray GC, Chesbrough KB, Ryan MAK, et al. The Millennium Cohort Study: a 21-year prospective cohort study of 140,000 military personnel. *Mil Med.* 2002;167:483–488.

6. Ryan MA, Smith TC, Smith B, et al. Millennium Cohort: enrollment begins a 21-year contribution to understanding the impact of military service. *J Clin Epidemiol.* 2007;60:181–191.

7. Dillman DA. *Mail and Telephone Surveys: The Total Design Method.* New York, NY: Wiley & Sons; 1978.

8. American Psychiatric Association. *Diagnostic and Statistical Manual of Mental Disorders*, 4th ed. Washington, DC: American Psychiatric Association, 1994.

9. Weathers FW, Huska JA, Keane TM. *The PTSD Checklist—Civilian Version.* Boston, MA: National Center for PTSD; 1991.

10. Terhakopian A, Sinaii N, Engel CC, Schnurr PP, Hoge CW. Estimating population prevalence of posttraumatic stress disorder: an example using the PTSD checklist. *J Traumatic Stress.* 2008;21:290–300.

11. Kroenke K, Spitzer RL, Williams JB. The PHQ-9: validity of a brief depression severity measure. *J Gen Intern Med.* 2001;16:606–613.

12. Spitzer RL, Kroenke K, Williams JB. Validation and utility of a self-report version of PRIME-MD: the PHQ primary care study. Primary Care Evaluation of Mental Disorders. Patient Health Questionnaire. *JAMA.* 1999;282:1737–1744.

13. Ware JE, Sherbourne CD. The MOS 36-Item Short-Form Health Survey (SF-36): conceptual framework and item selection. *Med Care.* 1992;30:473–483.

14. Ware JE, Kosinski M, Gandek B. *SF-36 Health Survey: Manual and Interpretation Guide.* Lincoln, RI: Quality Metric Incorporated; 2000.

15. Smith B, Wingard DL, Ryan MAK, et al. US military deployment during 2001–2006: comparison of subjective and objective data sources in a large prospective health study. *Ann Epidemiol.* 2007;17:976–982.

16. Smith TC, Smith B, Jacobson IG, et al. Reliability of standard health assessment instruments in a large, population-based cohort study. *Ann Epidemiol.* 2007;17:525–532.

17. Smith TC, Jacobson IG, Smith B, Hooper TI, et al. The occupational role of women in military service: validation of occupation and prevalence of exposures in the Millennium Cohort Study. *Int J Environ Health Res.* 2007;17:271–284.

18. Smith B, Chu LK, Smith TC, et al. Challenges of self-reported medical conditions and electronic medical records among members of a large military cohort. *BMC Med Res Methodol.* 2008;8:37.

19. Smith B, Leard CA, Smith TC, et al. Anthrax vaccination in the Millennium Cohort: validation and measures of health. *Am J Prev Med.* 2007;32:347–353.

20. Smith B, Smith TC, Gray GC, et al. When epidemiology meets the Internet: web-based surveys in the Millennium Cohort Study. *Am J Epidemiol.* 2007;166:1345–1354.

21. LeardMann CA, Smith B, Smith TC, Wells TS, Ryan MAK. Smallpox vaccination: comparison of self-reported and electronic vaccine records in the millennium cohort study. *Hum Vaccin.* 2007;3:245–251.

22. Cunradi CB, Moore R, Killoran M, Ames G. Survey nonresponse bias among young adults: the role of alcohol, tobacco, and drugs. *Subst Use Misuse.* 2005;40:171–185.

23. Littman AJ, Boyko EJ, Jacobson IG, et al. Assessing nonresponse bias at follow-up in a large prospective cohort of relatively young and mobile military service member. *BMC Med Res Methodol.* 2010;10:99.

24. Wells TS, Jacobson IG, Smith TC, et al. Prior health care utilization as a determinant to enrollment in a 22-year prospective study, the Millennium Cohort Study. *Eur J Epidemiol.* 2008;23:79-87.

25. Smith B, Wong CA, Smith TC, et al. Newly reported respiratory symptoms and conditions among military personnel deployed to Iraq and Afghanistan: a prospective population-based study. *Am J Epidemiol.* 2009;170:1433–1442.

26. Smith B, Wong CA, Boyko EJ, et al. The effects of exposure to documented open-air burn pits on respiratory health among deployers of the Millennium Cohort Study. *J Occup Environ Med.* 2012;54:708–716.

27. Office of Science Policy and Planning, Office of Science Policy, and the National Institutes of Health. *Iceland's Research Resources: The Health Sector Database, Genealogy Databases, and Biobanks*. Bethesda, MD: NIH; 2004.

28. UK Biobank. UK Biobank Website. http://www.ukbiobank.ac.uk/about-biobank-uk/. Accessed February 5, 2014.

29. Kaiser Permanente, Division of Research. *The Research Program on Genes, Environment, & Health: Building a Biobank.* http://www.dor.kaiser.org/external/DORExternal/rpgeh/index.aspx. Accessed February 5, 2014.

30. Kaufman D, Murphy J, Erby L, Hudson K, Scott J. Veterans' attitudes regarding a database for genomic research. *Genet Med.* 2009;11:329–337.

31. Kaufman D, Bollinger J, Dvoskin R, Scott J. Preferences for opt-in and opt-out enrollment and consent models in biobank research: a national survey of Veterans Administration patients. *Genet Med.* 2012;14:787–794.

32. US Department of Veterans Affairs. *National Center for Veterans Analysis and Statistics.* https://www.va.gov/vetdata/Veteran_Population.asp. Accessed February 5, 2014.

33. US Department of Veterans Affairs. *Office of Research & Development: Million Veteran Program—A Partnership With Veterans.* http://www.research.va.gov/MVP. Accessed February 5, 2014.

Chapter 32

NATIONAL HEALTH STUDY FOR A NEW GENERATION OF US VETERANS

AARON I. SCHNEIDERMAN, PhD, MPH, RN*

*Deputy Director, Epidemiology Program, Post-Deployment Health Group (10P3A), Office of Public Health, Veterans Health Administration, US Department of Veterans Affairs, 810 Vermont Avenue, NW, Washington, DC 20420

INTRODUCTION

The National Health Study for a New Generation of US Veterans (New Gen) is a 10-year longitudinal study designed to measure the health status of veterans who deployed to Operation Enduring Freedom (OEF) or Operation Iraqi Freedom (OIF). This study was also designed to compare their experience with nondeployed veterans who served in the military during the same time. Beginning with a sample size of 60,000, evenly split between deployed and nondeployed veterans, the New Gen study used a multimodal survey methodology to encourage participation through Web-based, paper-and-pencil, or telephone interviews. The survey is unique in deriving the sample from the entire universe of OEF/OIF veterans, not limiting selection to those who use services provided by the US Department of Veterans Affairs (VA). Assessing a variety of physical and mental health outcomes, as well as health risk behaviors, the study results will help provide a population-based understanding of health and illness among recent veterans to support and inform policy development and hypothesis generation for future research. The study is supported by the VA, Office of Public Health.

STUDY SAMPLE

The New Gen study established a permanent panel of 30,000 OEF/OIF veterans (*the deployed group*) and 30,000 non-OEF/OIF veterans who served in the military between October 2001 and June 2008 (*the contemporary military group*), including veterans in the Reserves or National Guard who had not separated from these military components. The sample population of deployed veterans was selected from data files provided to the VA by the US Department of Defense (DoD)/Defense Manpower Data Center and the VA/DoD Identity Repository (VADIR) database, a VA and DoD data-sharing initiative designed to consolidate data transfers between the DoD and VA. Members of the contemporary, nondeployed military cohort were selected from VADIR. The deployed and contemporary military groups were stratified by branch of service (Army, Air Force, Navy, and Marines), unit component (active duty, Reserves, or National Guard), and gender.[1]

This stratified random sampling design was intended to provide a representative sample of those who served in these recent conflicts and a comparator population. Military operations since September 11, 2001 have relied more heavily on the Reserve and National Guard components than in previous conflicts. Lengthy and multiple deployments have been a regular experience for many of these citizen soldiers. Women have also been integrated into the military's operations in ways not seen in previous decades. The increased participation of these groups made it essential that the sampling strategy ensure adequate representation to allow for statistically robust subgroup analyses.

TABLE 32-1

TOPICS COVERED IN THE NATIONAL HEALTH STUDY FOR A NEW GENERATION OF US VETERANS SURVEY

Health Risk Behaviors	Health Conditions	General Health	Health Care Utilization	Potential Exposures
Alcohol use	Anxiety	Functional status	Doctor visits	Accidents
HIV testing	Asthma	General health perception	Hospitalizations	Blasts
Motorcycle helmet use	Cancer	Pregnancy outcomes	Prescription drug use	Chemicals
Seatbelt use	Chronic diseases	Reproductive health	Use of complementary and alternative medicines	Dust/sand
Sexual behavior	Depression	BMI	VA facility use	Falls
Smoking	Heart disease			Head injuries
Speeding	Hypertension			Military sexual trauma
	Irritable bowel syndrome			Smoke
	Migraines			Vaccinations
	Pain			
	PTSD			
	TBI			

BMI: body mass index; HIV: human immunodeficiency virus; PTSD: posttraumatic stress disorder; TBI: traumatic brain injury; VA: US Department of Veterans Affairs

Data source: US Department of Veterans Affairs. *Health Study for a New Generation of US Veterans*. VA website. http://www.publichealth.va.gov/newgenerationstudy/index.asp. Accessed February 11, 2014.

STUDY QUESTIONNAIRE

The 16-page, 72-item questionnaire was developed based on lessons learned from previous studies of Gulf War era veterans and input on current interests from VA content experts in deployment health, women's health, infectious disease, mental health, and behavioral health. Survey questions addressed a broad array of topics on health status and conditions, health risk behaviors, use of healthcare services, and deployment-related exposures (Table 32-1).

Many questions and scales came from government agencies and from previously fielded surveys, such as the

- Centers for Disease Control and Prevention (Atlanta, GA),
- National Center for Health Statistics (Atlanta, GA),
- National Health Interview Survey,
- DoD Post-Deployment Health Assessment, and
- VA Longitudinal Health Study of Gulf War Era Veterans.

Specific mental health items include the Posttraumatic Stress Disorder Check List (PCL) and the Patient Health Questionnaire-9 (PHQ-9), scales used to identify symptoms and functional impairment associated with depression. The Medical Outcomes Study-Short Form 12 (MOS-SF12) was also included to assess the physical and emotional components of functional health status.[1]

STUDY IMPLEMENTATION AND FUTURE PROGRESS

Data for the study were collected following a sequential mailing protocol modeled on a modified "tailored design method."[2] Sequential mailings to sampled veterans detailed two options for completing the survey: (1) complete the survey online using a secure access portal or (2) respond to the paper version. All nonresponders to the Web and postal surveys were approached to participate in a computer-assisted telephone interview (CATI) that assessed reasons for nonresponse and attempted to complete the survey. Data collection began in August 2009 and continued through 2010, with the last surveys accepted in January 2011.

The overall response rate for the study was 34%, with approximately 55% of responders from the deployed sample. The response from female panel members was 21%, satisfying the sampling goal of 20%. Web-based surveys were predominant over paper surveys, but moderately with 49% to 45%, respectively, of the responses. The CATI protocol realized an additional 6% of the overall response.

The first article reporting on respiratory-specific data collected by the New Gen study was published in the March 2014 issue of *Military Medicine*. Barth et al[3] investigated the prevalence of three self-reported respiratory diseases—(1) asthma, (2) bronchitis, and (3) sinusitis—occurring in deployed and nondeployed veterans before and after 2001. The deployed veterans had a lower prevalence of all three diagnoses before 2001. Although both deployed and nondeployed veterans had higher self-reported prevalence rates for all three diagnoses after 2001, in a model adjusting for demographic variables and smoking status, only sinusitis had a statistically significant adjusted odds ratio (1.30) among the deployed veterans (95% confidence interval: 1.13–1.49).[3]

Future analyses of the New Gen study data pertinent to respiratory health will investigate potential associations between other risk factors for disease, including the history of self-reported environmental exposures such as burning trash/feces, smoke from oil well fires, dust and sand, and industrial pollution. As noted previously, respondents to the New Gen survey may not be users of VA healthcare services. However, there may be a sufficient number of VA health system users among the survey respondents to enable analyses that link survey responses to healthcare records. Such analyses could

- provide additional understanding to the natural history of disease among deployed individuals,
- provide information on the healthcare needs of individuals who are ill or symptomatic, and
- generate additional research questions to further elucidate the relationships between risk factors and respiratory disease.

The New Gen study is currently developing the follow-up survey of the panel that is scheduled for field implementation in 2015. Plans include augmenting the panel with an additional sample to capture individuals whose service ended after the close of the previous sampling period: June 2008. By extending the sample forward in time, we hope to add people who may have had slightly different experiences in the conflict regions under study.

The survey will retain many of the same scales used in the initial survey. However, in recognition of the increased attention and understanding of the issues associated with airborne hazards and burn pits, new questions concerning military and occupational exposures and additional items about respiratory disease will be included. The items are derived from efforts that supported development of the Airborne Hazards and Open Burn Pit Registry as mandated in section 201 of Public Law 112-260. This unified approach to data collection will provide another comparison for data on respiratory outcomes collected by the complementary efforts represented by the epidemiological survey and the clinical registry.

SUMMARY

The New Gen study is designed to track the changes in health status over time for a representative population of recent veterans and provide a broad range of information regarding the effects of combat deployment on health. In addition to being a population-based study, it includes both VA users and nonusers, and provides a more accurate description of the entire OEF/OIF veteran population.

REFERENCES

1. Eber S, Barth S, Kang H, et al. The National Health Study for a New Generation of United States Veterans: methods for a large-scale study on the health of recent veterans. *Mil Med*. 2013;178:966–969.

2. Dillman DA. *Mail and Internet Surveys: The Tailored Design Method*. 2nd ed. Hoboken, NJ: John Wiley & Sons,Inc.;2007.

3. Barth SK, Dursa EK, Peterson MR, Schneiderman AI. Prevalence of respiratory diseases among veterans of Operation Enduring Freedom and Operation Iraqi Freedom: results from the National Health Study for a New Generation of U.S. Veterans. *Mil Med*. 2014;179:241–245.

Chapter 33

DISCUSSION SUMMARY: WORK GROUP E—STRATEGIC RESEARCH PLANNING

DAVID A. JACKSON, PhD*; and MICHAEL R. PETERSON, DVM, MPH, DrPH†

*Director, Pulmonary Health Program, US Army Center for Environmental Health Research, 568 Doughten Drive, Fort Detrick, Maryland 21702-5010
†Chief Consultant, Post-Deployment Health, Office of Public Health, Veterans Health Administration, 810 Vermont Avenue, NW, Washington, DC 20420

INTRODUCTION

Since early in Operation Iraqi Freedom (OIF) and Operation Enduring Freedom (OEF), it has been clear that service members in southwest Asia (SWA) are exposed to extremely high levels of geogenic airborne particulate matter (PM). Data from the Army's Enhanced Particulate Matter Surveillance Program (EPMSP), which sampled ambient PM at 15 locations over 18 months throughout SWA, indicate that ambient levels of PM in the region far exceed US Environmental Protection Agency (Washington, DC) environmental levels, National Institute of Occupational Safety and Health (Atlanta, GA) and Occupational Safety and Health Administration (Washington, DC) occupational levels, and military exposure guidelines.[1] Both peer-reviewed publications and reports in the popular press[2] have suggested that deployment to SWA might be associated with an increase in respiratory symptoms[3,4] and lung disease.[5] Concerns have also been raised both in the press and in Congressional testimony[6] that exposure to combustion products from large-scale waste burning at military facilities might play a role in the development of chronic disease. However, formal studies[6,7] have not found clear associations between disease and exposure.

The US Army Center for Health Promotion and Preventive Medicine (now the US Army Public Health Command [USAPHC; Aberdeen Proving Ground, MD]) commissioned an evaluation of the EPMSP by the Committee on Toxicology (COT) of the National Research Council (Washington, DC).[8] The US Department of Veterans Affairs (VA; Washington, DC) charged the Institute of Medicine (IOM) with providing an independent assessment of health risks associated with burn pit exposure.[9] Neither of these reviews was able to draw clear conclusions about health risks associated with exposure to ambient PM or burn pit combustion products because of numerous data gaps in both the nature and extent of exposure; and the lack of understanding of how young, fit military populations might respond to airborne hazards. However, both study groups did express concern that exposures to high levels of ambient PM, burn pit combustion products, and other types of air pollution might result in chronic or long-term disease in service members who had been deployed to SWA. The COT and IOM recommended several efforts to ascertain the prevalence, severity, and causality of service-related disease that might have resulted from exposure to airborne hazards in SWA, including more thorough and extensive environmental monitoring and studies of service members and veterans who had been exposed or not to burn pit combustion products.

To facilitate the development of a comprehensive 5-year strategic research plan to assess possible health risks associated with exposure to natural and man-made airborne hazards during deployment to SWA, approximately 20 participants in the 2012 VA/US Department of Defense (DoD) Airborne Hazards Symposium (held in Washington, DC) assembled on the second day of the symposium (as Work Group E) to discuss the substance and structure of such a plan. Participants were asked to consider a number of programmatic and scientific factors during their discussions of the strategic plan and

- identify critical research questions;
- quantify the risk associated with exposure and development of respiratory disease;
- identify enabling technologies, competencies, and infrastructure that may need to be developed or acquired to address research questions;
- prioritize research questions based on the relevance for evaluating risks and feasibility;
- maximize payoff by coordinating VA and DoD research efforts in the design and implementation of short- and long-term plans ensuring collaboration throughout;
- integrate, where feasible, toxicological, clinical, epidemiological, and modeling data to effectively address different questions or aspects of the same question;
- include veterans in appropriate stages of research ("participatory research"); and
- recognize the need for ongoing effective communications with stakeholders throughout planning and implementation of studies.

Participants were also encouraged to think beyond current research efforts that have tended to focus on pulmonary injury following inhalational exposures to PM. The work group (WG) was reminded that health risks associated with other routes of exposure, other types of hazardous material (as well as mixtures of materials), and injuries to other organ systems might also be important for evaluating both short- and long-term health risks for service members. Thus, the WG was asked to consider other routes of exposure (eg, transdermal), injuries to other organ systems (eg, cardiovascular), and exposure to gases and vapors, in addition to PM.

Although the WG did not produce a 5-year plan, exchanges among the participants revealed a number of areas of concern related to airborne hazards and suggested methods for addressing them. The themes, nevertheless, present a body of concern held by professionals in relevant fields that should prove useful to policy makers and research managers in the VA and the DoD as they develop responses to the potential airborne occupational hazards experienced by service members in SWA.

As a side note, there was a cultural difference between participants with operational military backgrounds and participants from the research, clinical, and compensation communities. Participants from the operational world were highly focused on understanding environmental health risks with the aim of preventing injury through improved operational management, environmental risk assessment, and environmental surveillance. Other participants tended to focus on causal links between potential hazards and disease, severity of disease, and associated disability. Different perspectives were understandable, given the difference between carrying out operational activities, supplying medical care to veterans and service members, and providing compensation where appropriate.

Major areas of concern and highlights of the discussion are summarized in the next section.

OUTCOMES OF THE DISCUSSION

Prevalence and Severity of Deployment-Related Lung Disease

The fundamental issue that emerged from the conversation of the WG participants was whether or not deployed service members have had or are experiencing exposures to airborne hazards. The VA and USAPHC commissioned independent reports on health risks associated with burn pits in SWA from the IOM and the National Research Council COT on the value and quality of EPMSP. Both reports addressed evidence for associations between disease states in service members deployed to SWA. The COT[8] and IOM[9] reports, additional published data, and other data presented during the symposium provide a confusing picture of the prevalence and severity of pulmonary and other disease(s) that have been ascribed to deployment to SWA. For example, although analysis of self-reported respiratory symptoms taken from the Millennium Cohort Study[4] suggests that there may be an increase in respiratory symptoms associated with deployment, the observation does not seem to be supported by the clinical data presented by Dr Michael Morris[7] during this symposium. Case clusters of acute eosinophilic pneumonia[10] and constrictive bronchiolitis[5] have also been reported, but these involve few individuals. It has been difficult to assess to what extent these rare events might be harbingers of long-term risks or reflective of inapparent disease in the deployed cohort. A limited number of studies of the toxicity of natural PM from SWA have been performed and although these studies do not support the interpretation that the dusts are unusually toxic, the studies have all used single or short-term exposures that do not model the exposures that service members experience while deployed.[11]

The WG discussed a number of approaches to clarifying the relationship between exposures to airborne hazards and disease. These included studies of SWA populations. It is uncertain how much or what data might be extant, and it is unclear how to establish a relationship with SWA authorities that would permit either protocols relying on historical records or clinical studies. Successfully undertaking such studies might require the involvement of agencies other than the DoD and VA (eg, US Agency for International Development, Washington, DC), as well as mechanisms for providing benefit to the study population. Participants noted that, in the past, the DoD had performed studies of local populations in the region of the former Yugoslavia.

Participants were also concerned that the granularity of available exposure data was not fine enough to capture the actual exposures that service members received. Currently, exposure data are chiefly captured in terms of broad geographic localization or Military Occupation Specialty codes. In practice, in deployed settings, it is likely that neither of these variables can be relied on to capture exposure information with any degree of precision.

The WG supported continuing epidemiological survey studies through the efforts of the USAPHC,[12,13] the Millennium Cohort Study,[14] the Armed Forces Health Surveillance Center (Silver Spring, MD),[6] and the National Health Study for a New Generation of US Veterans.[15] However, because the occurrence of deployment-related disease from exposure to airborne hazards appears to be rare in the short term, a possible approach built on focused clinical studies of groups of service members or veterans reporting respiratory systems or disease might be informative for determining the range of diseases associated with deployment. A cohort of particular interest is a group of approximately 40 patients diagnosed with constrictive bronchiolitis by lung biopsy at Vanderbilt University Medical Center (Nashville, TN).[5] The limited number of known causes for constrictive bronchiolitis and the severity of the disease have made these patients a cohort of intense interest. Although a few of these patients may have been exposed to sulfur dioxide while fighting the sulfur fire at the Al-Mishraq sulfur plant near Mosul, Iraq, in 2003, the majority of them do not report exposures known to have clear associations with constrictive bronchiolitis.

However, it may be possible to capture a broader array of diseases by performing clinical follow-ups on service member and veteran participants in the Millennium Cohort Study and the National Health Study for a New Generation of US Veterans who self-report respiratory symptoms or disease. Although a number of caveats apply to both studies, their large number of participants, the mix of deployed and nondeployed present and former service members, and the ability to follow veterans over long periods would provide a strong foundation for informative epidemiological studies in their own right or for focused clinical follow-on work. Approaches that have not yet been taken but that could provide leads to deployment-related illness include examining the reasons for service member separation and comorbidities associated with traumatic brain injury and posttraumatic stress disease. Because disease states may be progressive, it was also important to perform baseline studies of veterans that would establish the baseline health of the population.

Other populations that might prove to be sources for follow-up studies include patients within the VA medical system; firefighters who fought the sulfur fire at Al-Mishraq; and service members who were not actively involved in firefighting activities, but who were deployed within the radius of the fire's plume.

As noted previously, the toxicity of geogenic PM and burn pit combustion products have not been well studied. In particular, there is a lack of chronic studies and comparative toxicity assessment of PM from different localities. The WG considered that ascertaining the adverse outcomes resulting from exposures to these materials in animals could effectively highlight possible disease states in the service member and veteran populations.

Finally, the committee members were in accord with the IOM report[9] on burn pit exposures. Although the emphasis to date has been on exposures to geogenic dusts and burn pit combustion products, other exposures singly and in combination may also increase the risk of disease in the deployed population.

Environmental Sampling for Health Surveillance

A second major discussion theme was whether and how environmental sampling and surveillance in theater could be improved and better utilized. Whereas the current procedures have limitations and are restricted to sampling for potentially hazardous materials that are known or plausibly expected to be present, a vast amount of data is currently being gathered. Participants were concerned that these data were not readily available for data mining and decision-making because of data storage practices. Participants averred, for example, that not all data were routinely digitized. If data were more accessible, the distribution of analytes of interest could be better linked to troop movements for risk assessment and exposure evaluation. It was also suggested that increasing the availability of sampling data from previous conflicts might enhance epidemiological studies.

The discussants considered the issue of gases and volatile organic compounds that are ubiquitous in military occupational environments. Many solvents are highly volatile; and burning waste, cooking, and vehicle operation produce gases and volatile organics. Many of these chemicals have established toxicities, but are not routinely sampled. These compounds are difficult to capture in exterior environments (eg, near burn pits). There is no inventory of such compounds generated in common activities in the deployed environment, thus representing a significant data gap. With respect to burn pits, it will be difficult to generate such an inventory without better understanding the types of materials that were incinerated. Improved sampling equipment and protocols will probably be required to refine capture and analysis of these materials.

There was some discussion, as well, of whether sampling could be improved with better-trained personnel and better equipment. The value of unmanned aerial vehicles and personal sampling devices similar to radiation badges was also discussed. Although the availability of personal dosimeters is not likely to occur in the near term, the WG considered whether monitoring exposures at the small group level might be a useful intermediate term tactic. An interesting approach that was briefly considered was the use of either wild or domesticated animals present in the local environment as sentinels.

Improved Procedures and Methods for Diagnosis and Screening for Environmental Injury

A third recurrent topic of discussion among the participants was the need for improved procedures and methods for diagnosing and screening environmental, especially pulmonary, injuries. There was some question about whether there was a sufficient benefit to warrant spirometric screening for service members with conventional methods. Also, there was a question concerning whether a better solution might be the development of technology that would allow self-capture of respiratory data for frequent respiratory function testing without requiring a large increase in the number of pulmonary function technicians.

Discussants also raised the issue of whether it would be possible to develop improved diagnostic measures and tools. One aspect of this discussion was improved functional physiological testing, and another was the development of a new generation of biochemical biomarker tests in exposure and disease in blood and urine. The WG participants also suggested that there is value in archiving biosamples for both the individual health record and the historical investigation of delayed health effects. This topic flowed into a brief consideration of whether current archival procedures and technologies were adequate.

There was also a very brief consideration of whether there might be value in using genetic profiling to identify individuals at high risk for adverse responses to exposure and limiting their exposure to relevant hazards.

The WG also devoted some discussion to the appropriateness of the current generation of survey instruments for capturing exposures following deployment. There was concern that service members might not truthfully report exposures because they feared it could affect redeployment or leave. There was also concern that service members might not recognize exposures that should be reported.

Mitigating the Risks of Exposure

The fourth topic of discussion was improvements in mitigating the risks of exposure. There was consensus that combatant commanders did not willingly make decisions that put service members at risk; but that lack of policy, planning, and training might leave them unprepared to mitigate risks to the fullest extent possible. For example, exposures to burn pits might have been avoided or reduced if the locations of the burn pits had been considered earlier during operations. Participants suggested that both improved methods for reducing the volume of the waste stream and disposing of waste will be necessary in the future because it is unlikely that the burn pits can be eliminated in the short term.

The WG also suggested that, particularly if new tools for health screening come on line, it may be necessary to update or improve training for commanders so that they can take these new data into account. A significant concern of the participants was the difficulty of predicting what the relevant exposures might be for future deployments and how to prepare to deal with them. The WG suggested that improved methods, training, and policy for proactively dealing with exposure threats were desirable.

Finally, participants proposed that it might be necessary to develop improved personal protective equipment for high-level ambient exposures, such as the airborne PM present in SWA. Available respirators are uncomfortable and clog rapidly.

Other Topics

The WG also discussed some specific issues that do not fit cleanly into the categories as previously described. These issues included research into better methods for preventing tobacco use and promoting and aiding tobacco use cessation. There was also concern that the services did not have a solid understanding of the risks and prevalence of berylliosis in service members, given the increasing use of beryllium in electronics and other materiel.

Members of the VA WG were concerned about how to integrate clinical measures into disability determinations. Appropriate biomarkers of exposure would have great utility in establishing whether disability applicants had grounds for consideration. Because disability determinations depend on how much capacity the applicant veteran has lost, there is a need to understand how the disease process affects the entire person.

SUMMARY

In general, the discussions by the WG were well-aligned with the recommendations in the IOM's *Long-Term Health Consequences of Exposure to Burn Pits in Iraq and Afghanistan*[9] (six key recommendations and discussion of current responses are included in the Attachment). Although they ranged over a wider field, they reflected the presence of operational, clinical, and exposure science experts in the WG. Perhaps the two broadest conclusions of the WG were (1) that effective resolution of the key research questions would require the cooperative efforts of the DoD and VA; and (2) that effective resolution of the question of whether respiratory or other disease(s) is associated with deployment to SWA. The deliberate pace of scientific investigation needs somehow to be accelerated, particularly when it is combined with the pace of the deliberative process in government, the risk that decisions regarding compensation and the causality of injury may be made by the court of public opinion rather than by objectively weighing the evidence. Such decisions have an impact on every phase of occupational health decision-making and affect service members and veterans in all arenas, from the development of risk mitigation strategies to compensation award.

REFERENCES

1. Engelbrecht JP, McDonald EV, Gillies JA, et al. Characterizing mineral dusts and other aerosols from the Middle East—part 1: ambient sampling. *Inhal Toxicol.* 2009;21:297–326.

2. Peeples L. Gulf war syndrome, other illnesses among veterans may be due to toxic environments. *The Huffington Post.* http://www.huffingtonpost.com/2013/02/07/gulf-war-syndrome-veterans_n_2634838.html. Accessed February 22, 2013.

3. Szema AM, Peters MC, Weissinger KM, Gagliano CA, Chen JJ. New-onset asthma among soldiers serving in Iraq and Afghanistan. *Allergy Asthma Proc.* 2010;31:67–71.

4. Smith B, Wong CA, Smith TC, et al. Newly reported respiratory symptoms and conditions among military personnel deployed to Iraq and Afghanistan: a prospective population-based study. *Am J Epidemiol.* 2009;170:1433–1442.

5. King M. Constrictive bronchiolitis in soldiers returning from Iraq and Afghanistan. *N Engl J Med.* 2011;365:222–230.

6. US Armed Forces Health Surveillance Center, the Naval Health Research Center, and the US Army Public Health Command. *Epidemiological Studies of Health Outcomes Among Troops Deployed to Burn Pit Sites.* Silver Spring, MD: Defense Technical Information Center (DTIC); 2010.

7. Morris MJ. *Study of Active-Duty Military for Pulmonary Disease Related to Environmental Dust Exposure (STAMPEDE).* Presented at: VA/DoD Airborne Hazards Symposium. Washington, DC: VA/DoD; August 2012.

8. National Research Council. *Review of the Department of Defense Enhanced Particulate Matter Surveillance Program Report.* Washington, DC: The National Academies Press; 2010.

9. Institute of Medicine of the National Academies. *Long-Term Health Consequences of Exposure to Burn Pits in Iraq and Afghanistan.* Washington, DC: National Academies Press; 2011: 1–9, 31–44, 117–129.

10. Shorr AF, Scoville SL, Cersovsky SB, et al. Acute eosinophilic pneumonia among US military personnel deployed in or near Iraq. *JAMA.* 2004;292:2997–3005.

11. Jackson DA. *Research Studies and Future Directions.* Presented at: VA/DoD Airborne Hazards Symposium. Washington, DC: VA/DoD; August 2012.

12. Abraham JH, Baird CP. A case-crossover study of ambient particulate matter and cardiovascular and respiratory medical encounters among US military personnel deployed to southwest Asia. *J Occup Environ Med.* 2012;54:733–739.

13. Baird CP, DeBakey S, Reid L, et al. Respiratory health status of US Army personnel potentially exposed to smoke from 2003 Al-Mishraq Sulfur Plant fire. *J Occup Environ Med.* 2012;54:717–723.

14. The Millennium Cohort Study. The Millennium Cohort Study website. http://www.millenniumcohort.org/. Accessed April 12, 2013.

15. US Department of Veterans Affairs. National Health Study for a New Generation of U.S. Veterans website. http://www.publichealth.va.gov/newgenerationstudy/. Accessed April 12, 2013.

ATTACHMENT: FUTURE RESEARCH—RECOMMENDATIONS FROM THE INSTITUTE OF MEDICINE'S 2011 REPORT ON THE LONG-TERM CONSEQUENCES OF EXPOSURE TO BURN PITS IN IRAQ AND AFGHANISTAN

Introduction

The Institute of Medicine (IOM) made a number of recommendations for an integrated research effort ascertaining the health risks associated with burn pit exposures. They are cited herein with brief descriptions of relevant studies that could be leveraged, are in the planning stages, or are under way.

Institute of Medicine Recommendation 1

> A pilot [feasibility] study should be conducted to ensure adequate statistical power, ability to adjust for potential confounders, to identify data availability and limitations and develop testable research questions and specific objectives.[1(p126)]

A formal statement of research goals, structure, pilot, and feasibility studies will help minimize the overall risk of not achieving the stated research goals. Three studies (the US Department of Defense [DoD] Millennium Cohort Study,[2] the DoD Armed Forces Health Surveillance Center Cohort,[3] and the US Department of Veterans Affairs [VA]/DoD's National Health Study for a New Generation of US Veterans[4]) are investigating the relationship between deployment and long-term health effects, including potential respiratory effects.

The IOM recommends pilot studies to

> address issues of statistical power and develop design features for specific health outcomes.[1(p124)]

Physical examination on a population basis is necessary to determine individual variability as it relates to health outcomes, such as lung function over time. Care for veterans in the immediate postdeployment period cannot wait for long-term outcome studies to determine final disease states for those with postdeployment symptoms. Early markers of disease in the respiratory system should be a component of a research-based physical examination. Results of this research could help to inform veteran care and healthcare policy.

IOM also commented that

> More research is needed to identify useful, meaningful, reliable and implementable biomarkers.[1(p119)]

Epigenetics is an evolving discipline to detect the human effects of exposures. The VA's Million Veteran Program, an Office of Research and Development (ORD)-supported genomics research project within the Cooperative Studies Program (CSP), has the ability to administer health-related questionnaires and collect specimens. However, it is limited in its ability to understand burn pit exposures across the entire deployed population due to its nonrandom selection of participants and lack of physical examinations. The Million Veteran Program may offer insights to the background epigenetic variations as they relate to common exposures of daily nondeployed life. The CSP, which also supports Gulf War veteran studies, will be a logical resource to perform a study-by-study analysis to determine what modifications are necessary to meet gaps in burn pit (airborne hazards) research.

Institute of Medicine Recommendation 2

> An independent oversight committee ... should be established to provide guidance and to review specific objectives, study designs, protocols and results from the burn pit emissions research programs that are developed.[1(p126)]

Existing independent advisory bodies may potentially provide the recommended level of external oversight. The ORD has an extensive peer-review process for the VA researchers through its standing review committees (composed of experts from inside the VA, as well as those from academia, other government agencies, and industry). These committees review research applications, specific objectives, study designs, protocols, and all other aspects of proposed research in a structure modeled after the Center for Scientific Review at the National Institutes of Health (Bethesda, MD).

In the past, various work groups (WGs) were formed to address subsets of the respiratory issue. In 2005, the Assistant Secretary of Defense for Health Affairs formed the Joint Particulate Matter Work Group to investigate the composition of particulate matter (PM) across the Central Command Area of Responsibility (CENTCOM AOR), the Middle East, thus resulting in the Enhanced Particulate Matter Surveillance Program that has been reviewed by the National Academies.[5] In 2010, the Pulmonary Work Group was formed under the auspices of the Military Operational Medical Research Program of the US Army Medical Research and Materiel Command (Fort Detrick, MD). This WG has identified research gaps and priorities in the area of toxicology, epidemiology, and clinical studies.[6] It is critical to monitor the clinical course of case series, such as the US Army Study of Active Duty Military for Pulmonary Disease Related to Environmental Dust Exposure (STAMPEDE).[7] Under the auspices of the Joint Executive Council and Health Executive Council, the DoD/VA Deployment Health Work Group continues to collaborate and support many of these activities.

Institute of Medicine Recommendation 3

> A cohort study of Veterans and active duty military should be considered to assess potential long-term health effects related to burn pit emissions in the context of other ambient exposures at the JBB [Joint Base Balad].[1(p127)]

The VA Office of Public Health is developing an overarching research study to provide continuity and resources for the extended period (likely decades) necessary to address the potential long-term health effects. This multisite study is a collaborative effort with the VA CSP and is intended to examine the health of all veterans prospectively. Ongoing studies also continue to address the research goals as a whole. Three current studies continue to evolve and focus on health concerns of Operation Enduring Freedom (OEF), Operation Iraqi Freedom (OIF), and Operation New Dawn (OND). Efforts of the Millennium Cohort Study,[8] sponsored by the DoD, has evolved from its Gulf War origins to include additional deployment exposure questions related to OEF, OIF, and OND. The VA is partnering with DoD on the Millennium Cohort Study to facilitate the use of VA clinical data to confirm self-reported outcomes. First, this collaboration is likely to improve the validity of the Millennium Cohort Study and improve the understanding of health effects related to deployment. Second, the VA's National Health Study for a New Generation of US Veterans[4] has completed its first data collection and is now in the analysis phase. A paper on the prevalence of respiratory conditions has been submitted for publication. Self-reported exposure questions consistent with the Millennium Cohort Study questionnaire are included. Third, the Armed Forces Health Surveillance Center (Silver Spring, MD) followed deployed personnel for 36 months.[3] Clinical diagnoses from electronic databases were used, but did not allow for adjustment of known confounders (eg, smoking). These initial postdeployment health outcome studies, as well as those conducted by the Naval Health Research Center (San Diego, CA) with cohorts from locations in the CENTCOM AOR with burn pits, were cited by IOM as evidence of feasibility. These studies are ongoing and will be continued for many years.

Institute of Medicine Recommendation 4

> An exposure assessment for better source attribution and identification of chemicals associated with waste burning and other pollution sources at JBB [Joint Base Balad] should be conducted ... to help the VA determine those health outcomes most likely to be associated with burn pit exposures.[1(p127)]

Sampling and risk assessments were done at various times at Joint Base Balad (JBB), but individual sampling was not performed. The burn pit at JBB was closed in 2009 when incinerators were operational and no further real-time exposure measurements were possible. Although the IOM suggested further characterization of the JBB soil dioxin level to evaluate dispersion, soil turnover and covering have occurred, as well as a significant reduction in military presence in Iraq. The US Army Public Health Command (Aberdeen Proving Ground, MD) is currently analyzing the existing four earlier rounds of air sampling data to identify spatial and temporal trends.

Additional burn pits continue to operate in Afghanistan. DoD plans to perform personal monitoring of service members stationed in Bagram, Afghanistan. In addition, DoD plans to perform ambient monitoring for PM and volatile organic compounds. On occasion, deployed preventive medicine personnel collect ambient PM samples in and around burning operations (typically either every sixth day, or every 1 or 2 days when visiting remote forward operating bases). These data may help inform further studies on the association of exposure to airborne hazards and adverse health effects.

Institute of Medicine Recommendation 5

Exposure assessment should include detailed deployment information including distance and direction individuals lived and worked from the JBB [Joint Base Balad] burn pit, duration of deployment, and job duties.[1(p127)]

The VA relies on DoD to provide deployment data. A recently signed DoD/VA Data Transfer Agreement will expedite the transfer of data between both organizations, and increase the timeliness and completeness of future studies.

Various respiratory exposures should be considered. Burn pit exposures may have been highest in nonveteran populations (eg, US government contractors) working in proximity to the burn pits. The exposure assessment suggested by IOM will require individuals to complete exposure assessment questionnaires with specific questions related to location, duration, and duties.

Institute of Medicine Recommendation 6

Assessment of health outcomes is best done collaboratively using the clinical informatics systems of the DoD and VA.[1(p127)]

Current electronic health records are limited in their ability to capture exposure data and view complete healthcare outcomes across delivery systems. The VA plans to link outcome data with self-reported questionnaire data from the DoD's Millennium Cohort Study (which has a sizable veteran population). The Office of Public Health and ORD are also actively working to embed two or three VA personnel in the Millennium Cohort Study office to conduct joint DoD/VA research and provide VA chart reviews of conditions self-reported from veterans participating in the Millennium Cohort Study.

Summary

Approximately 20 participants in the DoD/VA Airborne Hazards Symposium participated in a multidisciplinary WG to formulate a comprehensive 5-year strategic research plan to assess possible health risks associated with exposure to natural and man-made airborne hazards during deployment to southwest Asia. The potential risks and solutions were sufficiently diverse that the WG did not develop such a plan. Nevertheless, deliberations of the WG converged on several areas of concern that may serve to inform research efforts by the VA and DoD. These areas included a very incomplete understanding of the prevalence and severity of deployment-related lung disease, thus

- improving the scope and effectiveness of environmental sampling for health surveillance,
- improving procedures and methods for diagnosis and screening for environmental injury, and
- mitigating the risks of exposure.

References

1. Institute of Medicine of the National Academies. *Long-Term Health Consequences of Exposure to Burn Pits in Iraq and Afghanistan*. Washington, DC: National Academies Press; 2011: 1–9, 31–44, 117–129.

2. Smith B, Wong CA, Smith TC, et al. Newly reported respiratory symptoms and conditions among military personnel deployed to Iraq and Afghanistan: a prospective population-based study. *Am J Epidemiol*. 2009;170:1433–1442.

3. US Armed Forces Health Surveillance Center, the Naval Health Research Center, and the US Army Public Health Command. *Epidemiological Studies of Health Outcomes Among Troops Deployed to Burn Pit Sites*. Silver Spring, MD: Defense Technical Information Center (DTIC); 2010.

4. Baird CP, DeBakey S, Reid L, et al. Respiratory health status of US Army personnel potentially exposed to smoke from 2003 Al-Mishraq Sulfur Plant fire. *J Occup Environ Med*. 2012;54:717–723.

5. National Research Council. *Review of the Department of Defense Enhanced Particulate Matter Surveillance Program Report*. Washington, DC: The National Academies Press; 2010.

6. The Millennium Cohort Study. The Millennium Cohort Study website. http://www.millenniumcohort.org/. Accessed April 12, 2013.

7. Morris MJ. *Study of Active-Duty Military for Pulmonary Disease Related to Environmental Dust Exposure* (*STAMPEDE*). Presented at: VA/DoD Airborne Hazards Symposium. Washington, DC: VA/DoD; August 2012.

8. US Department of Veterans Affairs. National Health Study for a New Generation of U.S. Veterans website. http://www.publichealth.va.gov/newgenerationstudy/. Accessed April 12, 2013.

APPENDIX A

A Self-Reporting Tool to Collect Individual Data for Respiratory Health Effects and Military Airborne Exposures

Veronique Hauschild, MPH
Environmental Scientist, Injury Prevention Program, Epidemiology and Disease Surveillance Portfolio, Army Institute of Public Health, US Army Public Health Command, 5158 Blackhawk Road, Aberdeen Proving Ground, Maryland 21010-5403

Jessica Sharkey, MPH
Epidemiologist, Environmental Medicine Program, Occupational and Environmental Medicine Portfolio, Army Institute of Public Health, US Army Public Health Command, 5158 Blackhawk Road, Aberdeen Proving Ground, Maryland 21010-5403

Although self-reported data has its limitations, questionnaires or survey tools are incorporated into many aspects of public health research, clinical settings, and medical registries. Several of the initiatives described in previous chapters of this book have made use of some form of a questionnaire. Whereas different applications (eg, research vs clinical) may require different questions, there is often overlap of certain topics. The concept of a single standardized set of questions for US Department of Defense (DoD) and US Department of Veterans Affairs (VA) users to draw upon has been recommended by various entities.[1-4]

PURPOSE

This appendix describes the basis for the set of standardized questions provided in Appendix B (Respiratory Health and Exposure Questionnaire). These questions could be used to collect more consistent and detailed information from individual service members or veterans regarding their deployment exposure experiences and health conditions or symptoms that might be associated with respiratory illness. Questions regarding history of smoking, physical fitness, work activities, and hobbies are also included to help evaluate the influence of potentially critical confounding risk factors. Information obtained through use of these questions could substantially enhance future evaluation of the relationship between deployment exposures and respiratory health. Specific questions provided in this appendix are proposed as the initial start to a larger "standardized reference library" of exposure and health-related questions that could be used by various DoD and VA researchers, clinicians, and public health experts. The questions may be used in their entirety (eg, as the full set provided) or in part (only selected questions), depending on the user's application, an individual's (eg, patient's) experiences and concerns, and/or the time available.

BACKGROUND: A TWO-STAGE EFFORT

The questions in this appendix resulted from combining two separate, but related, questionnaires that evolved from a US Army Public Health Command (USAPHC; Aberdeen Proving Ground, MD) project initiated in 2010.[5] These questionnaires helped to improve two areas of variability that have contributed to the limitations of studies completed thus far regarding postdeployment respiratory health: (1) exposure variability and (2) diagnostic variability. The studies to date evaluate population health with limited sensitivity to individual health, exposures, and risks factors. Because the health outcomes of concern are not clearly evident at the broadest population levels, attempts to minimize individual variability are warranted.

The project started with the Deployment Airborne Respiratory Exposure (DARE) questionnaire. The DARE questionnaire was designed as a tool to help obtain individual exposure information about potentially hazardous constituents in the air that personnel may have inhaled during their deployment(s). Because exposure history is such a critical component in evaluating environmental associations to health outcomes, the DARE questionnaire was designed to illicit responses that could be used to represent individual service member exposure variability. Specifically, questions regarding the frequency, duration, and intensity of identified exposures would yield responses that could be used to characterize exposures in a semiquantified manner (eg, by grouping those exposed to more severe conditions, those exposed for longer periods, and/or those exposed more frequently). Although exposure variability is acknowledged as a potential key factor in exposure characterization (see Chapter 5, Future Improvement to Individual Exposure Characterization for Deployed Military Personnel), existing reviewed questionnaires have not addressed this variability.

Whereas several reviewing clinicians and researchers applauded the DARE questionnaire, they noted that an additional set of questions to collect standardized information regarding associated clinical and health-related questions was needed to help reduce the potential for diagnostic variability (see discussions in Chapter 5 [Future Improvements to Individual Exposure Characterization for Deployed Military Personnel] and Chapter 11 [Discussion Summary: Basic Diagnosis and Workup of Symptomatic Individuals]). Therefore, the USAPHC drafted the Clinical Evaluation of Respiratory Conditions (CERC) questionnaire. The CERC questionnaire focused on questions regarding symptoms, medical history, conditions, and health status. Although this initiative was focused on a clinical application, reviewers also provided input for use in research applications.[5]

Subsequent reviews of the DARE and CERC by DoD, VA, and academia clinicians, epidemiologists, public health experts, statisticians, questionnaire/survey developers, and those involved in a limited USAPHC military personnel beta test lead to the eventual composite set of questions provided in Appendix B.

WHY A QUESTIONNAIRE IS SO CRITICAL

The lack of detail regarding a service member's individual exposure experiences and personal risk factors has prevented studies from evaluating individual conditions that may result in higher risk of a chronic respiratory health outcome (see Chapter 5).[1-9] This was the original impetus for USAPHC's effort to create a standardized deployment exposure questionnaire. Reviewers of early versions of the questionnaires noted that these same data gaps were also problematic for clinical applications. The importance of a questionnaire for each application is summarized in the following section.

Public Health Research Needs

As discussed in Chapter 2 (Background of Deployment-Related Airborne Exposures of Interest and Use of Exposure Data in Environmental Epidemiology Studies) and Chapter 5, ambient environmental data has been of limited use to researchers who are trying to analyze the relationship between deployment exposures and individual pulmonary conditions. Instead, most research studies have used deployment status to southwest Asia as a proxy for exposure.[3,10] This assumes that all persons deployed to this area have had the same exposure experiences, ignoring the potentially significant differences in individuals' exposure experiences that can be affected by the individual's assigned tasks, activities, unique durations, frequencies, and intermittent peak exposures at specific locations at specific times. In addition, without confounding risk factor data from individuals (smoking status, aerobic physical fitness, and activities), research is not able to determine potential higher risk groups. Despite limitations and the lack of a standardized, official DoD- and VA-endorsed reference source of questions, questionnaires and survey tools continue to be used as a critical source of data in many, if not most, of the past studies and ongoing studies that are described in previous chapters of this book. With a library of approved questions, researchers could select questions most pertinent to study objectives. A standardized set of questions across services and the VA would help ensure more consistent and, thus, comparable data, improving transparency of future epidemiological studies and allowing for study comparisons.[3,4,10,11]

Clinical Applications

Upon return from deployment to southwest Asia, military personnel are required to complete a Post-Deployment Health Assessment (PDHA) and Post-Deployment Health Reassessment (PDHRA) (Tables A-1 and A-2).[12] These forms include

TABLE A-1

SUMMARY OF PUBLISHED MILITARY QUESTIONNAIRES REVIEWED

Questionnaire	Purpose
Pre-Deployment Health Assessment (DD Form 2795) Post-Deployment Health Assessment (DD Form 2796) Post-Deployment Health Reassessment (DD Form 2900)	Required forms for assessing state of health prior to determining medical deployability (PDHA-2795) and then status after deployment (PDHA-2796) within 30 days and then by 6 months (PDHRA). The form must be completed in an electronic or web-enabled form following service-specific directives and using one of the following service-specific data systems: Army MEDPROS, Air Force PIMR or AFCITA, or Navy / Marine Corps EDHA. *(Accessed December 2012 at http://fhp.osd.mil/pdhrainfo/sm_fam/sm_fam_Army.jsp)*
Depleted Uranium Questionnaire (DD Form 2872 test, February 2004) Health Survey (DD Form 2872-1 test, February 2004)	Required forms if patient indicates DU exposure on PDHA. Providers complete the DoD DU Questionnaire and Health Survey with the assistance of the patients being assessed for DU exposure. The DU form is used to obtain exposure information, and the health survey is a short measure of health-related functioning comprised of 36 questions asking the patient to describe physical or emotional problems over the past 4 weeks. *(Accessed December 4, 2012. Questionnaire at http://www.dtic.mil/whs/directives/infomgt/forms/eforms/dd2872t.pdf and survey at http://www.dtic.mil/whs/directives/infomgt/forms/eforms/dd2872t1.pdf. Other information at http://www.pdhealth.mil/downloads/OIF_DU_Med_Mgmt_Supp.pdf)*
Medical Record—Post-Deployment Medical Assessment (DD Form 2844 test, March 2002)	Established as a test form in response to Persian Gulf War deployment exposure concerns. Prescribed form used when evaluating patient with postdeployment health concerns when referred for care subsequent to screening using DD Form 2796 or when self-referred to facilitate outpatient treatment documentation by cueing patients and providers to note key aspects in the assessment, management, and treatment of patients with deployment-related health concerns. As a test form that has not been updated in more than 10 years, it is no longer considered an active form.
Asbestos Exposure Part 1 — Initial Medical Questionnaire (DD Form 2493-1, January 2000)	Borrows questions from the ATS Respiratory Disease Questionnaire. *(Accessed December 4, 2012 at http://www.dtic.mil/whs/directives/infomgt/forms/eforms/dd2493-1.pdf)*
Medical Examination Respirator Use Questionnaire (Example DA 470)	Questions focused on health status to be able to wear respiratory equipment without adverse health outcome. *(Blank form accessed December 4, 2012 at http://armypubs.army.mil/eforms/pdf/A4700.PDF)*
Persian Gulf Registry Code Sheet (VA Form 10-9009a(RS))	In 2002, the VA and DoD established the Persian Gulf Registry and the Clinical Comprehensive Evaluation Program for troops that deployed during Operation Desert Shield / Operation Desert Storm. The program is a now primarily the VA Gulf War Registry. This VA code sheet is similar to the questionnaire used by DoD. *(Accessed December 4, 2012 at http://www.gulflink.org/gwr/10-9009a.pdf. Related information at http://www.gulflink.org/gwr/registry.htm and http://www.publichealth.va.gov/exposures/gulfwar/registry_exam.asp)*
PTSD Check List–Military Version (PCL-M)	Self-administered questionnaire with 17 questions for assessing trauma-related stress. Three different versions are available. *(Accessed December 4, 2012 at http://www.pdhealth.mil/guidelines/appendix4.asp)*
Post-Deployment Clinical Assessment Tool (May 20, 2003)	Form consisting of an array of brief standardized illness-specific screens and assessments to assess and follow-up patients with postdeployment health concerns and illnesses. Measures patient status in the following areas: somatic symptoms; PTSD; depression; anxiety and panic; functional status; alcohol use; frequency of healthcare visits; social support; and satisfaction with healthcare. *(Accessed December 4, 2012 at http://www.pdhealth.mil/downloads/PDCAT_v7.pdf)*

(Table A-1 *continues)*

Table A-1 *continued*

MVP's Long-Form Survey Questionnaire	MVP is a national, voluntary research program of the VA Office of Research & Development. The goal of MVP is to partner with veterans in the VA Healthcare System to study how genes affect health. Data collected will be stored anonymously for research on diseases like diabetes and cancer, and military-related illnesses (ie, PTSD). *(Accessed December 4, 2012 at http://www.research.va.gov/MVP/)*

AFCITA: Air Force Complete Immunization Tracking Application; ATS: American Thoracic Society; DA: Department of the Army; DD: Department of Defense; DoD: US Department of Defense; DU: depleted uranium; EDHA: Electronic Deployment Health Assessment; MEDPROS: Medical Protection System; MVP: Million Veteran Program; PCL-M: PTSD Check List-Military; PDHA: Pre-Deployment Health Assessment / Post-Deployment Health Assessment; PDHRA: Post-Deployment Health Reassessment; PIMR: Preventive Health Assessment and Individual Medical Readiness; PTSD: posttraumatic stress disorder; VA: US Department of Veterans Affairs

Note: This is not a completely exhaustive list of all questionnaires found, but represents primary tools considered that have been implemented and are available for public viewing. (Many questionnaires cited in the study literature are not contained as part of the book and are not readily available.)

basic questions regarding overall and mental health status, symptoms, and a list of potential environmental deployment exposures. They are intended to be a screening tool for healthcare providers to identify potential postdeployment physiological and mental conditions. Providers are expected to ask patients appropriate follow-up exposure history questions. The DoD does provide for follow-up questionnaires to address concerns regarding depleted uranium (DU) exposures.[13] Yet, despite a growing number of patients who have postdeployment chronic respiratory conditions, there is no official required set of DoD or VA exposure history and medical/symptom questions for all clinicians to consistently use. This is problematic, especially because many patients with exposure concerns may be interacting with providers who are not specialists in environmental or occupational medicine. Data collected are inconsistent and may be inadequate, especially because most environmental and occupational diseases either manifest as common medical problems (eg, headache, rashes, asthma) or have nonspecific symptoms. Yet, consideration of environmental exposures does not often factor into most clinicians' history-taking or diagnosis.[14] As a result, clinicians may miss opportunities to make correct diagnoses or may fail to associate disease with past exposure. In an attempt to ensure that environmental exposures are adequately considered in the specialty cases they receive, the VA War Related Illness and Injury Study Centers have been developing a series of standardized questions that include several of those contained in this appendix. These questions, however, need to be vetted and incorporated more broadly across agencies and services. In addition, response data need to be collected in a retrievable electronic system. Currently, patient exposure history information, as documented in medical records, is not readily accessible for public health research applications.

Registry Needs

As discussed in Chapter 22 (Discussion Summary: Methodological Considerations to Design a Pulmonary Case Series and a National, Broad-based Registry for Veterans of Operation Iraqi Freedom and Operation Enduring Freedom), Chapter 25 (Toxic-Embedded Fragment Registry: Lessons Learned), and Chapter 26 (Lessons Learned From Self-Selected Registries [Agent Orange Registry]), the DoD and VA have established certain registries of past military exposure settings and incidents. The development and implementation of questionnaires are a critical component of registries (eg, the Gulf War Registry).[8] As future registries (eg, burn pit registry) may be established, the use of a questionnaire to collect individual information will likely be required. Although every operation and exposure incident may require some unique questions, the establishment of a consistent "library" of questions to draw on would facilitate implementation of registries and provide a better mechanism for use of responses in public health research applications.

EXISTING PRECEDENCE

Despite the recognized limitations of self-reported data from questionnaires (eg, recall and self-reporting bias),[9,11] there is substantial precedence for using such data to address gaps in "individual data." Tables A-1 and A-2 describe publically available questionnaires or tools that have been implemented by the military, other US or inter-

TABLE A-2

SUMMARY OF PUBLISHED UNITED STATES OR INTERNATIONALLY RECOGNIZED QUESTIONNAIRES AND SURVEYS REVIEWED

Questionnaire	Purpose
FOH Medical Surveillance Management Program—Health History and Physical Examination Form (FOH 5, Rev April 21, 2010)	Preoccupational assessment tool used by providers to document exposure and health history and determine duty fitness and respiratory fitness (for respirator use). *(Accessed December 4, 2012 at http://co.gloucester.nj.us/Pdf/Emergency/Medical%20Surveillance.pdf)*
ATS—Recommended Respiratory Disease Questionnaires for Use With Adults and Children in Epidemiological Research (ATS-DLD-78-A)	A critical internationally recognized instrument designed to support epidemiological research of respiratory diseases. Initially, a questionnaire was devised in the early 1950s in Great Britain after realization that the clinical assessment of subjects in epidemiological studies was plagued by uncontrollable biases. In 1969, the ATS published a version of its questionnaire in a document titled *Standards for Epidemiologic Surveys in Chronic Respiratory Disease*. A later version was expanded to address smoking history, family history, and occupational exposures history; this was endorsed by the MRC. The Division of Lung Diseases of the National Heart, Lung, and Blood Institute (which was funded by ATS) published the 1978 version that is still used today. Different groups have used the ATS Questionnaire, in part or in its entirety, to develop other surveys for various respiratory outcomes (eg, the European Community Respiratory Health Survey Questionnaire). *(Accessed December 4, 2012 and http://www.thoracic.org/statements/resources/archive/rrdquacer.pdf and www.ecrhs.org)*
IUATLD Bronchial Symptoms Questionnaire, 1984	The IUATLD Bronchial Symptoms Questionnaire was originally developed for use in studies of asthma. Its reliability has been evaluated and determined to be a useful tool for many applications (eg, distinguishing between bronchial asthma and chronic bronchitis) and for response to histamine. It has been a foundation for many other international respiratory questionnaires and protocols over the years, including that of the WHO. *(Accessed December 4, 2012 at http://site.theunion.org/download/asthma/Asthma_questionnaire.doc)*
OSHA 1910.1043 Subpart: Z, Toxic and Hazardous Substances; Cotton Dust; Appendix B Respiratory Questionnaire(s)	Appendix B-I: Respiratory Questionnaire. Appendix B-II: Respiratory Questionnaire for nontextile workers for the cotton industry. Appendix B-III: Abbreviated Respiratory Questionnaire. *(Accessed December 4, 2012 at http://www.osha.gov/pls/oshaweb/owasrch.search_form?p_doc_type=STANDARDS&p_toc_level=1&p_keyvalue=1910)*
USEPA BASE Indoor Air Quality Questionnaire (EPA 402-C-06-002, January 2006)	To provide baseline information from typical buildings to compare during "sick building" assessments, USEPA conducted the BASE study that covers three major areas: (1) environmental and comfort measurements; (2) building HVAC systems characterization; and (3) building occupant demographics, symptoms, and perceptions. *(Accessed December 4, 2012 at http://www.epa.gov/iaq/base/pdfs/2003_base_protocol.pdf[Appendix F])*

(Table A-2 *continues)*

Table A-2 *continued*

NHANES III: NCHS Questionnaire(s) (asthma / respiratory conditions, smoking questionnaires)	The NHANES is a program of studies designed to assess the health and nutritional status of adults and children in the United States. The survey is unique in that it combines interviews and physical examinations. Interviews use several questionnaires for different topics. (*Accessed December 4, 2012. Guidance at http://www.cdc.gov/nchs/data/nhanes/nhanes3/cdrom/nchs/manuals/fieldint.pdf*) • *Asthma/respiratory questions at http://www.cdc.gov/asthma/survey/NHANES.pdf* • *Physical activity/fitness questions at http://www.cdc.gov/nchs/data/nhanes/nhanes_09_10/mi_paq_f.pdf* • *Smoking questions at http://www.cdc.gov/nchs/data/nhanes/nhanes_09_10/ai_smq_f.pdf*
California Flavoring Respiratory Questionnaire	This questionnaire helps healthcare providers monitor the health of workers in companies that manufacture food flavorings. It was developed to address concerns associated with bronchiolitis obliterans, a severe lung disease identified in workers who make microwave popcorn. (*Accessed December 4, 2012 at http://www.cdph.ca.gov/HealthInfo/discond/Pages/FlavoringLungDisease.aspx. Related information at www.dhs.ca.gov/ohb/flavorings.htm*)
IMCA	The IMCA is an international consensus product of clinicians and researchers in the field of respiratory diseases, representatives from international organizations (ie, WHO Europe), and scientific societies on a set of indicators to monitor COPD and asthma in all EU member states as part of an effort to build a "European system of information and knowledge concerning major chronic diseases." (*Accessed December 4, 2012 at http://www.imca.cat*)
Borg Perceived Exertion Scale	The CDC website describes use of the Perceived Exertion Scale. Original source: Borg, G. Perceived exertion as an indicator of somatic stress. *Scand J Rehabil Med*. 1970;2:92–98. (*Accessed December 4, 2012 at http://www.cdc.gov/physicalactivity/everyone/measuring/exertion.html*)
MRC Breathlessness Scale	Original source: Stenton C. The MRC breathlessness scale. *Occup Med (Lond)*. 2008;58:226–227.

ATS: American Thoracic Society; BASE: Building Assessment Survey and Evaluation; CDC: Centers for Disease Control and Prevention; COPD: chronic obstructive pulmonary disease; DLD: Division of Lung Disease; EU: European Union; FOH: Federal Occupational Health; HVAC: heating, ventilation, and air-conditioning; IMCA: indicators for monitoring COPD and asthma; IUATLD: International Union Against Tuberculosis and Lung Disease; MRC: Medical Research Council; NCHS: National Center for Health Statistics; NHANES: National Health and Nutrition Examination Survey; OSHA: Occupational Safety and Health Administration; Rev: revised; USEPA: US Environmental Protection Agency; WHO: World Health Organization

Note: This is not a completely exhaustive list of all questionnaires found, but represents primary tools considered that have been implemented and are available for public viewing. (Many questionnaires cited in the study literature are not contained as part of the book and are not readily available.)

national organizations, and/or research entities. Although most have not been definitively validated, some have been repeatedly studied and are considered to meet validation criteria in certain controlled occupational settings and populations.[15–23] Even though validation of tools used to help characterize military exposures may be impossible, the use of questions borrowed from well-established tools is considered a reasonable basis for precedent.

The military's use of questionnaires to address Gulf War assessment needs, as well as the detailed exposure and health history questionnaires of data for the DoD's DU Medical Surveillance Program, also indicate the feasibility of systematic self-reported data collection.[13,14,22] The program uses the PDHA/PDHRA as a screening tool to identify personnel needing to answer more detailed follow-up questions. This concept could be paralleled to address individuals with airborne exposure and respiratory health concerns. Specifically, those who identify health concerns in the PDHA electronic system could be flagged for a more detailed exposure and health questionnaire in the follow-up healthcare provider evaluation.

SUMMARY AND NEXT STEPS

Given other available options, and the many precedents for using questionnaires to collect self-reported exposure and relevant health status information, a standardized set of questions is considered a very viable solution to filling individual-level data gaps. Whereas the resulting set of questions are detailed and complex, they provide critical individual data that have not been available despite more than a decade of substantial and costly resources used to collect ambient environmental data. As previously noted, because the respiratory health outcomes of concern are not demonstrated in a larger population, attempts to minimize individual exposure and diagnostic variability are warranted. Despite concerns that use of such questions may be too difficult or time-consuming in research or clinical settings, a small internal beta test and lessons from other past examples, including the DoD DU program, suggest that administration of these questions is feasible in both research study and certain clinical applications. Of course, not all questions need to be used in all cases; the questions may be tiered or adjusted for specific applications and personnel. For example, clinical applications may not use the full set of questions unless a previously deployed patient presents with respiratory symptoms or a condition. Although specific implementation and use of such questions have not been determined, ideally an electronic system could be instituted to collect and archive responses in a database for broader public health use.

REFERENCES

1. National Research Council. *Review of the Department of Defense Enhanced Particulate Matter Surveillance Program Report.* Washington, DC: The National Academies Press; 2010.

2. Institute of Medicine. *Long-Term Health Consequences of Exposure to Burn Pits in Iraq and Afghanistan.* Washington, DC: The National Academies Press; 2011.

3. Smith TC, Millenium Cohort Study Team. Linking exposures and health outcomes to a large population-based longitudinal study: the Millenium Cohort Study. *Mil Med.* 2011;176(suppl 7):56–63.

4. Rose C, Abraham J, Harkins D, et al. Overview and recommendations for medical screening and diagnostic evaluation for postdeployment lung disease in returning US Warfighters. *J Occup Environ Med.* 2012;54:746–751.

5. Tinklepaugh C, Hauschild V. Survey tools to support analyses of deployment exposures and respiratory health outcomes. Presented at: 1st Annual Scientific Symposium on Lung Health after Deployment to Iraq and Afghanistan. New York, NY: School of Medicine/Health Sciences Center, State University of New York at Stony Brook; February 13, 2012.

6. Mallon TM. Progress in implementing recommendations in the National Academy of Sciences reports: "protecting those who serve: strategies to protect the health of deployed U.S. Forces." *Mil Med.* 2011;176(suppl 7):9–16.

7. Jollenbeck LM. Medical surveillance and other strategies to protect the health of deployed U.S. forces: revisiting after 10 years. *Mil Med.* 2011;176(suppl 7):64–70.

8. Brix K, O'Donnell FL. Panel 1: medical surveillance prior to, during, and following potential environmental exposures. *Mil Med.* 2011;176(suppl 7):91–96.

9. Glass DC, Sim MR. The challenges of exposure assessment in health studies of Gulf War veterans. *Philos Trans R Soc Lond B Biol Sci.* 2006;361(1468):627–637.

10. US Department of the Army. *Summary of Evidence Statement: Chronic Respiratory Conditions and Military Deployment.* Aberdeen Proving Ground, MD: US Army Public Health Command; 2011. Factsheet 64-018-1111.

11. Samet JM. A historical and epidemiologic perspective on respiratory symptoms questionnaires. *Am J Epidemiol.* 1978;108:435–446.

12. US Department of Defense. *Post Deployment Health Assessment.* Washington, DC: Assistant Secretary for Defense (Health Affairs); March 2005. DoD Memorandum.

13. U.S. Department of Defense. *Supplemental Information and Clinical Guidance for DoD Depleted Uranium (DU) Medical Management Program*. Deployment Clinical Health Center; April 2012. https://www.pdhealth.mil/downloads/DU_supplemental_info_and_clinical_guide.pdf . Accessed April 25, 2013.

14. Agency for Toxic Substances and Disease Registry (ATSDR). *Taking an Exposure History: What Role Can Primary Care Clinicians Play in Detecting, Treating, and Preventing Disease Resulting from Toxic Exposures?* Atlanta, GA: ATSDR; May 2011.

15. US Department of the Army. *Health Assessment of 2003 Qarmat Ali Water Treatment Plant Sodium Dichromate Incident Status Update: May 2010*. Aberdeen Proving Ground, MD: US Army Public Health Command (Provisional); 2010. Factsheet 64-012-0510.

16. Bellia V, Pistelli F, Giannini D, et al. Questionnaires, spirometry and PEF monitoring in epidemiological studies on elderly respiratory patients. *Eur Respir J*. 2003;40(suppl):21s–27s.

17. Liard R, Neukirch F. Questionnaires: a major instrument for respiratory epidemiology. *Eur Respir Mon*. 2000;15:154–166.

18. Hanania NA, Mannino DM, Yawn BP, et al. Predicting risk of airflow obstruction in primary care: validation of the lung function questionnaire (LFQ). *Respir Med*. 2010;104:1160–1170.

19. Burney PGJ, Luczynska C, Chinn S, Jarvis D. The European Community Respiratory Health Survey. *Eur Respir J*. 1994;7:954–960.

20. Ravault C, Kauffmann F. Validity of the IUATLD (1986) questionnaire in the EGEA study. International Union Against Tuberculosis and Lung Disease. Epidemiological Study on the Genetics and Environment of Asthma, Bronchial Hyperresponsiveness and Atopy. *Int J Tuberc Lung Dis*. 2001;5:191–196.

21. Doherty DE, Belfer MH, Brunton SA, et al. Chronic obstructive pulmonary disease: consensus recommendations for early diagnosis and treatment. *J Fam Pract*. 2006;55(suppl):1s–8s.

22. Borg G. Perceived exertion as an indicator of somatic stress. *Scand J Rehabil Med*. 1970;2:92–98.

23. Proctor SP. *Development of a Structured Neurotoxicant Assessment Checklist (SNAC) for Clinical Use in Veteran Populations*. Boston, MA: Department of Veterans Affairs, VA Boston Healthcare System; 2006.

APPENDIX B

Respiratory Health and Exposure Questionnaire

This questionnaire was developed by past and present members of the Environmental Medicine Program, Occupational and Environmental Medicine Portfolio, US Army Public Health Command (Aberdeen Proving Ground, MD), including Joseph Abraham, ScD; Coleen Baird, MD, MPH (Program Manager); Deanna Harkins, MD, MPH; Veronique Hauschild, MPH; Charles McCannon, MD, MPH, MBA; Jessica Sharkey, MPH; Jeremiah Stubbs, MD, MPH (currently at Walter Reed National Military Medical Center, Bethesda, MD); and Carole Tinklepaugh, MD, MBA. Other developmental contributions also came from Michael J. Falvo, PhD, New Jersey War Related Illness and Injury Study Center (East Orange, NJ); Michael Hodgson, MD, MPH, Occupational Safety and Health Administration (Washington, DC); and Michael Morris, MD, Brooke Army Medical Center (Fort Sam Houston, TX).

Note: The appropriate and current laws and rules designed to protect (patient/personal) privacy and confidentiality and related protected personal information are to be followed and complied with at all times.

This questionnaire was reproduced with minor changes from the US Army Public Health Command's Respiratory Health and Exposure Questionnaire (combined version of Deployment Airborne Respiratory Exposures [DARE] and Clinical Evaluation of Respiratory Conditions [CERC] Questionnaires).

Abbreviations used—AFG: Afghanistan; Avg: average; CBRN: chemical, biological, radiological, nuclear; FOB: Forward Operating Base; hrs: hours; MOS: Military Occupational Specialty; N/A: not applicable; Nat: national; NEC: Navy Enlisted Classification; Ops: operations; PT: physical training; Recon: reconnaissance; wk: week

QUESTIONNAIRE FOLLOWS ON PAGE 340

Respiratory Health and Exposure Questionnaire

The following questions resulted from the US Army Public Health Command's 2010–2012 development of the Deployment Airborne Respiratory Exposures (DARE) and Clinical Evaluation of Respiratory Conditions (CERC) Questionnaires. The questions are posed as the start of a "reference library" of standardized questions. The full set or only selected questions may be used for different applications.

Today's date (mm/dd/yyyy): __ __/__ __/__ __ __ __

Section A-1: PERSONAL INFORMATION *(not to be released - for internal study use only)*

Name: First [ ] **Last** [ ]
Social Security Number: __ __ __-__ __ -__ __ __ __
Email 1 *(optional)* [ ] **Email 2** *(optional)* [ ]
Phone #1 *(optional)* [ ] **Phone #2** *(optional)* [ ]
Mailing Address: APT/Street/PO Box [ ]
City [ ] State __ __ ZIP __ __ __ __ __ Country [ ]

Section A-2: DEMOGRAPHICS

Gender: ❑M ❑F **Date of Birth** (mm/dd/yyyy): __ __/__ __/__ __ __ __ **Age:** [ ] years old
Race/Ethnicity: ❑Hispanic/Latino ❑American Indian or Alaska Native ❑Asian
❑Hawaiian Native or other Pacific Islander ❑Black or African-American ❑White

Section A-3: FAMILY HISTORY

a. Indicate lung conditions that a doctor told either of your biological parents they had:

	FATHER			MOTHER		
	No	Yes	Don't know	No	Yes	Don't know
Chronic bronchitis	❑	❑	❑	❑	❑	❑
Emphysema	❑	❑	❑	❑	❑	❑
Asthma	❑	❑	❑	❑	❑	❑
Lung cancer	❑	❑	❑	❑	❑	❑
Other chest conditions?*	❑	❑	❑	❑	❑	❑

**If other chest conditions, describe:* [ ]

b. Indicate if your parents are currently living or deceased; if deceased, age of death and cause:

FATHER: ❑Living ❑Deceased at age [ ] *Describe cause* [ ]
MOTHER: ❑Living ❑Deceased at age [ ] *Describe cause* [ ]

Section A-4: CURRENT HEALTH STATUS

a. Are you currently limited in any way in any activities because of a breathing, lung, chest, rash, or allergy-related health problem?

❑No ❑Yes *If yes, describe:* [ ]

b. Indicate all events that have occurred during your military service *as a result of health problems*:

❑My military duty has never been impacted by a health problem *(skip to Section B)*
❑Evacuation out of area of operation *Describe (dates, reason):* [ ]
❑Hospitalization *Describe (dates, reason):* [ ]
❑Medically boarded *Describe (dates, reason):* [ ]
❑Permanent profile *Describe (dates, reason):* [ ]
❑Change of MOS/NEC *Describe (dates, reason):* [ ]
❑Medically discharged *Describe (dates, reason):* [ ]
❑Other *Describe (dates, reason):* [ ]

Section B: SYMPTOMS

Identify SYMPTOMs you have ever experienced (not related to common cold/flu) and answer follow-on questions:

B1	**Stuffy, itchy, runny nose** *(not related to a common cold/flu)*	❑ Never *(skip to B2)* ❑ Rarely ❑ Sometimes ❑ Often ❑ Very often	How many years have you had stuffy itchy runny nose symptoms? [ ] years *Check all "triggers" for your nose symptoms or indicate:* ❑None ❑Unknown ❑ Pollen/plants ❑ Cold air ❑ Work environment: *Describe* [ ] ❑ Animals/feathers ❑ While exercising ❑ Dusty environment ❑ After exercising ❑ Other: *Describe* [ ] ❑ Moldy environment Have your nose symptoms changed over time? ❑No ❑Yes–better ❑Yes–worse *If yes, describe reason:* ❑None known [ ] Have you experienced these nose symptoms in the last 12 months? ❑No ❑Yes Are you currently taking medication(s) for your stuffy, itchy, or runny nose symptoms? ❑No ❑Yes *If yes, specify:* [ ]
B2	**Watery, itchy eyes** *(not related to a common cold/flu)*	❑ Never *(skip to B3)* ❑ Rarely ❑ Sometimes ❑ Often ❑ Very often	How many years have you had watery or itchy eye symptoms? [ ] years *Check all "triggers" for your eye symptoms or indicate:* ❑None ❑Unknown ❑Pollen/plants ❑ Cold air ❑ Work environment: *Describe* [ ] ❑Animals/feathers ❑ While exercising ❑Dusty environment ❑ After exercising ❑ Other: *Describe* [ ] ❑Moldy environment Have your eye symptoms changed over time? ❑No ❑Yes–better ❑Yes–worse *If yes, describe reason:* ❑None known [ ] Have you experienced these eye symptoms in the last 12 months? ❑No ❑Yes Are you currently taking medication(s) for your watery, itchy eye symptoms? ❑No ❑Yes *If yes, specify:* [ ]
B3	**Throat tightness** *(not related to a common cold/flu)*	❑ Never *(skip to B4)* ❑ Rarely ❑ Sometimes ❑ Often ❑ Very often	How many years have you had episodes of throat tightness? [ ] years *Check all "triggers" for your throat tightness or indicate:* ❑None ❑Unknown ❑ Pollen/plants ❑ Cold air ❑ Work environment: *Describe* [ ] ❑ Animals/feathers ❑ While exercising ❑ Dusty environment ❑ After exercising ❑ Other: *Describe* [ ] ❑ Moldy environment Have you experienced these throat symptoms in the last 12 months? ❑No ❑Yes Are you currently taking medication(s) for your throat symptoms? ❑No ❑Yes *If yes, specify:* [ ]
B4	**Hoarseness or change in voice** *(not related to a common cold/flu)*	❑ Never *(skip to B5)* ❑ Rarely ❑ Sometimes ❑ Often ❑ Very often	How many years have you experienced hoarseness or change in voice? [ ] years *Check all "triggers" for your hoarseness/voice change or indicate:* ❑None ❑Unknown ❑ Pollen/plants ❑ Cold air ❑ Work environment: *Describe* [ ] ❑ Animals/feathers ❑ While exercising ❑ Dusty environment ❑ After exercising ❑ Other: *Describe* [ ] ❑ Moldy environment Has your hoarseness changed over time? ❑No ❑Yes–better ❑Yes–worse *If yes, describe reason:* ❑None known [ ] Have you experienced hoarseness/voice change in the last 12 months? ❑No ❑Yes Are you currently taking medication(s) for your hoarseness? ❑No ❑Yes *If yes, specify:* [ ]

B5	**Coughing episodes** *(not related to a common cold/flu)*	❑ Never *(skip to B6)* ❑ Rarely ❑ Sometimes ❑ Often ❑ Very often	How many years have you had coughing episodes? [ ] years Have you ever coughed up blood? ❑No ❑Yes *If yes, describe circumstances:* ❑[ ] *Check all "triggers" for your coughing episodes or indicate:* ❑None ❑Unknown ❑ Pollen/plants ❑ Cold air ❑ Work environment: *Describe* ❑ Animals/feathers ❑ While exercising [ ] ❑ Dusty environment ❑ After exercising ❑ Other: *Describe* ❑ Moldy environment [ ] Have your coughing episodes changed over time? ❑No ❑Yes–better ❑Yes–worse *If yes, describe reason:* ❑None known [ ] Do you usually cough 4 or more days a week? ❑No ❑Yes Have you coughed for 3 or more consecutive months in a year? ❑No ❑Yes Have you ever been short of breath while coughing? ❑No ❑Yes Have you experienced coughing episodes in the last 12 months? ❑No ❑Yes Are you currently taking medication(s) for your coughing episodes? ❑No ❑Yes *If yes, specify:* [ ]
B6	**Productive cough with phlegm (or sputum) from chest** *(not related to a common cold/flu)*	❑ Never *(skip to B7)* ❑ Rarely ❑ Sometimes ❑ Often ❑ Very often	How many years have you had productive cough with phlegm? [ ] years What color is the phlegm typically? ❑Clear ❑Green ❑Yellow ❑Other [ ] Do you bring up phlegm from your chest 4 or more days a week? ❑No ❑Yes Have you had this productive cough with phlegm for 3 or more consecutive months in a year? ❑ No ❑ Yes Have you experienced these phlegm symptoms in the last 12 months? ❑No ❑Yes Are you currently taking medication(s) for your phlegm symptoms? ❑No ❑Yes *If yes, specify:* [ ]
B7	**Wheezing or whistling noise in your chest** *(not related to a common cold/flu)*	❑ Never *(skip to B8)* ❑ Rarely ❑ Sometimes ❑ Often ❑ Very often	How many years have you experienced chest wheezing or whistling? [ ] years *Check all "triggers" for your wheezing symptoms or indicate:* ❑None ❑Unknown ❑Pollen/plants ❑Cold air ❑Work environment: *Describe* ❑Animals/feathers ❑While exercising [ ] ❑Dusty environment ❑After exercising ❑Other: *Describe* ❑Moldy environment [ ] Does your chest wheezing primarily occur when you breathe: ❑In ❑Out ❑Both Have you ever been short of breath while wheezing? ❑No ❑Yes Has your chest wheezing changed over time? ❑No ❑Yes–better ❑Yes–worse *If yes, describe reason:* ❑None known [ ] Have you experienced these wheezing symptoms in the last 12 months? ❑No ❑Yes Are you currently taking medication(s) for your chest wheezing episodes? ❑No ❑Yes *If yes, specify:* [ ]

B8	**Tightness in chest** *(not related to a common cold/flu)*	❑ Never *(skip to B9)* ❑ Rarely ❑ Sometimes ❑ Often ❑ Very often	How many years have you experienced episodes of chest tightness? [ ] years *Check all "triggers" for your chest tightness or indicate:* ❑None ❑Unknown ❑ Pollen/plants ❑ Cold air ❑ Work environment: *Describe* [ ] ❑ Animals/feathers ❑ While exercising ❑ Dusty environment ❑ After exercising ❑ Other: *Describe* [ ] ❑ Moldy environment Have you ever been short of breath while experiencing chest tightness? ❑No ❑Yes Has your chest tightness changed over time? ❑No ❑Yes–better ❑Yes–worse ❑No ❑Yes *If yes, describe reason:* ❑None known [ ] Have you experienced chest tightness symptoms in the last 12 months? ❑No ❑Yes Are you currently taking medication(s) for your chest tightness? ❑ No ❑ Yes *If yes, specify:* [ ]
B9	**Unusual attacks of shortness of breath or difficulty breathing**	❑ Never *(skip to next section)* ❑ Rarely ❑ Sometimes ❑ Often ❑ Very often	How many years have you experienced these breathing problems? [ ] years *Check all "triggers" for your breathing problems or indicate:* ❑None ❑Unknown ❑ Pollen/plants ❑ Cold air ❑ Work environment: *Describe* [ ] ❑ Animals/feathers ❑ While exercising ❑ Dusty environment ❑ While at rest ❑ Other: *Describe* [ ] ❑ Moldy environment ❑ After exercising How many times have you had emergency care/hospitalization for these breathing problems? [ ] times *Check all that you have ever experienced with your shortness of breath:* ❑ Inability to fill the lungs or take a satisfying breath ❑ Numbness and/or tingling around mouth, arms, and/or legs ❑ Trembling of the hands ❑ Palpitations ❑ Severe anxiety or fear ❑ Frequent sighing or yawning ❑ Lightheadedness or dizziness Have your breathing problems changed over time? ❑No ❑Yes–better ❑Yes–worse *If yes, describe reason:* ❑None known [ ] Have you experienced shortness of breath in the last 12 months? ❑No ❑Yes Are you currently taking medication(s) for your shortness of breath? ❑No ❑Yes *If yes, specify:* [ ] *Check all statements that apply to your experience(s):* ❑ I am troubled by shortness of breath when hurrying on the level or walking up a slight hill ❑ I walk slower than people my age because of breathlessness ❑ I sometimes have to stop for breath when walking my own pace on the level ❑ I sometimes have to stop for breath after level walking for ~100 yards or a few minutes ❑ I am too breathless to leave my house or breathless on dressing/climbing a flight of stairs ❑ I have been awakened by an attack of breathing difficulty

Section C: DIAGNOSED MEDICAL CONDITIONS

Indicate the conditions that a healthcare provider has told you that you have/have had and answer the follow-on questions. *NOTE: Medications include medically prescribed and over-the-counter (OTC) nasal sprays, inhalers, nebulizers, tablets, capsules, liquids, injections, suppositories, or supplemental oxygen.

C1	**Hay fever, allergic rhinitis, and nasal allergies**	❑No (skip to C2) ❑Yes	At what age did you first have allergies?	[ ] years old
			Have your allergies changed over time? *If yes, describe any particular event or time that you noticed a change or say "**None**"*	❑No ❑Yes–better ❑Yes–worse *If yes, list any known reason:* [ ]
			Have you had allergies in the last 12 months?	❑No ❑Yes
			Are you currently taking medication(s)* for allergies?	❑No ❑Yes *If yes, specify:* [ ]
C2	**Asthma**	❑No (skip to C3) ❑Yes	At what age were you first diagnosed with asthma?	[ ] years old
			Has your asthma changed over time? *If yes, describe any particular event or time that you noticed a change or say "**None**"*	❑No ❑Yes–better ❑Yes–worse *If yes, list any known reason:* [ ]
			Have you had attacks in the last 12 months?	❑No ❑Yes
			Are you currently taking medication(s)* for asthma?	❑No ❑Yes *If yes, specify:* [ ]
C3	**Pneumonia**	❑No (skip to C4) ❑Yes	How many times have you been diagnosed with pneumonia?	[ ] # times
			At what age were you first diagnosed with pneumonia?	[ ] years old
			Have you had pneumonia in the last 12 months?	❑No ❑Yes
			Are you currently taking medication(s)* for pneumonia?	❑No ❑Yes *If yes, specify:* [ ]
C4	**Bronchitis**	❑No (skip to C5) ❑Yes	How many times have you been diagnosed with bronchitis?	[ ] # times
			At what age were you first diagnosed with bronchitis?	[ ] years old
			Has your bronchitis changed over time? *If yes, describe any particular event or time that you noticed a change or say "**None**"*	❑No ❑Yes–better ❑Yes–worse *If yes, list any known reason:* [ ]
			Have you had bronchitis in the last 12 months?	❑No ❑Yes
			Are you currently taking medication(s)* for bronchitis?	❑No ❑Yes *If yes, specify:* [ ]
C5	**Chronic bronchitis** *(this is a form of chronic obstructive pulmonary disease or "COPD")*	❑No (skip to C6) ❑Yes	At what age were you first diagnosed with chronic bronchitis?	[ ] years old
			Has your chronic bronchitis changed over time? *If yes, describe any particular event or time that you noticed a change or say "**None**"*	❑No ❑Yes–better ❑Yes–worse *If yes, list any known reason:* [ ]
			Are you currently taking medication(s)* for chronic bronchitis?	❑No ❑Yes *If yes, specify:* [ ]

C6	**Emphysema** *(this is a form of chronic obstructive pulmonary disease or "COPD")*	❑No (skip to C7) ❑Yes	At what age were you first diagnosed with emphysema?	[______] years old
			Has your emphysema changed over time? *If yes, describe any particular event or time that you noticed a* change or say "**None**"	❑No ❑Yes–better ❑Yes–worse *If yes, list any known reason:* [______________________]
			Are you currently taking medication(s) or treatments* for emphysema?	❑No ❑Yes *If yes, specify:* [______________________]
C7	**Other chest or lung illness or injury**	❑No (skip to next section) ❑Yes	*Describe condition, date(s) diagnosed:*	[______________________]
			Has this condition changed over time? *If yes, describe any particular event or time that you noticed a* change or say "**None**"	❑No ❑Yes–better ❑Yes–worse *If yes, list any known reason:* [______________________]
			Are you currently taking medication(s) or treatments* for this condition?	❑No ❑Yes *If yes, specify:* [______________________]

SECTION D FOLLOWS ON PAGE 346

Section D: MEDICAL PROCEDURES

Indicate any of the following medical procedures you have ever had and provide requested details. If you had more than one of the same procedures, please indicate "yes" and describe them all in follow-on questions.

D1	**Chest x-rays**	❑No (skip to D2)	How many times have you had this procedure?	[_____] # times
			What year(s) did you have this procedure?	_ _ _ _ _ _ _ _ _ _ _ _ _ _ _ _
		❑Yes	Description of finding(s) [ ]	
			Diagnosis(es) [ ]	
			Other comments [ ]	
D2	**CT scan of chest**	❑No (skip to D3)	How many times have you had this procedure?	[_____] # times
			What year(s) did you have this procedure?	_ _ _ _ _ _ _ _ _ _ _ _ _ _ _ _
		❑Yes	Description of finding(s) [ ]	
			Diagnosis(es) [ ]	
			Other comments [ ]	
D3	**Breathing tests (spirometry)**	❑No (skip to D4)	How many times have you had this procedure?	[_____] # times
			What year(s) did you have this procedure?	_ _ _ _ _ _ _ _ _ _ _ _ _ _ _ _
			Description of finding(s) [ ]	
		❑Yes	Diagnosis(es) [ ]	
			Other comments [ ]	
D4	**Methacholine or other broncho-provocation tests**	❑No (skip to D5)	How many times have you had this procedure?	[_____] # times
			What year(s) did you have this procedure?	_ _ _ _ _ _ _ _ _ _ _ _ _ _ _ _
		❑Yes	Description of finding(s) [ ]	
			Diagnosis(es) [ ]	
			Other comments [ ]	
D5	**Chest operations, including lung biopsy**	❑No (skip to D6)	How many times have you had this procedure?	[_____] # times
			What year(s) did you have this procedure?	_ _ _ _ _ _ _ _ _ _ _ _ _ _ _ _
		❑Yes	Description of finding(s) [ ]	
			Diagnosis(es) [ ]	
			Other comments [ ]	
D6	**Other diagnostic chest studies**	❑No (skip to next section)	Year _ _ _ _ Description of test [ ] Diagnosis(es) [ ] Description/comments [ ]	
		❑Yes	Year _ _ _ _ Description of test [ ] Diagnosis(es) [ ] Description/comments [ ]	

Section E: AEROBIC PHYSICAL FITNESS

E1 **Indicate the category that best describes your *current* level of aerobic fitness:**

- ❑ Not fit
- ❑ Average fitness
- ❑ Very fit/competitive
- ❑ Professional/elite

E2 **If you were asked to walk briskly for 100 yards (length of a football field) up a slight incline, what would your exertion level be:**

- ❑ No exertion at all
- ❑ Very light
- ❑ Light
- ❑ Somewhat hard (a little heavy breathing, but okay to continue and complete); light
- ❑ Hard (heavy breathing)
- ❑ Very hard (very strenuous, heavy breathing, tired; really would have to push self)
- ❑ Maximal exertion (too strenuous/tired or difficulty breathing to complete)

E3 **a. Indicate the best description of the change in your aerobic fitness *within the last 12 months:***

❑ No change *(skip to E4)* **or:** ❑ Slightly improved ❑ Very improved ❑ Slightly worse ❑ Much worse

b. What factor(s) do you attribute the change in your physical fitness?

❑ Don't know *OR check as many as apply:*

❑ Weight gain ❑ Deconditioning ❑ Injury/illness/shortness of breath *Specify:* [ ]

❑ Weight loss ❑ Conditioning ❑ Other *Describe:* [ ]

c. Over what period of time (in months) did the change in your aerobic fitness occur? [ ] months

d. Was there any specific life change prior to the change in fitness *(work, home location, hobbies, smoking)?*

❑ No ❑ Yes *If yes, specify:* [ ]

E4 *IF APPLICABLE:* **Starting with the most recent, describe the type of your past aerobic military physical fitness tests, times in minutes, and dates of tests.**

Test types: 1.5-mile run, 2-mile run, 3-mile run, swim, bike, elliptical, other – Describe: [ ]

Test type *Describe* [______________] Time 1 (min) [______] Date (mm/yyyy) __ __/__ __ __ __
Test type *Describe* [______________] Time 2 (min) [______] Date (mm/yyyy) __ __/__ __ __ __
Test type *Describe* [______________] Time 3 (min) [______] Date (mm/yyyy) __ __/__ __ __ __
Test type *Describe* [______________] Time 4 (min) [______] Date (mm/yyyy) __ __/__ __ __ __
Test type *Describe* [______________] Time 5 (min) [______] Date (mm/yyyy) __ __/__ __ __ __
Test type *Describe* [______________] Time 6 (min) [______] Date (mm/yyyy) __ __/__ __ __ __

Section F: TOBACCO SMOKE EXPOSURE HISTORY

F1	**Did you grow up in a household with one or more smokers?** ❑No ❑Yes
F2	**Have you smoked more than 100 cigarettes, 20 cigars, and/or 20 ounces of pipe tobacco in your lifetime?** ❑No *(If no, go to Section G)* ❑Yes
F3	**Over the entire time you have smoked, indicate the amount that best represents the average number that you smoked *for each type of product used*:**
F4	**How old were you when you started smoking regularly?** [ ] years old
F5	**Do you still smoke?** ❑No *If no, please answer a and b* ❑Yes **a.** How old were you when you stopped? [ ] years old **b.** Why did you stop? ❑Personal decision ❑Medical reason *Describe:* [ ]

F3 response options:

Cigarettes	Cigars	Pipe	Other (e.g., hookah)
❑ 0 (none)	❑ 0 (none)	❑ 0 (none)	❑ 0 (none)
❑ 1–2 cigarettes per day or occasional	❑ <7 per week	❑ <7 per week	❑ <7 per week
❑ 3–10 (up to half a pack) per day	❑ 7–14 per week	❑ 7–14 per week	❑ 7–14 per week
❑ 11–20 cigarettes (up to a pack) per day	❑ >14 per week	❑ >14 per week	❑ >14 per week
❑ 21–40 cigarettes (1–2 packs) per day			
❑ >40 cigarettes (>2 packs) per day			

Section G: NONMILITARY DUTIES AND HOBBIES

Deployment exposures affect people differently, in part because of other exposure experiences one may have had to dusts, vapors, or fumes in ***nonmilitary work duties or hobbies.*** ****For this study, this would be if you had a job(s) or hobby(s) in which you routinely breathed dust in or had dust on your clothes, skin, or hair, or that you breathed in fumes or had a lasting smell on your clothes, skin, or hair.*** *Describe your overall history of these exposures. Do NOT include occasional or rare exposure events.*

G1. Have you had nonmilitary occupational/hobby-related exposures to dusts, vapors, or fumes?*

❑**No** *If no, go to Section H*

❑**Yes** *If yes, complete table and questions below*

	FREQUENCY *Number of years that you experienced the exposure*	**DURATION** *Amount of time each day that you experienced exposure*	**EFFECT(S)** *Health effects you experienced that you considered related to the specified exposure*	
	0 = Not exposed* **1** = 1–5 years **2** = 6–10 years **3** = 11–15 years **4** = 16–20 **5** = 21+ years **if "0," then skip → and instead go down to next listed exposure type*	**1** = <1 hour/day **2** = 1–2 hours/day **3** = 3–5 hours/day **4** = 6–8 hours/day **5** = >8 hours/day	**1** = No health effects or symptoms **2** = Mild effects or symptoms that did not affect ability to conduct physical activities. Examples: mild eye or throat irritation, strange odors **3** = Moderate effects or symptoms that had some affect on physical activity. Examples: notable coughing or eye irritation; mild difficulty breathing, dizziness, or nausea **4** = Severe effects to include those described above, but that were so debilitating, they severely impaired physical activity and/or required medical treatment	
			AVERAGE Intensity *Effects experienced during most typical exposure conditions*	**PEAK Intensity** *Effects from any unique short-term incidents of higher than usual exposures; if no unique incidents, use same score as for average*
Dust from: baking flours, grains, wood, cotton, plants, or animals	0 1 2 3 4 5	1 2 3 4 5	1 2 3 4	1 2 3 4
Dust from: rock, sand, concrete, coal, asbestos, silica, or soil	0 1 2 3 4 5	1 2 3 4 5	1 2 3 4	1 2 3 4
Chemical gases or vapors from: solvents, paints, cleaning products, glues, and acids	0 1 2 3 4 5	1 2 3 4 5	1 2 3 4	1 2 3 4
Metal fumes from: welding/soldering	0 1 2 3 4 5	1 2 3 4 5	1 2 3 4	1 2 3 4
Exhaust fumes: from **vehicle, heavy machinery, or diesel engines**	0 1 2 3 4 5	1 2 3 4 5	1 2 3 4	1 2 3 4
Other: *Describe:* [__________]	0 1 2 3 4 5	1 2 3 4 5	1 2 3 4	1 2 3 4

G2. Provide specific job title/description or hobby name(s) for above exposures:

List: [ ]

G3a. Have you ever been advised to wear respiratory protection for any of these nonmilitary jobs/hobbies?
❑No ❑Yes *If yes, describe:* [ ]

b. Did any of these occupational or hobby exposures require medical evaluation or medical treatment?
❑No ❑Yes *If yes, describe:* [ ] **# of times in life** and *Describe type of exposure(s), health effects:*
[ ]

c. Have you ever been put on a nonmilitary work restriction or received disability or workers' compensation relating to an exposure to a hazardous substance?
❑No ❑Yes *If yes, describe type of exposure(s), health effects:*
[ ]

Section H: MILITARY SERVICE HISTORY

a. Service Affiliation(s) – *List start and separation dates (**or "NS"** if not yet separated) and all primary and secondary assigned occupations (e.g., MOS(s)) and last Rank/Pay Grade (e.g., E5, O4, W3)*

	Start Date *mm/yyyy*	**Separation** *mm/yyyy or NS*	**Your Assigned Job Descriptions/MOS** if secondary not applicable, use "NA"		**Last Rank/ Pay Grade**
			Primary	**Secondary**	
Army	__/____	__/____			
Army Reserves	__/____	__/____			
Army Nat Guard	__/____	__/____			
Air Force (AF)	__/____	__/____			
AF Reserves	__/____	__/____			
Air Nat Guard	__/____	__/____			
Navy	__/____	__/____			
Navy Reserves	__/____	__/____			
Marine Corps (MC)	__/____	__/____			
MC Reserves	__/____	__/____			
Coast Guard (CG)	__/____	__/____			
CG Reserves	__/____	__/____			

b. List total number of your deployments [_____] # times ***(if "0," you have completed the questionnaire)***
Otherwise, continue to next section

Sections H-1 and H-2: DEPLOYMENT LOCATIONS, EXPOSURES, AND ACTIVITIES

There are 3 parts to Section H that ask detailed questions regarding each of your deployments.

If you have been deployed more than once, please complete a separate Section H for each deployment.

In Section H-1, you are asked to describe an overall deployment and list all unique locations where you were during that deployment that you consider to have been a uniquely different exposure setting.

Please note that for each unique location that you list for each deployment (1-01, 1-02, etc.), you are asked to complete separate Sections H-2 and H-3.

If you feel your overall exposure experiences were similar at all the locations where you were during a specific deployment, or if you moved around frequently and do not recall any specific camp or location names, you may group them together as a single general location in Section H-1 (eg 1-01). Therefore, you will only complete a single Sections H-2 and H-3 for that deployment.

Examples:

- *A maintenance person deployed to Afghanistan primarily spends time at FOB Bravo. (General Country Location – AFG; 1 key location = FOB Bravo)*
- *An engineer unit, normally located at a single Base Camp Charlie in Iraq, is detailed for 3 weeks to assist with controlling a fire at an industrial site near City Z, over 100 km away (Country Location – Iraq; 2 key locations = Base Camp Charlie, City Z)*
- *A security unit assigned to Base Camp Delta in Iraq spent a lot of their time in convoys to distant locations and then short-term facility security in different cities (Country – Iraq; 1 key location = Base Camp Delta)*

SECTION H-1: DEPLOYMENT SUMMARY TABLE

Operation Code (*e.g., Operation Iraqi Freedom = OIF, if unknown = UNK*) [ ]

Start date: (mm/yyyy) __ __/__ __ __ __ **End date:** (mm/yyyy) __ __/__ __ __ __

Country/Location Code (*e.g., Iraq = IRQ or description if unknown*) [ ]

Deployment Location Reference Number	**Name That Represents Key Location(s) Where You Were*** (base camp/FOB name, city/area; ship)	**Key Activity (Activities)/Mission** (e.g., transport, medical, flight line maintenance, security)	**Location Arrival** (mm/yyyy)	**Location Departure** (mm/yyyy)
♦[ ]-01			__ __/__ __ __ __	__ __/__ __ __ __
♦[ ]-02			__ __/__ __ __ __	__ __/__ __ __ __
♦[ ]-03			__ __/__ __ __ __	__ __/__ __ __ __
♦[ ]-0_			__ __/__ __ __ __	__ __/__ __ __ __

SECTION H-2: LOCATION-SPECIFIC EXPOSURE AND ACTIVITIES INFORMATION – DEPLOYMENT H♦ [#____]

Please complete Section H-2 (questions H2-1 through H2-7) and the table in Section H-3 for ***each unique deployment location*** that you identify in *Section H-1. EXAMPLE: for Deployment #1, if you listed 2 unique locations, then you would complete a Section H-2 and a Section H-3 for location (1-01) and a separate one for location (1-02). Complete an additional "Section H" for your other deployments and any associated unique exposure locations.*

List Deployment Location (e.g., *#1-01***):** [ ]

H2-1a. Check all items that describe your primary duty type(s) while at this location:

❑Maintenance
❑Security
❑Logistics
❑CBRN
❑Medical
❑Planning/Ops/Base Command
❑Engineering construction: *Check type:* ❑General ❑Mechanic ❑Electrical ❑Steelworker ❑Welder ❑Other[ ]
❑Transportation: *Check type:* ❑Air ❑Ground ❑Other [ ]
❑Field/Forward Ops (e.g., Recon/Surveillance/Infantry)
❑Other *Describe* [ ]

b. Were you monitored or assessed while at this location as part of any occupational health program?
❑No
❑Yes *If yes:* ❑Respiratory Protection Program ❑Medical Surveillance Program ❑Other *Describe*[ ]

c. Level of physical activity required for your daily work duties at this location:
❑Not very physical; mostly sedentary
❑Light: limited physical activity
❑Moderate: some strenuous/hard breathing
❑Heavy: many hours strenuous/hard breathing

d. While at this location, were your work duties primarily inside or outside?
❑Inside
❑Outside
❑About equal (inside and outside)

e. Did your assigned duties at this location involve hazardous substances (*e.g., specific chemical fumes in a maintenance facility or welding shop*)
❑No ❑Yes *If yes, describe* [ ]
❑Don't know

f. Did your duties at this location include tasks associated with trash-burning operations *(e.g., bulldozing at pit, operating a burn box, security near pit)?*
❑No ❑Yes *If yes, indicate average hours per week* **#[**]

g. While at this location, did you typically spend more than 20 hours a week in convoy?
❑No ❑Yes *If yes –* Estimate time in convoy per week **#[**] Avg hrs/wk and *Describe details of your typical convoy duties and experience (e.g., type of duty, vehicle, where you sat)* [ ]

H2-2a. While at this location, how often did you wear a N95, M40, or other respirator?
[ ] of days while at location *(if "0," skip to Question H2-3)*

b. *Describe the type(s) of respirator/mask(s), associated job duty(ies), and duration(s) worn*
[ ]

H2-3. While at this location, how often did you wear a cravat to minimize air exposures?
[ ] of days while at location

H2-4. While at this location, how many days was air quality so bad that it was a "no-fly day" or day that most outdoor missions were halted because of lack of visibility?
[ ] of days while at location

H2-5a. While at this location, how often did you smoke tobacco products?
[ ] of days per week *(if "0," skip to Question H2-6)*

b. What kind of tobacco did you smoke *(Check all that apply)*:
❑US supplied cigarettes ❑Cigars ❑Other [ ]
❑Iraqi/local cigarettes ❑Hookah

c. Did you start smoking for the first time while at this location?
❑No ❑Yes

d. If you smoked prior to this deployment, did the frequency/amount change at this location?
❑N/A – *did not smoke prior deployment*
❑Stayed the same
❑Increased
❑Decreased

H2-6a. Check the best description of your aerobic activities (e.g., physical training and sports) at this location:
❑Rarely to never
❑Light: 1–2 aerobic activities/week
❑Moderate: 3–4 aerobic activities/week
❑Heavy: Greater than 5 aerobic activities/week

b. Was your PT carried out primarily inside or outside?
❑Inside
❑Outside
❑About equal (inside and outside)

c. Was your level of physical activity level impacted by the quality of the air?
❑Not impacted
❑Decreased – command required
❑Decreased – voluntarily reduced

H2-7a. While at this location, how many times (if any) did you *seek* medical evaluation for a problem *that you thought was caused by something in the air*?
[ ] of times while at location ***(if "0," skip to next Section H-3)***

b. How many times (per B-7a) were you not able to *receive* the medical evaluation for this problem?
[ ] of times while at location *Describe reason, if known:* [ ]

c. When you received treatment, how many times were you assigned to sick quarters for more than 24 hours?
[ ] of times while at location

d. Briefly describe the type of health problem(s) that you attributed to air exposures that you sought help for:
❑Severe coughing
❑Trouble breathing
❑Asthma/asthma-like attack
❑Other *Describe*[ ]

SECTION H-3: SPECIFIC DEPLOYMENT LOCATION EXPOSURE SUMMARY TABLE – DEPLOYMENT H♦ [#____]

*Please complete the table below to summarize your overall air exposures **at each unique deployment location** that you identified in Section H-2. EXAMPLE: for Deployment #1, if you listed 2 unique locations, then complete two separate tables: one for location (#1-01) and one for location (#1-02). Continue to use additional tables for your other deployments and any associated unique exposure locations (such as deployment location #2-01).*

The following table pertains to my experiences at: [ ]

EXPOSURE TYPE	FREQUENCY	DURATION	EFFECT(S)	
	Number of days over which you experienced the exposure at this location	*Amount of time each day that you experienced exposure at this location*	*Health effects you experienced that you considered related to the specified exposure*	
	0 = Not exposed* **1** = Seldom/few days **2** = Occasionally up to about half of time **3** = Majority of the days at location **4** = Every day spent at this location **If "0" then skip → and go to next listed exposure type*	**1** = Few hours (3 hrs or less) **2** = Several hours (4–12 hrs) **3** = Majority, but not all of day (13–20 hrs) **4** = All day continuously (>20 hrs)	**1** = No health effects or symptoms **2** = Mild effects or symptoms that did not affect ability to conduct physical activities; *Examples*: mild eye or throat irritation, strange odor **3** = Moderate effects or symptoms that had some affect on physical activity; *Examples:* notable coughing or eye irritation; mild difficulty breathing, dizziness, or nausea **4** = Severe effects to include those described above but that were so debilitating, they severely impaired physical activity and/or required medical treatment	
			AVERAGE Intensity *Effects experienced during most typical exposure conditions*	**PEAK Intensity** *Effects from any unique short-term incident of higher than usual exposures – if no unique incidents, use same score as for average*
Sand and dust *from wind, digging, vehicles, sandstorms*	0 1 2 3 4	1 2 3 4	1 2 3 4	1 2 3 4
Smoke from burning trash *from burn pits, burn boxes, incinerators*	0 1 2 3 4	1 2 3 4	1 2 3 4	1 2 3 4
Exhaust and diesel fumes *from generators, vehicles*	0 1 2 3 4	1 2 3 4	1 2 3 4	1 2 3 4
Industrial air pollution *from local factories*	0 1 2 3 4	1 2 3 4	1 2 3 4	1 2 3 4
Pesticides *from during or after applications*	0 1 2 3 4	1 2 3 4	1 2 3 4	1 2 3 4
Unique chemicals used *in military duties – such as maintenance, fueling, construction* *Describe:* [ ]	0 1 2 3 4	1 2 3 4	1 2 3 4	1 2 3 4
Other – *Describe:* [ ]	0 1 2 3 4	1 2 3 4	1 2 3 4	1 2 3 4
Other – *Describe:* [ ]	0 1 2 3 4	1 2 3 4	1 2 3 4	1 2 3 4

APPENDIX C

Proposed Evaluation of Patients With Normal Spirometry

EVALUATION FOLLOWS ON PAGE 356

Proposed Evaluation of Patients With Normal Spirometry

Normal Spirometry	Considerations
Spirometry Post-BD	Review spirometry for reduction in FEV_1; 12% increase post-BD diagnostic of AHR
Spirometry w/ Symptoms	Intermittent nature of asthma may require repeat spirometry when patients are symptomatic
Chest Radiograph	Will be normal in most patients; helpful to eliminate pulmonary infiltrates, effusions, or mediastinal disease
Complete Blood Count	Rule out anemia, especially in females
Inspiratory FVL	Review the inspiratory FVL on all spirometry examinations for truncation or flattening
Exercise Larynoscopy	Presence of abnormal FVL or history of inspiratory wheezing or noisy breathing; diagnostic for vocal cord dysfunction
Bronchoprovocation Testing	With normal spirometry, important to rule out underlying airway reactivity, such as EIB
Methacholine	Most common test used for AHR, with good negative predictive value; diagnostic for EIB with associated exercise symptoms
Mannitol	Newest modality with equivalence to methacholine; requires 15% decrease in FEV_1
Eucapnic Hyperventilation	Equivalent to methacholine for diagnosing AHR, but requires a 15% decrease in FEV_1
Exercise Spirometry	Poor predictability compared with other methods and may not reproduce symptoms in laboratory setting
Impulse Oscillometry	Newer modality that measures airway resistance and may identify AHR based on reduction in post-BD values
High-Resolution CT	May identify subclinical lung disease, airway trapping, or bronchiectasis; low diagnostic yield in this population
Cardiopulmonary Exercise Testing	Primarily used to assess patient's ability to exercise and measure VO_{2max}; given limited reference values and low suspicion for cardiac disease, it may not identify specific cause
Allergy Evaluation	Consideration for allergy testing in patient with other atopic symptoms, such as atopic dermatitis and allergic rhinitis
Cardiology Evaluation	Very low likelihood of cardiac disease in a younger population; referral should be based on physical examination findings
Electrocardiogram	Numerous nonspecific changes found in younger population and are rarely diagnostic
Echocardiogram	In the absence of physical findings, it is not routinely warranted unless there are concerns for valvular disease or PH

Proposed evaluation of patients with normal spirometry. There is no single approach to evaluating the young patient with dyspnea and normal spirometry. Most consideration should be given to establishing the presence or absence of airway hyperactivity and upper airways disorders (eg, vocal cord dysfunction), and ruling out parenchymal lung disease.

AHR: airway hyperresponsiveness; BD: bronchodilation; CT: computed tomography; EIB: exercise-induced bronchospasm; FEV_1: forced expiratory volume in 1 second; FVL: flow volume loop; PH: pulmonary hypertension; VO_{2max}: maximal oxygen consumption; w/: without

Illustration: Reproduced with permission and minor changes from Zanders TB, Lucero PF, Bell DG, et al. San Antonio Military Medical Center (SAMMC): standardized evaluation of post-deployment dyspnea. Presented at: CHEST 2012 Centers of Excellence, Atlanta, GA, October 22–25, 2012.

APPENDIX D

Airborne Hazards Joint Action Plan

This document was reproduced with permission from the US Department of Veterans Affairs/US Department of Defense Deployment Health Working Group (Washington, DC).

VA/DoD Deployment Health Working Group
Airborne Hazards Joint Action Plan
In Support of the VA/DoD Joint Executive Council Strategic Plan

April 2013 (Initial Version)

Terry J. Walters, MD, MPH
(VHA Co-Chair)
Deputy Chief Consultant, Post-Deployment Health
Office of Public Health
Veterans Health Administration

Kelley Brix, MD, MPH
(DoD Co-Chair)
Deputy Director for Defense Medical Research and Development Program
Force Health Protection and Readiness
Office of the Assistant Secretary of Defense for Health Affairs

Contents

Pages 4 and 5 intentionally omitted from this section.

Mission[1]

To improve the quality, efficiency, and effectiveness of post-deployment health services to Veterans, service members, and military retirees with health concerns related to airborne hazards through a partnership between the Department of Veterans Affairs (VA) and the Department of Defense (DoD).

Vision Statement

A world-class partnership that promotes seamless, cost-effective, quality post-deployment health care policy to beneficiaries and value to our nation

Guiding Principles

COLLABORATION – to achieve shared goals through mutual support of both our common and unique mission requirements

STEWARDSHIP – to provide the best value for our beneficiaries and the taxpayer

LEADERSHIP – to establish clear policies and guidelines for a VA/DoD partnership, to promote active decision-making, and to ensure accountability

6

1. Derived from VA/DoD Joint Executive Council Strategic Plan FY 2009-2011.

Pages 1 and 2 intentionally omitted from this section.

Background

Numerous concerns on the part of active duty Service members and veterans, the media, and the Congress have been raised regarding possible long-term health effects associated with exposures to burn pit smoke and the elevated levels of airborne particulate matter common to Southwest Asia. For example, specific concerns among Operation Iraqi Freedom Veterans were expressed to SECVA in 2009 in letters from Senator Akaka and Congressman Bishop, along with six co-signers. The letters solicited VA's plans to track and evaluate possible long-term health problems among troops exposed to hazardous materials from open waste burn pits. Burn pit waste disposal at the Joint Air Base Balad (JBB), located in northern Iraq, and elsewhere in Iraq and Afghanistan has been a focus of health concerns among Servicemembers, Veterans, and their families, as evidenced by multiple news articles, Congressional hearings, and other inquiries. Joint Balad Air Base, which at one time had the largest burn pit in Iraq, housed up to 30,000 U.S. Servicemembers at one time with frequent turnover, with hundreds of thousands of Servicemembers assigned to, or passing through, this location.

VA requested that the Institute of Medicine (IOM) review the long-term health impact of burn pit exposure in Iraq or Afghanistan after reports of increasing health concerns by Veterans and other stakeholders coupled with media reports and scientific studies. The IOM Study started in November 2009. The review was inconclusive as to the long-term health consequences of burn pit exposure (IOM, 2011).

Reports of airborne exposures in Iraq are not limited to burn pits. In the spring of 2003, during the early portion of Operation Iraqi Freedom, up to 800 U.S. Service members were potentially exposed to hexavalent chromium dust, recognized as a cause of lung cancer, while guarding a former Iraqi industrial water treatment plant. In another instance, soldiers near the city of Mosul, Iraq were potentially exposed to sulfur dioxide when involved in firefighting operations at a sulfur mine (USAPHC, May 2010). Sulfur dioxide is a known respiratory irritant with a potential to cause long-term adverse health effects (Baird, 2012 54;6). DoD and VA programs were initiated to identify and ascertain the status of their health. Concerns over airborne particulate matter (PM) (e.g., blowing geologic dusts and industrial pollution) prompted DoD to consult with the National Institute for Occupational Safety and Health (NIOSH) in 2005 and to conduct more extensive air sampling throughout the U.S. Central Command (CENTCOM) Area of Responsibility, including Afghanistan (Desert Research Institute) This sampling activity was reviewed in a report by the National Research Council (NRC) of the National Academies of Science (NAS). NRC was unable to determine whether the airborne particulate matter posed a long-term health risk and commented, "The committee recognizes the difficulty of performing sampling and health studies in an active theater. However, it also recognizes that exposure sources in this environment are more complex and potentially more toxic than in the United States and Europe, where health studies are traditionally conducted." (NRC, 2010).

DoD and VA are working closely together to address environmental health concerns of U.S. Servicemembers and Veterans who served in recent conflicts in Iraq and Afghanistan. These concerns include potential exposure to airborne hazards associated with open waste burning pits (burn pits) commonly used for trash disposal during deployment. Veterans of the 1991 Gulf War also expressed significant adverse health effect concerns from exposure to smoke from burn pits, as well as oil well fires. The Gulf War concerns were discussed in the National Academy of Sciences (NAS) Institute of Medicine (IOM), "Gulf War and Health" series of reports (IOM, 2006).

IOM Committee Findings

- **Limited/Suggestive evidence of an association between exposure to combustion products and reduced pulmonary function [Note: not respiratory disease] in the surrogate populations studied**
- **Inadequate/insufficient evidence of an association between exposure to combustion products and cancer, respiratory diseases, circulatory diseases, neurologic diseases, and adverse reproductive and developmental outcomes in the [surrogate] populations studied**

Discussion of Findings

The IOM report, "Long-Term Health Consequences of Exposure to Burn Pits in Iraq and Afghanistan," was a special report requested by the VA and was not required by law. This report was requested in order to address both Veterans' concerns and the uncertainties in exposure assessment and risk assessment drawn from field monitoring and health outcome data. For this report, the IOM Committee used a wide range of data sources to include peer-reviewed literature, government reports, raw environmental monitoring data, public comment, and other government documents.

The IOM first assessed the "types and quantities of materials burned during the time of pit use." It next analyzed air monitoring data collected at JBB during 2007 and 2009. It then examined "anticipated health effects from exposure to air pollutants found at JBB" and studies of health effects in similar populations with similar exposures, grading the quality of those studies as key or supportive. The Committee then performed a synthesis of key information on potential long-term health effects in military personnel potentially exposed to burn pits and developed design elements and feasibility considerations for an epidemiologic study.

The Committee's synthesis on potential long-term health effects of burn pit exposure resulted in two conclusions and several recommendations for further research. Importantly, the IOM recognized that burn pits may not be the main cause of long-term health effects related to Iraq and Afghanistan deployment. The report states, "service in Iraq or Afghanistan--that is, a broader consideration of air pollution than exposure only to burn pit emissions--might be associated with long-term health effects, particularly in susceptible (for example, those who have asthma) or highly exposed subpopulations (such as those who worked at the burn pit). Such health effects would be due mainly to high ambient concentrations of PM from both natural and anthropogenic sources, including military sources." IOM suggested the need for studies of those who deployed regardless of burn pit exposure.

Overview: VA/DoD Health Executive Council (HEC) Deployment Health Working Group (DHWG) Response and Action Plan

After careful review of the findings of the IOM report, "Long-Term Health Consequences of Exposure to Burn Pits in Iraq and Afghanistan," and consideration of other working group efforts, the HEC Deployment Health Working Group arrived at the following objectives (linked to the HEC DHWG Activities and Milestones in the FY 2011-2013 Joint Strategic Plan, see Appendix B). These objectives respond to post-deployment health concerns related to airborne hazards and the IOM Committee's conclusions on long-term health effects of burn pit exposure. Appendix C provides a prioritized list of these objectives. Appendix D links the IOM's recommendations for future research to the objectives of this Joint Action Plan and Appendix E and F provide summaries of pertinent completed, ongoing and planned research.

Activity 1: Follow-up Medical Care of Deployed Populations

Supports HEC DHWG Activity and Milestone 1

Discussion

Servicemembers and Veterans with respiratory symptoms, such as dyspnea on exertion (DOE), may have multiple causes for these symptoms. These causes may include prior disease, deconditioning, and both occupational or life-style exposures to known pulmonary irritants, such as tobacco smoke. The impact of these symptoms on individual Servicemembers and Veterans would be expected to vary and requires evaluation.

Objectives

1.1 (Protocols) – Joint DoD/VA Clinical Assessment Protocols

Case definitions and clinical evaluation protocols should be standardized across DoD and VA. The DoD-VA Deployment Health Working Group (DHWG), chartered through the Health Executive Council (HEC), should be tasked to develop expert consensus on elements of the evaluation protocols, such as standardized clinical questionnaire(s), case definitions, diagnostic algorithms and medical coding guidance. An initial effort began with the February 2010 work from the National Jewish Health Workshop, Denver, CO (established by DoD with VA participation). More recently, the Army's Public Health Command (USAPHC) drafted the Clinical Evaluation of Respiratory Conditions (CERC) questionnaire and an algorithm for evaluation of dyspnea on exertion (DOE). DoD and VA's current information systems should be utilized to record the standardized evaluation protocols.

1.2 (Transitions) – Improved Care Transitions from DoD to VA and VA to DoD with Expanded Exposure Assessment

Existing post-deployment exposure assessments (DoD Form DD2796 and DD2900) are screening level questionnaires intended to trigger follow-up evaluations. More specific task-oriented exposures are being considered for use within the DoD and VA health care systems. The DoD US Army Public Health Command's (USAPHC) Deployment Assessment of Respiratory Exposures (DARE) is one potential survey tool being evaluated. If assessments are determined to be beneficial, the tools will likely require modification for differing contexts (such as self-assessments, primary care, and specialty clinics). VA's "My Health-E-Vet" is being updated to include an exposure self-assessment with health risk communication. DoD's AHLTA and VA's VISTA Electronic Health Record should allow access to exposure assessments by clinicians.

Activity 2: Outreach and Health Risk Communication Products

Supports HEC DHWG Activity and Milestone 1

Discussion

The science and understanding of long-term health effects is expected to evolve. As new findings and opportunities for Servicemember and Veteran participation occur, outreach should be provided.

Objectives

2.1 (Stakeholders) – Improving Servicemember, Family and Veteran Knowledge of Potential and Known Health Effects

Many resources are currently available to educate Servicemembers, Veterans and their families on some of the known and potential airborne hazards associated with deployment. Resources are available via the internet on sites managed by VA's Office of Public Health (OPH), the Army Public Health Command (USAPHC), Naval and Marine Corps Public Health Center (NMCPHC) and other government entities. As information becomes available, VA and DoD should work to ensure that it is provided to the public in a format that is optimal for understanding and addresses the issues and concerns of these audiences.

In addition to posting information on websites and the use of social media, another approach will be corresponding with individuals who may have been directly affected.

2.2 (Health Care Team) – Improving Health Care Provider Understanding of Potential and Known Health Effects of Military Service

In order to ensure that the health needs of all Servicemembers and Veterans returning from deployment can be met, health care providers must be armed with the best possible information on their potential concerns. For example, the VA is working to improve post-deployment training efforts by launching a national awareness campaign to increase the visibility of their products on topics such as environmental exposures, post-traumatic stress disorder, and traumatic brain injury. These products include information on treatment, ideas to communicate to patients, and other resources to consult for further information. Additionally, to directly improve care for Veterans that may have been exposed to airborne hazards, VA will distribute a pocket card and do a number of seminars to instruct frontline providers on steps to take when seeing patients with exposure concerns.

DoD's USAPHC, which is the DoD Executive Agent for Deployment Environmental Health Surveillance, should continue its current educational efforts. For example, the Environmental Medicine Clinical Consult Service offers direct physician-to-physician consults for patients with exposure concerns and develops factsheets for providers to communicate with Service members. DoD should continue to partner with VA where possible. DoD and VA should sponsor a joint Airborne Hazards Symposium to bring together subject matter experts, inform health care teams and develop joint action products to implement joint approaches. The symposium should occur on an annual basis as needed.

8

Activity 3: Surveillance

Supports HEC DHWG Activity and Milestone 3

Discussion

The IOM's strongest health finding of "Limited/Suggestive evidence of a decrement in pulmonary function" relates to a physiologic change, which by itself is not sufficient to diagnose a specific disease or impairment. The specific impact upon an individual is likely to vary based on an individual's fitness levels, and any pre-existing illness, predispositions and the magnitude and types of exposure. In light of a recent published case-series of post-deployment dyspnea on exertion (DOE), and self-reported increases in respiratory symptoms in those who deployed, further investigation of short-term and long-term respiratory effects is warranted (King, 2011 365) (Smith, 2009 170;11). In addition, a more general surveillance is warranted to monitor for the wider range of organ system effects possible from exposure to airborne hazards (pollution).

Objectives

3.1 (Cases) – Post-deployment DOE Case Finding

A VA/DoD wide approach to enhanced case finding and assessment of post-deployment DOE and other respiratory symptoms and illnesses is the highest priority effort to better understand the scope and impact of deployment on respiratory function. DoD and VA should continue participating in joint workgroups with academia, where possible, to study and report case findings (Special Issue, 2012 Vol 54;6).

Research activities ongoing and proposed within the Military Operational Medicine Research Program (MOMRP) of U.S. Army Medical Research and Materiel Command (MRMC) are key efforts to meeting this objective. Specifically the STAMPEDE studies (Study of Active Duty Military for Pulmonary Disease related to Environmental Dust Exposure) require continued financial support. Clinical and histopathological case-series should include long-term follow-up to monitor changes in respiratory and functional status. Cases should also be followed for other potential organ effects, especially cardiovascular abnormalities. (See Appendix D for more details on these studies.)

3.2 (Cohort) – Long-Term Cohort Study of Post-Deployment Airborne Hazard Health Effects

DoD and VA should continue to support efforts to monitor all potential health effects of deployment, with particular emphasis on airborne hazards and pulmonary and cardiovascular systems. Both short and long-term (e.g. respiratory cancer) effects should be monitored.

Study objectives should encompass all potential long-term health effects of inhalational hazards (including reproductive effects). Designs should include statistical power to detect burn-pit effects, as well as, other potential airborne hazards. Pilot and feasibility studies should consider the three-tiered recommendation of the IOM in their power calculations. Focus areas should be consistent with the Environmental Protection Agency Integrated Science Assessment for Particulate Matter in 2009 [EPA/600/R-08/139F]. As more knowledge is gained, specific issues could be studied in "spin-off" studies. A nested cohort should include physical exams to look for early markers of disease and understand normal variations in the organ systems to be studied. The preferred approach is to develop an overarching cohort study. DoD and VA should work jointly to support this effort.

As recommended by the IOM, the proposed study design should be reviewed by an independent advisory body, as currently exists in the VA research program (via peer-review and the National Research Advisory Committee) and in the DoD (via the Defense Health Board).

Current studies were cited by IOM as evidence of feasibility and should be continued to address the breadth of potential health effects. First, the Millennium Cohort Study (MilCo), sponsored by DoD, includes deployment exposure questions and is investigating methodologies to determine exposure intensity around the JBB burn pit. MilCo is also investigating the feasibility of serum biomarkers as measures of exposure. VA is partnering with DoD on the MilCo to facilitate the use of VA clinical data to confirm self-reported outcomes. This collaboration is likely to improve the validity of the MilCo and the knowledge of various health effects (e.g., behavioral health) related to deployment. Second, the VA's "National Health Study for a New Generation of U.S. Veterans" has completed its first data collection and is now in the analysis phase. Self-reported exposure questions consistent with the MilCo questionnaire are included. Third, in May, 2010, the Armed Forces Health Surveillance Center (AFHSC) published a 36 month follow-up study of personnel who had been assigned to burn pit locations examining their health outcomes. The AFHSC is in the process of completing similar studies with a longer follow-up period of 48 months to identify any latent health effects that have become evident and intends to update this study annually and pursue collaboration with the VA to minimize losses to follow-up. Adjustment was made for age and previous respiratory diagnosis but the administrative data source did not allow for adjustment of smoking history. (See Appendix D for more details on these studies.)

Activity 4: Research Initiatives

Supports HEC DHWG Activity and Milestone 4

Discussion

The IOM Committee recommends further research into potential deployment-related, long-term health effects of inhalational exposures from multiple sources including pollution, dust, burn pits, and other potential toxic exposures.

IOM's conclusion was derived from long-term health studies in similar populations. There are limitations inherent in drawing conclusions about the potential health effects of deployment-related exposures from studies of non-deployed, non-military subjects. These limitations can only be addressed through studies of deployed populations and a consideration of additional potential exposures. IOM's statement that other pollution sources (e.g., PM) are of concern leads this Working Group to recommend continuing the study of airborne exposures in general and not limiting these studies to burn pit exposures. Variation in the composition of PM may impact its toxicology and should be assessed.

Objectives

4.1 (Markers) – Markers of Early Disease or Injury

The evolving science of imaging, physiologic testing, and biomarkers may be of significant value over the course of the decades during which long-term health effects should be studied. Population norms for some of these test modalities do not yet exist. Data points and samples should be taken from a subset of the planned cohort studies in order to allow retrospective data analysis of repeated samples during an individual's lifetime. Feasibility studies will be essential for less mature markers.

4.2 (Exposure) – Validated Exposure Assessment Tools

Due to the immediate need for improved exposure assessment tools, current development must rely on expert consensus between DoD, VA, and external bodies. A strategic approach is needed to identify feasible approaches to develop validated tools considering the limitations imposed by sparse or non-existent environmental sampling in prior deployments. Ongoing deployments offer a short window to perform field validation, although retrospective validation through exposure modeling is also of value.

4.3 (Toxicology) – Animal and Toxicological Studies

A wealth of information regarding the long-term effects of airborne exposures related to deployment can be gained through laboratory research using animal and alternative model systems. VA and DoD may collaborate with external research authorities to study the mechanisms of action and subsequent health outcomes of chronic exposures to hazards encountered during deployment, such as those highlighted in the IOM study (e.g. PM, dioxins, etc). Studies in model organisms will be helpful especially in determining the cancer-causing risks of these hazards, since manifestation of the disease in humans may take a number of years. (See Appendix E for more details on these studies.)

4.4 (Modeling) – Exposure Modeling

DoD should continue to lead exposure modeling efforts with a focus on validated models based on field measurements. The continued operations of burn pits in Afghanistan offer a window of opportunity to obtain additional exposure data points.

Appendix A: References

Baird, C. (2012 54;6). Respiratory Health Status of US Army Personnel Potentially Exposed to Smoke From 2003 Al-Mishraq Sulfur PLant Fire. *J Occ Envir Med* , 717.

Department of Veterans Affairs Notice: Initial Research on the long-Term Health Consequences of Exposure to Burn Pits in Iraq and Afghanistan, Federal Register, Vol 78. No 23, Monday February 4, 2013

Desert Research Institute. *DoD Enhanced Particulate Matter Surveillance Program Final Report* . Reno, NV.

IOM. (2006). *Gulf War and Health Volume 3: Fuels, Combustion Products, and Propellants.* Washington, DC: National Academies Press.

IOM. (2011). *Long-term health consequences of exposure to burn pits in Iraq and Afghanistan.* Washington, DC: The National Academies Press.

King, M. (2011 365). Constrictive bronchiolitis in soldiers returning from Iraq and Afghanistan. *New Eng J Med* , 222-230.

NRC. (2010). *Review of the Department of Defense Enhanced Particulate Matter Surveillance Program Report.* Washington, DC: National Academies Press.

Smith, B. (2009 170;11). Newly Reported Respiratory Symptoms and Conditions Among Military Personnel. *Am J Epi* , 1433-1442.

Special Issue. (2012 Vol 54;6). *Health Effects of Deployment to Afghanistan and Iraq.* J Occup Envir Med.

USAPHC. (May 2010). *Health Assessment of 2003 Qarmat Ali Water Treatment Plant Sodium Dichromate Incident Status Update.* US Army.

Appendix B: FY 2011-2013 Joint Strategic Plan Strategic Goal 2.1 – (Quality)

HEC DHWG SMART Objective:

Coordinate joint efforts to increase health surveillance information sharing, review relevant literature on hazardous environmental exposures, and share Servicemember and Veteran health information between DoD and VA, so that situations in theater, which place these populations at risk, are identified at the earliest stage possible and DoD and VA responses are appropriately coordinated.

Activities and Milestones

1. Review DoD's identification of major environmental and occupational exposure incidents in theater, DoD's provision of data to VA, and development of appropriate DoD and VA follow-up activities, including outreach to Servicemembers and Veterans, while providing an assessment to the HEC and to other relevant stakeholders, by September 30th annually.

2. Develop and coordinate a Data Transfer Agreement for interagency approval, which will provide two-way data exchange between the DoD and VA to facilitate the identification of deployment-related hazards that could lead to long-term adverse health effects, by September 30, 2012.

3. Evaluate the 2011 Institute of Medicine report on the potential health effects of exposure to burn pits and provide an assessment of lessons learned to the HEC, related to future health surveillance, research, and possible preventive measures for future deployments, by January 1, 2012.

4. Analyze relevant research literature and government reports on deployment-related environmental exposures and provide strategic recommendations to the HEC, to mitigate and prevent the potential health effects of hazardous exposures, by September 30th annually.

Appendix C: High Priority Action Plan Objectives

Objective Number - Description	Supporting Efforts/Studies
3.1 (Cases) – Post-deployment DOE Case Finding	US Army Study of Active Duty Military for Pulmonary Disease related to Environmental Dust Exposure (STAMPEDE), NJ War Related Illness and Injury Study Center (WRIISC)
3.2 (Cohort) – Long-Term Cohort Study of Post-Deployment Airborne Hazard Health Effects	Proposed VA Office of Public Health (OPH) Study, DoD Millennium Cohort Study (MilCo), VA Study for a New Generation of Veterans (New Gen), DoD Armed Forces Health Surveillance Center (AFHSC) Cohorts
(Protocols) – Joint DoD/VA Clinical Assessment Protocols	Deployment Health Working Group with US Army Public Health Command (USAPHC), VA Office of Public Health (OPH)
2.2 (Health Care Team) – Improving Health Care Provider Understanding of Potential and Known Health Effects	Deployment Health Working Group with US Army Public Health Command (USAPHC), VA Office of Public Health (OPH)
4.2 (Exposure) – Validated Exposure Assessment Tools	US Army Public Health Command (USAPHC)

C-1

Appendix D: IOM Recommendations for Future Research with Supporting Action Plan Objectives

"A pilot [feasibility] study should be conducted to ensure adequate statistical power, ability to adjust for potential confounders, to identify data availability and limitations and develop testable research questions and specific objectives."

3.2 (Cohort) – Long-Term Cohort Study of Post-Deployment Airborne Hazard Health Effects,
4.1 (Markers) – Markers of Early Disease or Injury

"An independent oversight committee... should be established to provide guidance and to review specific objectives, study designs, protocols and results from the burn pit emissions research programs that are developed."

3.2 (Cohort) – Long-Term Cohort Study of Post-Deployment Airborne Hazard Health Effects

"A cohort study of Veterans and active duty military should be considered to assess potential long-term health effects related to burn pit emissions in the context of other ambient exposures at the JBB [Joint Base Balad]."

3.2 (Cohort) – Long-Term Cohort Study of Post-Deployment Airborne Hazard Health Effects,
4.1 (Markers) – Markers of Early Disease or Injury

"An exposure assessment for better source attribution and identification of chemicals associated with waste burning and other pollution sources at JBB should be conducted... to help the VA determine those health outcomes most likely to be associated with burn pit exposures."

4.2 (Exposure) – Validated Exposure Assessment Tools
4.3 (Toxicology) – Animal and Toxicological Studies
4.4 (Modeling) – Exposure Modeling

"Exposure assessment should include detailed deployment information including distance and direction individuals lived and worked from the JBB burn pit, duration of deployment, and job duties"

4.2 (Exposure) – Validated Exposure Assessment Tools

"Assessment of health outcomes is best done collaboratively using the clinical informatics systems of the DoD and VA."

(Protocols) – Joint DoD/VA Clinical Assessment Protocols
3.1 (Cases) – Post-deployment DOE Case Finding
3.2 (Cohort) – Long-Term Cohort Study of Post-Deployment Airborne Hazard Health Effects
4.1 (Markers) – Markers of Early Disease or Injury

Appendix E: Select Completed, Current and Planned Deployment Health Studies in Humans

Agency	Study Name and Brief Summary	Study Population	Study Design	Information Collected	Status
VA OPH	National Health Study for a New Generation of U.S Veterans (NewGen) Research Aims 1. Do veterans of OIF/OEF have an increased prevalence of health problems and behavioral risk factors following deployment in combat theaters relative to non-deployed veterans? 2. Are some health problems among deployed veterans associated with a specific exposure or experience in combat theaters?	-30,000 OIF/OEF Veterans and 30,000 Veterans who served elsewhere during same period (October 2001-June 2008) -representative of each branch -representative for component -oversample women for 20%	-Prospective Cohort -Three follow up surveys over ten years. -Self Report Survey -Medical records review of 1,000 subjects	-Health Risk Behaviors (ETOH, HIV, sexual behavior, helmet use, seatbelt use, smoking, speeding) -Health Conditions (anxiety, asthma, cancer, depression, chronic disease, CVD, IBS, PTSD, TBI, pain, migraines) -General Health (functional status, general health perception, pregnancy outcomes, reproductive health) -Health Care Utilization (doctor visits, hospitalizations, prescription drug use, CAM, VA facility use) -Potential Exposures (accidents, blasts, burn pits, chemicals, dust/sand, falls, head injury, MST, smoke, vaccinations)	-Active -22,000 participated in first wave.

Agency	Study Name and Brief Summary	Study Population	Study Design	Information Collected	Status
VA ORD	Million Veteran Program (MVP)	-1,000,000 Veterans (ideally) -Volunteer	-Prospective cohort	-Demographics (race, ethnicity, ancestry, education, marital status, income) -Family information (structure, vital status of biological family members, family medical history) -Medical history (CV, ID, MH, GI, neurological, and musculoskeletal) -Functional health status (SF-12) -Frequency of physical activity -ETOH and tobacco consumption -History of military service (period of service, location, exposure to selected deployment related agents) -Physical features -Healthcare utilization (hospitalizations, prescription use, VA usage) -Biological specimen (blood) -Past medical records	Currently enrolling

Agency	Study Name and Brief Summary	Study Population	Study Design	Information Collected	Status
DOD NHRC	Millennium Cohort Study (MilCo) Largest prospective health study in military history, designed to assess the long term health effects of military service.	-Active Duty (deployed and non deployed), Reserve, and Guard -To date 151,596 have been enrolled (still have one more panel to sample) -Oversampled for females, Marines, Married, Prior deployers (SWA, Bosnia/Kosovo after 8/97), and National Guard/Reserves -57% of sample has deployed in support of Iraq/Afghanistan since 2001 -12% include GWV -33% of sample has separated	-Prospective cohort: 21 years -Began in 2001 -Questionnaire every three years through 2022	Questionnaire includes: -Demographics -Medical conditions (including asthma, chronic bronchitis, and emphysema, shortness of breath) -Depression -Anxiety -Eating disorders -PTSD -Physical activity -Chronic pain -Health status changes -CAM -Anthrax vaccine history -ETOH use/abuse -Smoking -Deployment exposures -Occupational hazards -Job code -Does not have specific base camp information, just deployment country -Linkage to medical and military records with data on demographics, occupation, deployment, separation, vaccinations, health care utilization, pharmacy prescriptions, lost work days, employability, and mortality	On-going: 3 yr questionnaires Link to Abstract More than 30 Articles on Military Health Proposed: Examine effect of PTSD or anxiety disorder symptoms and diagnosis on respiratory symptoms and diagnoses Geographic area evaluations Explore linkages between the Millennium Cohort Study and individual exposure data; determine feasibility Examine the prognosis of incident respiratory symptoms reported by land-based deployers using the 2011-2012 survey cycle data Investigate the impact of respiratory symptoms post-deployment, including at self-reported assignment locations

Agency	Study Name and Brief Summary	Study Population	Study Design	Information Collected	Status
DOD, USAPHC	Mishraq Sulfur Fire Cohort Research Aim To assess whether or not exposure to chemicals released during the 2003 Mishraq Sulfur Fire may have caused or exacerbated any adverse health conditions among exposed personnel during or after OIF deployment	-6,532 Exposed Active Duty composed of 191 Army firefighters who extinguished the fire and 6,341 Soldiers assigned, attached to, or co-located with units that were located within 50km of Mishraq Sulfur plant during active burning-1 Jun 2003-21 Aug 2004. Majority were members of 101 DIV, either 1st Brigade Combat Unit of 326th Engineering Unit -4,153 Unexposed Active Duty Time based: 1,869 OIF/OEF Soldiers who were deployed during the year prior to or following the exposure period according to DMDC Location based: 2,284 Soldiers who were deployed for at least 1 day to Q-West area (largest established camp in that area) 14 to 24 months after burn period ended, and were not in either of the other two groups 10,685 total	Historical cohort	-Self reported health status before and after deployment (DD 2795 and 2796) -Medical encounter data	Completed. Link to Abstract Findings: -The two exposed groups had significantly more frequent self reports of fair or poor health -Exposed groups significantly more often referred for further care, significantly more reports of health concerns and exposure concerns -Exposed groups had significantly more frequent reports of runny nose, difficulty breathing, rash, tearing, and coughing during deployment. -Both exposed and unexposed had a significant increase in the percent reporting poorer health post deployment compared to pre-deployment -Incidence of respiratory diagnoses encounters decreased from pre to post deployment, but not significant. -Incidence of encounters for acute respiratory infections decreased from pre to post deployment period-and was significant in each of the groups

Agency	Study Name and Brief Summary	Study Population	Study Design	Information Collected	Status
DOD USA	A Database Registry of Military Personnel Diagnosed with Post-Deployment Chronic Pulmonary Disease Research Aim To examine the relationship between onset of chronic pulmonary disease and deployment history 2005-2009-any active duty with any disease, anyone seen at any MTF, and any back at deployment. Also, do they really have it (b/c coding is bad)?	Current number=80,000+	Retrospective database registry	Diagnoses included in this database: -asthma (those undergoing a Medical Evaluation Board (MEB) and new onset) -COPD (COPD, emphysema, chronic bronchitis) -sarcoidosis - other pulmonary interstitial/infiltrative disorders (pulmonary fibrosis, constrictive bronchiolitis) -No information on where person was stationed	MEB, COPD complete

E-5

Agency	Study Name and Brief Summary	Study Population	Study Design	Information Collected	Status
DOD USA	STAMPEDE Registry of Deployment Related Lung Disease <u>Research Aim</u> Establish a centralized database registry of patients diagnosed with lung disease related to deployment to OIF/EIF/OND from DOD medical treatment facilities.	Projected N=3,000 Likely members of this cohort are also members of the other STAMPEDE cohorts and other studies at Brooke Army Medical Center (most subjects are Army)	Prospective registry (with ten year follow-up).	Enrolls all patients seen at an MTF with diagnosed chronic lung disease related to deployment, including: -asthma -emphysema -chronic bronchitis -COPD -bronchiectasis -sarcoidosis -pulmonary fibrosis -constrictive bronchiolitis -other pulmonary interstitial/infiltrative disorders -Will collect clinical data for 10 years post-diagnosis -Has information on where the subject was stationed	On going

E-6

Agency	Study Name and Brief Summary	Study Population	Study Design	Information Collected	Status
DOD USA	Pre- and Post-Deployment Evaluation of Military Personnel for Pulmonary Disease Related to Environmental Dust Exposure (STAMPEDE-II) Research Aims Evaluate active duty military pre and post deployment for the development of lung disease measured by chest imaging and PFTs.	Deploying Soldiers from Ft. Hood (Predominately Army) N=1500	Prospective Study	Chest radiography, standard spirometry and impulse oscillometry pre and post deployment	First year funding obtained.
DOD USA	Study of Active Duty Military for Pulmonary Disease related to Environmental Dust Exposure (STAMPEDE) Research Aim To evaluate military personnel who have recently returned from OIF/EIF for evidence of lung disease related to prolonged environmental dust exposure in the current theaters of operation	N=50 Subjects recruited from units returning from deployment to Fort Hood (Army) within past six months with primary complaints of dyspnea.	Prospective Study	Detailed history Physical exam Risk factor assessment Complete pulmonary evaluation: -chest radiograph -high resolution CT of chest -full pulmonary function testing -impulse oscillometry -methacholine challenge testing -bronchsopy with bronchoalveolar lavage Location of unit during deployment.	Ongoing

E-7

Agency	Study Name and Brief Summary	Study Population	Study Design	Information Collected	Status
DoD/ USA DOI/ USGS/ National Jewish Health	Development of a Morphometric Approach to Quantification of Small Airways Disease and a Particulate Matter Exposure Profile in Lung Biopsies of Deployed US Military Personnel	US Military Personnel	Case-Control	Independent Pathological review of biopsy specimens and measurement of pathological features for objective diagnosis; characterization of PM in lungs	Ongoing
DoD JPC	Histopathological and chemical analytical evaluation of pulmonary specimens from US military Operation Iraqi Freedom and Enduring Freedom veterans	US Military Personnel	Case Series	Histopathology physico-chemical characterization of inhaled PM	Approved by IRB
Iraqi Military	Baseline spirometry Values for Iraqi National Military: The Impact of Chronic Dust Exposure. Study conducted by Iraqi doctor, not a DOD funded or sponsored study	Iraqi military personnel	Cross-sectional	Pulmonary questionnaire and baseline spirometry to determine baseline pulmonary function in a sample of the native population	Results will be shared with Dr. Morris

E-8

Agency	Study Name and Brief Summary	Study Population	Study Design	Information Collected	Status
DoD AFHSC	Epidemiologic studies of Health Outcomes among Troops deployed to Burn Pit Sites	Active component service members of the US Army and US Air Force who were deployed to one of four locations in CENTCOM (two with a burn pit and two without),or Korea compared to a never deployed CONUS based population	Retrospective cohort	Health care encounters during and following deployment; responses on post deployment health assessment form (2796, 2900)	Initial report (36 month follow-up) completed. Report: Link: Burn_Pit_Epi_Studies.pdf 48 month follow-up and improvement on comparison population and increased specificity of outcome definitions completed and is being drafted for release. Additional yearly follow-up of these cohorts is planned.
DoD AFHSC	Incidence of respiratory conditions among all deployers to OIF/OEF/OND	Active component service members, all services, with a deployment of >30 days where the operation was OEF/OIF/OND and a CONUS based comparison cohort	Retrospective cohort	Health care encounter with an ICD-9 coded diagnosis for a disease of the respiratory system (460-519) or a sign, symptom or ill-defined condition involving the respiratory system.	Completed; Results under preparation for publication
DoD AFHSC	Epidemiologic studies of Health Outcomes among Troops deployed to Kabul and Bagram	Active component service members deployed to one of two bases located near Kabul and Bagram, AF	Retrospective cohort	Location, electronic medical record administrative data	Currently working with DMDC to identify cohorts
DoD NHRC	Birth Outcomes Among Military Personnel After Exposure to Documented Open-Air Burn Pits Before and During Pregnancy	Active duty women and men within a 3-mile radius of select open-air burn pits	Retrospective cohort	Live births and infant health outcomes	Complete J Occ Envir Med, Vol 54;6:689-697

Agency	Study Name and Brief Summary	Study Population	Study Design	Information Collected	Status
VA OPH NJ WRIISC	Effects of Deployment Exposures on Cardiopulmonary and Autonomic Function Research Aims: 1 – Evaluate cardiopulmonary function (i.e. exercise gas exchange and spirometry) in deployed OEF/OIF Veterans versus those deployed elsewhere. 2- Determine whether deployment-related exposures alter cardiovascular autonomic control.	-OEF/OIF/OND Veterans deployed to Iraq or Afghanistan and age/gender matched Veterans of the same time period deployed elsewhere	Case-control	Physiological Assessments: 1 –Exercise Challenge 2 – Spirometry 3 – Autonomic battery Questionnaires: 1- Exposure assessment 2 – DARE 3 – CERC 4 – Health history 5 – Military history 6 – Physical activity history	Data Collection

E-10

Appendix F: Select Non Human and Toxicological Studies

Agency	Study Name and Brief Summary	Study Population	Study Design	Information Collected	Status
VA/USAF Military Working Dog Center/DoD Joint Pathology Center	Military Working Dogs (MWD) as sentinels for human disease: examining health records to identify diseases common to deployed military personnel and deployed MWDs Research Questions: These dogs were exposed to the same environmental hazards as military personnel and therefore may serve as sentinels for adverse health effects in humans	MWDs deployed to the Gulf and other regions	Cohort	MWD health records and MWD necropsy/biopsy results	Preliminary discussion with partners
DOD/USACEHR/HHS/NIOSH	Effects of Pulmonary Exposure of Rats to Airborne Particulate Matter from Iraq	Rat	Toxicology: Intratracheal instillation of fine PM from Camp Victory	histopathology, biochemical and immunological markers of injury in lung lavage	Ongoing; limited toxicity of aerosol fine PM collected at Camp Victory

F-1

Agency	Study Name and Brief Summary	Study Population	Study Design	Information Collected	Status
DOE/Pacific Northwest Labs/ Institute for Systems Biology	Biomarkers for Pulmonary Injury Following Deployment (microRNA and protein biomarkers in lung lavage fluid and serum from rats	NIOSH rat study	Toxicology	microRNA and protein biomarkers in lung lavage fluid and serum	Ongoing
DoD/NAM RUD/USA & NC State	Biological Responses in Rats Exposed to Cigarette Smoke and Middle East Sand (Dust)	Rats	Toxicology: Inhalational exposure to Camp Victory soil:	Biochemical and immunological markers of disease in lung lavage fluid, lung gene expression, serum and lung lavage proteomics, behavioral measures, PFTs	Completed. Inhalation Toxicology, 2012; 24(2): 109–124 Limited toxicity of Camp Victory soil.
DoD/NAM RU-D	The Acute and Long-Term Effects of Middle East Sand Particles on the Rat Airway Following a Single intratracheal Instillation	Rat	Toxicology	toxicity of Camp Buehring (Kuwait) dust	Completed. J Toxicol Environ Health A. 2011;74(20):1351-65 Limited toxicity of Camp Buehring (Kuwait) dust
DoD/NAM RU-D	Studies of composition of plume from reconstituted burn-pit	Cultured cells	Toxicology	toxicity of plume to cells in culture; toxicity of plume to rats pending, chemical composition of plume	Ongoing
DoD/NAM RU-D	In vitro toxicity of SWA soils, toxicity of instilled extracts of soils	Cultured cells	Toxicology	Cell viability	Manuscript in preparation

F-2

APPENDIX E

Frequently Asked Questions About Military Exposure Guidelines

This document was reproduced with permission from the US Army Public Health Command (Provisional). *Environmental Health Risk Assessment and Chemical Exposure Guidelines for Deployed Military Personnel.* Aberdeen Proving Ground, MD: USAPHC (Prov); June 2010 Revision.

FREQUENTLY ASKED QUESTIONS FOLLOW ON PAGE 388

US Army Public Health Command (Prov)
Technical Guide 230
June 2010 Revision

What are military exposure guidelines?

Military exposure guidelines (MEGs) are decision aids used to assess health risk to deployed forces from chemical exposures in the environment. The MEGs are designed specifically for use within the risk management framework (Field Manual 5-19) supporting the Commander's decision making process.

A MEG is a chemical concentration in air, water, or soil that represents an exposure threshold. There are several types of thresholds that refer to an increasing potential for mission-related health effects within the entire exposed military population. These thresholds are specifically linked to one part of the military risk management framework in FM 5-19.

Each MEG is an estimate of the exposure level above which certain types of health effects may begin to occur in individuals within the exposed population after an exposure of the specified duration. The severity of the health effects and percentage of the exposed population that might demonstrate the health effects may increase as concentrations increase above the MEG. The degree to which severity and/or incidence of health effects increase as exposure increases above a MEG is chemical-specific. Some of the MEGs are "screening levels" below which certain health effects would not be expected to occur within a deployed population under reasonable worst-case exposure conditions.

The MEGs are population-based; therefore, they are not designed for predicting health effects in specific individuals. The MEGs provide the basis for more detailed evaluation by appropriate health experts—they are not stand-alone action levels. They are often based on other U.S. Federal standards, such as unsafe levels use for emergency response planning or safe levels in the workplace as prescribed by the U.S. Occupation Safety and Health Administration. They are either the same values as U.S. federal agency standards or guidelines or they are adjusted to match the unique exposure scenarios or subpopulations of the deployed forces.

The MEGs have been developed for many chemicals; some chemicals have MEGs for different media (e.g., air, water, and soil) and for different exposure conditions and timeframes (e.g., for short-term exposures of 1 hour or 1 day, as well as for long-term, continuous 1-year exposures). The MEGs are designed to assess a variety of military exposure scenarios, such as a single release of large amounts of a chemical, temporary exposure conditions lasting hours to days, or for continuous ambient environmental conditions, such as a regional pollution.

What kind of MEGs are available and what does 'exceedance of a MEG' mean?

The currently available set of MEGs includes values for air, water, and soil for several different exposure durations arranged along differing military hazard severity levels from Negligible to Catastrophic (see Field Manual 5-19). For example, for a given chemical, there are four possible Air MEG values for the 1-hour exposure duration. The following table presents the standard interpretation and use of the MEGs.

Example of the Potential Types of Air MEGs for the 1-Hour Exposure Duration for a Hypothetical Chemical and the Standard Interpretation of the Hazard Severity Level Associated with Various Field Exposures

Exposure Estimate*	MEG Name	MEG Value	Hazard Severity Designation ‡
† 5 – 29 mg/m^3	1-hour Negligible MEG	5 mg/m^3	Negligible
30 – 149 mg/m^3	1-hour Marginal MEG	30 mg/m^3	Marginal
150 – 339 mg/m^3	1-hour Critical MEG	150 mg/m^3	Critical
≥ 340 mg/m^3	1-hour Catastrophic MEG	340 mg/m^3	Catastrophic

* This exposure estimate represents an average 1 hour exposure. Analytical error associated with measurements at the boundaries of the categories (e.g., 29 vs. 30 mg/m^3) must be acknowledged.
† Field exposures < 5 milligrams per cubic meter (mg/m^3) would not be considered to be a deployment hazard and would not be evaluated in a formal risk assessment.
‡ In reality, hazard severity blends together at the margins between each category, which reflects a graded series of health responses as exposure increases. For example, there is no practical measurement and toxicological distinction between 29 and 30 mg/m3 even though the selected severity categories will be different. The risk assessment method addresses exposures near the borders of the categories.

This standard approach for setting hazard severity levels within a risk assessment sets a useful framework, but it does not highlight the chemical-specific knowledge and the scientific uncertainties associated with the underlying data for any given assessment. The USAPHC (Prov) TG 230 provides additional details on what data the MEGs are based on and what it means to exceed a MEG (i.e., where a field exposure is greater than a MEG).

The fact that a chemical concentration measured in the field is greater than a MEG should never, by itself, be interpreted to mean there is a notable or definitive risk of a specific health effect in an exposed individual. The MEGs are not stand-alone action levels. The MEGs are decision tools used within a risk assessment which informs decision makers about the potential need for actions for adjustments to military operations, potential medical treatment, long-term health surveillance. Because MEGs are derived from protective 'threshold' estimates that often have low confidence, exceeding a MEG only indicates a potential for specified health effects increase among some members of the exposed military population. However, the significance of the increased risk (i.e., type of health effects, severity, and number or personnel) will depend on many factors. These factors include chemical-specific, dose-response relationships, exposure-time profiles, and the frequency of human susceptibility factors (underlying illnesses, health behaviors (e.g., smoking) and at-risk genes) within the exposed population that may predispose certain individuals to certain effects.

What types of health effects are considered when developing a MEG?

When short-term MEGs are generated, health effects that may develop immediately or shortly after an exposure are considered. Generally speaking, acute/short term effects occur after single relatively brief or short-term exposures (minutes to days). Reversible and irreversible health effects are considered when developing these MEGs. Some of the short-term MEG categories also consider increased risk for developing cancer.

When long-term MEGs are generated, health effects that may develop or continue post-deployment (e.g., months or years later) are considered. In general, the long-term Negligible MEGs are protective of both cancer and the most sensitive health endpoints other than cancer that have been identified in toxicological or epidemiological studies.

How accurately does a MEG estimate a threshold for the possibility of health effects?

The quantity and quality of the health effects and toxicological data upon which the MEGs are based varies substantially across the chemicals. Since existing toxicological databases and health criteria were utilized to develop the MEGs, the quality and extensiveness of toxicological and epidemiological information underlying these guidelines is comparable and as variable as that used by other Federal agencies for worker and civilian applications.

The overall confidence that certain kinds of health effects will not occur within a population when field exposures are below a MEG is generally high. The overall confidence that effects will occur in the population when exposures are above a MEG ranges from low to moderate for most chemicals and health effects. In most cases, some type of margin of safety has been built into a MEG value to address the uncertainty resulting from gaps in toxicological data. This means that MEGs typically reflect levels that are lower than effect levels determined in scientific studies. The amount lowered (safety margin) depends on the extent of scientific uncertainties for that chemical and effect. Some MEGs, especially those for long-term exposures and health effects, have a safety margin that is several orders of magnitude lower than what would be considered safe for the animals studied in the laboratory.

What is a "screening-level" MEG?

The most commonly used MEG is the long-term (1-year) Negligible MEG, which is the lowest MEG concentration for a chemical. This 1-year Negligible MEG is often used as a "screening level" in that it addresses the worst case deployment exposure conditions (most frequent and continuous long-term exposure conditions, e.g. soldiers continuously exposed "on-the-job" 24 hours a day, 7 days a week, for 1 whole year). The screening-level MEG is used as the initial basis to compare field sampling data to determine if there is a potential hazard. As long as sample data for a detected chemical is below the screening level MEG, then there is no hazard and, thus, no operational risk. If concentrations are above the 1-year Negligible MEG, then a chemical exposure may pose a military hazard and it requires further assessment, to include comparison to the other available MEGs for that chemical.

How are MEGs used?

Within the context of a health risk assessment, MEGs are used to determine the significance of field exposures to the military mission at a specific location or for a specific operation. The MEGs are used to rank the hazard severity of the exposure. See the section called "*What kind of MEGs are available and what does 'exceedance of a MEG' mean?*" to understand how severity is ranked.

The severity rank is then combined with estimates of hazard probability to estimate the operational risk of the field exposure (the hazard). Risk is estimated using the following risk matrix.

Military Risk Assessment Matrix

HAZARD SEVERITY	HAZARD PROBABILITY				
	Frequent (A)	Likely (B)	Occasional (C)	Seldom (D)	Unlikely (E)
Catastrophic (I)	Extremely High	Extremely High	High	High	Moderate
Critical (II)	Extremely High	High	High	Moderate	Low
Marginal (III)	High	Moderate	Moderate	Low	Low
Negligible (IV)	Moderate	Low	Low	Low	Low

Source: Army Field Manual 5-19

Can MEGs be used to estimate the number of personnel that will develop certain health effects?

The MEGs are not designed for determining casualty estimates. In general, there will not be adequate toxicity data, exposure data, and modeling to support the development of casualty estimates for most chemicals and pollutants. While the severity of the health effects and percentage of personnel potentially demonstrating health effects will generally increase as concentrations increase above the MEG, it is not considered reasonable to estimate the number of individuals that will have specific effects using the MEGs.

The MEGs are preventive medicine guidelines designed for use in determining a qualitative level of risk posed to an exposed military population. The qualitative risk rank is specified in terms that are derived from the military risk management model (see Field Manual 5-19). The MEGs cannot be used as a planning tool for estimating the loss of effectiveness of personnel to perform daily duties due to incapacitation or other health effects without knowing the actual level and duration of exposure to a specified chemical.

Can MEGs be used to determine which personnel will develop health effects?

The MEGs are population-based and are not designed for predicting health effects in specific individuals. While it is true that for many chemicals there are certain types of human susceptibility factors or underlying health conditions that may predispose persons to develop effects, the available information is inadequate to predict specific cases with certainty. Many, if not most, MEGs are based on civilian health criteria designed to address certain key susceptible subgroups in the civilian population (e.g., asthmatics). Even though these subgroups make up a small fraction of any given military population, the intent in using these guidelines was to ensure protective estimates that would address these Service members.

The general human factors that play a role in susceptibility to chemical exposures include the following:

- Gender: For example, females are more susceptible to effects from exposures to benzene and nerve agents.
- Underlying heath conditions: For example, asthmatics (estimated 2-5 percent of troops) are more susceptible to effects from exposure to PM matter as well as other air pollutants and certain acid gases.
- Other health factors: For example, susceptibility generally changes with age, fitness level, dehydration, fatigue, nutritional status/anemia, tobacco use, and so forth.

Why were MEGs developed for Soldiers instead of using U.S. civilian health standards?

While there are some specific exceptions, in general, civilian exposure standards and guidelines are not sufficient for the military Force Health Protection mission for several reasons. For example, those guidelines are not specific to the exposure scenarios faced by deployed personnel. In general, deployed personnel can experience exposure rates (for example, amount of air inhaled, amount of water consumed) that are higher than their civilian counterparts. While an existing civilian exposure standard or guideline can often form the basis for a MEG value, the MEG development process often makes population-specific adjustments to address different exposure rates or exposure durations.

In addition, civilian standards and guidelines are generally not aligned to the military risk management hazard severity levels used to rank risks for Commanders. The MEG development process takes adjusted-civilian guidelines and aligns them according to the severity levels of Negligible, Marginal, Critical, and Catastrophic. These categories are used by preventive medicine personnel to rank risks according to mission and force health protection metrics.

Notably, U.S. short-term emergency response guidelines, such as the AEGLs and ERPGs, are examples of civilian guidelines that do align with aligned to the military risk management hazard severity levels. When available, these are used as MEGs.

Who should use MEGs? When should MEGs be used?

The MEGs (and USAPHC (Prov) TG 230) are designed for preventive medicine and medical personnel trained in the identification and evaluation of environmental health hazards. Within the Army, these individuals function at or above the Health Service Support Level II, according to DA Pam 40-11 Section 3–2 (DA Pam, 2006). The MEGs are designed for use in the context of a health risk assessment for use within the military risk management framework (see FM 5-19, 2006). The DOD (DoDI 6490.03, 2006) and Joint Staff (CJCS 2007) policy states that MEGs are to be used to assess environmental chemical exposures that occur during military deployments. Since MEGs have been specifically developed for military deployment conditions, unless otherwise indicated, they should be used in place of other civilian or occupational standards during deployments.

The risk assessment guidance provided in USAPHC (Prov) TG 230 serves as an objective base from which to make educated determinations within this framework. Risk assessors should have a basic understanding of the underlying toxicological and health basis for the MEGs. They should be familiar with basic methods of exposure assessment for chemicals in the environment. Finally, it is necessary that the risk assessor appreciate the uncertainties associated with sampling and with the assumptions used for estimating representative exposure levels and possess a high degree of understanding of basic risk communication principles. This guidance does not replace the need for basic technical training in these areas; nor does it provide guidance for sample planning or collection.

Where can I learn more?

The USAPHC (Prov) TG 230 provides risk assessment guidance on how to interpret field data using the MEGs. Also, USAPHC (Prov) RD 230 provides methodological details on how the MEGs were developed. These reference materials and guidance can be obtained electronically at: http://phc.amedd.army.mil/tg.htm.

F-6

APPENDIX F

Executive Summary: Screening Health Risk Assessment, Burn Pit Exposures, Balad Air Base, Iraq

This document was reproduced with permission from the US Army Center for Health Promotion and Preventive Medicine (USACHPPM; Aberdeen Proving Ground, MD), *Report No. 47-MA-08PV-08*/Air Force Institute for Operational Health (AFIOH; Brooks City-Base, TX), *No. IOH-RS-BR-TR-2008-0001*; May 2008.

EXECUTIVE SUMMARY FOLLOWS ON PAGE 396

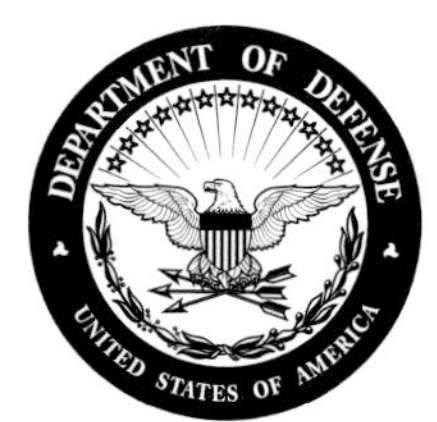

EXECUTIVE SUMMARY
SCREENING HEALTH RISK ASSESSMENT
BURN PIT EXPOSURES
BALAD AIR BASE, IRAQ
USACHPPM REPORT NO. 47-MA-08PV-08/
AFIOH REPORT NO. IOH-RS-BR-TR-2008-0001
MAY 2008

1. PURPOSE. This report documents the results of ambient air sampling conducted at Balad Air Base, Iraq by on-site military environmental health personnel. The ambient air sampling was intended to collect multiple classes of pollutants expected to be emitted by the Air Base municipal waste open burn pit, which operated 24 hours (hrs), 7-days per week. The results of the ambient air sampling will provide the foundation for a screening health risk assessment (HRA) of military personnel located at the site and likely exposed to these pollutants. The ambient sampling relied upon for this report was performed 2 January 2007 through 21 April 2007, prior to the operation of on-site incinerators. Subsequent air sampling will be conducted following the installation and operation of multiple municipal waste incinerators. No incinerators were operational during this sampling period.

2. CONCLUSIONS.

a. The U.S. Army Center for Health Promotion and Preventive Medicine (USACHPPM) and the U.S. Air Force Institute for Operational Health (AFIOH) have jointly developed a screening HRA documenting the current understanding of the health risk from burn pit operations at Balad Air Base, Iraq. Findings indicate that measured exposure levels from burn pit operations are not routinely above deployment military exposure guidelines (MEGs) for exposures up to 1 year. The MEGs, as published in USACHPPM Technical Guide (TG) 230, (*Chemical Exposure Guidelines for Deployed Military Personnel*), represent chemical concentrations above which certain types of health effects may begin to occur in individuals within an exposed population after a continuous, single exposure of specified duration. The MEGs are not designed for determining casualty estimates but are instead used as preventive guidelines. The occupational and environmental health (OEH) risk estimate for exposure to all substances sampled for in the ambient air (except particulate matter particles of 10 micrometers or less (PM_{10}) at Balad Air Base indicates adverse health risks are unlikely. These levels are not likely to cause short-term onset health effects.

b. In addition, a human HRA was performed under guidance outlined by the U.S. Environmental Protection Agency (U.S. EPA). Cancer (carcinogenic) and non-cancer (or non-carcinogenic, which means any health effect other than cancer) risk estimates were developed. These results indicate an "acceptable" health risk for both cancer and non-cancer long-term health effects. This methodology and resulting estimates do not indicate an absolute measure of an individual's probability of an adverse health effect. Instead, the results indicate the likelihood

ES-1

that such outcomes (longer term/delayed cancer or non-cancer health effects) might occur under very specific exposure conditions.

c. Dioxins were evaluated separately for non-cancer risks since they do not have the "toxicity value" from U.S. EPA needed for that methodology. Using a model to estimate body-burden level (build up of dioxins in the body), the burn pit has minimal impact on body-burden level. A pilot serum study supports this finding.

d. A software error resulting from an improperly programmed access database in the initial reporting of sample results for dioxin congeners produced results which were 1,000 times greater than the measured value. Consequently, initial draft reports, to include a document released on 3 December 2007 titled "Balad Burn Pit Interim Report—Executive Summary," significantly overestimated the carcinogenic risk to personnel. As noted above, revised estimates for carcinogenic and non-carcinogenic effects find the health risk levels "acceptable" by U.S. EPA guidelines for long-term exposure. These results reflect conditions through June 2007, upon which two incinerators became operational and are expected to reduce contaminant levels.

e. This report is based on the results of a comprehensive air sampling effort conducted by U.S. Air Force Bioenvironmental Engineering and U.S. Army preventive medicine personnel in the first four months of 2007. The air sampling study targeted expected emissions from the burn pit to include particulate matter, volatile organics, metals, polycyclic aromatic hydrocarbons, and polychlorodibenzodioxins/furans (hereafter called "dioxins" and "furans"). Sampling locations were selected to represent typical and maximum exposure levels for the general population serving at Balad Air Base. The samples were also collected over multiple 24-hour periods to account for some of the operational and meteorological variability in exposure levels. A total of 163 samples were collected, resulting in 4811 individual analyte results. The 1-year MEGs were exceeded in 52 samples, to include 50 samples for particulate matter less than 10 (PM_{10}) microns in size and two samples for volatile organic compounds. Particulate matter levels were typical of what would be expected in the region and similar to background levels. Testing results do not indicate that PM_{10} was significantly increased by burn pit operations. Particulate matter exposure in the U.S. Central Command (USCENTCOM) region has been previously identified as a potential health concern and is being addressed in other studies. Results from the particulate matter were not evaluated as part of this assessment.

f. Despite the comprehensive sampling effort, there is significant uncertainty about actual exposure levels and the associated health risk estimates for those who currently are or have been assigned to Balad Air Base. Therefore, the exposure scenario was performed using a worse-case scenario approach and most individual exposures and resulting risks are expected to be less than predicted. Contaminant concentrations and related exposure levels are highly variable due to changing meteorological conditions (such as, wind direction and speed), differences in amount and type of material burned, as well as the temperature at which the material is burned. The risk assessment in this report conservatively assumed air sample results were representative of daily exposure, continuous, and stable burn pit operations and that the base population remained constant.

g. Continued work by preventive medicine personnel in the U.S. Air Force and U.S. Army will be aimed at protecting the health of all Service members and reducing the level of uncertainty in these estimates. Any significant refinement that improves the precision of the estimate will be shared with Balad Air Base and USCENTCOM leadership as they are obtained.

3. RECOMMENDATIONS. The following recommendations should be considered in the development of an action plan to reduce any future burn pit exposures at Balad Air Base and at other locations in USCENTCOM area of responsibility. These include the following:

a. Reduce or eliminate the open burning of plastic materials. The main source of ambient levels of dioxins and furans is low-temperature burning plastic materials, especially in the presence of metal catalysts. These conditions typify open pit burning operations.

b. Assess effectiveness of control measures. Assess air pollution levels at Balad Air Base after controls are implemented. Air sampling should be performed to ensure that recommended control measures for reducing exposure levels to personnel are implemented and working.

c. Develop a risk communication plan. A risk communication plan, to include both information products and open discussion opportunities, should be developed. Appropriate risk communication products, such as fact sheets for Service members and commanders, should be disseminated to communicate the results of any HRAs and potential plans for determining the meaning of the results. While information products can be helpful in increasing understanding, open discussion opportunities are proven to help minimize unnecessary concerns by outwardly reinforcing leadership focus on Force Health Protection; clarifying misinformation/ misperceptions; and by ensuring that decision makers remain cognizant of nonexperts' interests, values, and concerns.

d. Conduct a policy review. Recommend Force Health Protection and Readiness, Joint Staff, and Under Secretary of Defense (Acquisition, Technology and Logistics) conduct a comprehensive policy review concerning proper use of burn pits and develop new policies to fill any gaps.

e. Force Health Protection and Readiness coordinated with the Defense Health Board (DHB) to review the updated USACHPPM/AFIOH Balad screening health risk assessment and corresponding calculations for health risks for individuals deployed to Balad Air Base. The DHB remarks were documented in a Memorandum, Defense Health Board (DHB), subject: Defense Health Board Findings Pertaining to Final "Draft Health Risk Assessment, Burn Pit Exposures, Balad Air Base, Iraq". The Board concluded "given the data available, the screening risk assessment provides an accurate determination of airborne dioxin exposure levels for service members deployed to Balad Air Base. Based on the information provided, no dioxin-associated significant short- or long-term, health risks or elevated cancer risks are anticipated among the personnel deployed to Balad, Iraq."

ES-4

APPENDIX G

Executive Summary, Addendum 2: Screening Health Risk Assessment, Burn Pit Exposures, Balad Air Base, Iraq

This document was reproduced with permission from the US Army Center for Health Promotion and Preventive Medicine (USACHPPM; Aberdeen Proving Ground, MD), *Report No. 47-MA-08PV-08*/Air Force Institute for Operational Health (AFIOH; Brooks City-Base, TX), *No. IOH-RS-BR-TR-2008-0001*; May 2008.

EXECUTIVE SUMMARY FOLLOWS ON PAGE 402

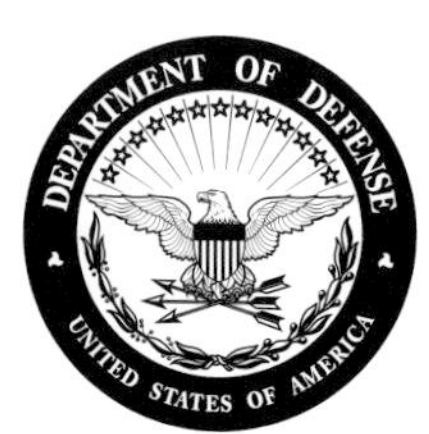

EXECUTIVE SUMMARY
ADDENDUM 2
SCREENING HEALTH RISK ASSESSMENT
BURN PIT EXPOSURES
BALAD AIR BASE, IRAQ
USACHPPM REPORT NO. 47-MA-08PV-08/
AFIOH REPORT NO. IOH-RS-BR-TR-2008-0001
MAY 2008

1. PURPOSE. This report documents the results of ambient air sampling conducted at Balad Air Base, Iraq (now known as Joint Base Balad, Iraq; the current name is used throughout this addendum) by on-site military environmental health personnel in Fall 2007 as a follow-up to ambient air sampling conducted in January through April 2007. The ambient air sampling was intended to collect multiple classes of pollutants expected to be emitted by the Air Base municipal waste open burn pit, which operated 24 hours (hrs) per day, 7 days per week. Although burn pit emissions were noted as the primary concern amongst site personnel, other air pollution sources including flight operations, vehicular emissions, generators, and off-site sources were present and likely contributing to the pollutant levels found during this sampling effort. The results of the ambient air sampling provide the foundation for a screening health risk assessment (HRA) of military personnel located at the site and likely exposed to these pollutants. The ambient air sampling relied upon for this assessment was performed 18 October 2007 through 25 November 2007, after two on-site incinerators had begun operation and waste segregation practices had commenced. Additional air sampling will be conducted to increase knowledge of airborne contaminants and their potential health risk to deployed personnel.

2. CONCLUSIONS.

a. The U.S. Army Center for Health Promotion and Preventive Medicine (USACHPPM) and the U.S. Air Force School of Aerospace Medicine (USAFSAM) have jointly developed a screening HRA documenting the current understanding of the health risk from exposure to the ambient air at Joint Base Balad, Iraq. Though it is primarily focusing on burn pit operations and changes since the installation and operation of 2 incinerators, many sources as discussed above were contributors to ambient air. The two primary methods used to assess risk were the military occupational and environmental health (OEH) risk estimate and the Screening HRA.

b. Using Composite Risk Management (CRM) risk estimate methodology to complete the OEH risk estimate, findings indicate that measured chemical exposure levels are not routinely above deployment military exposure guidelines (MEGs) for exposures up to 1 year. The MEGs, as published in USACHPPM Technical Guide (TG) 230, (*Chemical Exposure Guidelines for Deployed Military Personnel*), represent chemical concentrations above which certain types of health effects may begin to occur in individuals within an exposed population after a continuous, single exposure of specified duration. The MEGs are not designed for determining casualty estimates but are instead used as preventive guidelines. The OEH risk estimate for exposure to all substances sampled for in the ambient air (except particulate matter with aerodynamic diameters of 10 micrometers or less (PM_{10})) at Joint Base Balad indicates long-term adverse health effects are unlikely. The PM_{10} was excluded because it is being addressed in other studies.

c. In addition, a screening human HRA was performed under guidance outlined by the U.S. Environmental Protection Agency (U.S. EPA). Cancer (carcinogenic) and non-cancer (or non-carcinogenic, which means any health effect other than cancer) risk estimates were developed. This methodology and its resulting estimates do not indicate an absolute measure of an individual's probability of an adverse health effect. Instead, the results indicate the likelihood that such outcomes (longer term/delayed cancer or non-cancer health effects) might occur under very specific exposure conditions. The results from this sampling effort indicate an "acceptable" health risk for cancer long-term health effects. For non-cancer health effects the hazard index exceeded 1.0 due to a combination of respiratory irritants. A hazard index greater than 1.0 indicates there is a potential for non-cancer health effects under the specific exposure conditions chosen. It does not indicate that a health effect will occur; however, the safety margin for protection is being breached so further evaluation is necessary.

d. Similar results were obtained from the previous sampling effort, conducted from January through April 2007. The initial and recalculated OEH risk estimates for exposure to all substances sampled for in the ambient air, excluding PM_{10}, indicated long-term adverse health effects were unlikely. Using U.S. EPA methodology the cancer risk for all receptors was within or below the U.S. EPA's acceptable cancer risk range. For non-cancer health effects the hazard index was initially calculated to be less than 1.0 as reported in the initial Screening Health Risk Assessment. These calculations did not incorporate estimated values for chemicals detected at levels less than the laboratory reporting limit. This was discovered during analysis of the Fall 2007 sampling data. The hazard index was recalculated for the January through April 2007 results to include the estimated values. The recalculated hazard index slightly exceeded the protective level of 1.0 due to a combination of respiratory irritants. This indicated the safety margin for protection is being breached and there is potential for non-cancer health effects under the specific exposure conditions chosen. However, it does not indicate that long-term health effects will occur.

e. This addendum is based on the results of an air sampling effort conducted by U.S. Air Force Bioenvironmental Engineering and U.S. Army preventive medicine personnel in October and November 2007. The air sampling study targeted expected emissions from the burn pit to include particulate matter, volatile organics, metals, polycyclic aromatic hydrocarbons, and polychlorinated dibenzo-p-dioxins/furans (hereafter called "dioxins" and "furans"). Sampling locations were selected to represent typical and maximum exposure levels for the general population serving at Joint Base Balad. The samples were also collected over multiple 24-hour periods to account for some of the operational and meteorological variability in exposure levels. A total of 107 samples were collected, resulting in 3079 individual analyte results. The 1-year MEGs were exceeded in 32 samples, to include 29 samples for particulate matter less than 10 microns in size (PM_{10}) and three samples for volatile organic compounds. Particulate matter levels were typical of what would be expected in the region and similar to background levels.

Testing results do not indicate that PM_{10} was significantly increased by burn pit operations. Particulate matter exposure in the U.S. Central Command (USCENTCOM) region has been previously identified as a potential health concern and is being addressed in other studies. Results from the particulate matter were not evaluated as part of this assessment

f. Despite the comprehensive sampling effort, there is significant uncertainty about actual exposure levels and the associated health risk estimates for those who currently are or have been assigned to Joint Base Balad. Therefore, the exposure scenario was performed using a worst-case scenario approach and most if not all individual exposures and resulting risks are expected to be less than predicted. Contaminant concentrations and related exposure levels are highly variable due to changing meteorological conditions (such as, wind direction and speed), differences in non-burn pit operations, differences in amount and type of material burned, as well as the temperature at which the material is burned. The risk assessment in this report conservatively assumed air sample results were representative of daily exposure, continuous and stable burn pit operations occurred, and that the base population and operations remained constant.

g. Continued work by preventive medicine personnel in the U.S. Air Force and U.S. Army will be aimed at protecting the health of all Service members and reducing the level of uncertainty in these estimates. Any significant refinement that improves the precision of the estimate will be shared with Joint Base Balad and USCENTCOM leadership as they are obtained.

3. RECOMMENDATIONS. The following recommendations should be considered in the development of an action plan to reduce future exposures to airborne pollutants at Joint Base Balad and at other locations in USCENTCOM area of responsibility. These include the following:

a. Continue to minimize the open burning of plastic materials and waste cooking grease through source reduction and recycling as well as incineration. The low-temperature burning of plastic materials and cooking grease, especially in the presence of metals that acts as catalysts, generates dioxins, furans, polycyclic aromatic hydrocarbons, and other organic chemicals of potential concern. These conditions typify open pit burning operations. Also, consider relocation of the burn pit to a predominantly downwind location.

b. Assess effectiveness of control measures. Assess air pollution levels as additional controls and countermeasures are implemented. Air sampling should be performed to ensure that recommended control measures for reducing exposure levels to personnel are working. Continue to seek improved monitoring and analytical procedures.

c. Refine the risk communication plan. A risk communication plan, to include both information products and open discussion opportunities, should be refined to reflect new and changing information on site conditions. Appropriate risk communication products, such as fact sheets for Service Members and commanders, should be disseminated to communicate the results of any HRAs and potential plans for determining the meaning of the results. While information products can be helpful in increasing understanding, open discussion opportunities are proven to help minimize unnecessary concerns by outwardly reinforcing leadership focus on Force Health Protection; clarifying misinformation/ misperceptions; and by ensuring that decision makers remain cognizant of non-experts' interests, values, and concerns.

d. Conduct a policy review. Recommend Force Health Protection and Readiness, Joint Staff, and Under Secretary of Defense (Acquisition, Technology and Logistics) conduct a comprehensive policy review concerning proper use of burn pits and develop new policies to fill any gaps.

e. Implement administrative controls when practical to reduce exposures to the ambient air during periods of observed poorer air quality, such as during an inversion, dust storm, or large scale convoy operation. Controls could include moving indoors, using alternate outdoor locations for an activity, or altering the physical training schedule.

f. Submit this addendum to the Defense Health Board for an independent, third-party review. Ensure that the results of this review are communicated and used to further improve surveillance, risk assessment, and risk mitigation.

Abbreviations and Acronyms

A

ACOEM: American College of Occupational and Environmental Medicine
AEGL: Acute Exposure Guideline Level
AFCITA: Air Force Complete Immunization Tracking Application
AFHSC: Armed Forces Health Surveillance Center
AHLTA: Armed Forces Health Longitudinal Technology Application
AHR: airway hyperresponsiveness
AIT: allergy immunotherapy
AOR: adjusted odds ratio
ATP: adenosine triphosphate
ATS: American Thoracic Society
A-VO_2: arterial-venous oxygen difference

B

BAL: bronchoalveolar lavage
BALF: bronchoalveolar lavage fluid
BAMC: Brooke Army Medical Center
BASE: Building Assessment Survey and Evaluation
BC: bradycardia
BMI: body mass index
BPT: bronchoprovocation testing

C

CATI: computer-assisted telephone interview
CB: constrictive bronchiolitis
CBPR: community-based participatory research
CDC: Centers for Disease Control and Prevention
CENTCOM AOR: Central Command Area of Responsibility
CERC: Clinical Evaluation of Respiratory Conditions
CHAMPS: Career History Archival Medical and Personnel System
CI: confidence interval
CIA: Central Intelligence Agency
CL: confidence limit
CLa: absolute confidence limit
CLr: relative confidence limit
CO: cardiac output
CONUS: continental United States
COP: cryptogenic organizing pneumonia
COPD: chronic obstructive pulmonary disease
COT: Committee on Toxicology
CPET: cardiopulmonary exercise testing
CPRS: Computerized Patient Record System
CSP: Cooperative Studies Program
CT: computed tomography
CTR-EMED: Combat Trauma Registry Expeditionary Medical Encounter Database
CXR: chest X-ray

D

DA: Department of the Army
DARE: Deployment Airborne Respiratory Exposure
DAV: Disabled American Veteran
DD: Department of Defense
DEERS: Defense Enrollment Eligibility Reporting System
DHB: Defense Health Board
Dis: disease
DLCO: diffusing capacity of the lung for carbon monoxide
DLCO/VA: diffusing capacity of the lung for carbon monoxide corrected for alveolar volume
DLD: Division of Lung Disease
DMDC: Defense Manpower Data Center
DMSS: Defense Medical Surveillance System
DNA: deoxyribonucleic acid
DoD: US Department of Defense
DoDSR: Department of Defense Serum Repository
DOEHRS: Defense Occupational and Environmental Health Readiness System
DU: depleted uranium
DVA: US Department of Veterans Affairs

E

EDHA: Electronic Deployment Health Assessment
EIB: exercise-induced bronchospasm
Endo: endocrine
EPMS: enhanced particulate matter sampling/surveillance
EPMSP: Enhanced Particulate Matter Survey Program
ERS: European Respiratory Society
EU: European Union

F

FEV_1/FEV1: forced expiratory volume in 1 second
FMEF: forced midexpiratory flow
FOB: fiberoptic bronchoscopy
FOH: Federal Occupational Health
FRC: forced residual capacity
FVC: forced vital capacity
FVL: flow volume loop

G

G6PD: glucose-6-phosphate dehydrogenase
GenISIS: Genomic Information System for Integrated Sciences
GMP: Genomics Medicine Program
GMPAC: Genomics Medicine Program Advisory Committee

H

H_2S: hydrogen sulfide
HEAR: Health Enrollment Assessment Review
HIPAA: Health Insurance Portability and Accountability Act
^{1}H-NMR: proton nuclear magnetic resonance
HRCT: high-resolution computed tomography
HVAC: heating, ventilation, and air conditioning

I

IARC: International Agency for Research on Cancer
ICD: *International Classification of Diseases*
ICD-9: *International Classification of Diseases*, Ninth Revision
ICD-9-CM: *International Classification of Diseases, Ninth Revision, Clinical Modification*
ID: identification
IEHR: integrated electronic health record
IgE: immunoglobulin E
ILD: interstitial lung disease
ILER: individual longitudinal exposure record
IMCA: indicators for monitoring COPD and asthma
IOM: Institute of Medicine
IR: incidence rate
IRR: incidence/incident rate ratio
IUATLD: International Union Against Tuberculosis and Lung Disease

J

JBB: Joint Base Balad/Joint Air Base Balad
JMeWS: Joint Medical Workstation
JPMWG: Joint Particulate Matter Work Group
JTTR: Joint Theater Trauma Registry

K

Kt: kiloton

L

LLD: limit of longitudinal decline
LLDa: absolute limit of longitudinal decline
LLDr: relative limit of longitudinal decline
LLN: lower limit of normal

M

Max HR: maximal heart rate
MCS: Millennium Cohort Study
MCT: methacholine challenge test
MEDPROS: Medical Protection System
MEGs: Military Exposure Guidelines
MEP: maximum expiratory pressure
MESL: Military Exposure Surveillance Library
Metab: metabolism
MHS: Military Health System
MIP: maximum inspiratory pressure
MOMRP: Military Operational Medicine Research Program
MOS-SF12: Medical Outcomes Study-Short Form 12
MRC: Medical Research Council
MRMC: US Army Medical Research and Materiel Command
MS: musculoskeletal
MTF: military treatment facility
MVP: Million Veteran Program

N

NAMRU-D: Naval Medicine Research Unit-Dayton
NCHS: National Center for Health Statistics
NewGen: National Health Study for a New Generation of US Veterans
NHANES: National Health and Nutrition Examination Survey
NHANES III: Third National Health and Nutrition Examination Survey
NHLBI: National Heart, Lung, and Blood Institute
NHRC: Naval Health Research Center
NIEHS: National Institute of Environmental Health Sciences
NIOSH: National Institute for Occupational Safety and Health
NMCB-17: Naval Mobile Construction Battalion SEVENTEEN
NRC: National Research Council
Nutrit: nutrition

O

OEF: Operation Enduring Freedom
OIF: Operation Iraqi Freedom
OND: Operation New Dawn
ORD: Office of Research and Development
OSHA: Occupational Safety and Health Administration

P

PACT: Patient Aligned Care Team
PAH: polycyclic aromatic hydrocarbon
PBD: postbronchodilator
PCL: Posttraumatic Stress Disorder Check List
PCL-M: PTSD Check List-Military
PDF: Portable Document Format
PDHA: Post-Deployment Health Assessment/Pre-Deployment Health Assessment
PDHRA: Post-Deployment Health Reassessment
PDTS: Pharmacy Data Transaction System
PFT: pulmonary function test/testing
PHQ-9: Patient Health Questionnaire-9
PIMR: preventive Health Assessment and Individual Medical Readiness
PM: particulate matter
PM_{10}: particulate matter with an aerodynamic diameter less than or equal to 10 µm; particulate matter level 10
$PM_{2.5}$: particulate matter with an aerodynamic diameter less than 2.5 µm; particulate matter level 2.5
PPV: positive predictive value
pred: predicted
Proj: projected
PTSD: posttraumatic stress disorder
PVNTMED: preventive medicine

Q

QG: quality grade

R

RADS: reactive airways dysfunction syndrome
REF: reference value
Regr: regression
Rep: repeatability
Resp: respiratory
Rev: revised
RNA: ribonucleic acid
RR: respiratory rate
RV: residual volume

S

SADR: Standard Ambulatory Data Record
SD: standard deviation
SE: standard error
Seabee: member of the US Navy Construction Battalion (CB); the term "Seabee" is derived from "CB"
SIDR: Standard Inpatient Data Record
SO_2: sulfur dioxide
Sp: absolute within-person variation
SPIROLA: Spirometry Longitudinal Data Analysis (software)
SPOD/E: Shuaiba Port of Debarkation/Embarkation
Sr: relative within-person variation
SSIC: Standard Subject Identification Codes
STAMPEDE: Study of Active-Duty Military for Pulmonary Disease Related to Environmental Dust (or Deployment) Exposure
Sw: within-person variation
SWA: southwest Asia
Swr: relative within-person variation
Sys: system

T

TAIHOD: Total Army Injury and Health Outcomes Database
TBLB: transbronchial lung biopsy
TC: tachycardia
TCDD: 2,3,7,8-tetrachlorodibenzo-*p*-dioxin
TED: TRICARE Encounter Data
TEFSC: Toxic Embedded Fragment Surveillance Center
TGV: thoracic gas volume (performed by plethysmography)
TIC/TIM: toxic industrial chemical/toxic industrial material
TLC: total lung capacity
TO: toxic organic

U

95% UCL: 95% upper confidence limit
US: United States
USAPHC: US Army Public Health Command
USCENTCOM: US Central Command
USEPA: US Environmental Protection Agency
USPM: US urban particulate matter

V

VA: US Department of Veterans Affairs/Veterans Affairs
VAD IR/VADIR: VA/DoD Identity Repository
VAMC: Veterans Affairs Medical Center
VATS: video-assisted thoracoscopic surgery
VC: vital capacity
VCD: vocal cord dysfunction
VCO_2: carbon dioxide production
V_E: minute ventilation
VF: ventricular fibrillation
VHA: Veterans Health Administration
VO_2: oxygen uptake/oxygen consumption
VO_{2max}: maximal oxygen consumption
VOC: volatile organic compound

W

WG: working group
WHO: World Health Organization
WRIISC: War Related Illness and Injury Study Center
WTC: World Trade Center

Y

y: year

INDEX

A

B

C

D

E

F

G

H

I

J

L

M

Q

R

S

T

U

V

W